T0141804

Pelvic Floor Dysfunction and Pelvic Surgery in the Elderly

David A. Gordon • Mark R. Katlic

Editors

Pelvic Floor Dysfunction and Pelvic Surgery in the Elderly

An Integrated Approach

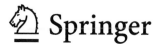

Editors
David A. Gordon
Division of Pelvic NeuroScience
Department of Surgery
The Sinai Hospital of Baltimore
Baltimore, MD, USA

Mark R. Katlic
Sinai Center for Geriatric Surgery
Department of Surgery
Sinai Hospital
Baltimore, MD, USA

ISBN 978-1-4939-8235-6   ISBN 978-1-4939-6554-0   (eBook)
DOI 10.1007/978-1-4939-6554-0

© Springer Science+Business Media New York 2017
Softcover reprint of the hardcover 1st edition 2017
This work is subject to copyright. All rights are reserved by the Publisher, whether the whole or part of the material is concerned, specifically the rights of translation, reprinting, reuse of illustrations, recitation, broadcasting, reproduction on microfilms or in any other physical way, and transmission or information storage and retrieval, electronic adaptation, computer software, or by similar or dissimilar methodology now known or hereafter developed.
The use of general descriptive names, registered names, trademarks, service marks, etc. in this publication does not imply, even in the absence of a specific statement, that such names are exempt from the relevant protective laws and regulations and therefore free for general use.
The publisher, the authors and the editors are safe to assume that the advice and information in this book are believed to be true and accurate at the date of publication. Neither the publisher nor the authors or the editors give a warranty, express or implied, with respect to the material contained herein or for any errors or omissions that may have been made.

Printed on acid-free paper

This Springer imprint is published by Springer Nature
The registered company is Springer Science+Business Media LLC
The registered company address is: 233 Spring Street, New York, NY 10013, U.S.A.

Preface

As geriatric surgeons, we are in the midst of dramatic changes in the demographic structure of the United States. Currently, almost 25% of the population is over the age of 65 years and the fastest-growing cohort within this group will be those people over 75 years. This aging of the US population presents potentially significant challenges to our healthcare system. In addition, it raises the question about whether it can support the needs of older people and enable them to live healthy, independent, and productive lives.

As the population ages, there is a natural enhancement in the development of medical technology which diffuses into many aspects of daily life. This includes all forms of minimally invasive operative technologies, health-monitoring devices, and computers exhibiting artificial intelligence which are being used to perform a variety of tasks, from the most routine to the most complex. To meet these challenges, we may actually have to *redefine* what it means to be "older." So, does *old* mean 65 years or 75 years or even 80 years of age? Newspapers, television, and the Internet are replete with stories about octogenarian triathletes, mountain climbers, and fountain-of-youth aficionados. These elderly individuals are increasingly unwilling to accept a shortened life span, much less the prospect of disability or even inconvenience.

Physicians understand far better than most that the concept of *time on tissue* is a prescription for physical breakdown and deteriorating disease. Having said that, pelvic *surgeons*, as anatomic scientists, like Galileo and Newton before them, are intimately aware of the complications that can occur when one adds *gravity* to time and tissue. Consequently, those physical defects within the anatomic pelvis that ultimately lead to socially unacceptable clinical conditions such as urinary and/or fecal incontinence will be absolutely intolerable to a healthier, more diverse, and better-educated population of centenarians that continue to exhaustively pursue active lives in a fashion unparalleled to the previous generations.

The editors, while surgeons, embody a combined half century of interest in the elderly. One of us (DAG) is fellowship trained and board certified in Pelvic Reconstruction/Neurourology and established one of the first Geriatric Pelvic Medicine fellowships. The other (MRK) published his paper "Surgery in Centenarians" in 1985 and his first book, *Geriatric Surgery*, in 1990. Our chapter authors represent the best of the multidisciplinary spectrum of those focused on the pelvis, from radiology and gastroenterology to urology and colon and rectal surgery. No book to date has brought together in one volume their combined expertise. All of us who care for the elderly—geriatricians, family physicians, surgeons, nurses, and many others—will learn something that will help us care for this burgeoning group. So, read the volume cover to cover or, more likely, read chapters of particular interest. All of our terrific patients, veterans of wars and other intense life experiences, will benefit.

Baltimore, MD, USA

David A. Gordon
Mark R. Katlic

Contents

Contributors

Andrea Chao Bafford Department of Surgery, University of Maryland Medical Center, Baltimore, MD, USA

Brian L. Bello Medstar Washington Hospital Center, Colorectal Surgery Program, Washington, DC, USA

Jennifer L. Bennett Johns Hopkins University, School of Medicine, Baltimore, MD, USA

Ray Bologna Department of Urology, Cleveland Clinic Akron General, Akron, OH, USA

Linda Cardozo Department of Urogynaecology, Kings College Hospital, London, UK

Arif R. Chaudry Department of Surgery, Sinai Hospital of Baltimore, Baltimore, MD, USA

John Cmar Department of Medicine, Sinai Hospital of Baltimore, Baltimore, MD, USA

JoAnn Coleman Sinai Center for Geriatric Surgery, Department of Surgery, Sinai Hospital, Baltimore, MD, USA

Chirag Dave Department of Urology, Beaumont Hospital, Royal Oak, MI, USA

Jonathan E. Efron Ravitch Division, Department of Surgery, Johns Hopkins University, Baltimore, MD, USA

Michael Ehlert Department of Urology, Beaumont Hospital, Royal Oak, MI, USA

Askin Erdogan Division of Gastroenterology and Hepatology, Augusta University, Augusta, GA, USA

Daniel Galante Department of Surgery, Sinai Hospital, Balitmore, MD, USA

Veerabhadram Garimella Royal Stoke University Hospital, Stoke on Trent, UK
Center for Colon and Rectal Surgery, Florida Hospital Medical Group, Orlando, FL, USA

Susan L. Gearhart Department of Surgery, Johns Hopkins Medical Institution, Baltimore, MD, USA

David A. Gordon Division of Pelvic NeuroScience, Department of Surgery, The Sinai Hospital of Baltimore, Baltimore, MD, USA

Rohit Gossein Department of Internal Medicine, Sinai Hospital of Baltimore/John's Hopkins University, Baltimore, MD, USA

Mikel Gray Department of Urology, University of Virginia, Charlottesville, VA, USA

Caitlin W. Hicks Department of Surgery, The Johns Hopkins University, Baltimore, MD, USA

Okechukwu A. Ibeanu Gynecologic Oncology, Johns Hopkins University, Baltimore, MD, USA
Alvin and Lois Lapidus Cancer Institute, at Sinai Hospital, Baltimore, MD, USA
Alvin and Lois Lapidus Cancer Institute, at Northwest Hospital, Randallstown, MD, USA

Jessica Jackson Department of Urology, University of Virginia, Charlottesville, VA, USA

Megan Kahn-Karen Department of Food and Nutrition, Sinai Hospital of Baltimore, Baltimore, MD, USA

Mark R. Katlic Sinai Center for Geriatric Surgery, Department of Surgery, Sinai Hospital, Baltimore, MD, USA

Johannes Koch Digestive Disease Institute, Virginia Mason Medical Center, Seattle, WA, USA

Pooja Lakshmin Department of Psychology, Rutgers, The State University of New Jersey, Newark, NJ, USA

Otto S. Lin Digestive Disease Institute, Virginia Mason Medical Center, Seattle, WA, USA

Tisha N. Lunsford Department of Internal Medicine, University of Texas Health Science Center at San Antonio, San Antonio, TX, USA

Christopher Madsen Department of General Surgery, Sinai Hospital, Surgical Resident, Baltimore, MD, USA

Dean D.T. Maglinte Indiana University School of Medicine, IU Health – University Hospital, Indianapolis, IN, USA

John R.T. Monson Center for Colon and Rectal Surgery, Florida Hospital Medical Group, Orlando, FL, USA

Ashrit Multani Department of Medicine, Sinai Hospital of Baltimore, Baltimore, MD, USA

Ha Lam Department of Internal Medicine, University of Texas Health Science Center at San Antonio, San Antonio, TX, USA

Jennifer L. Ortiz Her Physical Therapy, Columbia, MD, USA

Haritha Pendli The Maryland Institute for Pelvic Neuroscience, Lutherville, MD, USA

Kenneth M. Peters Department of Urology, Beaumont Hospital, Oakland University William Beaumont School of Medicine, Royal Oak, MI, USA

Raymond Rackley Department of Urology, Cleveland Clinic, Cleveland, OH, USA

Priyamvada Rai Department of Medicine, Sylvester Comprehensive Cancer Center, University of Miami Health System, Miami, FL, USA

Navpreet Rana University of New England, Biddeford, ME, USA

Satish S.C. Rao Division of Gastroenterology and Hepatology, Augusta University, Augusta, GA, USA

Erica N. Roberson Oregon Health and Science University, Portland, OR, USA

Dudley Robinson Department of Urogynaecology, Kings College Hospital, London, UK

Ana Catarina A. Silva Department of Radiology, Unidade Local de Saúde de Matosinhos, EPE, Senhora da Hora, Portugal

Rupinder Singh Department of Geriatric Pelvic Medicine and Neurourology, Department of Internal Medicine, Sinai Hospital of Baltimore, Baltimore, MD, USA

Edward T. Soriano Pain Management Services, Sinai Hospital, Baltimore, MD, USA

Cari K. Sorrell Department of Internal Medicine, University of Texas Health Science Center at San Antonio, San Antonio, TX, USA

Sushma Srikrishna Department of Urogynecology, King's College Hospital, London, UK

Samantha Staley Department of Urology, Cleveland Clinic Akron General, Akron, OH, USA

Shane Svoboda Department of Surgery, Sinai Hospital, Baltimore, MD, USA

Ganesh Thiagamoorthy Department of Urogynecology, King's College Hospital, London, UK

Thai Lan Tran Department of Surgery, University of California, Irvine, Washington, DC, USA

Bruce R. Troen Division of Geriatrics and Palliative Medicine, Department of Medicine, Jacobs School of Medicine and Biomedical Sciences, Buffalo, NY, USA

Sandip Vasavada Department of Urology, Center for Female Pelvic Medicine and Reconstructive Surgery, Cleveland Clinic, Cleveland, OH, USA

Arnold Wald Division of Gastroenterology and Hepatology, University of Wisconsin School of Medicine and Public Health, Madison, WI, USA

Elizabeth C. Wick Department of Surgery, Johns Hopkins Hospital, Baltimore, MD, USA

Siegfried W.B. Yu Division of Gastroenterology and Hepatology, Augusta University, Augusta, GA, USA

Part I

General Physiology and Pelvic Floor Disorders

Anatomy, Neuroanatomy, and Biomechanics of the Pelvis

1

Christopher Madsen and David A. Gordon

Introduction

The pelvis, both in the female and male forms, proves to be one of the most complex anatomic and physiologic regions within the human body. Nowhere else in the body can one find the multitude of muscles, tendons, nerves, ligaments, blood vessels, organs and physiological functions tightly knit into such a compact structure (Fig. 1.1). *The pelvis is responsible for biped ambulation and support of the spinal column, sexuality,* reproduction, storage and elimination of urinary and fecal waste, and indeed represents the human body's foundation for both form and function.

A thorough and proper understanding of all of these structures and functions and how they integrate into one seamless anatomic box is of paramount importance for the surgeon operating within the pelvis. In order to be successful, the surgeon who operates within the pelvis must be disciplined and prepared, as along with its complexity, comes a great deal of risk. Often times it is resourcefulness and creativity that allows successful surgical operations here, and this can only be made possible with an appropriate fund of knowledge.

Perhaps one of the most fascinating aspects of the pelvis is its remarkable dynamic nature. From its embryological origins, through its fetal and adolescent development and into its adult maturation and finally senescent changes in older age, it truly embodies the point that the only thing that is constant is change. In addition to its evolution along the broader span of one's life span, it has only recently been truly recognized for its dynamic nature in daily activities.

C. Madsen
Department of General Surgery, Sinai Hospital, Surgical Resident, Baltimore, MD, USA

D.A. Gordon (✉)
The Division of Pelvic Neuroscience, Department of Surgery, The Sinai Hospital of Baltimore, 2401 W. Belvedere Ave, Baltimore, MD 21215, USA
e-mail: dgordon@lifebridgehealth.org

Much of the function of *the pelvic floor* derives from its ability to change both its form and function during various activities. This can be appreciated when one considers the changes necessary to accommodate straining, micturition, defecation, child birthing, intercourse, and even just standing there appearing to do nothing!

The focus of this chapter will be on the anatomic structure of the pelvis and some of the changes it experiences as it progresses with age. Particular attention will be paid to how these structures and functions relate to both the surgeon and the physiologist, and the relevance of significant changes that occur through adulthood and older age—though many of these will be addressed in specific chapters later in this text.

The Pelvis as a Unit

The *pelvis* (L. basin) is a term used loosely to identify *the region between the abdomen and the lower extremities*, a cavity bound by the pelvic girdle. It can be subdivided into the greater pelvis, a larger more superficial bowl protected by the alae of the ilia, and the lesser pelvis, a smaller bowl which lies below the pelvic brim and greater pelvis. The pelvic girdle consists of two large bones, the ossa coxae, and the sacrum, which provide mechanical support and muscular and fascial attachments for the thoraco-abdominal trunk, the lower legs, and the perineum. The lesser pelvis, or true pelvis, which is inferior to the pelvic brim, contains all of the organs related to micturition, reproduction, sexual activity, and defecation. The muscles and fascial attachments of the individual organs, as well as the pelvic diaphragm, support these structures and prevent herniation and prolapse. Externally, the pelvic cavity is bound by the muscular structures of the thigh and buttocks on each side, the anterior, lateral, and posterior abdominal wall superiorly, and the perineum inferiorly.

The term *perineum* is used to identify a specific anatomical group of structures that lie beneath the pelvis. In its most restrictive

© Springer Science+Business Media New York 2017
D.A. Gordon, M.R. Katlic (eds.), *Pelvic Floor Dysfunction and Pelvic Surgery in the Elderly*,
DOI 10.1007/978-1-4939-6554-0_1

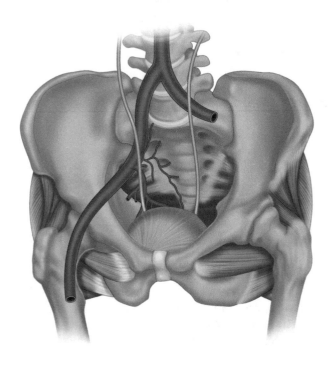

Fig. 1.1 Pelvis

definition, it refers to the soft tissue superficial to the perineal body, between the anus and the testicles or vagina. Some expand that definition to include the structures that can be found between the mons pubis, the coccyx and the thighs. However, the *Terminologia Anatomica* defines it as all of the structures which lie within the anal and urogenital triangles, including the deep structures all the way to the pelvic diaphragm.

Pelvic Osteology

Developmental Considerations

The lower limbs first appear during embryological development as ventrolateral mesenchymal outpocketings at the end of the fourth week of gestation. Complete sets of cartilage models of the pubis and ilium are seen by the end of the 6th week, and by the end of the 8th week of gestation, a homogenous cartilage model of both the right and left os coxae, including the ilium, ischium, and pubis is present [1]. Endochondral ossification of the ilium begins during the ninth week, with multiple primary and secondary ossification centers (Fig. 1.2). Haversian bone remodeling doesn't begin until late in fetal development, usually after the 28th week, but the finalization of fetal pelvis development is highly dependent on mechanical stimulation, namely gluteal muscle activity and pressure at the femoral head [2]. After birth, and even through childhood, the three bones of the coxae remain separated by the triradiate cartilage, which centers within the cup of the acetabulum.

The development of the sacrum occurs in a rudimentary, but similar fashion as that of the vertebral column, through migration, resegmentation, and fusing of sclerotomes beginning in the 4th week of gestation. By the 8th week, the sacrum and coccyx are recognizable structures, and the four pairs of sacral foramina are present. Fusion of the coccyx and the sacrum occur as processes which last throughout fetal development and early postnatal development, and even continue into adolescence and young adulthood.

The relationship between the sacrum and pubic bones forms as a result of a complex process which begins as early as they can be identified near the 6th week of gestation, with an "ilio-sacral connector" composed of fibrocytes embedded within a collagen and elastin matrix cord. The ala of the ilium rapidly elongates to meet the opposing sacral ala to unite the appendicular and axial skeletons. The sacroiliac joint forms uniquely when compared to most joints in the body, in a process termed secondary joint development, occurring much later in neonatal development.

The pelvis continues to develop and change throughout life, with continued ossification and growth during childhood and puberty. The ala of the ilium grows disproportionately to the pelvic bodies during the first 8 years of life, and the progression of sacral kyphosis continues until approximately 14 years of age when it reaches approximately 25° with an apex at the level of S3. The rotation and anteroposterior position of the sacrum relative to the spine and femur, measured by the pelvic incidence (PI), changes in a linear fashion throughout life (Fig. 1.3).

In addition to osteoporotic changes, as the pelvis ages, it collapses in a cephalo-caudal direction with concurrent widening of the pelvis in the anteroposterior plane, caused by posterior migration of the sacrum relative to the femoral head. The pelvis grows both in width and length during childhood, but has long been assumed to cease growth with skeletal maturity. More recent radiographic analyses suggest that the pelvis continues to widen throughout adulthood at a linear rate of about 1 mm every 3 years measured both at the trochanters and the iliac wings. Interestingly, the pelvic inlet does not change in dimensions over this same time period, and these observations are consistent in both men and women.

Site Specific Considerations

The Ossa Coxae

The right and left hip bones, or *os coxae*, are large irregularly shaped bones which form the foundation that unites the upper body with the lower body. Each is derived from the fusion of three separate bones, the *ilium*, the *ischium*, and the *pubis*. The fusion of the ilium, ischium, and pubis occurs during puberty, as the ossification of the triradiate cartilage molds the acetabulum into a single cohesive cup. The anatomic structures of the ossa coxae are illustrated in Fig. 1.4.

Fig. 1.2 (**a**) Lower extremity of an early 6-week embryo, illustrating the first hyaline cartilage models. (**b**, **c**) Complete set of cartilage models at the end of the 6th week and the beginning of the 8th week, respectively

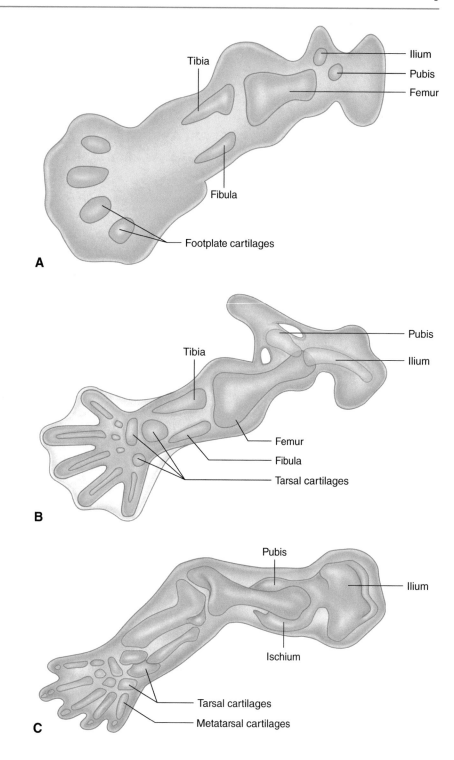

The *ilium* is the largest and most superior portion of the coxae. It is composed of a large fan-shaped region, the *ala* (wing), and the *body of the ilium*, to which the fan is attached. The *iliac crest* is the most superior portion of the pelvic girdle, and lies between the *anterior superior iliac spine* (ASIS), and the *posterior superior iliac spine* (PSIS). On the inside surface the iliac fossa can be found, bordered by the iliac crest superiorly, and the *arcuate line*, or pelvic brim, inferiorly. The posterior portion of the ilium is responsible for articulating with the sacrum, at the articular surface, which lies just below the ilial tuberosity and above the greater sciatic notch.

The *ischium* is the posteroinferior portion of the coxae and makes up the posterior wall of the obturator canal. The body of the ischium attaches to the body of the ilium, and together they form the majority of the acetabulum and are responsible for the greatest amount of load bearing and weight transference associated with the hip joint. The *ischial spine* projects from the posterior portion of the body, just

Fig. 1.3 Diagram showing
the sacral slope, pelvic tilt,
and pelvic incidence

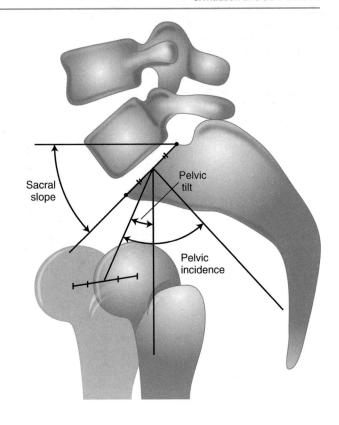

Fig. 1.4 Structures and
anatomic relationships of the
ossa coxae

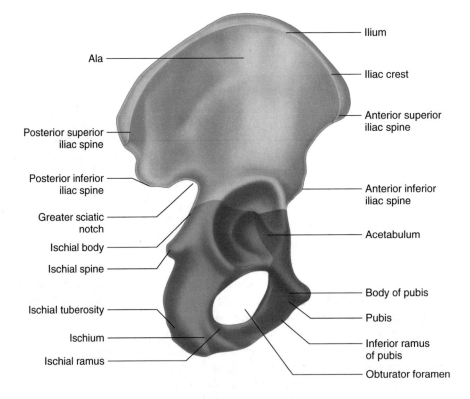

below which can be found the *lesser sciatic notch*. The *ischial tuberosity* and *ischial ramus* project inferiorly from the body of the ischium, and in turn, communicate with the pubic ramus to form the obturator canal.

The *pubis* makes up the last of three portions of the coxae, lying inferior to the ilium and anterior to the ischium. The body of the pubis attaches to the anterior portion of the body of the ilium. The arcuate line of the ilium continues through the pubis as the *pectineal line*, or *pectin pubis*, terminating at the *pubic tubercle*. The *superior pubic ramus* projects inferomedially from the pubic body to join the contralateral pubis at the *pubic symphysis*. The pubis symphysis is a secondary cartilaginous joint articulating medially at the symphyseal surface of each pubis. The joint is composed of an interpubic disc, strengthened by the superior and inferior pubic ligaments.

Significant differences are observed between men and women in the overall shape of the ossa coxae, and thus the pelvis itself (Fig. 1.5). Women tend to have more attenuated contours, less pronounced features and an overall lighter, more flattened pelvis. The female pelvis generally exhibits a larger pelvic outlet (distance measured between

ischial spines) with a concurrent wider and more circular pelvic inlet (the shortest distance measured between the most anterior portion of S1 and the pubis symphysis). The female ilia and iliac wings fan out laterally more than that of the male, and as a result do not project as far superiorly, which results in a lower iliac crest relative to the sacrum. The angle between the two opposing pubic bones, or pubic angle, in the female pelvis is much narrower when compared to the male, with pubic angles commonly >100° in females and <90° in males. Many of these anatomic differences are a result of adaptations to the physiologic stresses and loads placed by carrying the fetus during pregnancy as well as delivery of the fetus during childbirth.

The Sacrum and Coccyx

The *sacrum* is a large triangular shaped bone that consists of five individual vertebrae that fuse into a single cohesive unit early in life. Initially, the individual sacral vertebrae resemble the lumbar vertebrae; however, at the end of the first year of life ossification of the sacral ala occurs [3]. The process of sacral vertebral fusion begins during puberty with the lateral

Fig. 1.5 Differences between the male and female bony pelvis

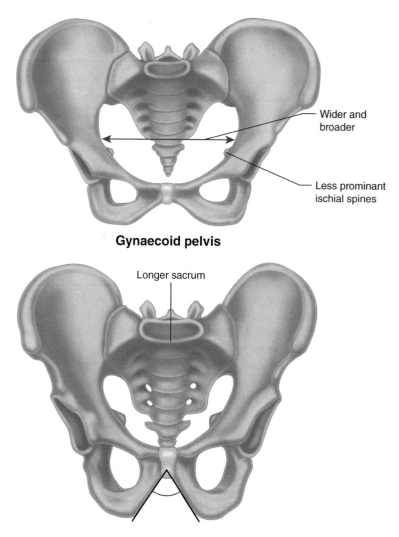

Gynaecoid pelvis

Android pelvis

costal elements, and it is not until the age of 18 that the vertebral bodies themselves begin to fuse, beginning caudally and advancing cranially [4]. Completion of sacral fusion does not occur until between the ages of 25 and 33 [5], and is a direct result of load bearing activity, as paraplegic children who do not bear weight will retain independent sacral vertebrae with incomplete fusion [6]. At birth, the sacral base and lumbar spine are angulated approximately 20° from the vertical axis, however this progresses consistently until it reaches approximately 60–70° in adulthood [4, 7]. The curvature of the sacrum itself is minimal in newborns but develops into a mean angle of approximately 65° by late adolescence (measured in the sagittal plane as the angle between the first and fifth sacral vertebra). The discrepant relationships that male and female sacrums have to the pelvis can be almost entirely accounted for by the sacral slope, or the angle that the fifth lumbar vertebral body rests on the sacrum, as the sacral curvature does not change significantly between men and women.

The *anterior sacral surface* forms a bowl-shaped concavity with four prominent ridges traveling in a transverse direction, each correlating with a neural foramen on either side (Fig. 1.6). These ridges are the remnants of the intervertebral discs that were obliterated in the process of sacral fusion. The four pairs of sacral foramina reside on either side of the transverse ridges, and are positioned in an anterolateral direction to allow the passage of the anterior divisions of their corresponding sacral nerves and lateral sacral arteries.

The *posterior sacral surface* forms the reciprocal exterior bowl shape of the sacrum, inheriting a convex shape and is primarily involved in muscle attachment for the posterior thigh and lower back. Similar to the anterior sacral surface, the posterior surface has a number of ridges that dominate its topography; however, on the posterior surface these ridges run longitudinally. The *median sacral crest* is the most pronounced posterior sacral ridge, a confluence of spinous processes most pronounced at the first sacral vertebra, diminishing with each level below and absent by the fourth or fifth sacral vertebrae. On either side of the median sacral crest are the *sacral grooves* which are longitudinal indentations within the underlying sacral laminae, and lateral to these are the fused articular processes that make up the *parallel intermediate crests* [4]. Similar to the anterior surface, the posterior surface houses four smaller, less regular pairs of neural foramina which are all located lateral to the intermediate crests and contain the posterior divisions of the sacral nerves. The transverse processes of the sacral vertebrae appear as a longitudinal series of tubercles lateral to the posterior foramina and are collectively termed the *lateral crests*. Inferiorly, the longitudinal crests and grooves of the posterior sacral surface terminate before that of the fused sacral vertebral bodies, creating an opening referred to as the sacral hiatus. The anterior and posterior sacral anatomy is illustrated in Fig. 1.6.

The *coccyx* develops as a primitive tail consisting of as many as ten somites, but regresses in a stepwise caudal to cranial fashion with resorption of as many as six of the distal most coccygeal vertebrae, along with their corresponding nerves and blood vessels [8, 9]. Approximately 75% of the population has 4 coccygeal vertebrae with a mean length between 3.0 and 3.3 cm [10]. Unlike the other named portions of the human spine, the coccyx has a wide range of "normal" angulations relative to the vertical axis and sacrum, and discrepant data exists on whether or not women have less of a curvature than men [11]. Interestingly, although the sacrum and coccyx both become fused osseous structures by age 30, the sacrococcygeal joint remains unfused and retains a mean degree of articulation of 9° in the sagittal plane, as measured between the standing and sitting position [12], and up to 12.5° between contraction and relaxation during defecation [13].

The Ligamentous Structure of the Pelvis

The osteologic form of the pelvis provides a tremendously strong infrastructure for the ligamentous support of the pelvis, its contents, as well as the lower extremities and torso and the forces they each apply. The fascial and ligamentous elements of the pelvis are composed of collagen and elastin matrices, as they are elsewhere in the body, and are prone to changes in relative distribution during pregnancy, maturation, and senescence. These changes often cause an increase in structural laxity of the pelvic support system, which can lead to urinary and fecal incontinence, urinary retention and constipation, and eventually organ prolapse.

Broadly speaking, the pelvis attaches to various ligaments and fascial layers externally to maintain its anatomic position relative to the torso and lower extremities, and internally to maintain the anatomic position of the organs within. The myofascial and ligamentous superstructure of the anterior pelvis is intimately associated with the musculature of the abdominal wall and the adductor muscle groups of the lower extremities [14]. The myofascial and ligamentous superstructure of the posterior pelvis contributes to a broader overall function, with attachments derived from the back and abdomen, the lower extremity and even the upper extremity [14].

External Ligamentous Support of the Pelvis

The *pubic symphysis* is a fibrocartilaginous joint that articulates between the bilateral pubic bones, and considered by most to be a static structure, although vertical displacement of up to 2 mm in addition to 1° rotation is commonly observed [14]. The articular surfaces that oppose each other have a thin layer of hyaline cartilage associated with them, which decreases with age; however, most do not consider the pubic symphysis to be

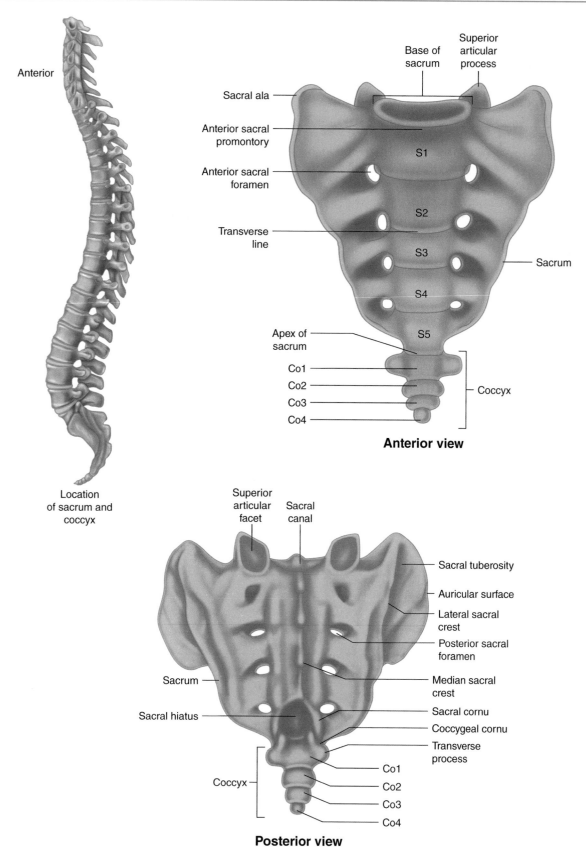

Fig. 1.6 Anterior and posterior views of the human sacrum and coccyx

a synovial joint [14]. The joint is reinforced by the *superior and inferior pubic ligaments*, as well as the *anterior and posterior pubic ligaments*. The anterior pubic ligament splays into an important aponeurosis that attaches to the rectus abdominis superiorly and the adductor longus muscle inferiorly.

The *sacroiliac joint* is a kidney bean shaped bicondylar joint associated with a multitude of both intrinsic and extrinsic ligaments. The anterior surface of the joint is composed of the smooth sacroiliac joint capsule that is firmly attached to the *iliolumbar ligaments* superiorly, and the *sacrospinous* and *sacrotuberous ligaments* inferiorly. The sacroiliac joint is reinforced posteriorly by the *short posterior sacroiliac ligaments* that span between the posterior superior iliac spine (PSIS) and the more superior lumbar vertebral spinous processes.

Similarly, the *long posterior sacroiliac ligaments* span between the PSIS and the more inferior lumbar vertebral spinous processes. The multifidus muscle influences the sacroiliac joint's motion posteriorly via attachments to the connective tissue fibers of the gluteus maximus near the midline and the biceps femoris muscle after it crosses the sacrotuberous ligament [10, 12, 14]. The ligaments of the sacrum are illustrated in Fig. 1.7.

Internal Ligamentous Support of the Pelvis

The internal ligamentous support of the pelvis is essentially derived from two sources; those associated with individual muscles of the pelvic floor and those that act as suspensory

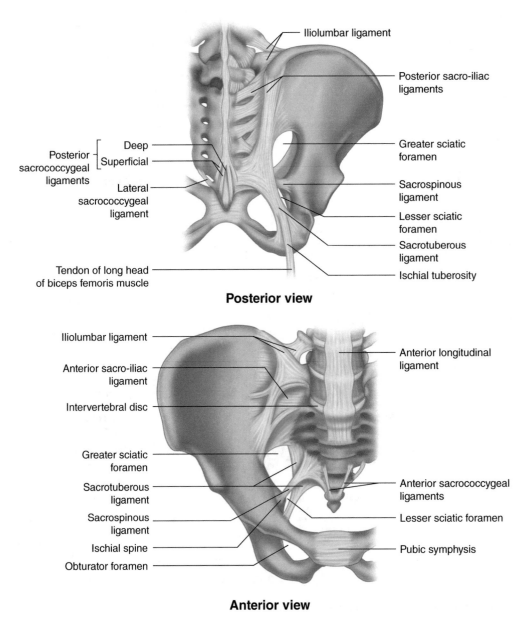

Posterior view

Anterior view

Fig. 1.7 Ligaments of the sacrum and pelvis

ligaments for individual organs. The internal anatomic form of the pelvis obviously differs a great deal between men and women with the additional organs and their supporting structures. The function and integrity of the organs within the pelvis rely completely upon the supporting ligaments, fascia and muscles, and without these structures, "normal" function would be impossible.

Female Specific Anatomy

Among the more important intrinsic pelvic ligaments involved in urethral suspension in females are the *pubourethral ligament* (PUL) and the external urethral ligament (EUL) [15]. The PUL originates from the posterior inferior edge of the pubis symphysis and splays into a fan-shaped structure to insert onto the midurethra, pubococcygeus muscle, and vaginal wall [15, 16]. The *external urethral ligament*, also known as the anterior pubourethral ligament, helps support the urethral meatus against the anterior surface of the pubic rami, and continues superiorly to the clitoris and inferiorly to the PUL [17]. The *pubovesical ligament* (PVL) serves as the major structural unit for the anterior wall of the bladder, originating from the posterior surface of the pubis and inserting onto the *transverse precervical Arc of Gilvernet*, a thickened portion of the PVL that maintains the anterior placement of the bladder and helps to prevent anterior collapse of the bladder wall during micturition [17]. The *cardinal ligaments*, as well as the *uterosacral ligaments* (USL), each attach to the cervical ring complex from just above the ischial spine, and

from the overlying fascia of S2–S4, respectively [17], and help to suspend the vagina and uterus. Additionally, the USL provides fixation points for the action of the levator plate and the longitudinal muscle of the anus. The internal ligamentous structure of the female pelvis is illustrated in Fig. 1.8.

The *arcus tendineus fascia pelvis (ATFP)* in women is a critical structure involved in vaginal suspension that has multiple important components. It is composed of a confluence of parietal fascia derived from the neighboring pubococcygeus and iliococcygeus portions of the levator ani mechanism and the obturator internus [18]. It courses along the pelvic sidewall between its origin approximately 1 cm lateral to the pubic symphysis. It inserts at each of the ischial spines, and has been divided into 3 distinct segments: anterior, middle and posterior—with the anterior and middle segments each approximately 3 cm in length and the posterior segment approximately 2.5 cm [18].

The most anterior segment attaches to the proximal urethra and anterior vaginal wall, the middle segment attaches to the anterolateral vaginal wall, and the posterior segment acts only to anchor the entire structure. The ATFP has two very important connections that insert at the point between the middle and posterior segments: the *arcus tendineus levator ani (ATLA)* and the rectovaginal fascia. *Interestingly, it has been noted that >96 % of parous women have an avulsion of the posterior segment of the ATFP from the ischial spines, but often do not experience prolapse until years later, if at all.*

Lateral vaginal fascial attachments to the ATFP ligaments span the length of the vagina and create a structure akin to a cloth army cot with metal bars on either side, on top of which

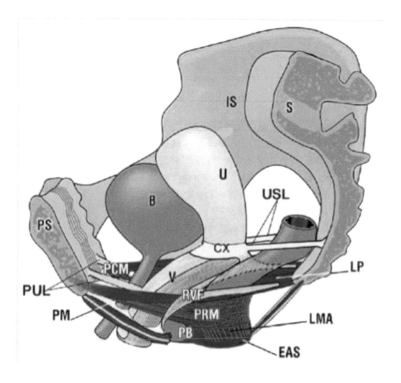

Fig. 1.8 The internal ligamentous structures of the female pelvis. *PS* pubis symphysis, *B* bladder, *U* uterus, *USL* uterosacral ligament, *PCM* pubococcygeus muscle, *V* vagina, *C* cervix, *LP* levator plate, *PUL* pubourethral ligament, *RVF* rectovaginal space, *PM* muscles of the perineal membrane, *PRM* puborectalis muscle, *LMA* longitudinal muscle of the anus, *PB* perineal body, *EAS* external anal sphincter

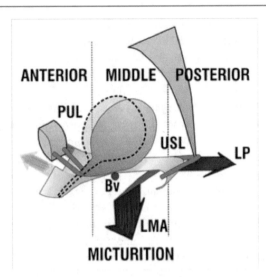

Fig. 1.9 Anterior, middle, and posterior segments of the ATFP ligament and its actions related to the LP and LMA mechanisms involved in micturition

the vagina rests. The bilateral ATFP ligaments are critical structures involved with not only vaginal suspension though, but indeed total pelvic support, and form anchor points for the action of multiple force vectors produced by the pelvic floor musculature, such as the *longitudinal muscle of the anus (LMA) and levator plate (LP)*. Relaxation of the LMA and LP mechanisms allow for the ATFP to close the urinary outflow tract by collapsing the rigid inferior portion of the *trigone* against the opposing side of the urethral canal, while flexion of the LMA and LP mechanisms allow for the opening of the urinary outflow tract by allowing the ATFP to pull open and splint the urethral canal open using the pubococcygeus muscle (PCM) (Fig. 1.9) [17].

Male Specific Anatomy

In males, the overall mechanism that suspends the urethra is a complex structure similar to that found in females and formed by a number of both discreet and visibly indiscreet ligaments (Fig. 1.10). This structure is a pyramidal shaped band inserting along the lateral aspects of the membranous urethra and originating from the pubic arch. It is made up of three ligaments that are found contiguous with one another: the *anterior pubourethral ligament*—a facial reflection of the perineal membrane which also acts partially to suspend the penis, *the intermediate pubourethral ligament*—composed of the arcuate and transverse ligaments, and the *posterior pubourethral ligament* (or "puboprostatic ligament") [19]. In addition to a specific urethral suspensory mechanism, the penis itself has its own important suspensory ligamentous structure that maintains its proper position over the pubis, particularly important during erection and sexual intercourse.

The penile suspensory mechanism is composed of three individual structures; the penile suspensory mechanism proper, the fundiform ligament, and the arcuate subpubic ligament (Fig. 1.11). The *penile suspensory ligament proper* spans between the pubis symphysis and the tunica albuginea which invests the corpus cavernosa [20]. The *fundiform ligament* is a thin superficial band that courses just anterior to the penile suspensory ligament proper but does not have a direct attachment to the tunica albuginea [20], and the *arcuate subpubic ligament* is a thick triangular arch that lies just posterior, spanning between the two inferior pubic rami underneath the pubic symphysis [21].

There are both true and false ligaments that support the bladder and prostate in the male (Fig. 1.12). The *lateral true ligaments* are fibroareolar ligaments derived from transversalis fascia (otherwise known as the tendinous arch of the endopelvic fascia) overlying the levator muscles that connect directly to the external muscular fascia of the bladder. The *posterior vesical ligaments* are formed by continuations of fibrous tissue derived from the posterior vesical venous plexus located laterally at the base of the bladder and drain into the internal iliac veins on either side. Similarly, the *lateral puboprostatic ligaments* also derive from tendinous arch of the endopelvic fascia derived from the transversalis fascia and insert onto the fibrous sheath of the prostate. The *medial puboprostatic ligaments* run from the inferior portion of the pubis and insert onto the anterior prostatic fibrous sheath.

The Trigone

The *vesical trigone* has historically been described as having embryological origins from the common nephric duct and ureter [22, 23], and possibly the detrusor muscle itself as well [24]. It is composed mainly of smooth muscle and forms a significant portion of bladder base that spans between the ureteral orifices and the urethral opening, and continues down the posterior wall of the urethra all the way to the external urethral meatus. Although the trigone is identified as a muscular structure, its action is akin to a rigid structure with more ligamentous properties than muscular. This rigid structure is then manipulated by bladder and endopelvic musculature to open the urethral orifice during micturition events (via the LMA and LP), and close the urethral orifice during continence (via the PCM) (Fig. 1.9).

Pelvic Myology

Embryologic Considerations

The embryologic development of the pelvic musculature occurs as a result of a complex orchestrated dance that involves the spinal column, the lower limbs, the abdominal wall, the

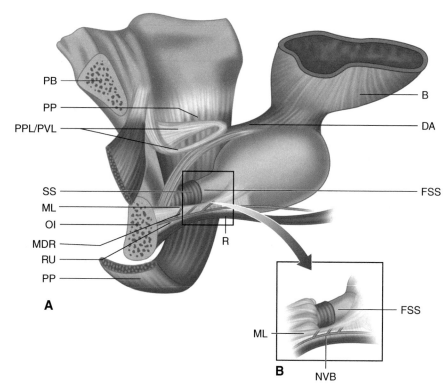

Fig. 1.10 Surgical anatomy of the urethral sphincter complex. (**a**) Fixation of the urethral sphincter; (**b**) Lateral aspect of the urethral sphincter after nerve sparing. *PPL* puboprostatic ligament, *PVL* pubovesicalis ligament, *PP* puboperinealis muscle, *DA* detrusor apron, *B* bladder, *FSS* fascia of the striated sphincter, *ML* Mueller's ligaments (ischioprostatic ligaments), *NVB* neurovascular bundle, *R* rectum, *MDR* medial dorsal raphe, *RU* rectourethralis muscle, *OI* Os ischiadicum, *SS* striated sphincter (rhabdosphincter), *PB* pubis bone

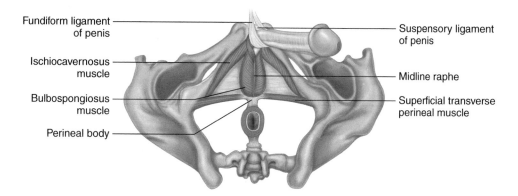

Fig. 1.11 Penile suspensory mechanism

peritoneal sac, the urogenital system, and the gastrointestinal tract. Muscular development within the pelvis occurs in a secondary process related to signaling that is derived from these many concurrently developing systems, and is largely outside the scope of this book. That being said, there are a few basic concepts that will be discussed that can lend to a better understanding of normal and variant pelvic anatomy.

During the 5th and 6th weeks of embryologic development, the distal hindgut, or cloaca, forms the allantoic diverticulum, which will later carry the umbilical vessels and eventually become the *median umbilical ligament* [25]. The urorectal septum forms within the dilated terminal hindgut that separates the cloaca into the ventral urogenital sinus, and the dorsal rectum.

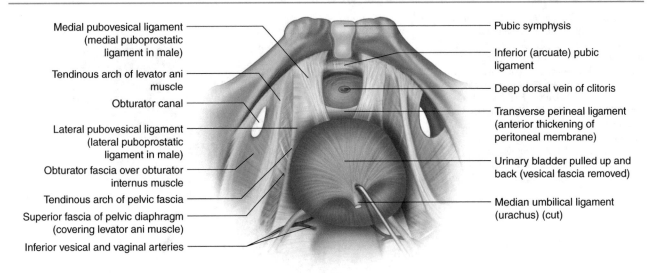

Fig. 1.12 Ligaments of the male and female pelvis associated with urethral and vesical suspension

During the 8th week, mesenchymal tissue that originates from the caudal eminence then migrates along the cloacal membrane to form the superficial perineum and its associated musculature that derives from the cloacal sphincter and innervated by the pudendal nerve [26]. This mesenchymal thickening divides itself into superficial and deep layers, which will become the superficial perineum and the deep perineum. The *superficial perineum* (or superficial perineal pouch) will later contain the superficial transverse perineal muscle, the bulbospongiosum, the ischiocavernosus, the crura of the penis and bulb of the penis in males, and the crura of the clitoris and vestibular bulbs in the female. The *deep perineum* (or deep perineal pouch) will develop into the external anal sphincter, the deep transverse perineal muscle, and the membranous (external) urethral sphincter.

After the 12th week, the cloacal sphincter divides into the ventral sphincter of the urogenital sinus and the more dorsal external anal sphincter. By the twentieth week, the *urogenital sinus* has further developed to include the superficial peroneal muscles and urethral sphincter, and deep peroneal muscles and anal sphincter [27]. Importantly, the levator ani and coccygeus muscles derive from mesenchymal tissue superior to where the perineum originates, and during embryonic development they descend into the pelvis.

Individual Considerations

The Psoas Major, the Psoas Minor, and the Iliacus

The muscles of the true pelvis do not include the psoas major, the psoas minor or the iliacus, nor do they include any of the muscles of the anterior abdominal wall. The *psoas major* arises from the lumbar vertebrae, is innervated by the nearby

ventral rami (L1–L3), and can be divided into deep (posterior) and superficial (anterior) portions. The deep psoas major originates from the lumbar transverse processes (L1–L4) and the superficial psoas major originates from the lateral portion of the vertebral bodies and intervertebral discs at similar levels (T12–L4), with the lumbar plexus running in between. The *psoas minor* muscle is a variably present structure in humans, and lies anterior and medial to the psoas major. It is a smaller, thinner muscle that follows the psoas major across the ilium and is innervated by the L1 ventral ramus, however it most commonly inserts onto the iliopubic eminence, whereas the psoas major crosses over the iliopubic eminence to insert onto the lesser trochanter of the femur.

The *iliacus muscle* is a broad fan-shaped muscle that sits within the iliac wing. It joins the psoas major muscle to become the iliopsoas, and also crosses over the iliopubic eminence to insert on the lesser trochanter. The iliacus is innervated by the femoral nerve (L2–L3). The psoas major, the psoas minor, and the iliacus all act as hip flexors to raise the leg and are illustrated in Fig. 1.13.

The Obturator Internus and Piriformis Muscles

The true pelvis is lined with muscles in much the same way that the *false pelvis* is lined by the iliacus and the iliopsoas. In the *true pelvis*, it is the obturator internus and the piriformis that are set against the sidewalls (Fig. 1.14).

The *obturator internus* is a broad based muscle that originates from the obturator membrane and surrounding ischium, travels posterior to cross out of the pelvis at the lesser sciatic foramen, and inserts onto the greater trochanter of the femur. Interestingly, this acute right-angle configuration of the obturator internus muscle belly and tendon is preserved all the way back to 6-week-old embryos—before even the anatomy

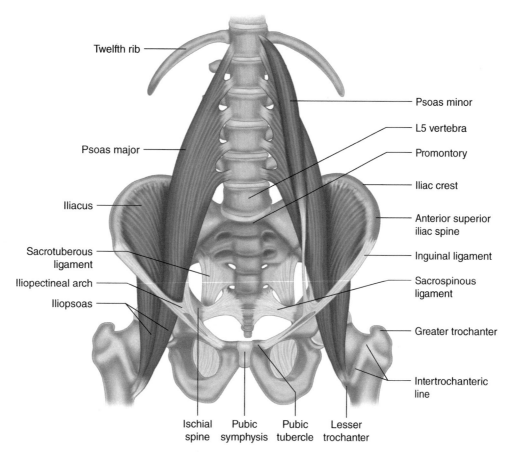

Fig. 1.13 The psoas major, psoas minor, and iliacus muscles

of the pelvic bones is determined [28]. The obturator internus is innervated by the nerve to the obturator internus,
derived from L5–S1, and acts to laterally rotate the thigh.
*The fascia overlying the obturator internus thickens to form
a strong band that spans between the ischial spine and pubis,
known as the arcus tendineus levator ani, (ATLA) which
anchors much of the pelvic diaphragm anteriorly.*

The *piriformis muscle* acts similarly to the obturator internus muscle. It originates from the anterior and lateral aspects
of the sacrum, with interdigitating fingers along the sacral
foramina. It passes out of the pelvis to cross over the greater
sciatic foramen and insert onto the greater trochanter—making it a lateral rotator of the hip as well. *Of clinical significance, the sciatic nerve passes between the obturator
internus and the piriformis muscles as it exits the pelvis to
course down the posterior thigh, and thus is a possible anatomic area for entrapment (Piriformis syndrome).* The piriformis nerve is derived from the ventral rami of S1-S2.

The Pelvic Diaphragm

Just as there are two major muscles that line the pelvic sidewalls, there are two major muscles that make up the floor of
the pelvis, i.e., the pelvic diaphragm. These two muscles are
the coccygeus and the levator ani (which can be divided into
the iliococcygeus, the pubococcygeus, and the puborectalis)
(Fig. 1.15).

The *coccygeus muscle* makes up the smaller, posterior
portion of the pelvic diaphragm. It is a broad fan-shaped
muscle of the pelvis that originates from the ischial spine and
sacrospinous ligament and inserts onto coccyx and anococcygeal body. The coccygeus muscle is innervated by the ventral rami of S4–S5.

The *levator ani* is a group of three muscles that comprises the majority of the muscular pelvic floor. The first,
the *iliococcygeus*, is the most posterior of the three and
originates from the medial side of the inferior ischium and
the obturator fascia and runs across the pelvic floor to the

Fig. 1.14 The obturator internus muscle, piriformis muscle, quadratus femoris muscle, and superior and inferior gemellus muscles

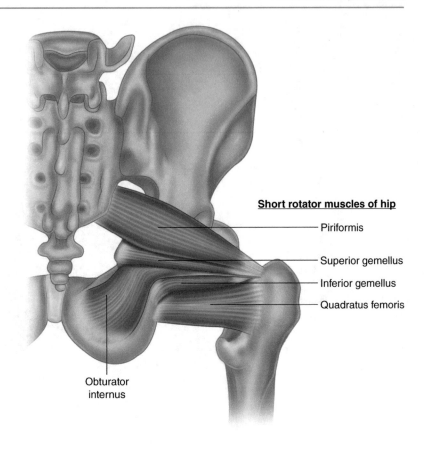

Short rotator muscles of hip

Piriformis

Superior gemellus

Inferior gemellus

Quadratus femoris

Obturator internus

Fig. 1.15 The levator ani and coccygeus muscles

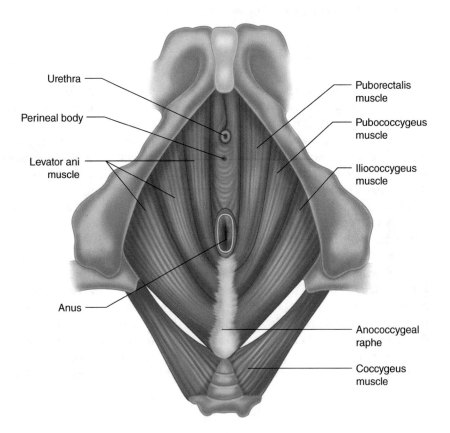

Urethra

Perineal body

Levator ani muscle

Anus

Puborectalis muscle

Pubococcygeus muscle

Iliococcygeus muscle

Anococcygeal raphe

Coccygeus muscle

anococcygeal body and coccyx. The iliococcygeus is commonly much less well developed when compared to the other components of the levator ani, and may be present only as a thick fibrous band. The *pubococcygeus* originates from the posterior inferior portion of the pubis and the arcus tendineus levator ani, and inserts onto the anococcygeal body and coccyx, and represents the majority of the levator ani musculature. The *puborectalis* muscle forms a sling around the rectum which aides in bowel continence. It originates from the posterior inferior portion of the pubis, medial to the pubococcygeal origin, and runs along either side of the rectum to unite with itself on the posterior side of the rectum.

Additional fibers from the pubococcygeus create sling mechanisms around the prostate (males) and vagina (females) and are appropriately termed the *puboprostatic*

and *pubovaginalis* muscles. The levator ani complex is chiefly innervated by the ventral rami of S4–S5, although it does receive some nerve fibers from the pudendal nerve.

Pelvic Myofascial Support

The fascial superstructure of the pelvis represents a complex web of fibrous support that derives from the lower extremities, the muscular torso, and many of the intra-abdominal organs. *The pelvic fascia can be divided into three distinct substructures—the inner stratum, the intermediate stratum, and the outer stratum* (Fig. 1.16).

The *inner stratum* is a subperitoneal fibrous layer investing the gastrointestinal tissue of the rectum. The rectal fascia forms the anterior lamella of Denonvilliers' fascia and covers the rectal arteries and nerves. The *intermediate stratum* is a layer that is contiguous with the renal fascia (Gerota's fascia) that has

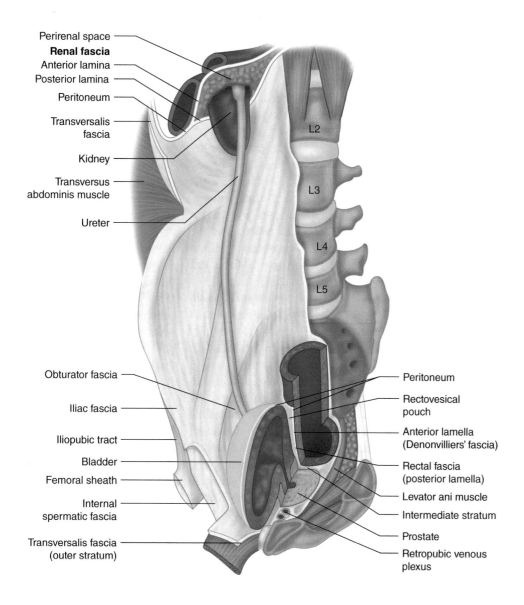

Fig. 1.16 The pelvic fascial layers

contributions from the anterior and posterior lamina of the renal fascia, the perirenal fat, and the ureteral sheath and continues inferiorly to make up the vesical and prostatic fascia. In the female, the intermediate stratum invests the uterus and the blood vessels supplying the uterus and vagina. The *outer stratum* consists of the transversalis fascia and its continuation throughout the pelvis, and is named regionally by the structures it covers, such as the iliac fascia, the psoas fascia, the iliacus fascia, the obturator fascia, and the pectineal fascia which continues down to form the posterior portion of the femoral sheath.

The endopelvic fascia, pelvic diaphragmatic fascia, and the lateral pelvic fascia are also continuous with the outer stratum, and thus, the transversalis fascia. This layer also forms the posterior portion of the inguinal ligament and the internal spermatic fascia. The tendinous arch of the pelvic diaphragm (ATFP) is a thickened band of fibrous tissue that runs from the pubis symphysis to either ischial spine, and is a distinct structure from that of the tendinous arch of the levator ani, which is a thickening of the obturator fascia and forms the wall of the ischiorectal fossa.

Peritoneal Reflections in the Male

The superior aspects of the pelvic organs are covered with a peritoneal lining much like a linen cloth draped over them, which creates multiple folds and pockets over and in between important anatomic structures. Deep in the pelvis lies the *rectovesical pouch,* commonly termed the "cul-de-sac," which is simply the pocket of space that lies between the bladder and rectum near the level of the seminal vesicles. The sacrogenital folds extend posteriolaterally from the bladder to the sacrum, marking the lateral boundary of the rectovesical pouch. There is a peritoneal depression on either side of the rectum that extends to the sacrogenital folds, this space is termed the *perirectal fossa* (Fig. 1.17).

The peritoneum near the bottom of the rectovesical pouch fuses early in life, creating a double layer of peritoneum, with resultant absorption of the peritoneal lining which leaves only a fibrous extraperitoneal connective tissue continuation that forms the *anterior lamella of Denonvilliers' fascia.*

As the peritoneum continues anteriorly and superiorly from the seminal vesicles and over the dome of the bladder, it forms three distinct folds that extend from the anterior abdominal wall. The *median umbilical fold* is in the midline and covers the urachus, which becomes the *median umbilical ligament.* Just lateral to this, on either side of the median umbilical fold, lies the *medial umbilical folds* that are composed of the obliterated umbilical arteries, and thus travel between the internal iliac arteries and the umbilicus. The *supravesical fossa* is found on either side in between the median and medial umbilical folds. The *lateral umbilical folds* cover the epigastric vessels and make up the lateral margins of the *median umbilical (paravesical) fossa,* with the lateral inguinal fossa on the lateral side (Fig. 1.18).

Peritoneal Reflections in the Female

The peritoneal coverings of the female pelvis are very much similar to that in the male, with the important differences relating to the presence of the uterus (Fig. 1.17). *The uterus lies between the bladder and the rectum within the female pelvis, and thus there is no rectovesical fossa. Rather, there is the recto-uterine fossa (pouch of Douglas),* which is much deeper than the rectovesical fossa in males, and extends nearly all the way to the anus. The *vesico-uterine fossa* is a much less developed recess between the female bladder and the uterus, and divided from the recto-uterine fossa by the broad ligaments.

The broad ligaments are covered by peritoneum derived from both anterior and posterior surfaces of the uterus.

The Perineum

The perineum is the anatomic term for a diamond shaped region superficial to the pelvic diaphragm that lies between the ischial tuberosities on either side, the pubis symphysis anteriorly and the coccyx posteriorly. By definition, the deep border of the perineum is the fascia of the levator ani. The *perineum* is commonly subdivided into anterior and posterior regions, the urogenital triangle and the anogenital triangle, as well as deep and superficial compartments. The *perineal membrane* divides the superficial and deep compartments. The urogenital triangle includes all of the structures anterior to the ischial tuberosities, and the anogenital triangle includes all of the structures posterior to the ischial tuberosities.

In the *male,* the deep perineal compartment contains the deep perineal muscles, external urethral sphincter and the bulbourethral glands; the superficial compartment contains the superficial perineal muscles, the ischiocavernosus, the bulbospongiosus, and the crura and bulbs of the penis (Fig. 1.19). In the *female,* the deep perineal compartment contains the deep perineal muscles, the compressor urethrae muscle, and the urethrovaginal sphincter; the superficial compartment contains the ischiocavernosus, the bulbospongiosus, the deep perineal muscles as well as the vestibular bulbs, Bartholin's glands, and the crura of the clitoris (Fig. 1.20).

The Anogenital Triangle

The *anogenital triangle* contains the anus, the external anal sphincter and the ischioanal fossa that lies on either side. Although there is no consensus on the matter, the external anal sphincter has historically been divided into three regions—the subcutaneous region, the superficial region, and the deep region. More recently, however, the subcutaneous and superficial regions have been combined, leaving just the superficial and deep compartments of the *external anal sphincter* [29]. The anal sphincter mechanism is composed of

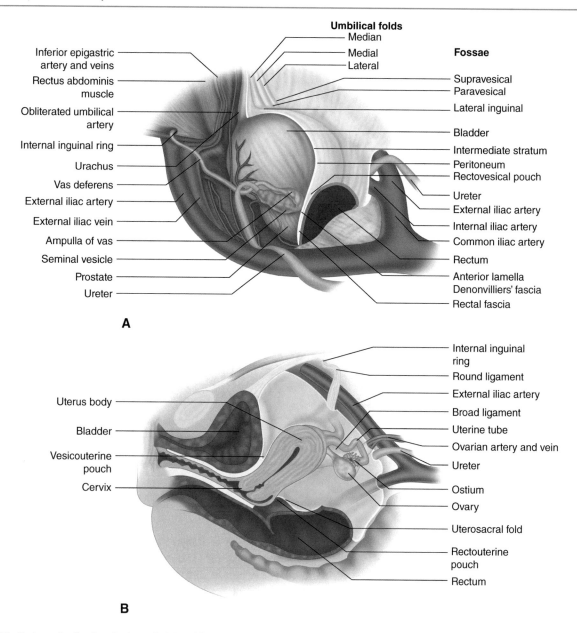

Fig. 1.17 Peritoneal reflections in the male (**a**) and female (**b**) pelvis

the external anal sphincter, the internal anal sphincter, and the puborectalis. The external anal sphincter is innervated by the pudendal nerve (S2–S4) and is made up of skeletal muscle under conscious control as well as tonic contraction with reflex activity as a result of increased intra-abdominal pressure. The details of the anal sphincter physiology and neuromodulation will be discussed in detail in a later chapter.

The Male Urogenital Triangle

The urogenital triangle in the male almost exclusively contains the structures associated with the base of the penis—the bulb and crura of the penis and its associated musculature

(Fig. 1.19). This includes the structures from the superficial perineal pouch (superficial perineal muscles, the ischiocavernosus, the bulbospongiosus, and the crura and bulbs of the penis), and the deep perineal pouch (deep perineal muscles, external urethral sphincter and the bulbourethral glands). The fascia overlying the rectus and external oblique muscles continues into the perineum to become the deep perineal fascia (Gallaudet's fascia) and is associated with the ischiocavernosus, the bulbospongiosus, and the superficial perineal muscles and continues further into the penis as the deep fascia of the penis (Buck's fascia). Similarly, Scarpa's fascia of the anterior abdominal wall continues into the perineum, renamed Colle's fascia, and further into the penis and scrotum as dartos fascia.

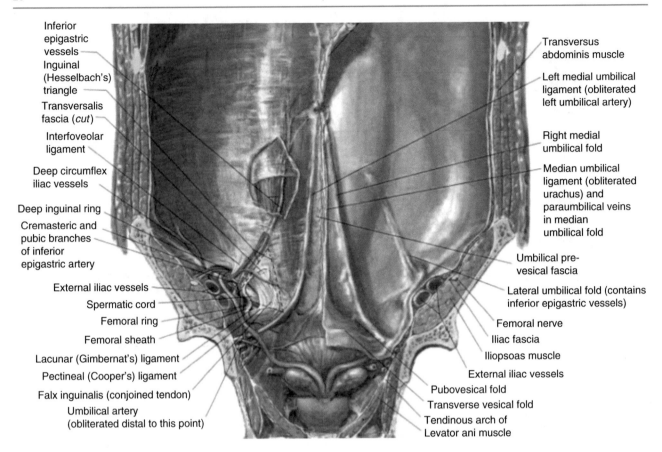

Inferior epigastric vessels

Inguinal (Hesselbach's) triangle

Transversalis fascia (*cut*)

Interfoveolar ligament

Deep circumflex iliac vessels

Deep inguinal ring

Cremasteric and pubic branches of inferior epigastric artery

External iliac vessels

Spermatic cord

Femoral ring

Femoral sheath

Lacunar (Gimbernat's) ligament

Pectineal (Cooper's) ligament

Falx inguinalis (conjoined tendon)

Umbilical artery (obliterated distal to this point)

Transversus abdominis muscle

Left medial umbilical ligament (obliterated left umbilical artery)

Right medial umbilical fold

Median umbilical ligament (obliterated urachus) and paraumbilical veins in median umbilical fold

Umbilical pre-vesical fascia

Lateral umbilical fold (contains inferior epigastric vessels)

Femoral nerve

Iliac fascia

Iliopsoas muscle

External iliac vessels

Pubovesical fold

Transverse vesical fold

Tendinous arch of Levator ani muscle

Fig. 1.18 Peritoneal reflections of the anterior abdominal wall in the male. The same peritoneal relationships of the abdominal wall are found in the female

The Female Urogenital Triangle

Just as can be found in the male, the female urogenital triangle is heavily dominated by the structures of the female genitalia. In addition to the mons pubis, the labia majora and minora, and clitoris, this includes the structures of the deep perineal compartment (deep perineal muscles, compressor urethrae muscle, and the urethrovaginal sphincter) and the superficial perineal compartment (the ischiocavernosus, bulbospongiosus, deep perineal muscles, as well as the vestibular bulbs and Bartholin's glands). The female superficial and deep fascial layers are the same as those found in the male as described above; however, by convention they retain the names superficial perineal fascia and deep perineal fascia.

The Blood Supply of the Pelvis

The bilateral common iliac arteries split from the abdominal aorta at the fourth lumbar vertebrae to course along the pelvic brim underneath the superior hypogastric nerve plexus and each of the ureters. Most commonly, the right common iliac artery is longer than the left, as the left internal iliac artery take-off is sooner than that of the right internal iliac. The common iliac veins run inferior and medial to their arterial counterparts, with the right common iliac artery coursing directly superior to the vein after it crosses the midline. The vascular structures of the pelvis are illustrated in Fig. 1.20).

The *internal iliac* arteries from either side provide the great majority of blood flow to the pelvis, and are commonly described as having anterior and posterior divisions. The external iliac arteries continue along the pelvic brim and medial border of the psoas to pass underneath the inguinal ligament and become the femoral arteries. The spermatic artery and vein, the vas deferens and the genital branch of the genitofemoral artery all pass over the external iliac vessels as they course through the pelvis into the leg. Only two arteries contributed to the pelvis from the external iliac system—the inferior epigastric artery of the anterior abdominal wall and the deep circumflex iliac artery that courses towards the ASIS to supply the lateral abdominal wall and even gluteal region. A great deal of variant blood vessel anatomy exists within the pelvis, and thus, by convention the branches of the internal iliac artery are named by the structure to which they travel and feed.

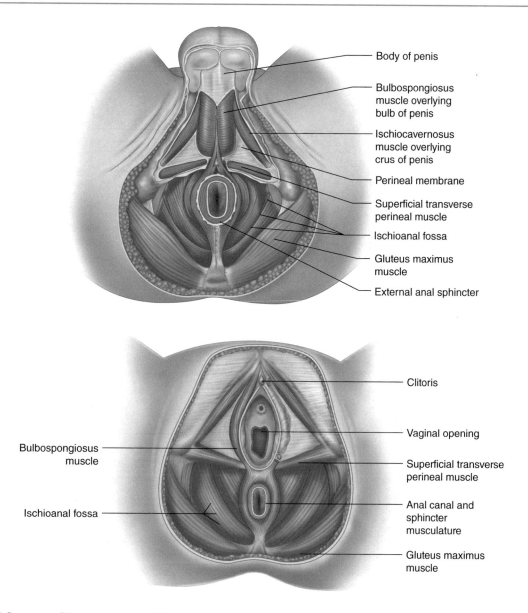

Fig. 1.19 (**a**) Structures of the male perineum. (**b**) Structures of the female perineum

Internal Iliac Vasculature

The internal iliac arteries divide into anterior and posterior divisions near the greater sciatic notch, with the posterior division having three main branches and the anterior division having three groups of three branches each (9 total). The divisions of the posterior branch of the internal iliac artery include the superior gluteal, lateral sacral, and iliolumbar arteries. The branches of anterior division of the internal iliac artery include three urinary branches (superior vesical, inferior vesical and the obliterated umbilical artery), the three visceral branches (middle rectal, and uterine artery and vaginal branches in the female, and three parietal branches (obturator, internal pudendal and inferior gluteal). As a general rule, the venous drainage of the pelvis mirrors

the arterial structure, and the vessels can be found as paired named vessels—though there tends to be multiple veins for each named artery.

Pelvic Venous Plexuses

There are a number of venous plexuses within the pelvis that are associated with either the pelvic viscera or the sacrum itself. In simple terms, there is a venous plexus associated with each of the major pelvic structures in both the male and female that receives blood from the veins of that particular structure (Fig. 1.21). The uterine, vaginal, and rectal plexuses drain into the internal iliac vein; however, these plexuses have free communications with the vesical and

Sagittal section

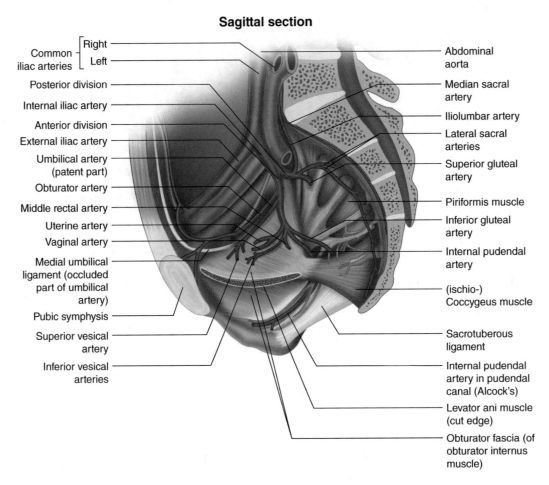

Common iliac arteries ⌈ Right
                     ⌊ Left
Posterior division
Internal iliac artery
Anterior division
External iliac artery
Umbilical artery (patent part)
Obturator artery
Middle rectal artery
Uterine artery
Vaginal artery
Medial umbilical ligament (occluded part of umbilical artery)
Pubic symphysis
Superior vesical artery
Inferior vesical arteries

Abdominal aorta
Median sacral artery
Iliolumbar artery
Lateral sacral arteries
Superior gluteal artery
Piriformis muscle
Inferior gluteal artery
Internal pudendal artery
(ischio-) Coccygeus muscle
Sacrotuberous ligament
Internal pudendal artery in pudendal canal (Alcock's)
Levator ani muscle (cut edge)
Obturator fascia (of obturator internus muscle)

Fig. 1.20 Major arterial branches of the pelvis

retropubic plexuses which drain directly into both the internal iliac vein and the internal pudendal vein. The larger prostatic venous plexus (of Santorini) in the male drains directly into the internal pudendal vein. The rectal plexus represents an important portosystemic venous anastomosis between the inferior rectal veins that drain through the iliac system, and the superior rectal veins that drain through the portal system.

The Lymphatic Drainage of the Pelvis

Similar to the venous drainage of the pelvis, the lymphatic drainage of the pelvis tends to follow the arterial inflow for the structure being drained. This can be simplified by grouping the lymph nodes by the major arteries that they follow, i.e., the common iliac, the external iliac and the internal iliac. The internal and external iliac lymph node basins drain into the common iliac lymph node chain, which in turn, drains into the para-aortic nodes (Fig. 1.22).

The *external iliac lymph node chain* is divided into three groups according to its position along the external iliac vessels. The three groups consist of the external chain, the middle chain

and the internal chain. The external chain lies lateral to the external iliac vessels, the middle chain lies anterior to the external iliac vessels, and the internal chain lies medial to the external iliac vessels. The external chain drains the deep and superficial inguinal nodes, the glans penis and clitoris, and the inferior portion of the anterior abdominal wall. The internal chain shares all of the same major drainage reservoirs with the external chain; however, it also drains portions of the bladder, prostate and urethera.

The *internal iliac lymph node chain* drains into the middle chain of the external iliac lymph node chain and most commonly has drainage patterns contiguous with the distribution of the anterior division of the internal iliac artery. The majority of pelvic lymphatic drainage occurs through this system.

The *common iliac lymph node chain* is divided into the same three groups that the external iliac is divided—the external chain, middle chain, and internal chain. These merely represent continuations of the same lymph channels of the external iliac, with one important difference. The internal chain receives additional lymphatic drainage from the bladder neck and prostate in males, and the uterus and vagina in females.

Fig. 1.21 Venous plexuses of the male pelvis. In the female, the prostatic plexus is replaced by the smaller vaginal venous plexus

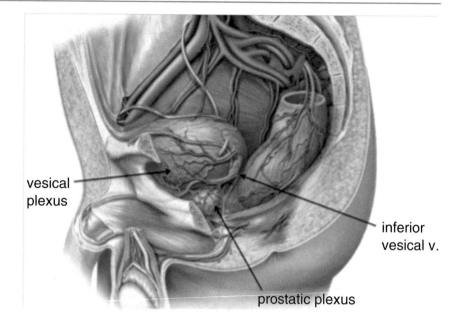

vesical plexus

inferior vesical v.

prostatic plexus

Fig. 1.22 Lymphatic drainage of the pelvis

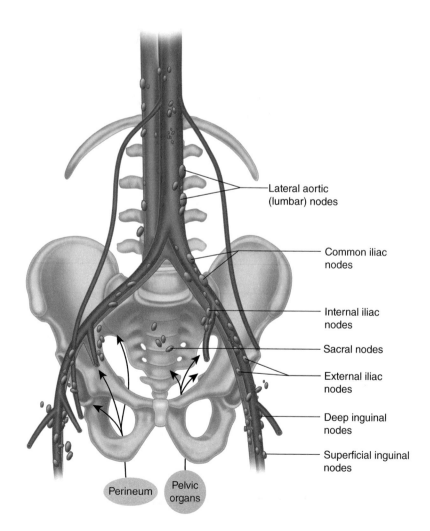

Lateral aortic (lumbar) nodes

Common iliac nodes

Internal iliac nodes

Sacral nodes

External iliac nodes

Deep inguinal nodes

Superficial inguinal nodes

Perineum

Pelvic organs

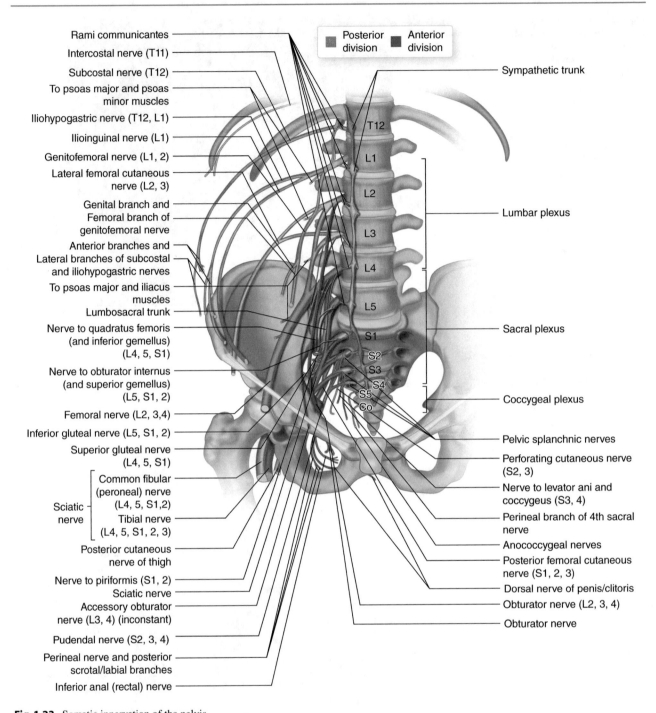

Fig. 1.23 Somatic innervation of the pelvis

The Innervation of the Pelvis

The nerves of the pelvis comprise of a complex network of somatic spinal nerves and autonomic sympathetic and parasympathetic nerve plexuses densely intertwined with each other and the other structures within the pelvis. In general, the somatic nerves (lumbar, sacral, and coccygeal plexuses) innervate the striated voluntary musculature of the pelvis and lower limb, and transmit sensory information back to the spinal cord. The sympathetic and parasympathetic nerves (pelvic splanchnic nerves) provide smooth muscle and glandular innervation via the pelvic, lumbar, and sacral splanchnic

nerves. Below is a (very) brief overview of pelvic neurology, as you will find in-depth discussions regarding specific nerves, muscles and conditions throughout this book as they pertain to each topic.

Somatic Innervation

The somatic nerves of the pelvis that comprise the sacral plexus derive from the ventral rami of the L4–5 and S1–4 nerve roots and course across the piriformis muscle and distribute throughout the pelvis (Fig. 1.23). The sciatic nerve and

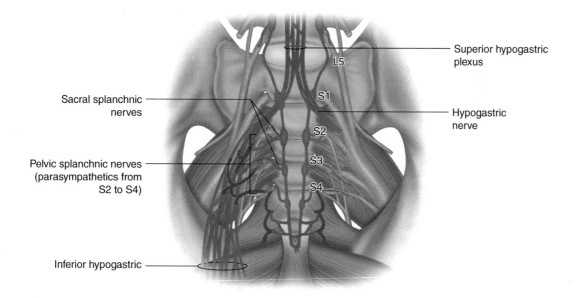

Fig. 1.24 Autonomic nervous plexuses of the pelvis

gluteal nerve branches exit the pelvis to innervate the lower leg and buttocks, respectively. The pudendal nerve (S2–S4) provides innervation for the skin of the perineum as well as the pelvic floor musculature. Historically, the pudendal nerve has also been attributed to at least partially innervating the levator ani, however, this has recently come into question [26]. The levator ani is, more definitively, innervated by the sacral nerve plexus (S2–S4) and the coccygeus muscle is innervated by the coccygeal nerve (S4–S5). The individual branches of the sacral plexus will be described in detail in later chapters.

Autonomic Innervation

The pelvic autonomic innervation derives from the aortic plexus which contains both sympathetic and parasympathetic fibers, and the pelvic splanchnic nerves (S2–S4) which contain parasympathetic and sympathetic fibers (Fig. 1.24). Parasympathetic fibers (S2–S4) within the pelvis act to contract detrusor smooth muscle, stimulate (vasodilate) erectile tissue, and inhibit contraction of the internal urethral sphincter and internal anal sphincter (promote waste excretion). Sympathetic fibers (T5–L2) within the pelvis act to mediate ejaculation and bulbourethral gland secretion (males) or Bartholin's gland secretion (females) and contract the internal urethral sphincter and internal anal sphincter (promote waste storage).

The superior hypogastric plexus is a continuation of parasympathetic and sympathetic fibers of the aortic plexus and resides within the extraperitoneal connective tissue on top of the sacral promontory and L5 vertebrae. This divides into the left and right inferior hypogastric nerves which descend into the pelvis on top of the sacral plexus and piriformis muscle. The right and left inferior hypogastric nerves then combine with the pelvic splanchnic nerves and branch to their final destinations. These include the vesical plexus, the uterovaginal plexus in females and the prostatic plexus in males, ureteric plexus, testicular plexus (males), and middle rectal plexus. The sacral nervous plexuses originate within the deep endopelvic fascia and will travel along this plane until closer to its target organ. Away from the pelvic sidewall, the majority of sympathetic fibers run just underneath the peritoneum whereas the parasympathetic fibers and organ specific plexuses lie within the loose areolar connective tissue (intermediate stratum). Care must be used when performing dissection within the pelvis, as often the synapses for autonomic innervation of specific structures lies away from the organ itself.

References

1. Sadler TW, Langman J. Langman's medical embryology. 10th ed. Philadelphia: Lippincott Williams & Wilkins; 2006.
2. Delaere O, Dhem A. Prenatal development of the human pelvis and acetabulum. Acta Orthop Belg. 1999;65(3):255–60.
3. Esses SI, Botsford DJ, Huler RJ. Surgical anatomy of the sacrum. A guide for rational screw fixation. Spine. 1991;16 Suppl 6:283–8.
4. Cheng JS, Song, JK. Anatomy of the Sacrum. Neurosurg Focus. 2003;15(2):25–50.
5. Agur AMR, Lee MJ, Boileau Grant JC. Grant's atlas of anatomy. 10th ed. Philadelphia: Lippincott Williams & Wilkins; 1999.
6. Abitbol MM. Evolution of the sacrum in hominoids. Am J Phys Anthropol. 1987;74:65–81.

7. Roussouly P, Gollogly S, Berthonnaud E, Dimnet J. Classification of the normal variation in the sagittal alignment of the human lumbar spine and pelvis in the standing position. Spine. 2005;30(3):346–53.

8. Donovan DJ, Pedersen RC. Human tail with noncontiguous intraspinal lipoma and spinal cord tethering: case report and embryologic discussion. Pediatr Neurosurg. 2005;41:35–40.

9. O'Rahilly R, Muller F, Meyer DB. The human vertebral column at the end of the embryonic period proper. 4. The sacrococcygeal region. J Anat. 1990;168:95–111.

10. Le Double A. Traite' des variations de la colonne verte'brale del'homme. Paris: Vigot fre'res; 1912. p. 501.

11. Woon JT, Stringer MD. Clinical anatomy of the coccyx: a systematic review. Clin Anat. 2012;25(2):158–67.

12. Maigne JY, Tamalet B. Standardized radiologic protocol for the study of common coccygodynia and characteristics of the lesions observed in the sitting position. Clinical elements differentiating luxation, hypermobility, and normal mobility. Spine. 1996;21:2588–93.

13. Grassi R, Lombardi G, Reginelli A, Capasso F, Romano F, Floriani I, Colacurci N. Coccygeal movement: assessment with dynamic MRI. Eur J Radiol. 2007;61:473–9.

14. Martini F, Ober WC. Fundamentals of anatomy and physiology. vol 1. Prentice Hall; 2001. ISBN 0130172928.

15. Petros PE. The pubourethral ligaments--an anatomical and histological study in the live patient. Int Urogynecol J Pelvic Floor Dysfunct. 1998;9(3):154–7.

16. Zacharin RF. The suspensory mechanism of the female Pelvis. J Anat. 1963;97:23–7.

17. The Female Pelvic Floor. The anatomy and dynamics of pelvic floor function and dysfunction. Berlin: Springer; 2007. p. 14–50. ISBN 978-3-540-33663-1.

18. Albright TS, Gehrich AP, Davis GD, Sabi FL, Buller JL. Arcus tendineus facia pelvis: a further understanding. Am J Obstet Gynecol. 2005;193(3 Pt 1):677–81.

19. Steiner MS. The puboprostatic ligament and the male urethral suspension mechanism: an anatomic study. Urology. 1994;44(4):530–4.

20. Li CY, Agrawal V, Minhas S, Ralph DJ. The penile suspensory ligament: abnormalities and repair. BJU Int. 2007;99(1):117–20.

21. Song DH, Neligan PC. Plastic surgery: vol 4: lower extremity, trunk and burns. 3rd ed. Elsevier Health Sciences; 2012. ISBN 1455740489.

22. Tanagho EA, Smith DR, Meyers FH. The trigone: anatomical and physiological considerations. 2. In relation to the bladder neck. J Urol. 1968;100:633–9.

23. Weiss JP. Embryogenesis of ureteral anomalies: a unifying theory. Aust N Z J Surg. 1988;58:631–8.

24. Meyer R. Normal and abnormal development of the ureter in the human embryo – a mechanistic consideration. Anat Rec. 1946;68:355–71.

25. Stamatiou D, Skandalakis J, Skandalakis LJ, Mirilas P. Perineal hernia: surgical anatomy, embryology, and technique of repair. Am Surg. 2010;76(5):474–9.

26. MacLennan G. Hinman's atlas of urosurgical anatomy. 2nd ed. Saunders; 2012. ISBN: 978-1-4160-4089-7.

27. Koch W, Marani E. Early development of the human pelvic diaphragm. Volume 192 of advances in anatomy, embryology and cell biology. Springer Science & Business Media; 2007. ISBN 3540680063.

28. Naito M, Suzuki R, Abe H, Rodriguez-Vazquez JF, Murakami GF, et al. Development of the human obturator internus muscle with special reference to the tendon and pulley. Anat Rec (Hoboken). 2015;298(7):1282–93.

29. Walters M, Karram M. Urogynecology and reconstructive pelvic surgery. 4th ed. Saunders; 2015.

Pelvic Floor Physiology: From Posterior Compartment to Perineal Body to Anterior Compartment

Shane Svoboda, Daniel Galante, Brian L. Bello, and David A. Gordon

Introduction

The primary physiologic function of the posterior pelvic floor is bowel continence and evacuation. The muscles of the pelvic floor act as both a supportive base for the abdominal viscera and provide mechanisms for continence. The bony pelvis provides the attachments for these muscles that surround the external orifices. These muscles are innervated by both the parasympathetic and sympathetic nervous systems.

Dysfunction of the pelvic floor contributes to morbidity and decreased quality of life in many patients, especially the geriatric population. Baseline pelvic floor muscle tone and neurologic integrity both play a role in the maintenance of fecal continence. In addition, there can be variation in the regulation of stool due to systemic disease, bowel motility, stool consistency, as well as cognitive and emotional factors. Understanding the anatomy, innervation, and reflexes of the pelvic floor and anal sphincters is the key to assessing disorders of continence and treating this patient population [1].

S. Svoboda • D. Galante
Department of Surgery, Sinai Hospital, Balitmore, MD, USA

B.L. Bello
Medstar Washington Hospital Center, Colorectal Surgery Program, Washington, DC, USA

D.A. Gordon (✉)
Division of Pelvic NeuroScience, Department of Surgery, The Sinai Hospital of Baltimore, 2401 W. Belvedere Ave, Baltimore, MD 21215, USA
e-mail: dgordon@lifebridgehealth.org

Posterior Pelvic Floor Physiology

Pelvic Floor and Anal Sphincters

The muscular pelvic floor consists of both superficial and deep muscles, both of which play a role in continence. The *superficial pelvic floor muscles* are most relevant to anal canal function are the (1) external anal sphincter, (2) perineal body, and the (3) puboperineal transverse muscles, which are considered. The *deep pelvic floor muscles* consist of the (1) pubococcygeus, (2) iliococcygeus, (3) coccygeus, and (4) puborectalis muscles (Fig. 2.1). These muscles originate at the pectinate line of the pubic bone and obturator internus fascia, and insert at the *coccyx*. The puborectalis muscle may be more accurately described as *located between* the superficial and deep layers. The muscle originates at the inferior pubic ramus, tracks posteriorly, wrapping around the rectum as it descends, and attaches to the contralateral pubic ramus.

The *internal anal sphincter (IAS)* and *external anal sphincter (EAS)* are the major constrictors of the anal canal. The *IAS* develops from a thickening of the circular colonic muscle layer (Fig. 2.2). As it progresses distally, it thickens and develops an increased number of muscle fibers. This makes the IAS histologically different from the upper colonic circular muscle layer. Involuntary, autonomic innervation is divided between sympathetic and parasympathetic nerves. *Sympathetic* nerves arise from the lower thoracic ganglia, creating the superior hypogastric plexus. *Parasympathetic* innervation arises from sacral nerves 2 through 4, forming the nervi erigentes and the inferior hypogastric plexus (Fig. 2.3). The IAS maintains a constant level of tone, preventing fecal incontinence. It is believed that the interstitial cells of Cajal (ICC) maintain this tone. Unlike the remainder of the gastrointestinal tract, where the interstitial cells of Cajal create rhythmic muscle contractions, studies using imatinib mesylate have shown that the ICCs create a constant level of tone in the IAS [2].

© Springer Science+Business Media New York 2017
D.A. Gordon, M.R. Katlic (eds.), *Pelvic Floor Dysfunction and Pelvic Surgery in the Elderly*,
DOI 10.1007/978-1-4939-6554-0_2

Fig. 2.1 Pelvic floor (*anterior* and *posterior*). With permission from Jorge JMN Habr-Gama A. Anatomy and Embryology of the Colon, Rectum, and Anus. In: Beck DE, Wexner SD, David E. Beck, Steven D. Wexner, Hull TL, Roberts PL, Senagore AJ, Stamos JM, Steele SR, eds. The ASCRS Manual of Colon and Rectal Surgery, 2nd Edn. Springer, New York, 2014; pp:1–25

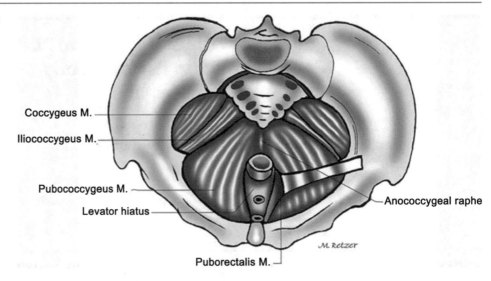

Fig. 2.2 Internal and external anal sphincter. With permission from Jorge JMN Habr-Gama A. Anatomy and Embryology of the Colon, Rectum, and Anus. In: Beck DE, Wexner SD,David E. Beck, Steven D. Wexner, Hull TL, Roberts PL, Senagore AJ, Stamos JM, Steele SR, eds. The ASCRS Manual of Colon and Rectal Surgery, 2nd Edn. Springer, New York, 2014; pp:1–25

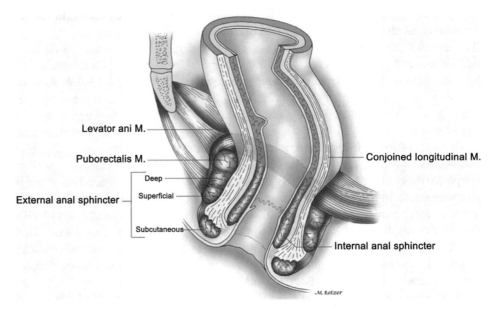

The inferior hypogastric plexus further divides to form the superior, middle, and inferior rectal nerves. These nerves synapse with the myenteric plexus of the rectal muscle to regulate tone. Sympathetic activation, via β-adrenergic receptors, creates and maintains internal anal sphincter tonicity, and thus involuntary continence. Parasympathetic innervation utilizes nitric oxide to cause sphincter relaxation [3].

The external anal sphincter (EAS) is comprised of three (3) muscular layers: (1) subcutaneous layer, (2) superficial layer, and (3) deep layer (Fig. 2.2). The subcutaneous portion lies distal to the internal anal sphincter, the superficial surrounds it, and the deep portion merges with the puborectalis muscle. Some consider the deep portion to be a part of the puborectalis muscle rather than a muscular component of the EAS muscle complex [4]. The EAS attaches to the perineal body and transverse perinei muscle anteriorly, and moves posteriorly to attach to the anococcygeal raphae. Laterally the EAS connects with the transverse perinei muscle. New MRI/ultrasound work has suggested that the EAS muscle complex is actually a purse-string morphology, rather than a "donut" configuration. In this purse-string arrangement, the EAS musculature continues (with the transverse perinei muscle) to the contralateral attachment [4]. The concept of this configuration is further supported by the fact that both the anorectal angle changes and the coccyx is pulled anteriorly during contraction of the external anal sphincter.

Comprised of voluntary muscle fibers with resting tonicity, the EAS is innervated by sacral motor neurons that arise in Onuf's nucleus and travel through the pudendal nerve (S2–S4). This monosynaptic reflex creates resting sphincter tone. This tone is abolished with spinal anesthesia and impaired in disorders such as diabetes. The fact that EAS tone can be over-

Fig. 2.3 Innervation of the posterior pelvic floor. With permission from Jorge JMN Habr-Gama A. Anatomy and Embryology of the Colon, Rectum, and Anus. In: Beck DE, Wexner SD, David E. Beck, Steven D. Wexner, Hull TL, Roberts PL, Senagore AJ, Stamos JM, Steele SR, eds. The ASCRS Manual of Colon and Rectal Surgery, 2nd Edn. Springer, New York, 2014; pp:1–25

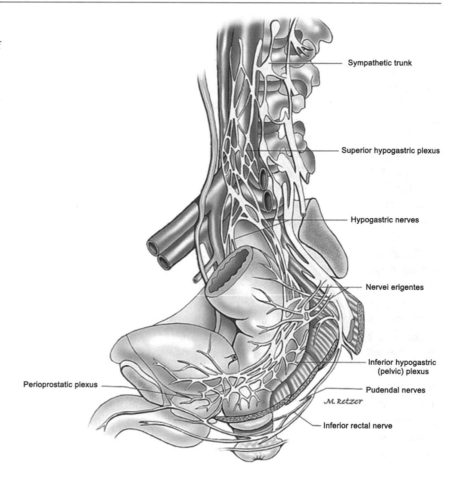

come by spinal anesthesia suggests that there may be a spinal reflex that helps to maintain external anal sphincter tone, and thus continence. A study by Broens et al. suggests that, in addition to previously documented reflexes and autonomic and somatic innervation, an "external sphincter continence reflex" exists, due to a spinal reflex that utilizes receptors in the mucosa and submucosa of the distal anal canal. The concept of this reflex was supported by the knowledge that the incidence of incontinence increases following mucosectomy and that patients with high spinal cord injuries (above the level of T5) can maintain some degree of continence [5].

The pudendal nerve (via S3-S4) innervates the puborectalis and levator ani muscles. In cases of severe pudendal nerve injury, such as a traumatic injury, both the EAS and pelvic floor musculature can be affected and fecal incontinence may result.

The sensory function of the rectum is a very important component to consider. This allows for the discrimination of solid, versus liquid, versus gas components of stool. These specialized cells and their attendant histologic arrangement are constructed within the distal rectum. The distal rectum extends from approximately 2.5–15 mm above the anal valves and can sense prick, light touch, hot and cold. Again, it is this sensory ability that helps discriminate between gaseous flatus and solid stool. Above this level, the rectum is only able to sense distention. The

inferior rectal branch of the pudendal nerve is responsible for this sensory ability in the lower rectum. Stretch receptors in the rectal wall and surrounding pelvic fascia, via S2-4 parasympathetic fibers, contribute to higher rectal sensation.

In addition to the musculature and neurologic components of continence, the physical orientation of the rectum and associated pelvic floor muscles creates an orientation, called the *Anorectal Angle* that ultimately develops a valve-like structure, believed to assist in continence. The puborectalis muscle, by nature of its attachments, pulls the rectum anteriorly. This causes apposition of the rectal mucosa. As intraabdominal pressure increases, pushing down on the rectum and contents, the anorectal angle becomes more acute, causing a tightening of the valve-structure. This development relies on the rectal reservoir to tolerate the rising volume of fecal material traveling into the rectum. These complex and mixed voluntary and involuntary movements facilitate the development of a stripping wave, which moves the stool from the rectum and relaxes the pelvic floor muscles and the anus resulting in stool evacuation [6, 7]. Figure 2.2 shows the anorectal angle at rest, constriction and defecation. There comes a point where rectal capacity will be reached, and overflow incontinence may ensue if defecation is not initiated voluntarily.

Anorectal Reflexes

There are multiple reflexes that assist in the maintenance of continence. The *cutaneous-anal reflex* is a contraction of the anal sphincter with scratching of the perianal skin. An S4 sensory and motor efferent and afferent from the pudendal nerve is responsible for this reflex. Due to the rapid fatigability of the anal sphincter, it is important to test this particular reflex early in sphincter testing proceedings. Patients suffering from cauda equina syndrome lack this reflex.

The *bulbocavernosus reflex* is the sensation of pelvic floor contraction with the squeezing of the glans of the penis or the clitoris. This reflex is perpetuated through the pudendal nerve (S2–S4).

The **R**ectal **A**nal **I**nhibitory **R**eflex (RAIR) is the act of IAS relaxation in response to distention of the rectum. RAIR plays an important role in fine adjustments of continence. The reflex starts with fecal material or flatus coming in contact with sensory receptors in the upper anal canal. These receptors sample the fecal contents and create a sense of awareness with regard to the contents (flatus versus stool). This reflex is responsible for one's ability to pass flatus and stool independently. This reflex is absent in patients with Hirschsprung's disease, and may be damaged by an overgenerous myotomy in a lateral internal sphincterotomy. While the relaxation of the IAS is a temporary phenomenon, thus preventing fecal incontinence, the IAS tone does not return fully to baseline, but rather a new "plateau pressure" which continues to maintain contraction of the sphincter complex [3].

The *Rectal Anal Excitatory Reflex*, in contrast, is the contraction of the EAS in response to rectal distention. This reflex prevents involuntary fecal incontinence, and is regulated by the splanchnic nerves (S2–S4 parasympathetic fibers). These splanchnic nerves may be considered to be associated with the pudendal nerve and as would follow, a pudendal nerve block will remove this reflex. The *cough reflex* is a polysynaptic reflex that develops in response to a rapid increase in intraabdominal pressure. This reflex causes contraction of the anal sphincters, thus preventing fecal incontinence during coughing, laughing, shouting, or any other activity causing a rapid increase in intraabdominal pressure.

Pelvic Floor Dysfunction

Physiology of the pelvic floor combines sensory input, anatomical variants, mechanical factors, and reflexes. Correlating physiologic properties with clinical pathology and patient symptoms has led to improvements in testing for specific defects. Pelvic floor dysfunctions (PFD) is common, affecting up to 10–15 % of the population with even higher incidence in women and the elderly, with significant impact on quality of life, emotional well-being, and ability to actively participate in society [8]. Etiologic risk factors for PFD include: (1) vaginal parity, (2) aging, (3) hormonal status, (4) pelvic surgery, (5) collagen diseases, (6) toilet training before complete myelination of the spinal tracts, and (7) depression. Clinical improvement requires a well-thought-out strategy. Definitive management and complete resolution of incontinence is rare and a combination of treatment options is essential for improving the quality of life in patients.

As with most clinical pathologies a complete history is essential in patients with pelvic floor dysfunction. Even more important is asking the right questions. Detailed questions about bowel habits may help to differentiate between pelvic floor dysfunction and other more concerning and immediate pathology such as obstruction due to cancer. Repeated visits to the bathroom with incomplete emptying, self-assistance in defecation with support of the perineum or posterior vaginal wall, and soiling in the absence of urge incontinence are all signs of pelvic floor pathology and are more chronic in nature. In addition, repeated questionnaires can be beneficial to systematically obtain history as well as provide quality of life information that may be followed through treatment modalities. There are multiple fecal incontinence scoring systems which are used to grade and categorize both the subjective and objective effects of incontinence.

Patients with pelvic floor dysfunction can usually be divided into one of two broad categories. The first and largest group is comprised of parous women suffering from long-term sequelae of pregnancy and childbirth. *The second* is men and nulliparous women who suffer from prior surgical intervention, connective tissue disorders, neuromuscular disorders, including adult neuromuscular sequelae of Hinman's syndrome or from more psychological and behavioral problems. The latter group tends to be misdiagnosed with irritable bowel syndrome (IBS) although significant life events such as physical or emotional abuse, eating disorders, and other psychological stress have been shown to have a strong association with pelvic floor dysfunction later in life. The most common conditions include constipation, obstructed defecation, fecal incontinence, and pelvic pain. Each of these can be very limiting to patient's ability to function normally in the world.

Immediate surgical intervention has lost appeal due to disappointing long-term improvement and morbidity. The 1980s utilized subtotal colectomy for slow transit constipation and postanal repair for incontinence. Therapeutic options have increased in the last decade with sacral nerve stimulation providing a tremendous option and preventing the need for a stoma or severely limiting conservative therapy. Surgical correction of rectal intussusception has also shown improvement in symptoms leading to further study on a perhaps unrecognized pathogenesis of incontinence. Providing patients with a multidisciplinary approach has shown improvements in quality of life. Early conservative management utilizes the assistance of a pelvic floor physiologist and specialist nurse to correctly diagnose underlying pathology. Even after a patient has been diagnosed with a defecatory problem, conservative treatment (increased dietary fibers, removal of constipating medications, increased fluid intake) should be attempted first. If this does not improve the patient's condition, then laxatives (both osmotic and stimulant) should be trialed. If the patient continues to suffer from dysfunctional defecation, then more testing should be performed [9]. Surgical input is recommended early from a colon and rectal surgeon and a radiologist with expert training in defecography and pelvic anatomy.

Constipation

Chronic constipation can be described as reduced frequency or difficulty of defecation. There are two major types of constipation: slow transit and outlet obstruction. Slow transit is associated with decreased motility of fecal material within the colon. Outlet obstruction occurs when the patient has difficulty evacuating contents from the rectum. The normal act of defecation includes performance of a Valsalva maneuver, with an increase in intra-abdominal and rectal pressures, as well as relaxation of the rectal and anal sphincters.

Functional constipation is related to slow transit colonic constipation, which is rather uncommon, and evacuation problems or a combination in which the motility of the colon slows over time secondary to difficulty in evacuation. Patients with slow transit or true colonic motility disorders do not experience the same urge or call to stool. Bloating, heaviness, and abdominal discomfort become more apparent. High-grade internal rectal prolapse has been chronically misdiagnosed as IBS with delayed surgical consultation. Most patients with a functional disorder have fecal incontinence, need for digitization, incomplete evacuation, and toilet revisiting [1].

There is a potential third type of constipation that is essentially a combination of anatomic obstructive constipation and functional constipation. Essentially, this type of patient exhibits characteristics of both. It is the patient with levator based hypertonic pelvic floor dysfunction, with the hypertonicity focused at the level of the "puborectalis muscle." Here, the hypertonicity of the puborectalis changes the anorectal angle and makes it more acute thereby creating a type of anatomic obstructive constipatory effect. This type of obstruction then can lead to an exaggerated beta III effect which in turns slows down colonic transit time and further precipitates constipation (Figs. 2.4, 2.5, and 2.6).

Fecal Incontinence

Fecal incontinence can be described as either associated with urgency or occur as a passive event. Incontinence is the inability to defer the passage of gas, liquid or solid stool until the desired time. Fecal urge incontinence (FUI or *active incontinence*) is the loss of stool despite efforts to control it. It may be associated with inflammatory changes in the rectum such as prostatitis as well as carcinoma, or may be associated with a problem with the external anal sphincter. Disastrous events of

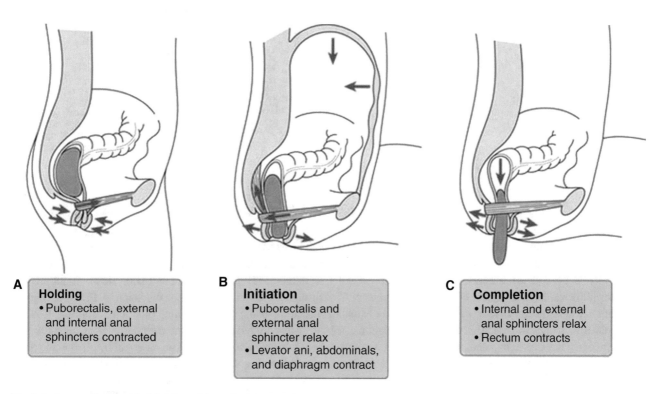

A   Holding
- Puborectalis, external and internal anal sphincters contracted

B   Initiation
- Puborectalis and external anal sphincter relax
- Levator ani, abdominals, and diaphragm contract

C   Completion
- Internal and external anal sphincters relax
- Rectum contracts

Fig. 2.4 Anorectal angle. Modified from Gianna Rodriguez, John C. King, Steven A. Stiens. Dysfunction and Rehabilitation. http://clinicalgate.com/neurogenic-bowel-dysfunction-and-rehabilitation/

Fig. 2.5 Perineal body with pelvic floor (*anterior* and *posterior*). Modified from http://teachmeanatomy.info

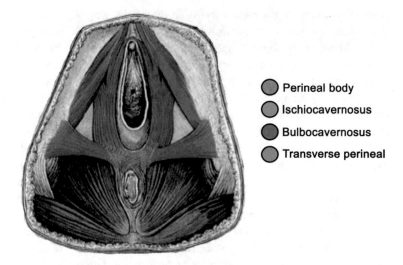

- Perineal body
- Ischiocavernosus
- Bulbocavernosus
- Transverse perineal

Fig. 2.6 Neuromuscular aspects of voiding

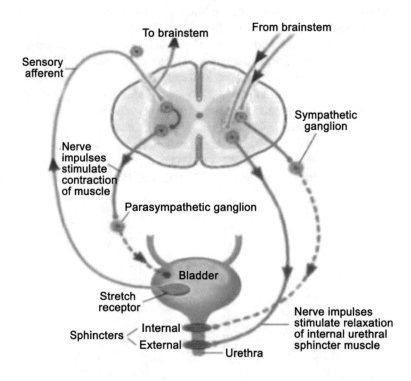

high volume incontinence can be socially crippling and associated with high levels of anxiety. Passive Incontinence is the loss of stool without awareness and is more often a physiologic outcome from a deficient internal anal sphincter or anatomic deformity. True anorectal prolapse or rectal intussusception results in a variable and unpredictable incontinence often resulting in underwear staining or release of small pellets rather than high volume. Abnormal rectal sensation can lead to incontinence due to hyperacute sensation in inflammatory pathology and blunted sensation leading to Overflow Incontinence.

Mixed symptoms may also occur as a consequence of passive loss of stool that is retained in the rectum or rectocele as a result of incomplete evacuation. This seems counterintuitive and results in misdiagnosis with only marginally reduced sphincter tone. These patients tend to benefit most from laparoscopic ventral rectopexy with improvement in continence.

Anal canal pressure is the major determinant of the strength of the anal continence mechanism. Pressures can be measured using anatomic and functional studies. Resting pressures are mostly related to the internal anal sphincter and voluntary squeeze pressure increase can be attributed to the external anal sphincter. At the same time, the anatomical location and association of the IAS, EAS, and puborectalis can be isolated based on pressure readings along the length of the anal canal. Pressure studies have found that fecal incontinence is rarely associated with an isolated dysfunction but rather the degree of incontinence is associated with a composite effect of damage to the three continence muscles. Biofeedback therapy has resulted in improvement of fecal incontinence symptoms associated with improvement in levator ani function, rather than improved contraction of the IAS or EAS.

Pelvic Pain

Chronic pelvic pain is a challenging frustrating and usually multidisciplinary clinical issue. The component part that make up the bulk of chronic pelvic pain syndromes are addressed in other chapters in this text. This includes a special chapter on the biology of chronic pelvic pain. Nevertheless, suffice it to say that most patients have been assessed by multiple specialists including urologists, gynecologists, and colon and rectal surgeons. They often seek assistance from pain management specialists with variable improvement on a socially limiting chronic condition. The original pathophysiologic source of their pain (endometriosis, prolapse, postpartum pain) may become lost in a long series of surgical interventions that if not treated with care, logic and sophistication may actually make the whole process worse. Please refer to the other sections in this book for more relevant details on the pathogenesis and treatment on chronic pelvic pain.

Physiologic Testing (Fecal Incontinence v. Constipation)

A variety of testing options now exist for definitive diagnosis of physiologic deficits leading to fecal incontinence and constipation. A combination of defects may contribute to the clinical symptoms, including fecal retention, prolapse, and incontinence. Less invasive testing methods are being developed with increased use of imaging modalities rather than direct physiologic testing with proven success. Diagnostic testing now includes:

1. Anorectal manometry
2. Balloon expulsion testing
3. Saline continence testing
4. Neurophysiologic testing
5. Pelvic floor imaging
6. Dynamic functional testing

Anorectal physiologic testing concentrates on two major areas: neurologic function and muscular function. If one or both of these is altered, clinical pathology occurs as retention, constipation, incontinence, or an array of symptoms. Muscles have a relatively simple function: they shorten from the insertion point towards the origin. In the case of the pelvic floor, the pubococcygeus, iliococcygeus, and ischiococcygeus

contracting result in the coccyx moving anteriorly (ventrally) toward the pubic bone, thus transforming a basin into a dome and lifting the contents of the abdomen, providing support. Laxity of this muscular support results in perineal descent and may lead to pelvic floor dysfunction [10].

Anorectal Manometry

The techniques for anorectal manometry have evolved drastically over the years. Such testing has progressed from balloons or water sacs to water perfusion and most recently microtransducers. Manometry measures the pressures within the anal canal and distal rectum that provides information about the function of the internal and external anal sphincters. Anal manometry testing is most useful in evaluation of fecal incontinence with suspected sphincter dysfunction. The testing involves an anorectal probe, pressure-recording device, balloon for inflation within the rectum, and a monitoring system. Stool evacuation or enema before the test is optimal to prevent interference of the recordings. Anal canal pressures are then measured using the pull-through technique that creates a reflex sphincter contraction. The probe begins measurements at 6 cm and is subsequently removed at one-centimeter increments from the rectum to the anal verge [11–14].

Pressures that may be recorded during anorectal manometry include squeeze pressure, which is attributed to an increase in pressure as the external anal sphincter is voluntarily contracted, as well as resting pressures. *Resting pressures* are usually around 40–70 mmHg and the majority comes from the IAS. If IAS is compromised, the mean pressure may be lower. *Squeeze pressures* are normally 2–3 times the baseline resting pressure and the EAS is the main contributor. Obstetric and traumatic defects can result in decreased squeeze pressure.

New 3D high definition anorectal manometry (3DHRAM) has the advantage of providing a pressure recording over the entire length and circumference of the anal canal, allowing a more useful physiological assessment of anorectal function. One study with 3DHRAM established normal values in asymptomatic volunteers. Increasing age was associated with lower maximum resting pressure, mean resting pressure, and maximum squeeze pressure [15]. This study also showed that there are significant gender differences concerning squeeze pattern—maximum squeeze pressure, residual anal pressure, and intrarectal pressure were significantly higher in males compared to females [15].

The *cough reflex* can be assessed with a rapid increase in intraabdominal pressure with associated increase in contraction of the EAS to maintain continence. A sphincter defect or innervation injury may result in a weaker cough reflex response. *Rectal sensation* can be measured by distending the rectal balloon and assessing the patient's response including first sensation of urge and maximal tolerable volume. This gives the clinician insight into the sensory perception of the patient. Rectal hypersensitivity is associated with fecal incontinence with increased frequency of defecation. Incontinent patients may have hyposensitivity and suffer from passive incontinence from overflow [16–20].

Balloon Expulsion Testing

Balloon expulsion testing can be used to evaluate rectal expulsion ability by inflation of a water-filled rectal balloon. This test, when performed correctly, should be able to uncover those patients who suffer with obstructed defecation. Normal patients should be able to expel a balloon containing 50–150 mL of water. Patients with enlarged rectums may have normal range of intrarectal pressure, but are unable to expel the balloon. This study may assist in evaluation of a patient with a hypertonic nonrelaxing pelvic floor muscle tone or even spasm in conjunction with other modalities [21, 22].

Saline Continence Testing

Saline continence testing evaluates the ability of the sphincters to remain continent during continuous infusion of saline into the rectum. Normal patients can accommodate approximately 1.5 L of saline without significant leakage. Patients with weak sphincter function or reduced rectal compliance can begin to leak with as little as 250–600 mL [7, 23–26].

Neurophysiologic Testing (PNTML & PFM EMG)

Neurophysiologic testing includes *Pudendal Nerve Terminal Motor Latency* (PNTML) and Pelvic Floor Muscle *Electromyography (PFM EMG)*. PNTML sends electrophysiologic impulses out to follow the course of the pudendal nerve and then return along its "reflex pathway," the Bulbocavernosus Reflex (BCR). The time course to complete this reflex is measured. The pudendal nerve innervates the EAS, urethral sphincter, perineal musculature, mucosa of the anal canal, and the perineal skin. Nerve conduction velocity can be measured with a disposable, finger-mounted electrode (the St. Mark's Electrode) placed in the rectum with stimulating and recording components placed near the ischial spine. The time for response at the level of the EAS is measured and is normally 2.0 ms. The other way to measure PNTML is to use a device that can electrophysiologically stimulate the more distal aspects of the pudendal nerve (the dorsal genital branches) and then follow the course through the sacrum and back to the recording electrodes anteriorly. Naturally, since the impulse is traveling a much longer distance, the time

course is also increased. Normal values for this more anterior testing scenario vary from 35 to 50 ms. It is important to remember that PNTML cannot be interpreted in a vacuum. This is a complementary tool in the physiologic evaluation of anorectal function especially in patients with known neuropathy or injury to the pudendal nerve [27, 28].

Pelvic Floor Muscle Electromyography (PFM EMG) samples activity of the striated pelvic floor muscles and is primarily used to identify EAS activity. Needle EMGs can provide information on nerve injury (denervation–reinnervation potentials) and aid in locating the muscle in the EAS although this has been largely replaced by endoanal ultrasound. Patients with fecal incontinence have high fiber density and longer motor unit potentials than in controls. EMG may be useful in locating the striated EAS muscles prior to surgical intervention in imperforate anus [29–32]. Many colon and rectal surgeons utilize EMG for functional information and endoanal ultrasound for anatomic information.

Pelvic Floor Imaging

Endo-anal ultrasound is useful for imaging the sphincters and detecting defects in the IAS and/or EAS. It is one of the diagnostic cornerstones for evaluation of patients with pelvic floor dysfunction, especially incontinence. This may aid in decisions regarding surgical repair and preoperative planning [33–36]. Ultrasonography has emerged as a simple technique that is subject friendly, inexpensive and may be performed in an office setting.

Advancements in pelvic floor imaging have allowed new insight into the function of the pelvic floor muscles. Through the use of MRI, CT, and 3D ultrasound, there is now a better understanding of the dynamic processes that occur during defecation. Changes seen in the size of the pelvic floor hiatus are related to the puborectalis muscle and reflect the constrictor function. Ascent and descent of the pelvic floor as well as craniocaudal movements of the anorectal angle are predominately related to the contraction and relaxation of the pubococcygeus, iliococcygeus, and ischiococcygeus muscles [1].

Dynamic Functional Testing (Defecography)

Dynamic functional testing can be achieved with fluoroscopic defecography or MR defecography. The latter has been shown to demonstrate more detailed anatomic information and be more accurate at diagnosis of intussusception although both may be useful in detection of anorectal angles, rectal emptying, rectal intussusception, rectal prolapse, and rectocele. During defecography, contrast is used to fill the rectum and is most useful for evaluation of outlet obstruction and prolapse. Patients may limit the study with false positive results due to embarrassment and inability to relax the pelvic floor. The ability to relax the puborectalis muscle and increase the anorectal angle from 75 to 90° at rest to 110–180° is necessary for evacuation [37–40].

Posterior Physiology: In Conclusion

The normal functioning of bowel continence relies on the complex interactions of various neural pathways with the rectum and anus and the pelvic floor. A thorough comprehension of these relationships is important in the diagnostic and therapeutic approach to the patients who have pelvic floor dysfunction.

The Perineum and Perineal Body

The perineum is a diamond shaped area between the coccyx posteriorly and the pubis anteriorly. This area is flanked by the ischial spines laterally. The diamond is further divided into two triangles, anterior and posterior. The anterior triangle is known as the urogenital triangle while the posterior triangle is known as the anal triangle. The perineal body, also known as the central tendon of perineum is a pyramidal fibromuscular mass of tissue located in the middle line of the perineum at the junction between the anterior and posterior triangles. The location of perineal body is different in males and females. In males, it is found between the bulb of the penis and the anus, while in females it is found between the vagina and anus, and about 1.25 cm in front of the latter. Most importantly, it must be noted that the perineal body is essential for the integrity of the pelvic floor musculature.

The pelvic floor musculature is integral in maintaining stability and functionality of the entire anterior abdominal wall with the posterior wall. Without an intact, strong pelvic floor muscular system our entire structure would fall apart. This strong, intact pelvic floor muscular system is made up of two (2) layers of expansive musculature with robust puborectalis muscle in between, almost making up a third layer. This large volume of musculature attaches to bone and ligaments anteriorly, posteriorly and laterally. However, for these large muscles to function well in both anterior and posterior positions there must be a central anchoring point. Obviously, an island of bone cannot really exist in that position. Consequently, a solid, strong, fibrous piece of tissue in the middle of the pelvis MUST exist. This tendinous center, or perineal body, is a median, fibromuscular mass between the urogenital and anal triangles. Several muscles and fasciae are anchored to it, including the levator ani and the external anal sphincter. Perineal body is essential for the integrity of the pelvic floor, especially in females. It provides attachment to the following muscles:

- EAS muscle
- Bulbospongiosus muscle
- Superficial transverse perineal muscle
- Levator ani muscle
- EUS
- Deep transverse perineal muscle

Understanding the relationships of its components is crucial for successful pelvic reconstructive surgical procedure. Now, the best way to understand this area from an anatomical perspective, as well as to help direct any surgical repair is to utilize MRI. Today in 2015, the use of advanced thin-slice MR images to identify structures within this region, define their 3 dimensional location, and provide a framework for visualizing this region's complex anatomy.

Anterior Pelvic Floor Physiology

Pelvic Floor and Urinary Sphincters

The muscular pelvic floor consists of both superficial and deep muscles, both of which play a role in continence. The superficial pelvic floor muscles most relevant to anal canal function are the (1) external anal sphincter, (2) perineal body, and the (3) puboperineal transverse muscles. The deep pelvic floor muscles consist of the (1) pubococcygeus, (2) iliococcygeus, (3) coccygeus, and (4) puborectalis muscles (Fig. 2.1). These muscles originate at the pectinate line of the pubic bone and obturator internus fascia, and insert at the coccyx. The puborectalis muscle may be more accurately described as located between the superficial and deep layers. The muscle originates at the inferior pubic ramus, tracks posteriorly, wrapping around the rectum as it descends, and attaches to the contralateral pubic ramus.

Lower Urinary Tract Physiology

The lower urinary tract is predominantly comprised of the bladder and the urethra. The nature of the bladder is essentially storage. In fact, it is the major storage organ for all liquid waste (urine) that is generated by our body's tissue. The base of the bladder begins to funnel into a **"bladder neck"** area which then segues into the urethra. It is this urethra that is a tubular conduit designed to facilitate the expulsion of urine. Now, at the bladder neck, there is a circular collar like smooth muscle known as the "internal urinary sphincter" (IUS). It is important to note here that the IUS is completely involuntary. There is no volitional control of continence at the bladder neck area. As one moves more distally down the urethra, there is a second collar like condensation of muscle tissue. The condensation of muscular tissue at this level is known as the external urinary sphincter (EUS). The EUS is more accurately described as a rhabdosphincter. This rhabdosphincter is composed in part of striated muscle. Moreover, a significant portion of this musculature is under volitional control. The bladder neck and proximal urethra down to the most distal portion of the EUS, which includes these two sphincter rich areas is known as the continence zone (CZ). If one looks at this area as a whole, that is, the bladder muscle and the CZ. If taken together, their function is twofold, (1) urine storage and (2) urine expulsion (voiding). The storage phase (of urine) requires low bladder pressure that does not exceed bladder outlet resistance. Voiding requires (1) intact neurological pathways which govern volitional triggers for voiding, combined with (2) autonomic bladder muscle contraction, (3) adequate bladder contractility, and possibly, the most important aspect of all which is (4) the coordinated relaxation of the bladder outlet and pelvic floor.

Physiology of Voiding

The basic process of micturition can be broken down into two broad categories or phases which are subsequently broken down into a total of six steps. The two phases are basically (1) urine storage and (2) bladder emptying. The six steps are as follows: (1) Urine is made at the kidneys and stored in the bladder. (2) The bladder fills with urine allowing for increasing volumes at low bladder pressures. (3) At a certain volume, the viscoelastic properties of the bladder wall muscle are met and a baroreceptor mediated sensory signal of fullness is generated. (4) The rhabdosphincter muscle voluntarily relaxes followed by the remainder of the CZ, (5) The bladder muscle (detrusor) then contracts in a coordinated fashion, (6) The bladder is emptied through the urethra and urine is removed from the body.

Now it is important to realize that even though we can break this process down into these six discreet steps as articulately, accurately, and logically as we have, that it is still over simplified. The physiology of voiding is an extremely complex process, beyond these six steps there are elaborate layers of control. The text below attempts to better explain the micturition process, and there is more depth in the graphic above.

The bladder is composed of bands of interlaced smooth muscle (detrusor). The innervation of the body of the bladder is different from that of the bladder neck. The body is rich in beta adrenergic receptors. These receptors are stimulated by the sympathetic component of the autonomic nervous system (ANS). Beta stimulation, via fibers of the hypogastric nerve, suppresses contraction of the detrusor. Conversely, parasympathetic stimulation, by fibers in the pelvic nerve, causes the detrusor to contract. Sympathetic stimulation accounts for baseline bladder muscle tone which is predominant during bladder filling, and the parasympathetic stimulation causes emptying.

The continence zone (CZ) which is composed of two sphincters control the bladder outlet. The internal sphincter is composed of smooth muscle like the detrusor and extends into the bladder neck. Like the detrusor, the internal sphincter is controlled by the ANS and is normally closed. The primary receptors in the bladder neck are alpha-adrenergic. Sympathetic stimulation of these alpha receptors, via fibers in the hypogastric nerve, contributes to urinary continence. The external sphincter is histologically different from the detrusor and internal sphincter. It is striated muscle. Like skeletal muscle, it's under voluntary control. It receives its innervation from the pudendal nerve, arising from the ventral horns of the sacral spinal cord. During micturition, supraspinal centers block stimulation by the hypogastric and pudendal nerves. This relaxes the internal and external sphincters and removes the *sympathetic* inhibition at the level of the detrusor to allow for unopposed parasympathetic tone via muscarinic receptor activation. The result is unobstructed passage of urine when the detrusor contracts.

Now bladder filling begins with the kidneys. Blood is filtered and urine is made at which point the urine is passed on to the ureters. The ureters then course down from the kidneys down along the ventral surface of the psoas and beneath the uterine pedicle to finally enter the bladder into the trigone via the intramural ureter between the layers of the detrusor. The ureters use its peristaltic activity to propel urine into the bladder. The bladder then passively expands to accommodate increasing volumes of urine at low pressures. As the bladder expands and intravesical pressure rises, the ureters are compressed between the layers of muscle, creating a valve mechanism. This valve mechanism limits the backflow of urine. The normal adult bladder can hold about 500 cc of urine. After emptying, the bladder may still retain about 50 cc residual volume. At about 150 cc of volume, stretch receptors in the detrusor begin signaling the CNS via afferent nerves; at 400 cc we are "seeking" an appropriate toilet.

Physiology of Urinary Continence

Now it is extremely important to understand the mechanism or process of urinary continence. Moreover, this process of urinary continence is *NOT* synonymous with the CZ as described above. The CZ is just one of the three major components required to maintain urinary continence. These are, respectively, (1) proximal urethral support, (2) the CZ, i.e. internal sphincter activity, and external sphincter function, (3) bladder muscle stability with intravesical pressure all contribute to continence. Any one alone may not be able to keep a patient dry. The pressures generated during a cough may easily overcome the internal and external sphincters closing powers, and the normal supportive mechanism works in such a way as to increase closure during increases in abdominal pressure. Normal support, conversely, is not sufficient in and of itself to maintain continence, and must have sufficient resting sphincteric activity along with bladder muscle stability to be effective. When one element is abnormal, the other mechanisms may be able to compensate and maintain continence. It is because there are these several interdependent parts of the continence mechanism that no single urodynamic parameter is predictive of continence. Each different etiologic type of incontinence reflects the malfunction of one of the anatomic or physiologic components of continence. Therefore, a knowledge of this mechanism's structure and function is fundamental to an understanding of this common clinical problem. Technologic advances in the neuro-diagnostic assessment of the lower urinary tract have allowed for a much more sophisticated understanding of the process and more importantly, the ability to create and effective interventional strategy to control urine leakage.

Anterior Physiology: In Conclusion

The normal functioning of bladder continence relies on the complex interactions of various neural pathways with the bladder, CZ, and the pelvic floor. In the normal condition, we are able to control where and when we void. This is largely because the CNS is able to suppress the sacral micturition reflex. If the sacral reflex is unrestrained, parasympathetic stimulation via the pelvic nerve causes detrusor contraction. Detrusor contraction is suppressed via the sympathetic side of the autonomic nervous system. More precisely, detrusor muscle stabilization is achieved with baseline *sympathetic* stimulation mediated through beta receptors via the hypogastric nerve. In response to afferent stimulation, the centers above the brainstem become aware of the need to void. If it is appropriate, the somatic and parasympathetic nervous system relaxes the external sphincter which in turn inhibits the sympathetic inhibitory effect on the bladder muscle. Finally, the end result is that the bladder contracts and urine is released.

References

1. Raizada V, Mittal RK. Pelvic floor anatomy and applied physiology. Gastroenterol Clin North Am. 2008;37(3):493–509. vii.
2. Lorenzi B, Brading AF, Mortensen NJ. Interstitial cells of Cajal modulate the tone of the human internal anal sphincter in vitro. Dis Colon Rectum. 2014;57(3):370–7.
3. Cheeney G, Nguyen M, Valestin J, Rao SS. Topographic and manometric characterization of the recto-anal inhibitory reflex. Neurogastroenterol Motil. 2012;24(3):e147–54.
4. Mittal RK, Bhargava V, Sheean G, Ledgerwood M, Sinha S. Purse-string morphology of external anal sphincter revealed by novel imaging techniques. Am J Physiol Gastrointest Liver Physiol. 2014;306(6):G505–14.
5. Broens PM, Penninckx FM, Ochoa JB. Fecal continence revisited: the anal external sphincter continence reflex. Dis Colon Rectum. 2013;56(11):1273–81.
6. Koh CE, Young CJ, Young JM, Solomon MJ. Systematic review of randomized controlled trials of the effectiveness of biofeedback for pelvic floor dysfunction. Br J Surg. 2008;95(9):1079–87.
7. Rao SS. American College of Gastroenterology Practice Parameters Committee. Diagnosis and management of fecal incontinence. American College of Gastroenterology Practice Parameters Committee. Am J Gastroenterol. 2004;99(8):1585–604.
8. Bharucha AE, Rao SS. An update on anorectal disorders for gastroenterologists. Gastroenterology. 2014;146(1):37–45.e2.
9. Bharucha AE, Wald A, Enck P, Rao S. Functional anorectal disorders. Gastroenterology. 2006;130(5):1510–8.
10. Mellgren A. Physiologic testing In: Beck DE et al., editors. The ASCRS textbook of colon and rectal surgery. 2nd ed. Springer, LLC; 2011. p. 49. 10.1007/978-1-4419-1584-9_4.
11. Lowry AC, Simmang CL, Boulos P, et al. Consensus statement of definitions for anorectal physiology and rectal cancer: report of the tripartite consensus conference on definitions for anorectal physiology and rectal cancer, Washington, DC, May 1, 1999. Dis Colon Rectum. 2001;44(7):915–9.
12. McHugh SM, Diamant NE. Anal canal pressure profile: a reappraisal as determined by rapid pull through technique. Gut. 1987;28(10):1234–41.
13. Rao SS, Hatfield R, Soffer E, Rao S, Beaty J, Conklin JL. Manometric tests of anorectal function in healthy adults. Am J Gastroenterol. 1999;94(3):773–83.
14. Rao SS, Azpiroz F, Diamant N, Enck P, Tougas G, Wald A. Minimum standards of anorectal manometry. Neurogastroenterol Motil. 2002;14(5):553–9.
15. Li Y, Yang X, Xu C, Zhang Y, Zhang X. Normal values and pressure morphology for three-dimensional high-resolution anorectal manometry of asymptomatic adults: a study in 110 subjects. Int J Colorectal Dis. 2013;28(8):1161–8.
16. Azpiroz F, Enck P, Whitehead WE. Anorectal functional testing: review of collective experience. Am J Gastroenterol. 2002;97(2):232–40.
17. Sun WM, Read NW, Miner PB. Relation between rectal sensation and anal function in normal subjects and patients with faecal incontinence. Gut. 1990;31(9):1056–61.
18. Sun WM, Read NW, Prior A, Daly JA, Cheah SK, Grundy D. Sensory and motor responses to rectal distention vary according to rate and pattern of balloon inflation. Gastroenterology. 1990;99(4):1008–15.
19. Chan CL, Scott SM, Williams NS, Lunniss PJ. Rectal hypersensitivity worsens stool frequency, urgency, and lifestyle in patients with urge fecal incontinence. Dis Colon Rectum. 2005;48(1):134–40.
20. Gladman MA, Scott SM, Chan CL, Williams NS, Lunniss PJ. Rectal hyposensitivity: Prevalence and clinical impact in patients with intractable constipation and fecal incontinence. Dis Colon Rectum. 2003;46(2):238–46.
21. Read NW, Timms JM, Barfield LJ, Donnelly TC, Bannister JJ. Impairment of defecation in young women with severe constipation. Gastroenterology. 1986;90(1):53–60.
22. Duthie GS, Bartolo DC. Anismus: The cause of constipation? results of investigation and treatment. World J Surg. 1992;16(5):831–5.
23. Lopez A, Holmstrom B, Nilsson BY, et al. Paradoxical sphincter reaction is influenced by rectal filling volume. Dis Colon Rectum. 1998;41(8):1017–22.
24. Pezim ME, Pemberton JH, Levin KE, Litchy WJ, Phillips SF. Parameters of anorectal and colonic motility in health and in severe constipation. Dis Colon Rectum. 1993;36(5):484–91.
25. Haynes WG, Read NW. Ano-rectal activity in man during rectal infusion of saline: a dynamic assessment of the anal continence mechanism. J Physiol. 1982;330:45–56.
26. Read NW, Haynes WG, Bartolo DC, et al. Use of anorectal manometry during rectal infusion of saline to investigate sphincter function in incontinent patients. Gastroenterology. 1983;85(1):105–13.

27. Cheong DM, Vaccaro CA, Salanga VD, et al. Electrodiagnostic evaluation of fecal incontinence. Muscle Nerve. 1995;18(6):612–9.

28. Wexner SD, Marchetti F, Salanga VD, Corredor C, Jagelman DG. Neurophysiologic assessment of the anal sphincters. Dis Colon Rectum. 1991;34(7):606–12.

29. Neill ME, Swash M. Increased motor unit fibre density in the external anal sphincter muscle in ano-rectal incontinence: a single fibre EMG study. J Neurol Neurosurg Psychiatry. 1980;43(4):343–7.

30. Rogers J, Levy DM, Henry MM, Misiewicz JJ. Pelvic floor neuropathy: a comparative study of diabetes mellitus and idiopathic faecal incontinence. Gut. 1988;29(6):756–61.

31. Womack NR, Morrison JF, Williams NS. The role of pelvic floor denervation in the aetiology of idiopathic faecal incontinence. Br J Surg. 1986;73(5):404–7.

32. Burnett SJ, Speakman CT, Kamm MA, Bartram CI. Confirmation of endosonographic detection of external anal sphincter defects by simultaneous electromyographic mapping. Br J Surg. 1991;78(4):448–50.

33. Tjandra JJ, Milsom JW, Schroeder T, Fazio VW. Endoluminal ultrasound is preferable to electromyography in mapping anal sphincteric defects. Dis Colon Rectum. 1993;36(7):689–92.

34. Fitz FF, Resende AP, Stupp L, Sartori MG, Girao MJ, Castro RA. Biofeedback for the treatment of female pelvic floor muscle dysfunction: a systematic review and meta-analysis. Int Urogynecol J. 2012;23(11):1495–516.

35. Enck P, von Giesen HJ, Schafer A, et al. Comparison of anal sonography with conventional needle electromyography in the evaluation of anal sphincter defects. Am J Gastroenterol. 1996;91(12): 2539–43.

36. Felt-Bersma RJ, Cuesta MA, Koorevaar M, et al. Anal endosonography: relationship with anal manometry and neurophysiologic tests. Dis Colon Rectum. 1992;35(10):944–9.

37. Ferrante SL, Perry RE, Schreiman JS, Cheng SC, Frick MP. The reproducibility of measuring the anorectal angle in defecography. Dis Colon Rectum. 1991;34(1):51–5.

38. Shorvon PJ, McHugh S, Diamant NE, Somers S, Stevenson GW. Defecography in normal volunteers: results and implications. Gut. 1989;30(12):1737–49.

39. Lamb GM, de Jode MG, Gould SW, et al. Upright dynamic MR defaecating proctography in an open configuration MR system. Br J Radiol. 2000;73(866):152–5.

40. Roos JE, Weishaupt D, Wildermuth S, Willmann JK, Marincek B, Hilfiker PR. Experience of 4 years with open MR defecography: pictorial review of anorectal anatomy and disease. Radiographics. 2002;22(4):817–32.

Cellular and Molecular Aging

Priyamvada Rai and Bruce R. Troen

with Introduction by David A. Gordon.

Every Day. You get a Little Older, that's the Law.

Butch Cassidy to the Sun Dance Kid.

Aging Seems to be the Only Available Way to Live a Long Life.

Daniel Francois Esprit Auber.

Introduction

As a clinical researcher whose area of expertise is Geriatric Pelvic Medicine, the physical changes that go along with increasing age is incredibly interesting to me. However, from a more practical perspective, the biology of aging, although fascinating, is not something that I would be pushed to address in a routine clinical or administrative situation. All that notwithstanding, questions, presumptions, and theories surrounding the definition of aging are inescapable. In fact, more often than I like to admit, I will find myself getting side tracked and drifting off into deep thought about what "aging really means," or what patients do I consider "old"? Are they really "old"? Which ones might I consider "young" and compare my assessments to their actual chronological age in years? Perhaps, the most frustrating piece of all, is that, almost invariably, after I come out of my intensely contemplative trance on" "aging," that I end up with more questions than answers.

Let's face it, when we discuss aging, there are so many issues to consider that it is difficult to get comfortable with some standard baseline. To complicate matters further, try to weigh all of the subtleties into the equation. So where do we begin? Perhaps the definition? Although everyone is familiar with the concept of aging, defining it is not so easy. In its simplest terms, aging signifies the passage of time. The passage of time, in and of itself, often carries a negative connotation. However, in a more global sense, *it is not always the case*, especially if we would *consider the presentation of wine*. Nevertheless, for the purposes of this book, we should look at aging in the context of senescence, more specifically, "cellular senescence" where the routine biologic processes necessary for normal life decline in functionality which is consistent with "growing older" in a phenotypic sense and a deleterious fashion.

How important is all of this. Well, let us first ask from a purely chronological perspective, what is old? Arbitrarily, many independent and governmental organizations consider 65 years as a reasonable number. So, let's look at the demographics. The older population, i.e. persons 65 years or older number close to 44.7 million in 2013. They represented 14.1% of the US population, about one in every seven Americans. By 2060, there will be about 98 million older persons, more than twice their number in 2013. People 65+ represented 14.1% of the population in the year 2013 but are expected to grow to be 21.7% of the population by 2040. The information in this section of the AoA website brings together a wide variety of statistical information about this growing population.

Considering all of the above, *if absolutely pressed for a definition, I would say that aging could be considered as a progressive decline in a cascade of complex biological processes, whose culmination is intrinsically related to a slowly*

P. Rai
Department of Medicine, Sylvester Comprehensive Cancer Center, University of Miami Health System, Miami, FL, USA

B.R. Troen
Division of Geriatrics and Palliative Medicine, Department of Medicine, Jacobs School of Medicine and Biomedical Sciences, Buffalo, NY, USA

© Springer Science+Business Media New York 2017
D.A. Gordon, M.R. Katlic (eds.), *Pelvic Floor Dysfunction and Pelvic Surgery in the Elderly*,
DOI 10.1007/978-1-4939-6554-0_3

but progressively changing phenotype which is less capable of responding to stress. Even if environmental factors do not cause aging, they certainly affect it. For example, overexposure to ultraviolet radiation accelerates the aging of the skin phenotype. Creating even more of a conundrum, different parts of the body may age at different rates. Two organisms of the same species can also age at different rates, so that biological aging and chronological aging are quite distinct concepts [1–71].

Before closing, let me say that I am proud Baltimorean (T.V. coverage, notwithstanding, it still is a beautiful town) and just like millions of Americans, the National Institute on Aging's (NIA) Baltimore Longitudinal Study of Aging (BLSA) approaches its 60th birthday in 2018. The study was the first to ask some important basic questions: **What is normal aging?** Thus far, two major conclusions can be drawn from the Baltimore study. **First, "normal" aging MUST be distinguished from disease.** Although people's bodies change and can in some ways decline over time, these changes do not inevitably lead to diseases such as diabetes, hypertension, or dementia. Remember, there are many disorders that typically occur as we get older, they are a result of disease processes, NOT a normal consequence of aging. **Second, there is NO single, universally accepted chronological timetable for human aging.** The bottom line is that we all age differently!

Life Span and Life Expectancy

The average/median life span (also known as life expectancy) is represented by the age at which 50 % of a given population survives, and maximum life span potential (MLSP) represents the longest-lived member(s) of the population or species. The average life span of humans has increased dramatically over time, yet the MLSP has remained approximately constant. For 99 % of our existence as a species, the average life expectancy for a human being was very short compared to the present. Daring the Bronze Age (circa 3000 BC), the average life expectancy was 18 years due to disease and accidents. Average life expectancy in 275 BC was still only 26 years. By 1900, improved sanitation helped to improve the average life expectancy at birth for humans to 47 years, but infectious disease was still a major killer. As of the new millennium (AD 2000), better diet, healthcare, and reduced infant mortality had results in an average life expectancy of 77.8 years. Today, in 2015, it has reached beyond 80 years. The increase in the average life expectancy has resulted in a compression of morbidity (a squaring of the mortality curve) towards the end of the life span. Of note, the longest-lived human for whom documentation exists was Jeanne Calment, who died at the age of 122 in August 1997. The longest-lived male was Christian Mortensen, who died

in 1998 at the age of 115. As causes of early mortality have been eliminated through public-health measures and improved medical care, more individuals have approached the maximum life span. Between 1960 and 2000, the population of these aged 85 years and over grew 356 %, whereas the elderly population in general rose 111 %, and the entire US population grew only 57 %.

A member of physiological functions begins a progressive decline from the fourth decade onward, including the cardiovascular, pulmonary, renal, and immune system. In women, this correlates with a decline in reproductive capacity. Interestingly, one study has shown that woman who are fertile in their forties are nearly four times as likely to survive to the age of 100 than woman who are not, suggesting that reproductive fitness later in life may be an indicator of longevity. The age of menopause has also been linked to life span. Controlling for socioeconomic factors, women who undergo menopause before the age of 40 are twice as likely to die before those who experience menopause after the age of 50. These findings hold true even when a history of estrogen replacement therapy is taken into account, suggesting that reduced estrogen alone is not responsible for the ostensible reduction in life span. Another study found that while late reproduction correlated with increased longevity in postreproductive Sinai women, maternal age at first birth a total fecundity did not appear to impact female longevity. In males, although spermatogenesis per ++ does not show a significant age-related decline, testosterone levels fall with advancing age, and a few studies have linked reduced bioavailability of testrone to age-related functional degeneration. Therefore, it would appear that there is a link between reproductive health, aging, and life span (see the disposable soma theory discussed below).

MLSP appears to be species-specific, implying a significant genetic component to the rate of aging. For example, humans have an MLSP 25- to 30-fold higher than mice. Some biodemographic estimates predict that elimination of most of the major killers such as cancer, cardiovascular disease, and diabetes would add no more than 10 years to the average life expectancy, but would not affect MLSP. This implies an upper limit to the MLSP. Some models suggest that genes operate by raising or lowering the relative risk of death by making cancer, coronary disease, or Alzheimer's disease more likely, rather than by fixing the life span. One mathematical model predicts that if participants in the Framingham Heart Study had been able to maintain the levels of 11 different risk factors similar to those of typical 30 year old, the men and women would have survived to an average age of 99.9 and 97.0 years, respectively.

There are three known regimens that can extend life span. The first two involve lowering ambient temperature and reducing exercise and are effective in poikilotherms (cold-blooded species). A 10 C drop or the elimination of a housefly's capacity to 8y extends the maximum life span approximately 250%. Both of these manipulations decrease the metabolic rate and are accompanied by decrease in free radical generation and oxidative damage to protein and DNA.

The third intervention is calorie restriction, which can extend life span in yeast worms, flies, grasshoppers, spiders, water fleas, hamster, mice, rats, and dogs. Dietary restriction without malnutrition can increase both the average and maximum life spans of mice and rats by more than 50%. Although calories are severely restricted (up to 40%), essential nutrients such as vitamins and minerals are maintained at levels equivalent to those found in ad libitum diets. The diet-restricted animals also exhibit a delay in the onset of physiological and pathological changes with aging. These include hormone and lipid levels, female reproduction, immune function, nephropathy, cardiomyopathy, osteodystrophy, and malignancies. Size, weight, fat percentage, and some organ weights are markedly less in calorically restricted animals. The specific metabolic rate, the amount of oxygen consumed per gram of tissues, decreased in rats subjected to caloric restriction. However, in one study, long-term food restriction did not alter the metabolic rate. This finding suggests that the specific metabolic rate may not be a critical determinant of longevity. To date, life span extension in mammals by dietary restriction has been most convincingly demonstrated in rodents. However, dietary restriction in primates and in humans does appear to improve a number of metabolic and cardiovascular disease risk parameters.

Characteristics of Aging

There is evidence supporting at least five common characteristics of aging in mammals:

1. Increased mortality with age after maturation: In the early nineteenth century, Gompertz first described the exponential increase in mortality with aging due to various causes, a phenomenon that still pertains today. In 2005, the death rate for all causes at the age of 25–34 was 104.4/100,000 and at the age of 35–44 was 93.3/100,000. Death rates at the age of 65–74, 75–84, and 85 and over were 2,137.1/100,000, 5,260.0/100,000, and 13,798.6/100,000, respectively: a greater than 130-fold increase from young adults to the oldest group. Indeed, the pattern of age related survival in similar across species, including invertebrates and single-cell organisms.
2. Changes in Biochemical Composition in Tissues with Age:
   There are notable age-related decreases in lean body mass and total bone mass in humans. Although subcutaneous fat is unchanged or declining, total fat remains the same [29]. Consequently, the percentage of adipose tissue increases with age. At the cellular level, many markers of aging have been described in various tissues from different organisms. Two of the first to be described were increases in lipofuscin (age pigment) and increased cross-linking in extracellular matrix molecules such as collagen. Recent studies have shown that DNA damage markers such as gamma-112AX and 53BPI are upregulated in tissues of aged primates and mice, presumably arising from DNA double-strand breaks (DSB) and/or dysfunctional chromosome ends called telomeres. Additional examples include age-related changes in both the rates of transcription of specific genes and the rate of protein synthesis and numerous age-related alterations in posttranslational protein modifications, such as glycation and oxidation. For instance, the p16INK4a gene product has been found to be upregulated in a number of tissues from aging individuals and animals.
3. Progressive decrease in physiological capacity with age: Many physiologic changes have been documented in both cross-sectional and longitudinal studies. Examples include declines in glomerular filtration rate, maximal heart rate, and vital capacity. These decreases occur linearly from about the age of 20; however, the rate of physiological decline is quite heterogeneous from organ to organ and individual to individual.
4. Reduced ability to respond adaptively to environmental stimuli with age: A fundamental feature of senescence is the diminished ability to maintain homeostasis. This is manifested not primarily by changes in resting or basal parameters, but in the altered response to an external stimulus such as exercise or fasting. The loss of "reserve" can result in blunted maximum responses as well as in delays in reaching a peak level and in returning to basal levels. For example, the induction of hepatic tyrosine aminotransferase activity by fasting is both attenuated and delayed in old rodents. The immune response also appears to be impaired in older individuals, leading to reduced ability to fight infections, less protection from vaccinations, higher incidences of autoimmunity, and impaired antigen affinity and class-switching by lymphocytes (reviewed by Dorshkind et al).
5. Increased susceptibility and venerability to disease: The incidence and mortality rates for many diseases increase with age and parallel the exponential increase in mortality with age. For the five leading causes of death for people over 65 years of age, the relative increase in death rates compared to people aged between 25 and 44 is: heart disease—92-fold, cancer—43-fold, stroke—>100-fold, chronic lung disease ->100-fold, and pneumonia and influenza—89-fold. The basis for these dramatic rises in mortality is completely understood but presumably involves changes in the function of many types of cells that lead to tissue/organ dysfunction and systemic illness. Interestingly, a retrospective study of centenarians dem-

onstrated that they live 90–95 % of their lives in very good health and with a high level of functional independence. The centenarians do suffer a 30–50 % annual morality at the end of their lives, but this represents a marked compression of morbidity towards the end of life and is close to the idealized survival curve.

Theories of Aging

- Developmental/genetic
- Antagonistic pleiotropy theory
- Longevity-associated genes
- Disposable soma theory
- Stochastic
- Free radical/oxidative stress
- Mitochondrial dysfunction theory
- DNA damage theory of aging

Development/Genetic Theories

A general framework for a plausible theory of aging begins with attempting to understand the evolutionary basis of senescence. Development-genetic theories consider the process of aging to be part of the genetically programmed and controlled continuum of development and maturation. Although this is an alternative motion, the diverse expression of aging effects is in sharp contrast to the tightly controlled and very precise process of development. Also, evolution selects for the optimization of reproduction; the effects of genes expressed in later life probably do not play a large role in the evolution of a species. This class of theories is supported by the observation that the maximum life span is highly species specific. As noted above, the maximum life span for humans is 30 times that of mice. In addition, studies comparing the longevity of monozygotic and dizygotic and dizygotic twins and noutwin siblings have shown a remarkable similarity between monozygotic twins that is not seen in the other two groups.

However, it is also likely that the interplay of genetic responses to extrinsic stresses may modulate the extent of aging. An interesting example of this theory comes from a study by Niedemhofer et al. who demonstrated that aging mice as well as normal adult mice treated with mitomycin C to elevate DNA damage levels showed a shift in gene expression that was very similar to that observed in a mouse model of XPF-ERCC deficiency, a novel genetic disorder associated with accelerated aging. The alterations in the transcriptome reflected enhanced antioxidant and anabolic pathways and reduced insulin growth factor (IGF-1) signaling (a known longevity assurance mechanism), suggesting a systemic shift of the "somatotropic axis from growth to maintenance under genotoxic stress. Thus, in the model of XFE/ERCC-progeroid syndrome, the phenotypic outcomes depend not just on DNA damaging stimuli, which likely cause a functional decline, but also on the genetic adaptive response to the damage mediated by the IGF metabolic pathway.

Stochastic Theories on Aging

Free Radical/Oxidative Stress

Denham Harman proposed one of the oldest and most enduring theories of aging over 50 years ago when he postulated that most aging changes are due to molecular damage caused by free radicals, which are incompletely reduced, highly reactive intermediates of oxygen. The term "free radical" is misleading because one of these intermediates is hydrogen peroxide, which contains no unpaired electrons and is therefore not a radical. The more accurate nomenclature for these intermediates is reactive oxygen species or ROS, and for the purposes of discussion herein and in the context of aging theories, we use the term free radical interchangeably with ROS, which likely is what Harman intended when he named his theory of aging.

Aerobic metabolism generates the superoxide radical (O_2^{-}) which is metabolized by superoxide dismutases to form hydrogen peroxide and oxygen. Hydrogen peroxide can go on to form the extremely reactive hydroxyl radical (OH). These oxygen-derived species can react with macromolecules in a self-percolating manner; they create free radicals out of subsequently attacked molecules, which in turn create free radicals out of other molecules thereby amplifying the effect of the initial free radical attack. ROS appear to play a role in regulating differential gene expression, cell replication, differentiation, and apoptotic cell death (in part by acting as second messengers in signal transduction pathways). In addition, nonradical pro-oxidants, for instance metals such as iron and copper that catalyze formation of the hydroxyl radical, as well as high concentrations of certain antioxidants can together generate a retrograde redox regenerative cycle, leading to homeostatic imbalance and oxidative stress.

In lower organisms, the role of antioxidants on life span extension is also complex. Increasing expression of the mitochondrial Mn-superoxide dismutase (aka SOD2) in flies has yielded confliction results, with one study reporting approximately 15 % extension in mean and maximum life span without changes in oxygen consumption and another reporting no significant effect on life span. However, SOD2 reduction in flies reduces life span and mimics aging related defects, progressive reeducation in SOD2 activity correlates with further shortening of life span. This dose dependent effect of SOD2 on life span is consistent with over expression of SOD2 in flies.

Overexpression of Cu, Zn-superoxide dismutase (aka SOD1), the cytosolic superoxide dismutase, has been reported to extend life span in flies by around 40–50 %; however, the significance of these results to the oxidative stress theory of aging is undercut by the facts that the majority of life extension was seen in the shortest-lived flies or by overexpressing SOD1 in tissues where there was a clear deficiency of the enzyme. In ant colonies, where large differences exist in life span between queens and workers, SOD1 activity correlates mostly negatively with life span with the shorter-lived males having higher SOD1 expression and activity compared to the long-lived queens. Over expression of catalase alone in transgenic flies also does not extend life span. Some transgenic flies with increased expression of both Cu/Zn-superoxide dismutase and catalase, which act in tandem to remove superoxide and hydrogen peroxide, respectively, exhibit up to a one-third extension of average and maximum life span. In addition, they exhibit increased resistance to oxidative damage and an increase in the metabolic potential (total amount of oxygen consumed during adult life per unit body weight). However, combinatorial over expression of the major antioxidants, SOD1, SOD2, catalase and thioredoxin reductase in relatively long-lived flies did not appear to enhance longevity. It has also been shown that over expressing glutathione reductase extends the life span of transgenic flies kept under hyperoxic or oxidant-treated conditions, but not under ambient conditions.

C. elegans is a model system in which a number of long lived mutants have been identified, the role of oxidants and antioxidants is similarly complicated. Although nutrient sensing pathways appear to be a dominant mechanism of life-span determination in C. elegans, a casual role for oxidative stress in their aging still has neither been validated nor disproved. In long-lived worms that overexpress daf-2, ROS production was higher than in wild type worms throughout the life-span, but protein carboxylation was reduced. The observed reduction in damage in the face of elevated ROS levels has been ascribed to compensatory protective effects due to enhanced enzymatic antioxidant activity from SOD proteins and glutathione's transferees. However, treatments of wild-type C. elegans strains with SOD and catalase mimetics failed to extend life span despite increasing antioxidant activity. Yet, the role of oxygen tension nevertheless appears to have an effect on life span and oxidative damage because worms kept 1 % oxygen have lower carbonyl levels and show approximately 24 % increase in life span relative to counterparts kept at ambient oxygen.

Production of ROS in the heart, kidney, and liver of a group of mammals was found to be inversely proportional to the maximum life span, although the activities of individual antioxidant enzymes were not consistently related to maximum life span. However, catalase overexpression targeted to the mitochondria does increase life span and improve functional health of the mice as they age. Transgenic mice that overexpress thioredoxin, another antioxidant protein, also exhibit about a 30 % improvement in mean life span. A series of studies have demonstrated that oxidative stress resistance of dermal fibroblasts correlates with the longevity of the species.

The studies discussed above illustrate the complexity behind the free radical theory of aging. Antioxidants, in general, only appear to have significant effect on life-span extension if their levels/function are limiting or under conditions of stress. Thus, over expression of enzymes that are already present to robust levels are not likely to have an effect on lifespan simply because increasing expression does not enhance catalytic efficiency of these enzymes, which are already operating at near optimal rates. Furthermore, given the importance of antioxidant enzymes, to survival of aerobically respiring organisms, there is a certain amount of redundancy between different antioxidants, and different tissues require their individual action to different extents. This heterogeneity and overlap of function may also be obscuring the effects of altering antioxidant levels in animal models of life-span extension. Thus, rather than overexpressing antioxidants alone, a more viable strategy of life-span extension perhaps needs to center on reducing production of ROS by modulating mitochondrial function or the prooxidant factors, which contribute to the deleterious effects of oxygen radicals.

Mitochondrial Dysfunction Theory of Aging

The mitochondrial DNA/oxidative stress hypothesis represents a synthesis of several theories and therefore comprises elements of both stochastic and developmental-genetic mechanisms of aging (see below). It is proposed that ROS contribute significantly to the somatic accumulation of mitochondrial DNA mutations, leading to the gradual loss of biogenetic capacity and eventually resulting in aging and cell death. Ozawa has dubbed this the "redox mechanism of mitochondrial aging." Mitochondrial DNA (mt-DNA) undergoes a progressive age-related increase in oxygen free radical damage in skeletal muscle, the diaphragm, cardiac muscle, and the brain. This exponential increase in damage correlates with the increase in both point and dilatational somatic mtDNA mutations seen with age. Interestingly, extrapolation of the curve to the point where 100 % of cardiac mtDNA exhibits deletion mutations gives an age of 129.

Mitochondrial DNA is maternally transmitted, continues to replicate throughout the life span of an organism in both proliferating and postmitotic (nonproliferation) cells, and is subject to a much higher mutation rate than nuclear DNA. This is due, in large part, to inefficient repair mechanisms and its proximity to the mitochondrial membrane where reactive oxygen species are generated. Defects in mitochondrial respiration are found not only in normal tissues but also in diseases that are increasingly manifested with age such as Parkinson's diseases. Alzheimer's disease, Huntington's Chorea, and other movement disorders. Diseases for which mtDNA mutations have been found include Alzheimer's, Parkinson's, and a large number of skeletal and cardiac myopathies. Apoptosis has also been associated with mtDNA fragmentation. As noted above, mitochondrial haplotype J is associated with human longevity. However, the role of inherited and somatic mutations in mitochondrial DNA during human aging is clearly complex, and additional studies are required to gain further insight.

The idea of mitochondrial involvement in aging postulates that accumulation of mtDNA damage leads to defective mitochondrial respiration, which in turn enhances oxygen free radical formation, leading to additional mtDNA damage. However, the reality appears not to be quite so simple. A mouse model has been developed to address the issue whether phenotypic aging of tissues depends on mitochondrial DNA mutations. These mice express an error-prone version of the major mitochondrial DNA polymerase, poly-gamma, generated by mutating the proofreading domain of the enzyme. The mutant mice show fairly uniform accumulation of both deletions and point mutations in the mitochondrial genomes of different tissues and an accelerated aging phenotype. The observations from the mutant poly-gamma mouse model mirror previous findings regarding the role of mitochondrial mutations in aging. On the surface, these observations fit well with the free radical/oxidative stress theory of aging, since mutations in mitochondrial genes coding for respiratory chain enzymes could in principle result in leakier election transfer, thus leading to increased accumulation of ROS. However, this does not appear to be the case in mouse embryonic lipolysis derived from the mutant mice that, despite impaired respiration, show neither augmentation of ROS production nor sensitivity to oxidative stress-medicated cell death. Lack of change in protein carboxylation levels is presented to support the idea that these mice suffer no elevation in oxidative stress, although these lesions may not be appropriate as the sole marker of cellular oxidative damage as they are detected only if they are present in a degradation-resistant state. Furthermore, since mitochondrial deletions in the pol-gamma mutant mice lead to linearized mitochondrial genomes, another possibility is that the premature aging phenotype observed in these mice is the result of a DNA damage response (DDR) (see below) rather than accruing directly due to mitochondrial dysfunction. Nevertheless, the pol-gamma mice provide an elegant and useful system in which to further explore the role of mitochondrial mutations and ROS in engendering the aging phenotype.

In humans, specific mutations, while increasing with age, seldom account for more than several percent of the total mtDNA. However, some studies suggest that the total percentage of mtDNA affected by mutations is much greater, as much as 85%, and increases with age. In addition, caloric restriction in mice retards the age-associated accumulation of mtDNA mutations. Agents that bypass blocks in the respiratory chain such as coenzyme Q10, tocopherol, nicotinamide, and ascorbic acid would be predicted to ameliorate some of the effects of mitochondrial disease and aging. Withdrawal of coenzyme Q from the diet of nematodes extends the life span by approximately 60%. Calorie restric-

tion can extend life span, reduces oxidative damage in primates. There are epidemiologic studies that appear to implicate dietary antioxidants in the reduction of vascular dementia, cardiovascular disease, and cancer in humans. However, results to date, in treatment of patients with myopathies, have been variably or only anecdotally successful. This suggests that a complex interaction exists between pro-oxidant and antioxidants forces in the cell and that regulation of the balance between the two may be the critical determinant in mitochondrial, and subsequently cellular and tissue integrity during aging.

An increasing number of studies have implicated mitochondrial biogenesis and efficiency as playing significant roles to enhance cellular fitness and organism longevity. Maintenance of energy production and prevention and/or amelioration of oxidative stress by mitochondria are key to healthy aging. As previously discussed, caloric restriction is the most reliable intervention to extend life span in a number of species, including mammals such as rodents, dogs, and rhesus monkeys. Multiple signals modulate PGC1cc activity and subsequent mitochondrial production and efficiency, such as AMP kinas, sirloins, and nitric oxide, all of which can be increased by caloric restriction. Furthermore, caloric restriction increases mitochondrial biogenesis in healthy humans. However, perhaps the best intervention to enhance mitochondrial production and function is exercise, which can at least partly normalize age related mitochondrial dysfunction and can significantly reverse age-related transcriptional alterations. Stochastic theories propose that aging is caused by random damage to vital molecules. The damage eventually accumulates to a level that results in the physiological decline associated with aging. The most prominent example is the somatic mutation theory of aging, which states that genetic damage from background radiation produces mutations that lead to functional failure and, ultimately, death. Exposure to ionizing radiation does shorten life span. However, analysis of survival curves of radiation-treated rodent populations reveals an increase in the initial mortality rate without an effect on the subsequent rate of aging. The life-span shortening is probably due to increased cancer and glomerulosclerosis rather than accelerated aging per??

DNA Damage Theory of Aging

Somatic Mutation, DNA Repair, Error Catastrophe

The DNA repair theory is a more specific example of the somatic mutation theory. Impairment of genomic maintenance has been strongly implicated as a major casual factor in the aging process. Defects in DNA repair mechanisms form the basis of a majority of human progeroid syndromes (see below). The ability to repair ultraviolet radiation-induced DNA damage in cell cultures derived from species with a variety of different life spans is directly correlated with the MI.SP. Unfortunately, there is not enough experimental support to conclude that these differences between species are a causative factor in aging. Although the prevailing belief has been that overall DNA repair capacity does not appear to change with age, several studies now indicate that repair of oxidative DNA damage lesions via base excision repair (BER) becomes more inefficient in aged mice. Calorie restriction can restore the age-related decline in BER. Repair of DNA double-strand breaks (DSRs) is also compromised in replica lively senescent human fibroblasts and in fibroblasts and lymphocytes taken from older humans.

Additionally, the site-specific repair of select regions of DNA appears to be important in several types of terminally differentiated cells. Biochemically, oxidative DNA damage has been shown to affect specific DNA sequences more than others, with the most affected sequences corresponding to conserved motifs in transcriptional elements involved in the regulation of stress response genes. Studies in cultured human neurons show that promoters of genes involved in memory, stress protection, and neuronal survival sustain selective oxidative stress-mediated DNA damage and exhibit reduced BER. Transcriptional profiling of the human frontal brain cortex reveals that the genes under the control of these promoter elements also show the most reduced function after the age of 40. Thus, DNA damage to specific areas of the neuronal genome appears to contribute to age-related cognitive decline. Future studies will need to focus upon repair rates of specific genes rather than indirect general measurements.

The error-catastrophe theory also centers on the role of DNA integrity in the aging process and proposes that random errors in synthesis eventually occur in proteins that synthesize DNA or other "template" molecules. Generally, errors occurring in proteins are lost by natural turnover and simply replaced with error-free molecules. Error-containing molecules involved in the protein-synthesizing machinery, however, would introduce errors into the molecules that they produce. This could result in amplification such that the subsequent rapid accumulation of error-containing molecules results in an "error catastrophic" that would be incompatible with normal function and life. Although there are numerous reports of altered proteins in aging, no direct evidence of age-dependent protein mis-synthesis has yet been reported. The altered proteins that do occur in aging cells and issues are, instead, due to posttranslational modifications such as oxidation and glycation. The increases in altered proteins appear to be due to decreased clearance in older cells.

Models of Aging

Accelerated Aging Syndromes in Humans

Although no disease exists that is an exact phenotypic copy of normal aging, several human genetic diseases including Hutchinson–Gilford syndrome (the "classic" early onset progeria seen in children), Werner's syndrome ("adult" progeria), Cockayne's syndrome or NFE syndrome (another childhood-onset progeroid disease), and Down's syndrome exhibit features of accelerated aging.

Hutchinson–Gilford Progeria Syndrome (HGPS) is an extremely rare autosomal recessive disease in which aging characteristics begin to develop within several years of birth. These include wrinkled skin, stooped posture, early hair loss, and growth retardation. HGPS patients suffer from advanced atherosclerosis, and myocardial infarction is the usual cause of death by the age of 30. However, unlike Werner's syndrome patients (see below), these patients do not typically suffer from cataracts, glucose intolerance, and skin ulcers. IIGPS is a laminopathy resulting from a single nucleotide substitution (1824 C> T) in the nuclear envelope, laminins A and C. The mutation leads to activation of a cryptic splice site and production of a transited version of the precursor protein, prelamin A, denoted progerin or LAA 50, which then leads to formation of abnormal nuclear lamina and delayed nuclear reassembly, as well as DNA damage and chromosomal abnormalities.

Werner's syndrome (WS) is an autosomal recessive inherited disease. Patients prematurely develop arteriosclerosis, glucose intolerance, osteoporosis, early graying, loss of hair, skin atrophy, and hypogonadism. However, patients do not typically suffer from Alzheimer's disease or hypertension. WS patients have an increased predisposition to cancer with a higher than unusual incidence of sacromatous (mesenchymal) tumors develop cataracts in the posterior surface of the lens, not in the nucleus as is usually seen in older people. In addition, they develop patients die before the age of 50, usually of myocardial infarction or cancer. The gene responsible for WS has been localized to chromosome 8 and appears to be a helicase, an enzyme involved in unwinding DNA. DNA helicases play a critical role in DNA replication and repair. Cells from WS patients display chromosomal instability, shortened telomeres, elevated rates of gene mutation, and non-homologous recombination. Furthermore, WS is characterized by hypersensitivity to the chemical carcinogen, 4-NQO, crosslinking agents, and the topoisomerase inhibitor, camptothecin, suggesting impairment of DNA repair mechanisms.

Cockayne's syndrome (CS) is a congenital autosomal recessive disorder characterized by stunted growth, extreme sensitivity to sunlight, retinopathy, deafness, nervous system abnormalities, and premature aging. This is a progressive disease that becomes apparent after 1 year of age and leads to mortality by 12 years of age. There are also more rare variants, one of which manifests at birth and another which presents milder symptoms and appears in late childhood CS results from mutations in the transcription-coupled repair (TCR) and global genomic (GG) repair proteins, ERCC6 and ERCC8, also known as Cockayne's Syndrome B (CSB) and Cockayne's Syndrome A (CSA), respectively. The CSA protein is a 396-amino acid protein with no known enzymatic activity and is part of a multicomponent ubiquitin ligase complex that also includes the DNA damage binding protein DDB. Not much is known about its specific role in producing the CS phenotype, CBS consists of 1493 amino acids and is a member of the SW12/SNF2 family of DNA-dependent ATPases. Although there is no phenotypic difference in disease whether it arises from mutations in CSA or mutations in CSB, approximately 80 % or CS cases have mutated CSB. Neither the site nor the specific nature of CSB mutations appears to correlate with severity of the disease, and in one patient, complete loss of the CSB gene product led to photosensitivity, but not CS, suggesting that there may be an environmental or epigenetic component to the disease. Surprisingly, unlike Werner's syndrome and other DNA repair defect diseases, Cockayne's syndrome patients do not have a significantly higher incidence of cancer unless they also suffer xeroderma pigmentosum (XP), which is linked to a strong predisposition to skin cancer.

People with Down's syndrome have trisomy or a translocation involving chromosome 21. They suffer from the early onset of vascular disease, glucose intolerance, hair loss degenerative bone and joint disease, and increased cancer. The life span is apparently 50–70 years (not as short as previously believed, since earlier mortality may have represented neglect of these individuals). Dementia occurs earlier and more often in patients with Down's syndrome than is the general population. Patients develop neuropathological changes similar to the changes seen in dementia of Alzheimer's type, including amyloid deposition and neurofibrillary tangles. This may be related to the presence of the B-amyloid gene on chromosome 21.

Although not strictly classified as progeroid syndromes, two diseases that bear mention are Fanconi's anemia (FA) and dyskeratosis congentita (DS). Fanconi's anemia is a rare autosomal recessive blood disorder, associated with multiple clinical symptoms. Classified as a developmental rather than progeroid disorder, FA is nevertheless characterized by several aspects of premature aging syndromes, including childhood onset bone marrow failure, susceptibility to squamous cell carcinomas, and congenital deformities. Furthermore, FA patients exhibit growth hormone and thyroid hormone deficiencies, glucose intolerance, and premature infertility. There are 13 FANC genes in which biallelic mutations lead to FA. Their protein products can aggregate into different core protein complexes in the muscles; one of the complexes acts as a ubiquitin ligase to modify another FANC complex, thereby facilitating its recruitment to chromatin foci in conjunction with the BRCAI, BRCA 2, and Rad51 DNA repair proteins. Not surprisingly, FA cells exhibit chromosomal instability and are highly susceptible to several forms of DNA damage, particularly inter-strand cross-links (ICL), therefore displaying acute sensitivity to cisplatin, mitomycin, and nitrogen mustard.

More significantly, cells derived iron FA patients are uniquely sensitive to ambient air and show a definitive effect of oxygen concentration on formation of chromosomal aberrations. Repeated hypoxia-reoxygenation cycles have been shown to induce premature senescence of bone marrow cells in a murine model of FA. Together, these observations suggest that the dramatic bone marrow dysfunction and chromosomal aberrations observed in FA likely stem from ROS-mediated DNA damage to hematopoietic cells. Additionally, there is evidence that multi-polymerization of FANC proteins and formation of nuclear complex 1 may be redox dependent, suggesting that the observed sensitivity to DNA damage may be compounded by an inability of mutated FANC proteins to facilitate recognition and repair of DNA damage. Thus, with its progeroid features and the mechanistic convergence of oxidative stress and DNA damage in its etiology, FA appears to be the only human model for the stochastic theories of aging.

Dyskeratosis congenital is a rare syndrome associated with severe bone marrow failure around the age of 30 years. In addition, DC patients suffer from aging-associated pathologies such as increased risk of cardiopulmonary failure and malignancy, early graying of hair, changes in skin pigmentation, brittle nails, and immune system failure which manifest itself as mucosal leukoplakia. DC is also characterized by chromosomal instability and telomere shortening at the cellular level. The X-linked version of DC results from mutations in the dyskerin gene DKC1 that appear to impair its association with TERC; the RNA component of telomerase, whereas the autosomal form arises from mutations in the TERC gene itself. Additionally, DC patients exhibit a uniform reduction in TERC itself. Thus, DC is unique in being the only human syndrome with progeroid features associated with telomere dysfunction, long considered a major causative biomarker of aging.

Consistent with the classic theories of aging, the human progeroid syndromes discussed above suggest that the critical determinants of aging are likely to be oxidative stress levels, accumulation of DNA damage/chromosomal instability, and nonfunctional or reduced DNA repair mechanisms. These three features have formed the basis of a number of animal and cellular models of aging, which are discussed below and which recapitulate the phenomenon of aging to varying degrees.

Cellular Senescence as a Model for Aging

The complexity of studying aging in organisms has led to the use of well-defined cell culture systems as models for cellular aging or senescence. Hayflick and Moorhead pioneered the model of replicative senescence and identified normal human diploid fibroblasts in culture as an experimental system for aging by observing an initial period of rapid and vigorous proliferation, invariably followed by a decline in growth rate and proliferation, invariably followed by a decline in growth rate and proliferative activity, finally leading to cessation of proliferation. This model proposed that aging is a cellular as well as an organismal phenomenon and that the loss of functional capacity of the individual reflected the summation of the loss of critical functional capacities of individual cells. It is important to note that populations of senescent cell types (although not all) are thought to be resistant to apoptosis medicated by caspase 3 and inhibited by bc1-2. In culture, they can be maintained for years in a post mitotic (nonproliferating) state with regular changes of culture medium.

Although a majority of studies on cellular senescence have been conducted on skin and fetal lung fibroblasts, limited in vitro life span has been reported for glial cells, keratinocytes, vascular smooth muscle cells, lens cells, endothelial cells, lymphocytes, and human breast epithelial cells (IIMEs). In vivo, serial transplants of normal somatic tissues, such as skin and breast, from old donor mice to young genetically identical recipients show a decline in proliferative activity and eventual failure of the graft. Similarly, skin from old donors retained an increased susceptibility to carcinogens whether transplanted to young or old recipients.

Do changes in cells in culture parallel changes in cells from aging organisms? The replicative life span of fibroblasts in culture is inversely related to the maximum life span of several diverse vertebrate species. Studies suggest that the replicative life span of cells in culture is inversely related to the age of the donor in both humans and rodents. This in-vivo/in-vitro relationship also hold for several different cell types, including skin fibroblasts, hepatocytes, keratinocytes, arterial smooth muscle cells, and T lymphocytes. However, in these cross-sectional studies, there is a great deal of variability, and the correlation coefficient, though statistically significant, is low. Cells cultured from healthy individuals do not appear to exhibit a consistent age-related proliferate capacity. Cells from people with Werner's syndrome do senesce more rapidly in culture than age-matched controls; however, a consistently similar relationship does not hold for cells from people with Hutchinson–Gilford syndrome. Thus, under some circumstances, the proliferative characteristics of cells during aging in vivo are maintained in culture. There are several studies that point to an accumulation of senescent cells in vivo with advancing age of both humans and primates.

The number of population doublings achieved before reaching a replicative limit is intrinsic to different cell types. Even more significantly, cells derived from animals that are the result of reproductive cloning via nuclear transfer show the same replicative proliferative capacity and rate of telomere shortening as the donor cells, suggesting an inherent mechanism of cellular life-span determination that occurs after nuclear transfer. The number of times the cells divide is more important in determining proliferative life span than the actual time the cells spend in culture. Cells continuously passaged in culture until the end of their proliferative life span achieve approximately the same number of population doublings (PDLs) as cells that are held in a stationary phase for an extended period (months) and then re-cultured until senescence. Therefore, under a given set of culture conditions, cells seem to possess an intrinsic mechanism that "counts" the number of divisions and not the time that passes.

However, suboptimal culture conditions or environmental stresses can adversely affect cellular replicative life span, leading to accelerated loss of proliferative capacity that is referred to as premature senescence or stress-induced premature senescence (SIPS). A number of acute exogenous stresses can lead to premature senescence, including, but not limited to, (1) oxygen radical producers, (2) extensive therapeutic radiation, (3) chemotherapeutic drugs, and (4) high oxygen tension culture. Additionally, creation of endogenous DNA damage due to failure of repair mechanisms and elevated ROS stemming from mitochondrial dysfunction or oncogene activation can also lead to rapid induction of a permanent proliferative arrest.

In morphological and biochemical respects, SIPS is almost identical to replicative senescence, leading to the idea that all exhaustion of replicative capacity may be form of stress-induced proliferative arrest. In accordance with this idea, one pervasive common denominator between replicative and SIPS appears to be induction of a DDR (and reviewed in). In fact, a persistent DDR and elevated intracellular ROS production appear to play a critical role not only in the induction of the senescent phenotype but also in its maintenance.

Products of the retinoblastoma (Rb) and p53 tumor suppressor genes have been identified as the major molecular pathways implicated in cellular senescence. The Tb gene product is not phosphorylated in senescent cells. Simian virus 40 large T antigen, which is bound by the p53 and Rb gene products, can facilitate escape from senescence. Furthermore, treatment with antioxidase oligonucleotides to the Rb and p53 tumor suppressor genes can extend the in vitro life span of human fibroblasts. The p21 CIP/WAF1 and p12 INK4a inhibitors of cyclin kinases (and therefore cell cycle progression) are overexpressed in senescent cells. The p21 protein appears to act by forming complexes with members of the family of E2F transcription factors in senescent cells (Rh/CDK2/cyclin E or with the Rb-related p107/CDK2/cyclin D), downregulating transcriptional activity, and thereby inhibiting progression through the cell cycle. Targeted disruption of the p21 gene delays the onset of senescence in fibroblasts derived from human lung. However, adrenocortical cells express high levels of p21 throughout their in vitro life span, up to and including senescence. Skin fibroblasts from patients with L1-Fraumeri syndrome are heterozygous for p53. These cells in culture lose the remaining p53 allele and in vitro aging, suggesting that p53 and p21 are not required for senescence. In senescent cells, p16 complexes to and inhibits both the CDK4 and CDK6 cell cycle kinases. Induction of expression of p16 by demethylation dependent pathways or of p21 by demethylation-independent pathways can induce senescence in immortal fibroblasts that do not express p53. Of genes whose expression is required for G1/S cell cycle progression, senescent fibroblasts express no cdk2 and cyclin A and reduced amounts of the G1 cyclins, C, D1, and E, compared to young cells. The expression of early G1 markers, but not late G1 markers, indicates that senescent cells may be blocked at a point in late G1.

The p53/p21 and the p16/Rb pathways are not induced to equivalent extents during cell senescence and do not contribute equally to the senescent phenotype the dominating pathway depends both on cell type and the nature of senescence-inducing stress. In general, the p53 pathway is activated in response to genotoxic stress, DNA damage, and telomere dysfunction, whereas the p16 arm of tumor suppression is engaged under conditions of oncogenic and other stresses. Skin fibroblasts typically enter senescence via the p53 pathway and have low levels of p16 event as they approach cellular senescence; in these cells, inhibition of the p53 pathway is sufficient to reverse the senescent phenotype. Lung fibroblasts, on the other hand, tend to show elevated levels of both tumor suppressor proteins in a senescing population as a whole, although individual cells may show one pathway is more dominant than the other. Even so, a mosaicism ahs been reported senescence programs are activated either in parallel or even jointly in individual cells.

The ras oncogene product can induce senescence that is accompanied by accumulation of p53 and p16. This occurs only in non-immortalized cells and may reflect a tumor-suppressive response of the cell to a transforming stimulus, as discussed below. However, it has been reported that the RAS onco-protein can only induce senescence in cells of DDR and senescence by increasing oxidized nucleotides and accompanying genomic DNA damage in human skin fibroblasts also leads to upregulated levels of both p53 and p16, but the senescence response can be rescued by abrogation of the p53 (but not the p16) pathway. In human mammary epithelial cells, there appear to be two different barriers to proliferation. After the initial four to live population doublings, these cells enter an early senescent-like arrest learned M0 that is medicated by p16, but a number of cells in a population are able to escape this proliferative barrier and continue to divide before reaching a p53-medicated senescence learned M1. In keratinocytes, abrogation of both p16 and p53 is needed to extend life span, but these cells still undergo senescence unless immortalized by introduction of hTERT. However, expression of hTERT alone does not immortalize these cells if one of the senescent pathways is still functional. Together, these observations emphasize the presence of complex and incompletely understood overlapping networks regulating cell cycle progression and proliferation. Depending upon the balance of positive and negative influences, cell proliferation can continue or senescence may ensue.

Although many biochemical, metabolic, and phenotypic differences have been reported between senescent cells and their early passage counterparts, several characteristics appear to be shared across a majority of cells that have entered senescence and can therefore be accurately referred to as markers of senescence. These include a lack of proliferation and response to proliferative stimuli, absence of DNA replication, a marked morphological change involving a flattened appearance, accumulation of stress fibers and vacuoles as well as nuclear abnormalities, upregulation of p53 and/or p16 proteins, and beta-galactosidase activity detected at an acidic pH. Senescent cells also exhibit auto-fluorescent globules of oxidized cellular proteins denoted as lipofuscin. Additionally, heterochromatic nuclear DNA foci called SAHSs (senescence associated heterochromatic foci) have been observed in cell types in which Rb/p16 signaling is the dominant molecular mechanism of senescence. These foci consist of a transcription-silencing variant macroH2A and various heterochromatic proteins and are believed to be formed by the action of chromatin regulator proteins, HIRA and ASF1a. They can be readily detected by their punctuate appearance during DAPI staining of cell nuclei. Formation of DNA double-strand break (DSB) foci via activation of the ATM/ATR pathway has also been reported as a senescence marker, both in senescent cells and aging mice and primates.

The senescence-associated (SA) beta-galactosidase activity, which is detected at pII 6.0, is commonly used in studies that assess induction of senescence both in cells and tissues. Despite its common usage, conflicting data exists regarding the status of SA beta-gal activity as a specific marker for senescence. For instance, in situ expression of beta-galactosidase exists in confluent quiescent pre-senescent cells and in cells undergoing crisis or terminal differentiation. The origin of SA beta-galactosidase activity appears to result from increases in lysosomal mass during the cellular aging process or under cellular stresses that can induce senescence. Fibroblasts from patients with the lysosomal disorder GM1-gangliodilosis (in which lysosomal beta-galactosidase is defective) do not show SA beta-galactosidase activity. Furthermore, beta-galactosidase activity at low pH is also observed in non-senescent cells with high lysosomal content such as vascular smooth muscle cells and endothelial cells. Thus, it would appear that SA beta-galactosidase activity is not a direct measure of senescence but a reflection of the lysosomal alterations that commonly occur as a consequence of senescence. Nevertheless, in general, for most cell types, beta-galactosidase activity is still a reliable nonspecific marker, although it is advisable to look for beta-galactosidase positively in conjunction with the other markers of senescence.

The three markers most commonly used to assess senescence in vivo are lack of proliferation (measured by K167 staining), SA beta-galactosidase activity, and levels of p16 protein. In particular, p16 protein is likely to be a good marker for in vivo aging as well because it has been reported to be strongly upregulated (sevenfold to eightfold) in aging human skin and in islet cells from aged humans, and in a number of tissues from aged rats and mice. Additionally, a DNA microarray screen of oncogenic-induced senescence in vitro identified three de novo markers of senescence which were validated in vivo, namely, p15INK4b. Dec 1, and DeR2.

Telomere length is another commonly used marker of senescence. The phenomenon of telomere shortening with aging represents a potential "clock" or counting mechanism for cellular lifespan. Telomeres are structures at the end of chromosomes that prevent degradation and fusion with other chromosomes ends. The average length of the terminal restriction fragment of chromosomes decreases with both in vitro and in vivo aging of fibroblasts and peripheral blood lymphocytes. Indeed, telomere length in lymphocytes progressively declines as a function of donor age from newborn to great-grandparents in their eighties. Immortalized and transformed cells and germ line cells express telomerase, which prevents shortening of the telomeres. However, some immortal cells exist without detectable telomerase, whereas stem cells and some normal somatic cells express telomerase, yet continue to experience telomeric shortening. Telomere length has been correlated with better health in centenarians. Interestingly, telomere length and frailty in an elderly cohort.

Shortened telomeres are associated with the progeroid pathology of dyskeratosis congenital and Werner's syndrome (see earlier discussion; reviewed by Lofer et al.) and also appear to lead to a form of premature aging in vivo mouse models. Mice lacking the RNA component of hTERT, TERC, do not show significant aging defects until the sixth generation. Transgenic mice that over express TERT exhibit increased tissue regeneration and a modest increase in maximal life span; however, these benefits are offset by the increased incidences of tumorigenesis suffered by these mice. Experimental non-enzymatic elongation of telomeres extends the life span of cell. Furthermore, reactivation of telomerase, via the introduction of the telomerase reverse transcriptase unit into normal human cells, increased telomere length and extends the life span of a number of different cell types without inducing morphological or pre-transformative abnormalities.

Furthermore, despite a clear ability to inhibit replicative senescence in a number of different cell types, telomerase cannot prevent or rescue many forms of SIPS, which are sometimes referred to as telomere-independent forms of senescence. However, it is not clear if telomeres are indeed not affected or whether telomerase is unable to heal certain types of damage to telomeres. Interestingly, while telomerase can readily immortalize adult long fibroblasts under ambient culture conditions, fetal lung fibroblasts can only be immortalized under 3 % oxygen and by addition of a number

of chemical antioxidants to the culture medium, suggesting either that the integrity of the telomerase complex or its function may be affected by oxidative stress or that oxidative damage to telomeres may alter telomeric structure in a way that inhibits recognition/healing by telomerase.

Telomeric shortening has been attributed to inefficient repair of DNA single-strand breaks, which are hallmark lesions of oxidative damage. Improvement of mitochondrial function, the major determinant of cellular ROS production, also slows down telomere shortening. Although irrefutable in vivo proof for a causal role for oxidative stress in generating senescence-inducing telomere dysfunction is still lacking, telomeres appear to be excellent candidates for the missing link between DNA damage and oxidative stress that will allow us to achieve a complete understanding of the mechanism behind the internal "clock" that governs cellular life span.

Using the markers of senescence discussed above, senescent cells have been detected in tissues from aged rodents, primates, and humans. Nevertheless, the question remains whether the in vivo presence of senescent cells in renewable tissue is coupled to any loss of organismal function. Presumably, such cells do not need to divide in vivo to the point of replicative exhaustion because they can be replenished by tissue progenitor cell populations. Thus, the role of cellular senescence in organismal aging, over and beyond its role as a tumor suppressor mechanism, may have greater functional relevance in stem cell population than in more differentiated cells. The self-renewal and differentiation of stem cells is critical for the maintenance of tissue function, repair, and homeostasis. Hematopoietic stem cells (HSC) from older mice, which have deficiencies in self-renewal, repopulating and homing mechanisms, accumulate high levels of p16 that impair their ability to undergo serial transplantation; HDCs displayed improved function and stress resistance in the absence of p16. There is also evidence to suggest that self-renewal ability of the lympho-hematopoietic stem cell system correlates with life span as a whole in mice (and reviewed by Geiger and Van Zant). Increasing p16 levels are also linked to decreased regenerative potential in pancreatic islet cells and reduced proliferation of progenitor populations in the mouse forebrain.

Nutrition and Metabolism, A Modern-Day Elixir of Life?

Nearly every culture and civilization has its own mythic search for the elixir of life, from the desperate pursuit of immortality by Gilgamesh in ancient Babylon and by the Chinese emperor Qin Shi Huang before 200 BC to the European alchemists' attempts at creating the longevity-conferring philosopher's stone and the Spanish conquistador Ponce de Leon's quest for the fountain of youth. With an improved understanding of the molecular and biochemical pathways behind the aging process and the advent of nutraceuticals, there has been resurgence in the interest to generate scientifically validated interventions that can extend life span while minimizing the systemic disadvantages of aging.

Mouse models of life-span extension can be broadly categorized as either embodying alterations in metabolic/nutrient responsive-pathways or in mitochondrial/oxygen responsive pathways. Most of these transgenic animal models exhibit a 15–30 % life-span extension, with varied improvements in functional aging, such as low damage levels, increased tissue function and stress resistance at later stages of life, and reduced incidences of cancer. However, few of these models have more than a modest impact on MLSP, and almost none show the broad gamut of improved physiologic function that would translate to significant improvement in human quality-of-life aging issues. A valid criticism leveled at murine models of aging is that most of these organisms are studied under laboratory controlled conditions that are unlikely to mimic the environmental vagaries that affect true aging. Therefore, while these model systems offer mechanistic insights into the processes that may impact aging, the actual effects of these proceeded need to be assessed in human beings in a systematic and noninvasive manner.

The confluence of oxygen metabolism and nutritional signaling on life span observed in animal models ranging from *C. elegans* to rodents suggests that dietary modifications are the most likely candidate for yielding maximal dividends when it comes to extending longevity and maintaining good health later in life. The ability to modulate diet is relatively simple, and accordingly, calorie restriction (CR) studies are at the forefront of life-span extension strategies. Calorie restriction in rhesus monkeys leads to reductions in body temperature and energy expenditure, consistent with changes seen in rodent studies in which aging is retarded by dietary restriction. Calorie restriction also increases high-density lipoprotein and retards the post maturational decline in serum dehydro-epiandrostenedione sulfate in the rhesus monkeys. Levels of the aging biomarker, p16NK4a, are reduced in tissue from aging rodents that fed a calorically restricted diet.

The Comprehensive Assessment of the Long-Term Effects of Reducing Intake of Energy (CALERIE) study is a randomized clinical trial to assess whether CR improves aging biomarkers in humans. After an initial 6-month of CR in 48 healthy men and women in their 40s and 50s, the study found an improvement in two biomarkers of longevity, namely reduction in fasting insulin levels and body temperature in groups that underwent dietary restriction. Other CALERIE studies have found that CR improves liver and cardiovascular health and increases muscle mitochondrial biogenesis and decreases oxygen consumption.

Population-based characterizations of aging have also identified diet and nutrition as likely major contributors to longevity. Long-lived human populations tend to share a few features in common, among them diets enriched in low-fat proteins such as fish and in fruits or beverages high in polyphenols and low in sugar and processed carbohydrates, often referred to as the Mediterranean Diet. Consumption of red wine is also believed to be conductive to a healthy life span. In Sardinia and the south-western regions of France, longevity of the local population has been correlated with the high vasoactive polyphenol contents of the locally produced red wine.

Polyphenols such as quercetin, epigallocatechin gallate (EGCG), and resveratrol (3, 5, 4′-trihydroxystilbene) are naturally occurring protective compounds found in dark-green vegetables, fruits, green tea, dark chocolate, and red wine currently being included in a number of studies of aging and aging related pathologies such as cancer and diabetes. Indeed, resveratrol is notable for its ability to activate physiologically sensitive nutrients and to increase maximum life span in lower organisms, such as yeast, worms, and flies. Resveratrol treatment improves the exercise capacity, insulin sensitivity, mitochondrial biogenesis, and survival of mice on a high fat, high calorie diet. Resveratrol can prevent diet-induced obesity concurrently with improved mitochondrial production, insulin sensitivity, and exercise endurance by activating SIRT1 and PGCa. Resveratrol treatment of mice can also delay age-related changes in physical performance, bone mineral density, inflammation, and the vasculature and concomitantly induces transcriptional profiles in as variety of tissues similar to those seen with dietary restriction. Consequently, there has been much interest in resveratrol as a supplement to enhance health and increase life-span in humans. However, resveratrol does not appear to extend the maximum life span of mice, but can increase the mean life span of mice with cardiovascular disease.

Although nutritional interventions may be able to significantly impact aging, it is likely that the genetic background of the individual will determine just how effective any particular modification is likely to be. Both calorically restricted and long-lived mice share common longevity assurance mechanisms when compared to progeroid mice, although the efficacy of such mechanisms varies widely in the two sets of mice.

References

1. Cutler RG. Evolutionary perspective of human longevity. In: Hazzard WR, Andres R, Bierman EL, et al., editors. Principles of geriatric medicine and gerontology. 2nd ed. New York: McGraw-Hill; 1985. p. 16.
2. Kung HC, Hoyert DL, Xu JQ, Murphy SL. Deaths: final data for 2005, vol. 56. Hyattsville: National Center for Health Statistics; 2008.
3. Perls TT, Alpert L, Fretts RC. Middle-aged mothers live longer. Nature. 1997;389(6647):133.
4. Yeap BB. Are declining testosterone levels a major risk factor for ill-health in aging men? Int J Import Res. 2008;21(1):24–36.
5. Sohal RS, Weindruch R. Oxidative stress, calorie restriction, and aging. Science 1996;273(5271):59–63.

6. Yu BP, Masoro EJ, McMahan CA. Nutritional influence on aging of Fischer 344 rats: I. Physical, metabolic and longevity characteristics. J Gerontol. 1985;40(6):657–70.
7. McCarter R, Masoro FJ, Yu IP. Does food restriction retard aging by reducing the metabolic rate? Am J Physiol. 1985;248(4 Pt 1):E488–90.
8. Lefevere M, Redman LM, Heibronn LK, et al. Calorie restriction alone with exercise improves CVD risk in healthy nonobese individuals. Atheroscirosis 2009;203(1):206–16.
9. Shock NW, Greation RC, Andres R, et al. editors. Normal human aging: the Baltimore longitudinal study of aging. Washington: U.S. Department of Health and Human Services; 1981.
10. Lefevre M, Redman LM, Heilbronn LK, et al. Caloric restriction and with exercise improves CVD risk in healthy non-obese individuals. Atherosclerosis. 2009;203(1):206–13.
11. Gompertz B. On the nature of the function expressive of the law of human mortality and on a new mode of determining life contingencies. Philos Trans R Soc Lond. 1825;115:513.
12. Shock NW, Greulich RC, Andres R, et al., editors. Normal human aging: the Baltimore longitudinal study of aging. Washington: U.S. Department of Health and Human Services; 1984.
13. Riggs BL, Melton III LJ. Involutional osteoporosis. N Engl J Med. 1986;314(26):1676–86.
14. Florini JR, editor. Composition and function of cells and tissues. In: Handbook of biochemistry in aging. Boca Raton: CRC Press; 1981.
15. Kirkwood TB. Human senescence. Bioessays. 1996;18(12):1009–16.
16. Kaeberlin M, Mcvey M, Guarente L. Using yeast to discover the fountain of youth. Sci Aging Knowl Environ. 2001.
17. Dudas SP, Arking R. A coordinate upregulation of antioxidant gene activities is associated with the delayed onset of senescence in a long-lived strain of Drosophilia. J Gerontol A Biol Sci Med Sci. 1995;50(3):B117–27.
18. Strehler BL. Time, cells, and aging. 2nd ed. New York: Academic; 1977.
19. Bjorksten J. Cross linkage and the aging process. In: Rothstein M, editor. Theoretical aspects of aging. New York: Academic; 1974. p. 43.
20. Kohn RR. Aging of animals: possible mechanisms. In: Principles of mammalian aging. 2nd ed. Englewood Cliffs: Prentice-Hall; 1978.
21. Herbig U, Ferreira M, Condel L, Carey D, Sedivy JM. Cellular senescence in aging primates. Science. 2006;311(5765):1257.
22. Jeyapalan JC, Ferreira M, Sedivy JM, Herbig U. Accumulation of senescent cells in mitotic tissue of aging primates. Mech Ageing Dev. 2007;128(1):36–44.
23. Sedelnikova OA, Horikawa I, Zimonjic DB, Popescu NC, Bonner WM, Barrett JC. Senescing human cells and ageing mice accumulate DNA lesions with unrepairable double-strand breaks. Nat Cell Biol. 2004;6(2):168–70.
24. Migliaccio E, Giorgio M, Mele S, et al. The p66shc adaptor protein controls oxidative stress response and life span in mammals. Nature. 1999;402(6759):309–13.
25. De Benedictis G, Rose G, Carrieri G, et al. Mitochondrial DNA inherited variants are associated with successful aging and longevity in humans. FASEB J. 1999;13(12):1532–6.
26. Ozawa T, Tanaka M, Ikebe S, Ohno K, Kondo T, Mizuno Y. Quantitative determination of deleted mitochondrial DNA relative to normal DNA in parkinsonian striatum by a kinetic PCR analysis. Biochem Biophys Res Commun. 1990;172(2):483–9.
27. Poulton J, Deadman ME, Ramacharan S, Gardiner RM. Germ-line deletions of mtDNA in mitochondria] myopathy. Am J Hum Genet. 1991;48(4):649–53.
28. Katsumata K, Hayakawa M, Tanaka M, Sugiyama S, Ozawa T. Fragmentation of human heart mitochondrial DNA associated with premature aging. Biochem Biophys Res Commun. 1994;202(1):102–10.
29. Ozawa T. Mitochondrial cardiomyopathy. Herz 1994;19(2):105–118, 125.
30. Trifunovic A, Wredenberg A, Falkenberg M, et al. Premature ageing in mice expressing defective mitochondrial DNA polymerase. Nature. 2004;429(6990):417–23.
31. Hart RW, Setlow RB. Correlation between deoxyribonucleic acid excision-repair and life-span in a number of mammalian species. Proc Natl Acad Sci U S A. 1974;71(6):2169–73.
32. Intano GW, Cho EJ, McMahan CA, Walter CA. Age-related -base excision repair activity in mouse brain and liver nuclear extracts. J Gerontol A Biol Sci Med Sci. 2003;58(3):B205–11.
33. Hanawalt PC, Gee P, Ho L. DNA repair in differentiating cells in relation to aging. In: Finch CE, Johnson TE, editors. Molecular biology of aging. UCLA symposia on molecular and cellular biology, vol. 123. New York: Alan R. Liss; 1990. p. 45.
34. Lu T, Pan Y, Kao S-Y, et al. Gene regulation and DNA damage in the ageing human brain. Nature. 2004;429(6994):883–91.
35. Orgel LE. The maintenance of the accuracy of protein synthesis and its relevance to aging. Proc Natl Acad Sci U S A. 1963;49:517.
36. Kristal BS, Yu BP. An emerging hypothesis: synergistic induction of aging by free radicals and Maillard reactions. J Gerontol. 1992;47(4):B107–14.
37. Brown WT. Genetic diseases of premature aging as models of senescence. Annu Rev Gerontol Geriatr. 1990;10:23–42.
38. Stevnsner T, Muftuoglu M, Aamann MD, Bohr VA. The role of Cockayne Syndrome group B (CSB) protein in base excision repair and aging. Mech Ageing Dev. 2008;129(7–8):441–8.
39. Cristofalo VJ, Allen RG, Pignolo RJ, Martin BG, Beck JC. Relationship between donor age and the replicative lifespan of human cells in culture: a reevaluation. Proc Natl Acad Sci U S A. 1998;95(18):10614–9.
40. Ressler S, Bartkova J, Niederegger H, et al. p16INK4A is a robust in vivo biomarker of cellular aging in human skin. Aging Cell. 2006;5(5):379–89.
41. Ozer HL, Banga SS, Dasgupta T, et al. SV40-mediated immortalization of human fibroblasts. Exp Gerontol. 1996;31(1–2):303–10.
42. Alcorta DA, Xiong Y, Phelps D, Hannon G, Beach D, Barrett JC. Involvement of the cyclin-dependent kinase inhibitor p16 (INK4a) in replicative senescence of normal human fibroblasts. Proc Natl Acad Sci U S A. 1996;93(24):13742–7.
43. Reznikoff CA, Yeager TR, Belair CD, Savelieva E, Puthenveettil JA, Stadler WM. Elevated p16 at senescence and loss of p16 at immortalization in human papillomavirus 16 E6, but not E7, transformed human uroepithelial cells. Cancer Res. 1996;56(13):2886–90.
44. Dechat T, Shimi T, Adam SA, et al. Alterations in mitosis and cell cycle progression caused by a mutant lamin A known to accelerate human aging. Proc Natl Acad Sci U S A. 2007;104(12):4955–60.
45. Liu B, Wang J, Chan KM, et al. Genomic instability in laminopathy-based premature aging. Nat Med. 2005;11(7):780–5.
46. Melov S, Hinerfeld D, Esposito L, Wallace DC. Multi-organ characterization of mitochondrial genomic rearrangements in ad libitum and caloric restricted mice show striking somatic mitochondrial DNA rearrangements with age. Nucleic Acids Res. 1997;25(5):974–82.
47. Larsen PL, Clarke CF. Extension of life-span in Caenorhabditis elegans by a diet lacking coenzyme Q. Science. 2002;295(5552):120–3.
48. Civitarese AE, Carling S, Heilbronn LK, et al. Calorie restriction increases muscle mitochondrial biogenesis in healthy humans. PLoS Med. 2007;4(3):e76.
49. Walburg HE. Radiation-induced life-shortening and premature aging. Adv Radiat Biol. 1975;5:145.
50. Capri M, Salvioli S, Sevini F, et al. The genetics of human longevity. Ann NY Acad Sci. 2006;1067:252–63.
51. Serrano M, Lin AW, McCurrach ME, Beach D, Lowe SW. Oncogenic ras provokes premature cell senescence associated with accumulation of p53 and p16INK4a. Cell. 1997;88(5):593–602.
52. Severino J, Allen RG, Balin S, Balin A, Cristofalo VJ. Is beta-galactosidase staining a marker of senescence in vitro and in vivo? Exp Cell Res. 2000;257(1):162–71.

53. Litaker JR, Pan J, Cheung Y, et al. Expression profile of senescence-associated beta-galactosidase and activation of telomerase in human ovarian surface epithelial cells undergoing immortalization. Int J Oncol. 1998;13(5):951–6.

54. Untergasser G, Gander R, Rumpold H, Heinrich E, Plas E, Berger P. TGF-beta cytokines increase senescence-associated betagalactosidase activity in human prostate basal cells by supporting differentiation processes, but not cellular senescence. Exp Gerontol. 2003;38(10):1179–88.

55. Harley CB. Telomere loss: mitotic clock or genetic timebomb? Mutat Res. 1991;256(2–6):271–82.

56. Bryan TM, Englezou A, Gupta J, Bacchetti S, Reddel RR. Telomere elongation in immortal human cells without detectable telomerase activity. EMBO J. 1995;14(17):4240–8.

57. Broccoli D, Young JW, de Lange T. Telomerase activity in normal and malignant hematopoietic cells. Proc Natl Acad Sci U S A. 1995;92(20):9082–6.

58. Woo J, Tang NL, Suen E, Leung JC, Leung PC. Telomeres and frailty. Mech Ageing Dev. 2008;129(11):642–8.

59. Rudolph KL, Chang S, Lee HW, et al. Longevity, stress response, and cancer in aging telomerase-deficient mice. Cell. 1999;96(5):701–12.

60. Lunetta KL, D'Agostiono Sr RB, Karasik D, et al. Genetic correlates of longevity and selected age –related phenotypes: a genome-wide association study in the Framingham Study. BMC Med Genet. 2007;8 Suppl 1:S13.

61. Di Bona D, Vasto S, Capurso C, et al. Effect of interleukin-6 polymorphisms on human longevity: a systematic review and metanalysis. Ageing Res Rev. 2009;8(1):36–42.

62. Hindorff LA, Rice KM, Lange LA, et al. Common variants in the CPR gene in relation to longevity and cause-specific mortality in older adults: the Cardiovascular Health Study. Atherosclerosis. 2008;197(2):922–30.

63. Partidge L, Gems D, Withers DJ. Sex and death: what is the connection? Cell. 2005;120(4):461–72.

64. Maisonneuve E, Ezraty B, Dukan S. Protein aggregates: an aging factor involved in cell death. J Bacteriol. 2008;190(18):6070–5.

65. Sedelnikova OA, Horikawa I, Redon C, et al. Delayed kinetics of DNA double-strand break processing in normal and pathological aging. Aging Cell. 2008;7(1):89–100.

66. d'Adda di Fagagna F, Reaper PM, Clay-Farrace L, et al. A DNA damage checkpoint response in telomere-initiated senescence. Nature 2003;426(6963):194–8.

67. Muller M. Cellular senescence: molecular mechanisms, in vivo significance, and redbox considerations. Antioxid Redbox Signal. 2009;11(1):59–98.

68. Partidge L, Gems D. Benchmarks for ageing studies. Nature. 2007;450(7167):165–7.

69. Pearson KJ, Baur JA, Lewis KN, et al. Resveratrol delays age-related deterioration and mimics transcriptional aspects of dietary restriction without extending life span. Cell Metab. 2008;8(2):157–68.

70. Wright WE, Brasiskyte D, Piatyszek MA, Shay JW. Experimental elongation of telomeres extends the lifespan of immortal x normal cell hybrids. EMBO J. 1996;15(7):1734–41.

71. Petersen S, Saretzki G, Zglinicki Tv. Preferential accumulation of single-stranded regions in telomeres of human fibroblasts. Exp Cell Res 1998;239:152–60.

Principles of Geriatric Surgery

4

Mark R. Katlic and JoAnn Coleman

Introduction

With a few obvious exceptions, those of us who are surgeons must become geriatric surgeons. The population as a whole is aging, with the most explosive growth in the over 85-year group, and the conditions that require surgery (atherosclerosis, cancer, arthritis, prostatism, cataract, pelvic floor disorders, and others) increase in incidence with increasing age. Improving our care of the elderly surgical patient will become progressively more important to all of us.

Admittedly, surgeons have always cared for the elderly, but the definition of "elderly" has changed. A threshold of 50 years was chosen for the 167 patients described in a paper in 1907 [1], and 20 years later influential surgeons still wrote that elective herniorrhaphy in this age group was not warranted [2]. Now, though, we are performing complex operations in octogenarians, nonagenarians, and occasionally centenarians [3–7]. In addition, the salutary results of such surgery can even influence general sentiment about medical care of the elderly. Linn and Zeppa's study [8] of junior medical students reported that the surgery rotation, in contrast to other clerkships, positively influenced the students' attitudes about aging regardless of the students' career choices, as the elderly surgical patients were admitted and treated successfully.

Surgery therefore has much to offer the geriatric patient, but that patient must be treated with appropriate knowledge and attention to detail. Discussions of pelvic physiologic changes in the elderly and results of specific operations comprise the bulk of this book and are not presented here. The authors' three decade study in this area, in addition to caring for an elderly oncology population, has led to a distillate of several general principles (Table 4.1) which are relevant to all who care for the aged. These principles are worthwhile chiefly for teaching purposes, as they cannot apply to every patient or every clinical situation. Some principles also apply to surgery in the young patient, but the quantitative differences in the elderly are significant enough to approach qualitative status. Risks of many emergency operations in the young, for example, are indeed greater than the risks of similar elective operations, but the differences are small compared to the threefold increase in the elderly. With respect to these principles the elderly need not be treated as a separate species but perhaps as a separate genus or order within the same larger group of surgical candidates.

Although our results have generally improved over the years (Fig. 4.1) [9, 10], This improvement has not been universal (Fig. 4.2) [11] and emergency surgery is still risky. Understanding these six general principles may help us improve our care of the elderly patient who requires pelvic surgery.

Principle I: Clinical Presentation

The clinical presentation of surgical problems in the elderly may be subtle or somewhat different from that in the general population. This may lead to delay in diagnosis.

Classic symptoms of appendicitis are present in a minority of elderly patients, as few as 26 % in Horattas' series over 20 years (Table 4.2) [12]. Rebound tenderness was present in fewer than half the patients in another [13] and leukocytosis in only 42.9 % in another [14]. Clouding the picture further, objective tests may suggest alternative diagnoses: one in six patients has an elevated bilirubin and one in four has signs of ileus, bowel obstruction, gallstones, or renal calculus on abdominal radiographs [15]. Even astute diagnosis may not prevent perforation, present in 42–60 % of elderly patients despite operation within 24 h of symptom onset [12, 14].

M.R. Katlic (✉) • J. Coleman
Sinai Center for Geriatric Surgery, Department of Surgery,
Sinai Hospital, 2401 West Belvedere Avenue,
Baltimore, MD 21215, USA
e-mail: mkatlic@lifebridgehealth.org

© Springer Science+Business Media New York 2017
D.A. Gordon, M.R. Katlic (eds.), *Pelvic Floor Dysfunction and Pelvic Surgery in the Elderly*,
DOI 10.1007/978-1-4939-6554-0_4

Biliary tract disease is the most common entity requiring abdominal surgery in the elderly, yet the diagnosis is often delayed. More than one-third of patients with acute chole-cystitis are afebrile, one-fourth are non-tender, and one-third are without leukocytosis [16–19]. Cholangitis may appear only as fever of unknown origin or as confusion [20]. Consequently, the elderly predominate in series of patients with complications of biliary disease (gallbladder perfora-tion, empyema, gangrene, gallstone ileus, cholangitis) [21], and the complication may result in the first apparent symp-tom [18, 22]. Saunders [23] reported that abdominal pain was a less prominent symptom and that the bilirubin level was nearly double in elderly patients presenting with bile duct carcinoma, compared to the findings in young patients seen during the same time period.

Peptic ulcer disease may present as confusion, malaise, anemia, or weight loss as opposed to pain [24]; even with

Table 4.1 Principles of geriatric surgery

I. The *clinical presentation* of surgical problems in the elderly may be subtle or somewhat different from that in the general population. This may lead to delay in diagnosis
II. The elderly handle stress satisfactorily but handle severe stress poorly because of *lack of organ system reserve*
III. Optimal *preoperative preparation* is essential, because of Principle II. When preparation is suboptimal the perioperative risk increases
IV. The results of elective surgery in the elderly are excellent in some centers; the results of emergency surgery are poor though still better than nonoperative treatment for most conditions. The risk of *emergency surgery* may be many times that of similar elective surgery because of Principles II and III
V. Scrupulous *attention to detail* intraoperatively and perioperatively yields great benefit, as the elderly tolerate complications poorly (because of Principle II)
VI. A patient's age should be treated as a *scientific fact, not with prejudice*. No particular chronologic age, of itself, is a contraindication to operation (because of Principle IV)

perforation, pain may be absent or minimal. Rabinovici [25] found a discrepancy between "severe intraoperative find-ings" and preoperative objective findings such as heart rate (mean 88/min), temperature (37.2 °C), and white blood cell count (10,900/dl). Some have suggested that the elderly and possibly their physicians become tolerant over the years to abdominal pain, loss of energy, and other symptoms, result-ing in a delay in diagnosis or an emergency presentation [26]. In Mulcahy's [27] series of patients with colorectal car-cinoma, for example, elderly patients were nearly twice as likely (18 %) as younger patients (11 %) to present emer-gently. Elderly patients with perforated diverticulitis are three times more likely to have generalized peritonitis at operation than young patients [28].

Gastroesophageal reflux disease in the elderly is less likely to cause heartburn and more likely to cause regurgitation or cough ($p=001$) [29]. In Pilotto's study of 840 consecutive patients [30], typical heartburn/acid reflux, pain, and indiges-tion were more likely in the young ($p<0.001$); older patients more often experienced dysphagia, anorexia, anemia, or vom-iting ($p<0.001$ each) or weight loss ($p<0.007$).

Head and neck disease may also present differently in the elderly. Sinusitis may lead to subtle signs such as delirium or fever of unknown origin [31, 32]; and head and neck cancers are less likely to be associated with smoking ($p<0.01$) [33] and alcohol use ($p<0.001$) [33, 34]. Hyperparathyroidism is more likely to cause dementia or skeletal complaints and less likely to cause renal stones [35]. In Thomas and Grigg's series [36] of patients with carotid artery disease, stroke was the most common indication for surgery in octogenarians and was the least common indication in younger patients. Unstable angina is as likely to present with dyspnea, nausea, or diaphoresis as it is with classic chest pain [37].

Even the eureka moments that keep us energized as diagnosticians [38] may be "subtler and less electric" [39] in the elderly.

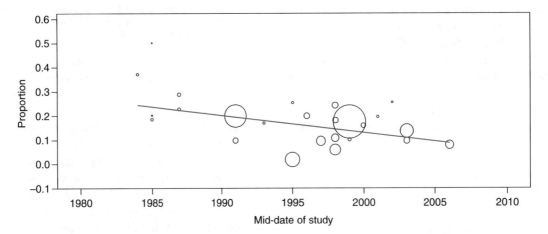

Fig. 4.1 Operative mortality for mitral valve surgery in octogenarians has improved over time. Scatter plot depicting odds ratios of operative mortality from mid-date of studies. From Biancari [10], with permission © Elsevier

Fig. 4.2 Operative mortality in the Medicare population has declined for some, but not all, procedures. Adjusted odds ratio and 95 % confidence intervals* describing the 6-year average effect (1994–1999) on operative mortality[†] in the national Medicare population. *Adjusted for age, gender, race, co-morbidities, admission acuity, income and hospital volume. Odds ratios[†] represent the average relative change in mortality over the study period, from 1994 to 1999. From Goodney [11] with permission © American College of Surgeons

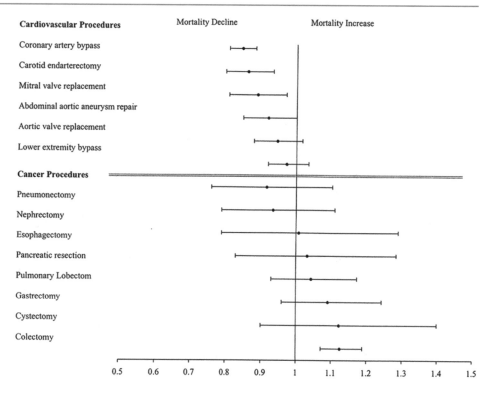

Table 4.2 Classic symptoms of appendicitis are present in a minority of elderly patients, resulting in perforation despite expeditious operation

Characteristic	1978–1988 (n = 96)	1988–1998 (n = 113)	1978–1998 (n = 209)
Classic presentation	(19) 20 %	(36) 30 %	(55) 26 %
Delayed presentation (>48 h)	(32) 33 %	(36) 30 %	(68) 33 %
Imaging			
AAS	(81) 84 %	(86) 76 %	(167) 80 %
Sensitivity	(22) 27 %	(22) 25 %	(44) 26 %
CT		(50) 44 %	
Sensitivity		(49) 90 %	
Correct admitting diagnosis	(49) 51 %	(52) 46 %	(101) 48 %
Surgery within 24 h	(80) 83 %	(97) 85 %	(177) 85 %
Perforation	(60) 72 %	(58) 51 %	(127) 61 %
Complications	(30) 32 %	(24) 21 %	(54) 26 %
Those with perforation	(25) 83 %	(15) 72 %	(40) 76 %
Deaths	(4) 4 %	(4) 4 %	(8) 4 %

Adopted from Storm-Dickerson [12]

The clinician who understands that classic presentations of surgical disease occur in a minority of elderly patients will maintain the high index of suspicion needed to minimize delay in diagnosis.

Principle II: Lack of Reserve

The elderly handle stress satisfactorily but handle severe stress poorly because of lack of organ system reserve.

Functional reserve may be considered the difference between basal and maximal function; it represents the capacity to meet increased demands imposed by disease or trauma. Although there is variability among individuals, this organ system reserve inexorably declines in one's seventies, eighties, and nineties. With excellent anesthetic and perioperative care the aged patient may tolerate the stress of even complex surgery—particularly if elective—but not the added stress of exceptional or emergency surgery.

The elderly patient with lung cancer, for example, can undergo routine pulmonary lobectomy with results nearly indistinguishable from those of the general population [40, 41], but the added stress of concomitant chest wall resection leads to a disparate increase in risk. In Keagy's series [42] the one death and two of the three respiratory failures were in patients who underwent the *en bloc* chest wall resection. An elderly patient, entering the operating room with decreased chest wall compliance and strength and decreased elastic recoil as a baseline, may tolerate lung resection but lacks the reserve to tolerate an extended operation. Other researchers have reported increased mortality in septuagenarians and octogenarians following pneumonectomy, especially right pneumonectomy or completion pneumonectomy [43–45].

On the other side of the spectrum, more limited procedures, such as video-assisted thoracic surgery, may decrease stress further by preserving respiratory muscle strength [46–49]. Yim [49] reported no deaths or pulmonary complications following thoracoscopic surgery in 22 patients over age 75 years, five with major resections; and Jaklitsch [47] found decreased mortality, length of hospital stay, and postoperative delirium after 307 video-assisted procedures in patients aged 65–90 compared to that associated with open thoracotomy. Video-assisted pulmonary lobectomy in half of a group of elderly lung cancer patients resulted in fewer complications ($p=04$) and decreased length of stay ($p<0.001$) compared to the half who underwent open (thoracotomy) lobectomy [50]. Patel [51] reported shorter hospitalization and similar late outcomes following endovascular thoracic aortic procedures in patients greater than 75 years, compared to open procedures. Endovascular repair of abdominal aortic aneuryms in the elderly had decreased all-cause and aneurysm related mortality compared to open repair [52]. Partial as compared to radical nephrectomy resulted in improved survival in elderly patients who were candidates for either procedure [53].

Left ventricular functional reserve assumes critical importance in elderly patients undergoing cardiac surgery. In general, results in the elderly diverge from those of young age groups only in the worst functional classes. Bergus et al. [54], for example, found that length of stay following aortic valve replacement was significantly longer ($p<0.05$) in septuagenarians in New York Heart Association class IV but not in class III, compared to patients under age 70. Patients over age 75 in Salomon's large series [55] had significantly higher mortality after coronary artery bypass grafting if they had suffered a myocardial infarction less than 3 weeks

preoperatively compared to more than 3 weeks (14.1 % vs. 5.2 %); there was much less difference in patients younger than age 75 (3.5 % vs. 2.3 %). When patients over age 70 years undergo a third coronary reoperation, only those in the worse Canadian Functional Class experience increased mortality, an increase not seen in young patients in a similar class [56]. Elayda [57] reported that mortality for isolated aortic valve replacement in patients over age 80 was acceptable (5.2 %), but addition of concomitant procedures increased this figure significantly (27.7 %). In cardiac surgery, too, a lesser procedure may be just as good in the elderly: contrary to a younger population, limited coronary revascularization appears to be acceptable in the high-risk elderly [58, 59].

Similar findings pertain to major abdominal surgery. Fortner and Lincer [60] found that the increased number of deaths among elderly patients undergoing hepatic resection for liver cancer were nearly all in the extended-resection group (i.e., extended right hepatectomy or trisegmentectomy), among whom 60 % of deaths were due to hepatic insufficiency. In another group of hepatic resections done for metastatic colon cancer, where cirrhosis and functional hepatic reserve are less important factors, there was no difference in mortality between young and old patients [61]. Even the addition of common duct exploration to open cholecystectomy significantly increased mortality in the elderly (3.5 % vs. 1.8 %, $p<0.05$) [62]. For some oncology cases (e.g., gastric cancer, lung cancer) a more limited operation in the elderly need not decrease survival [63–66].

The elderly can return to normal function after stressful operations (such as colectomy and hepatectomy) but after the most stressful operations (such as Whipple pancreaticoduodenectomy) it will take longer (Fig. 4.3) [67, 68].

With modern anesthetic and critical care management an elderly patient can tolerate the stress of even complex operations. However, if the most extended procedures are contemplated, a comprehensive preoperative evaluation of functional reserve is recommended.

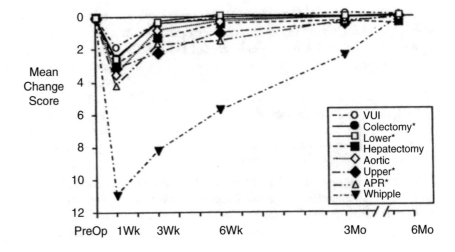

Fig. 4.3 Return to Activities of Daily Living after major surgery (function returns rapidly after stressful operations but not the most stressful, speaking to lack of reserve). From Lawrence [68] with permission © American College of Surgeons

Principle III: Preoperative Preparation

Optimal preoperative preparation is essential because of Principle II. When preparation is suboptimal the perioperative risk increases.

A patient's advanced age is immutable but some factors can be improved preoperatively, with benefits in excess of those to a younger patient. No universal threshold of blood hemoglobin applies to every patient, but correction of anemia and dehydration do assume greater importance in the elderly because of their general lack of reserve and particularly the physiology of the aged heart and kidney. Among the predictors of an overall good postoperative course in Seymour's series of 288 elderly general surgery patients were a hemoglobin level of more than 11.0 g/dl and absence of volume depletion [69]. Contrary to this, Dzankic found that routine blood testing in the elderly surgical patient rarely showed abnormal results and even when abnormal did not correlate with adverse postoperative outcome [70].

Few would argue that pulmonary problems are among the most common perioperative complications in the elderly, in part due to decreased respiratory muscle strength. Nomori [48] showed that following thoracotomy patients older than 70 years experience significant reductions in both maximum inspiratory and expiratory pressures, unlike their younger counterparts; this effect persists for 12 weeks (Fig. 4.4). Although few data exist to support the routine use of preoperative pulmonary conditioning or rehabilitation, most authors strongly advocate smoking cessation [71] and treatment of bronchitis and reactive airways disease such as asthma [72, 73]. Prophylaxis against deep vein thrombosis (DVT), clearly a risk in the elderly [74], and against pulmonary embolism should be routine [75].

The value of preoperative optimization of cardiac function (e.g., via placement of a pulmonary artery catheter) is controversial. Some authors have shown clear benefit [76], whereas others [77, 78], citing methodologic flaws in the former studies, reported no reduction in perioperative morbidity or mortality. These studies do not include exceptionally high risk or very elderly patients, who could well be helped by such treatment. Another unsettled issue concerns the value of aggressive preoperative screening for coronary and carotid artery disease, particularly in patients scheduled for peripheral vascular surgery. Leppo [79] considered age over 70 years one of several risk factors (the others being a history of angina, congestive heart failure, diabetes mellitus, prior myocardial infarction, and ventricular ectopy), which should trigger further cardiac assessment. Echocardiogram and dobutamine stress testing have been shown to bear incremental value over clinical evaluation [80].

There is some evidence that performance testing may hold value. Maximal oxygen consumption (VO2 Max) tests [81] may not be readily available in all hospitals, but reasonable surrogates—stair climbing [82–84], shuttle walk [85], long distance corridor walk [86], gait speed [87, 88], metabolic equivalent (MET)—have been shown to correlate. Weinstein [89] reported prolonged length of stay following thoracic cancer surgery in those patients with METs ≤4 (equating to calisthenics or walking briskly). The International Society of Geriatric Oncology has studied a standardized Preoperative Assessment in Elderly Cancer Patient (PACE); postoperative complications were associated with poor preoperative performance status and lower score on Instrumental Activities of Daily Living but major complications correlated only with American Society of Anesthesiologists (ASA) Physical Status ≤2 (Table 4.3) [90]. However, as Internullo recently concluded, "a practical and reliable individual risk assessment tool is still lacking." [91] We have termed this simple, reliable test to assess perioperative risk the Holy Grail of Geriatric Surgery [92].

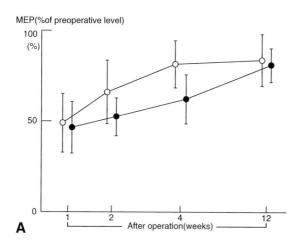
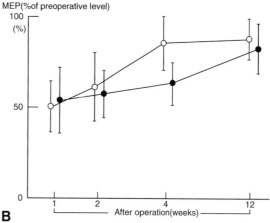
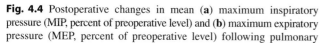

A   **B**

Fig. 4.4 Postoperative changes in mean (**a**) maximum inspiratory pressure (MIP, percent of preoperative level) and (**b**) maximum expiratory pressure (MEP, percent of preoperative level) following pulmonary resection in 36 patients younger than 69 years (*open circles*) and 12 patients older than 70 years (*closed circles*). From Nomori [48] with permission © Oxford Journals

Table 4.3 Components of preoperative assessment of cancer in the elderly (PACE)

Component of PACE	Any complication		Major complications	
	RR[a]	95 % CI	RR[a]	95 % CI
MMS Abnormal (<24)	1.23	0.81–1.88	1.08	0.48–2.44
ADL dependent (>0)	1.41	0.95–2.10	1.87	0.95–3.69
IADL dependent (<8)	*1.43*	1.03–1.98	1.65	0.88–3.08
GDS depressed (>4)	1.30	0.93–1.81	1.69	0.93–3.08
BFI moderate/severe fatigue (>3)	*1.52*	1.09–2.12	1.24	0.67–2.27
ASA abnormal (>1)	1.00	0.73–1.38	*1.96*	1.09–3.53
PS abnormal (>1)	*1.64*	1.07–2.52	1.97	0.92–4.23
Satariano's index (1)	1.11	0.78–1.59	1.29	0.68–2.44
Satariano's index (2+)	1.58	0.88–2.85	1.95	0.74–5.18

MMS mini mental status, *ADL* activities of daily living, *IADL* instrumental activities of daily living, *GDS* geriatric depression scale, *BFI* brief fatigue inventory, *ASA* American Society of Anesthesiologists physical status, *PS* eastern cooperative oncology group performance status
[a]Bold italics: significant relationship (*p* <0.05). Adapted from Audisio [90]

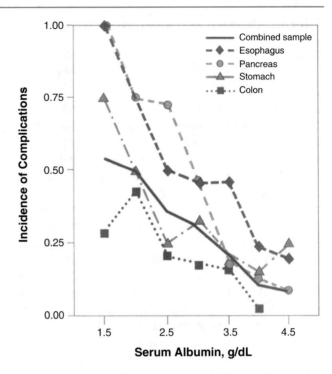

Fig. 4.5 Preoperative albumin level and major postoperative complications (by procedures). From Kudsk [98] with permission © Sage Publications

Preoperative antibiotics are not necessary for every type of elective surgery, but researchers agree that advanced age is a risk factor for nosocomial infection. Iwamoto [93] studied 4380 patients who underwent general anesthesia for thoracic, abdominal, or neurologic surgery and concluded that advanced age is a risk factor for nosocomial pneumonia, especially after thoracic surgery. Age greater than 70 years has been shown to be a risk factor for both positive bile cultures (*p* <0.001) [94] and septic complications of biliary surgery compared to younger patients [95]; antibiotic prophylaxis can reduce these complications [96].

Efforts to improve our elderly patients' preoperative nutritional state would seem desirable—even active, community-dwelling older adults manifest impaired recovery of strength after major surgery [97]—but it is unclear how to do this. Low levels of serum albumin, for example, correlate strikingly with postoperative problems [98], (Fig. 4.5) but cannot be improved to a great degree preoperatively. Souba [99] reviewed the literature on nutritional support and concluded that preoperative support should be reserved for severely malnourished patients scheduled to undergo major elective surgery and then should be provided for no more than 10 days.

In addition to those already cited, a number of surgeons have attributed their improved results in elderly patients to compulsive preoperative preparation. Bittner [100] believed that the significant decrease in mortality after total gastrectomy in septuagenarians (32.0 % in 1979 to 4.4 % in 1996) was the result of standardized perioperative antibiotics, thromboembolic prophylaxis, "a systemic analysis of risk factors and their thorough preoperative therapy," and nutritional support for the malnourished.

Hypovolemia is tolerated poorly by the elderly patient and it must be corrected. Smoking should stop. Treating other correctable aberrations such as anemia, bronchitis, and hypertension preoperatively increases the elderly patient's chance for a smooth postoperative course.

Principle IV: Emergency Surgery

> The results of elective surgery in the elderly are excellent in some centers; the results of emergency surgery are poor though still better than nonoperative treatment for most conditions. The risk of emergency surgery may be many times that of similar elective surgery because of Principles II and III.

Many centers have been able to achieve excellent results for elective surgery in the elderly, results indistinguishable from those in younger counterparts [101–103]. Coyle [104] reported the results of carotid endarterectomy in 79 octogenarians and summarized the results of five other series (634 total patients); mortality and morbidity were similar to those in a younger cohort. Maehara [105] had 0 % operative mortality in 77 patients over age 70 who underwent resection of gastric carcinoma, and Jougon's [106] results for esophagectomy in 89 patients aged 70–84 years were identical to those in 451 younger patients. An 85-year-old patient with lung cancer could anticipate mortality and survival after pulmonary lobectomy statistically identical to

Table 4.4 Predictive factors for operative mortality

Predictive factors	Odds ratio (95 % CI)	P value
Emergency operation	11.4 (4.7–27.5)	<0.0001
ASA classification: 1,2	0.1 (0.03–0.7)	0.0134
ADL impairment	3.2 (1.3–8.1)	0.0116
RVU	1.06 (1.009–1.103)	0.0176
Operative duration	1.17 (1.05–1.3)	0.0039
Hypertension	0.3 (0.1–0.6)	0.0019

Note power of emergency operation status. 80–103 years of age
Adapted from Turrentine [110]

that of younger patients with similar stage disease [72, 101, 107–109].

Identical operations performed emergently in the elderly, however, carry at least a threefold (and as much as a tenfold) increased risk (Table 4.4) [110]. Keller [111], for example, reported 31 % morbidity and 20 % mortality in 100 patients over age 70 who underwent emergency operations, which is significantly more ($p<0.0005$) than the 6.8 % morbidity and 1.9 % mortality following elective operation in 513 similar patients. Elective cholecystectomy can be performed in young and old with the risk of death approaching 0 % [22, 112, 113]; the risk of mortality for emergency cholecystectomy increases somewhat in the younger group (1–2 %) but increases greatly in the elderly (5–15 %) [22]. Surgical priority clearly affects cardiac surgery risk [114, 115]. Elective operative mortality for colorectal surgery is as low as 1.5–3.0 %, rising to over 20 % for emergency operation [116, 117].

A patient's advanced age therefore weighs in favor of commencing rather than deferring needed elective surgery.

Principle V: Attention to Detail

Scrupulous attention to detail intraoperatively and perioperatively yields great benefit, as the elderly tolerate complications poorly (because of Principle II).

Perioperative blood loss is the *bete noire* of geriatric surgery, as the elderly lack the responsive compensatory mechanisms necessary to restore equilibrium. Fong [61] reported that the only independent predictor of postoperative complications in 138 patients over age 70 who underwent pancreatic resection was intraoperative blood loss exceeding 2 l. This finding has been mirrored in reports from cardiac surgery and neurosurgery. Sisto [118] reported that six of 23 octogenarian coronary bypass patients who required reexploration for tamponade died; Logeais [119] found that reoperation for tamponade following aortic valve replacement placed the elderly patient at high risk for mortality ($p<0.001$). Hemostasis is exceptionally important in the elderly craniotomy patient, possibly because the elderly brain is less likely to expand to obliterate dead space: Maurice-Williams

[120] reported that postoperative bleeding following resection of meningioma occurred in 20 % of 46 elderly patients and 0 % of 38 young patients ($p<0.05$).

Meticulous surgical technique is important in any patient, but it becomes crucial in those of advanced age. Anastomotic leak after esophageal or gastric resection, a dreaded complication in any patient, embodies an exceptional risk of mortality in the elderly; [121] yet, this complication can be minimized by careful technique [122, 123]. Only one of Bandoh's [124] elderly patients who underwent gastrectomy for cancer experienced a leak, as did only 2 of 163 patients over age 70 in Bittner's series [100]. Despite having significantly greater preoperative co-morbidity, the elderly patients undergoing gastrectomy in Gretschel's series experienced no greater postoperative morbidity [64]. The elderly cardiac surgery patient may benefit from extra care when they have a calcified aorta (e.g., intraoperative ultrasound or modified clamping and cannulation technique) or a fragile sternum (e.g., additional or pericostal wires) [125]. Operative speed is less important than technique: in Cohen's series of 46 nonagenarians undergoing major procedures [7] the duration of operation did not correlate with mortality.

Perioperative monitoring is more important in the elderly, since they may manifest few signs or symptoms of impending problems (see Principle I above). Bernstein [126] credits intensive hemodynamic monitoring in his lack of mortality among 78 patients over age 70 who underwent abdominal aortic aneurysmectomy. Such monitoring and intensive care were also emphasized by Alexander [3], who reported excellent results for 59 octogenarians having major upper abdominal cancer operations, and by Lo [127] for 85 elderly patients undergoing adrenal surgery at the Mayo Clinic. Giannice [128] credits attention to perioperative care (DVT prophylaxis, antibiotics, monitoring, respiratory care, pain management, early mobilization) for his group's improved recent results in gynecologic oncology patients. Adequate resources such as skilled nursing facilities for the more complex patients are important [129].

We may continue to teach the surgical aphorism, "Elderly patients tolerate operations but not complications." (Table 4.5).

Principle VI: Age Is a Scientific Fact

A patient's age should be treated as a scientific fact, not with prejudice. No particular chronologic age, of itself, is a contraindication to operation (because of Principle IV).

Great biologic variability exists among the elderly, with some octogenarians and nonagenarians proving to be healthier than their sons and daughters. Even an 85-year-old patient has a life expectancy exceeding 5 years [130, 131], so why not offer him resection of his lung cancer? No other treatment

Table 4.5 Importance of postoperative complications in failure of octogenarians to return to normal function following major abdominal surgery

All cases	Odds ratio	95% Confidence interval
Emergency operation	2.7	0.99–7.24
ASA III or IV	1.0	0.29–3.56
Co-morbidity index >5	1.8	0.48–6.66
Dependence on activities of daily living	1.8	0.42–7.73
Preexisting cardiac disease	1.9	0.69–5.44
Preexisting chronic pulmonary disease	2.0	0.54–9.06
Preexisting cerebrovascular disease	2.0	0.43–9.06
Development of postoperative complications	24.5	3.08–194.88
Elective cases only:		
Co-morbidity index >5	11.2	1.08–116.26
Development of postoperative complications	10.6	3.08–194.88

Adapted from Tan [121]

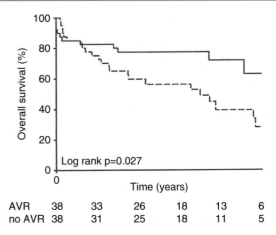

Fig. 4.6 Propensity score matched patients who refuse or are denied surgery for aortic valve diseased (*dashed line*) have decreased survival compared to those who undergo aortic valve replacement (*solid line*). From Pierard [151], with permission © Elsevier

is likely to give him those 5 years. Yet even in 2005 this does not always happen: prejudice against the elderly, so-called ageism exists.

Despite the fact that elderly patients treated for lung cancer have survival equal to their younger matched counterparts, Nugent [132] found that patients older than 80 years were significantly less likely ($p < 0.05$) to be treated surgically. In England the elderly are less likely to have histologic confirmation of their lung cancer and less likely to undergo anticancer treatment [133], although resection rates are increasing [134]. Kuo [135] also reported that octogenarian patients with lung cancer were more likely ($p < 0.01$) to receive only palliative care; when offered, they tolerate chemotherapy [136].

Elderly patients with ovarian cancer are less likely to undergo aggressive chemotherapy and surgery [137, 138] despite results equal to the young [139]. This has been reported with adjuvant treatment following pancreatic resection as well [67]. Older women with breast cancer were less likely to have had screening mammograms [140, 141] and were more likely to present in advanced stages than younger women [141]; once diagnosed, they tolerated surgery well [142, 143]. Guadagnoli [144] presented evidence against ageism in the treatment of early breast cancer, but Herbert-Croteau [145] found that only tamoxifen use was similar in women over and under age 70 ($p < 0.41$), while all other treatments (breast-conserving surgery, radiotherapy, axillary node dissection, chemotherapy) differed significantly ($p < 0.0001$). When elderly patients do receive chemotherapy for breast cancer they tolerate it [146] and they benefit from it [147]. Elderly patients with colon cancer are less likely to undergo extensive lymph node dissection ($p < 0.0001$) [148].

Selection bias in the elderly may also lead to delay in referral for abdominal aortic aneurysm surgery [149] and coronary artery bypass surgery [150].

When patients are denied surgery they often do poorly. In Pierard's [151] study of 163 octogenarians with severe aortic stenosis and clear indication for operation according to established guidelines, 40% either refused or were denied operation; this resulted in twofold excess mortality even after adjustment for co-morbidities (Fig. 4.6). In a study of pancreatic cancer patients across the USA those undergoing resection, regardless of age group into the 80s, were less than half as likely to die as the youngest group of unresected patients [152]. Owonikoko [153] noted, "Published evidence suggests that elderly patients are denied potentially beneficial treatment and participation in clinical trials solely because of chronologic age and because of physician perception that they are too frail to withstand treatment."

Some studies do report increased operative mortality [110, 154–157] (Fig. 4.7), increased complications [158, 159] (Fig. 4.8), and increased lengths-of-stay in the elderly [160–165], but overall results in many centers do not differ from the young for a wide variety of procedures: neurosurgery [120, 166]; head and neck surgery [33, 167, 168]; carotid endarterectomy [169, 170]; cardiac surgery [57, 125, 150, 171–175]; esophagectomy [91, 106, 122, 176–178] (Fig. 4.9); gastrectomy [3, 105, 179, 180] (Fig. 4.10); colectomy [181–183] (Fig. 4.11); hepatectomy [61, 184–187] (Fig. 4.12); pancreaticoduodenectomy [61, 67, 188, 189]; radical hysterectomy [190]; total knee/hip replacement [191–193]; microvascular free tissue transfer [194]; cardiac transplant [195–197]; lung transplant [198]; endovascular surgery [199]; gastric bypass [200]; laparoscopic colectomy [201];

Fig. 4.7 Increased mortality by age of aortoiliac aneurysm repair. From Tsilimparis [217], with permission © American College of Surgeons

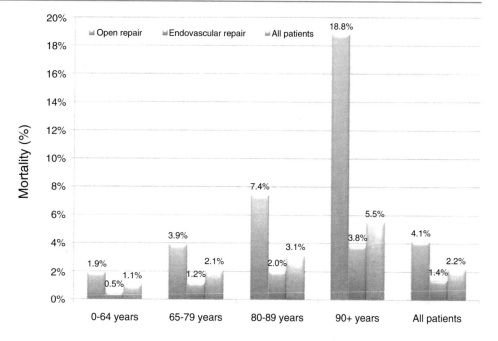

Fig. 4.8 Early postoperative neurologic complications after coronary artery bypass surgery and valve surgery in octogenarians (*RIND* reversible ischemic neurological deficit). From Ngaage [158] with permission © Oxford Journals

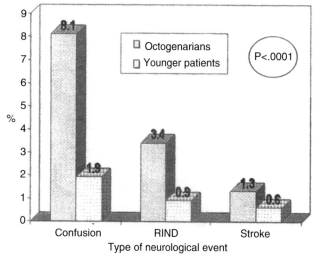

Fig. 4.9 Esophagectomy following neoadjuvant chemoradiation. Kaplan–Meier survival curves (including postoperative deaths) plotted for patients age <70 years versus ≥70 years. From Ruol [178] with permission © Springer

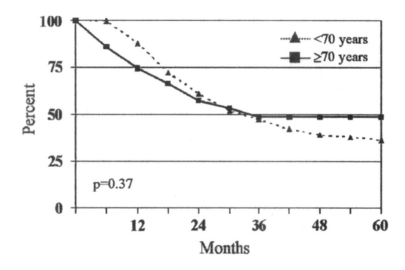

and hernia [202]. Return to preoperative quality of life (QOL) is gratifying after elective surgery for gastric or colorectal surgery [203], joint replacement [193], thoracic aneurysm [204] (Fig. 4.13), and aortic valve replacement [205, 206].

For most patients, general medical condition and associated medical problems are more important than age. Dunlop [207] studied 8889 geriatric surgical patients in Canada and concluded that severity of illness on admission was a much better predictor of outcome than was age; Akoh [208] had similar findings in 171 octogenarians undergoing major gastrointestinal surgery. Co-morbidities were a greater influence on survival than age in several series of elderly patients with lung cancer [40, 41, 209]. Mehta [210] reported that separation of mitral valve replacement patients into low, medium, and high risk medical groups was more important than stratification by age within these three groups. Within the American Society of Anesthesiologists (ASA) Physical Status system [211], the ASA status influences results more than age. For elderly patients undergoing surgery for cancer, the stage of the malignancy also influences outcome more than age [41, 212–215]. Ageism may even be detrimental for the ageist [216].

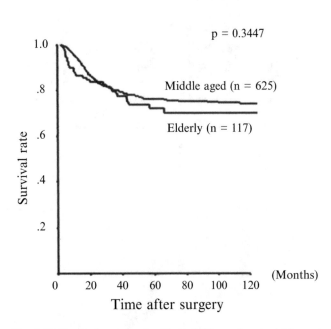

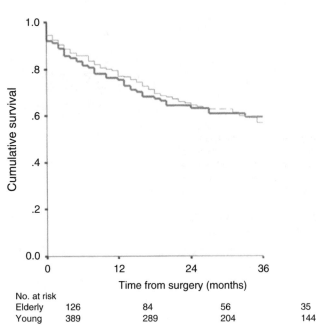

Fig. 4.10 Surgical outcome in elderly (≥75 years) and middle-aged (45–65 years) patients with gastric cancer. From Kunisaki [180] with permission © Elsevier

Fig. 4.12 Major hepatectomy. Overall survival for patients ≥70 years (*solid line*) and <70 years (*dashed line*), p=0.89; n=517. From Menon [187] with permission © American College of Surgeons

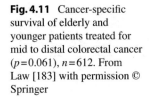

Fig. 4.11 Cancer-specific survival of elderly and younger patients treated for mid to distal colorectal cancer (p=0.061), n=612. From Law [183] with permission © Springer

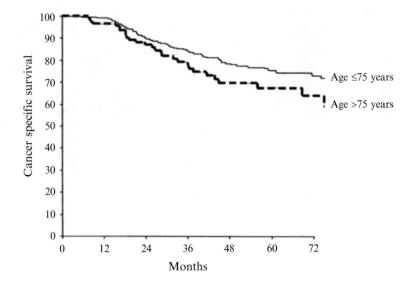

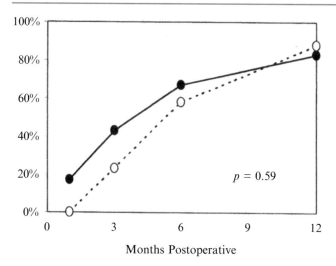

Fig. 4.13 Return to normal functional activity after thoracic aneurysm repair depending on age: <70 years (*solid circles*) and ≥70 years (*open circles*); *n* = 110. From Zierer [204] with permission © Elsevier

though still better than nonoperative treatment for m o s t conditions. The risk of *emergency surgery* may be many times that of similar elective surgery because of Principles II and III.

• Scrupulous *attention to detail* intraoperatively and perioperatively yields great benefit, as the elderly tolerate complications poorly (because of Principle II).

• A patient's age should be treated as a *scientific fact, not with prejudice*. No particular chronologic age, of itself, is a contraindication to operation (because of Principle IV).

Many geriatric surgery patients, including nonagenarians, have survival rates equal to those expected in the general population; even the sobering results of emergency surgery in the elderly are better than the results of nonoperative treatment for the same conditions. A patient's age should therefore be considered but not feared.

Conclusion

Surgical problems abound in the elderly and the numbers of elderly are increasing worldwide. Surgeons must become students of the physiologic changes that occur with aging and, guided by a few general principles, apply this knowledge to daily clinical care. The results of surgery in the elderly do not support prejudice against advanced age. We owe it to our elders to become good geriatric surgeons and in so doing we will become better surgeons to patients of all ages.

Key Points

• The *clinical presentation* of surgical problems in the elderly may be subtle or somewhat different from that in the general population. This may lead to delay in diagnosis.

• The elderly handle stress satisfactorily but handle severe stress poorly because of *lack of organ system reserve*.

• Optimal *preoperative preparation* is essential, because of Principle II. When preparation is suboptimal the perioperative risk increases.

• The results of elective surgery in the elderly are excellent in some centers; the results of emergency surgery are poor

References

1. Smith OC. Advanced age as a contraindication to operation. Med Rec (NY). 1907;72:642–4.
2. Ochsner A. Is risk of operation too great in the elderly? Geriatrics. 1967;22:121–30.
3. Alexander HR, Turnbull AD, Salamone J, Keefe D, Melendez J. Upper abdominal cancer surgery in the very elderly. J Surg Oncol. 1991;47(2):82–6.
4. Bridges CR, Edwards FH, Peterson ED, Coombs LP, Ferguson TB. Cardiac surgery in nonagenarians and centenarians. J Am Coll Surg. 2003;197(3):347–56. discussion 356–347.
5. Katlic MR. Surgery in centenarians. JAMA. 1985;253(21):3139–41.
6. Ullery BW, Peterson JC, Milla F, et al. Cardiac surgery in select nonagenarians: should we or shouldn't we? Ann Thorac Surg. 2008;85(3):854–60.
7. Cohen JR, Johnson H, Eaton S, Sterman H, Wise L. Surgical procedures in patients during the tenth decade of life. Surgery. 1988;104(4):646–51.
8. Linn BS, Zeppa R. Student attitudes about surgery in older patients before and after the surgical clerkship. Ann Surg. 1987;205(3): 324–8.
9. Thomas DR, Ritchie CS. Preoperative assessment of older adults. J Am Geriatr Soc. 1995;43(7):811–21.
10. Biancari F, Schifano P, Pighi M, Vasques F, Juvonen T, Vinco G. Pooled estimates of immediate and late outcome of mitral valve surgery in octogenarians: a meta-analysis and meta-regression. J Cardiothorac Vasc Anesth. 2013;27(2):213–9.
11. Goodney PP, Siewers AE, Stukel TA, Lucas FL, Wennberg DE, Birkmeyer JD. Is surgery getting safer? National trends in operative mortality. J Am Coll Surg. 2002;195(2):219–27.
12. Storm-Dickerson TL, Horattas MC. What have we learned over the past 20 years about appendicitis in the elderly? Am J Surg. 2003;185(3):198–201.
13. Elangovan S. Clinical and laboratory findings in acute appendicitis in the elderly. J Am Board Fam Pract. 1996;9(2):75–8.
14. Lau WY, Fan ST, Yiu TF, Chu KW, Lee JM. Acute appendicitis in the elderly. Surg Gynecol Obstet. 1985;161(2):157–60.
15. Horattas MC, Guyton DP, Wu D. A reappraisal of appendicitis in the elderly. Am J Surg. 1990;160(3):291–3.
16. Soroken C, Samaras N, Samaras D, Huber P. An unusual case of cholecystitis and liver abscesses in an older adult. J Am Geriatr Soc. 2012;60(1):160–61.
17. Adedeji OA, McAdam WA. Murphy's sign, acute cholecystitis and elderly people. J R Coll Surg Edinb. 1996;41(2):88–9.
18. Hafif A, Gutman M, Kaplan O, Winkler E, Rozin RR, Skornick Y. The management of acute cholecystitis in elderly patients. Am Surg. 1991;57(10):648–52.
19. Parker LJ, Vukov LF, Wollan PC. Emergency department evaluation of geriatric patients with acute cholecystitis. Acad Emerg Med. 1997;4(1):51–5.

20. Chen Y, Zheng M, Hu X, et al. Fever of unknown origin in elderly people: a retrospective study of 87 patients in China. J Am Geriatr Soc. 2008;56(1):182–4.

21. Stewart L, Grifiss JM, Jarvis GA, Way LW. Elderly patients have more severe biliary infections: influence of complement-killing and induction of TNFalpha production. Surgery. 2008;143(1):103–12.

22. Magnuson TH, Ratner LE, Zenilman ME, Bender JS. Laparoscopic cholecystectomy: applicability in the geriatric population. Am Surg. 1997;63(1):91–6.

23. Saunders K, Tompkins R, Longmire Jr W, Roslyn J. Bile duct carcinoma in the elderly. A rationale for surgical management. Arch Surg. 1991;126(10):1186–90. discussion 1190–1181.

24. Hilton D, Iman N, Burke GJ, et al. Absence of abdominal pain in older persons with endoscopic ulcers: a prospective study. Am J Gastroenterol. 2001;96(2):380–4.

25. Rabinovici R, Manny J. Perforated duodenal ulcer in the elderly. Eur J Surg. 1991;157(2):121–5.

26. Tong K, Merchant R. Nonacute acute abdomen in older adults. J Am Geriatr Soc. 2012;60(2):370–71.

27. Mulcahy HE, Patchett SE, Daly L, O'Donoghue DP. Prognosis of elderly patients with large bowel cancer. Br J Surg. 1994; 81(5):736–8.

28. Watters JM, Blakslee JM, March RJ, Redmond ML. The influence of age on the severity of peritonitis. Can J Surg. 1996;39(2):142–6.

29. Tedesco P, Lobo E, Fisichella PM, Way LW, Patti MG. Laparoscopic fundoplication in elderly patients with gastroesophageal reflux disease. Arch Surg. 2006;141(3):289–92. discussion 292.

30. Pilotto A, Franceschi M, Leandro G, et al. Clinical features of reflux esophagitis in older people: a study of 840 consecutive patients. J Am Geriatr Soc. 2006;54(10):1537–42.

31. Knutson JW, Slavin RG. Sinusitis in the aged. Optimal management strategies. Drugs Aging. 1995;7(4):310–6.

32. Norman DC, Toledo SD. Infections in elderly persons. An altered clinical presentation. Clin Geriatr Med. 1992;8(4):713–9.

33. Koch WM, Patel H, Brennan J, Boyle JO, Sidransky D. Squamous cell carcinoma of the head and neck in the elderly. Arch Otolaryngol Head Neck Surg. 1995;121(3):262–5.

34. Ehlinger P, Fossion E, Vrielinck L. Carcinoma of the oral cavity in patients over 75 years of age. Int J Oral Maxillofac Surg. 1993;22(4):218–20.

35. Chigot JP, Menegaux F, Achrafi H. Should primary hyperparathyroidism be treated surgically in elderly patients older than 75 years? Surgery. 1995;117(4):397–401.

36. Thomas PC, Grigg M. Carotid artery surgery in the octogenarian. Aust N Z J Surg. 1996;66(4):231–4.

37. Canto JG, Fincher C, Kiefe CI, et al. Atypical presentations among Medicare beneficiaries with unstable angina pectoris. Am J Cardiol. 2002;90(3):248–53.

38. Hellmann DB. Eurekapenia: a disease of medical residency training programs? Pharos Alpha Omega Alpha Honor Med Soc. 2003;66(2):24–6.

39. Durso SC. A bipolar disorder: eurekaphoria, then discouragement. Pharos Alpha Omega Alpha Honor Med Soc. 2004;67(3):49.

40. Birim O, Zuydendorp HM, Maat AP, Kappetein AP, Eijkemans MJ, Bogers AJ. Lung resection for non-small-cell lung cancer in patients older than 70: mortality, morbidity, and late survival compared with the general population. Ann Thorac Surg. 2003;76(6):1796–801.

41. Brock MV, Kim MP, Hooker CM, et al. Pulmonary resection in octogenarians with stage I nonsmall cell lung cancer: a 22-year experience. Ann Thorac Surg. 2004;77(1):271–7.

42. Keagy BA, Pharr WF, Bowes DE, Wilcox BR. A review of morbidity and mortality in elderly patients undergoing pulmonary resection. Am Surg. 1984;50(4):213–6.

43. Au J, el-Oakley R, Cameron EW. Pneumonectomy for bronchogenic carcinoma in the elderly. Eur J Cardiothorac Surg. 1994; 8(5):247–50.

44. Miller DL, Deschamps C, Jenkins GD, Bernard A, Allen MS, Pairolero PC. Completion pneumonectomy: factors affecting operative mortality and cardiopulmonary morbidity. Ann Thorac Surg. 2002;74(3):876–83. discussion 883–874.

45. Rostad H, Naalsund A, Strand TE, Jacobsen R, Talleraas O, Norstein J. Results of pulmonary resection for lung cancer in Norway, patients older than 70 years. Eur J Cardiothorac Surg. 2005;27(2):325–8.

46. Demmy TL, Plante AJ, Nwogu CE, Takita H, Anderson TM. Discharge independence with minimally invasive lobectomy. Am J Surg. 2004;188(6):698–702.

47. Jaklitsch MT, DeCamp Jr MM, Liptay MJ, et al. Video-assisted thoracic surgery in the elderly. A review of 307 cases. Chest. 1996;110(3):751–8.

48. Nomori H, Horio H, Fuyuno G, Kobayashi R, Yashima H. Respiratory muscle strength after lung resection with special reference to age and procedures of thoracotomy. Eur J Cardiothorac Surg. 1996;10(5):352–8.

49. Yim AP. Thoracoscopic surgery in the elderly population. Surg Endosc. 1996;10(9):880–2.

50. Cattaneo SM, Park BJ, Wilton AS, et al. Use of video-assisted thoracic surgery for lobectomy in the elderly results in fewer complications. Ann Thorac Surg. 2008;85(1):231–5. discussion 235–236.

51. Patel HJ, Williams DM, Upchurch Jr GR, et al. A comparison of open and endovascular descending thoracic aortic repair in patients older than 75 years of age. Ann Thorac Surg. 2008;85(5):1597–603. discussion 1603–1594.

52. Jackson RS, Chang DC, Freischlag JA. Comparison of long-term survival after open vs endovascular repair of intact abdominal aortic aneurysm among Medicare beneficiaries. JAMA. 2012;307(15):1621–8.

53. Tan HJ, Norton EC, Ye Z, Hafez KS, Gore JL, Miller DC. Long-term survival following partial vs radical nephrectomy among older patients with early-stage kidney cancer. JAMA. 2012;307(15):1629–35.

54. Bergus BO, Feng WC, Bert AA, Singh AK. Aortic valve replacement (AVR): influence of age on operative morbidity and mortality. Eur J Cardiothorac Surg. 1992;6(3):118–21.

55. Salomon NW, Page US, Bigelow JC, Krause AH, Okies JE, Metzdorff MT. Coronary artery bypass grafting in elderly patients. Comparative results in a consecutive series of 469 patients older than 75 years. J Thorac Cardiovasc Surg. 1991;101(2):209–17. discussion 217–208.

56. Lytle BW, Navia JL, Taylor PC, et al. Third coronary artery bypass operations: risks and costs. Ann Thorac Surg. 1997;64(5): 1287–95.

57. Elayda MA, Hall RJ, Reul RM, et al. Aortic valve replacement in patients 80 years and older. Operative risks and long-term results. Circulation. 1993;88(5 Pt 2):II11–6.

58. Mohammadi S, Kalavrouziotis D, Dagenais F, Voisine P, Charbonneau E. Completeness of revascularization and survival among octogenarians with triple-vessel disease. Ann Thorac Surg. 2012;93(5):1432–7.

59. Girerd N, Magne J, Rabilloud M, et al. The impact of complete revascularization on long-term survival is strongly dependent on age. Ann Thorac Surg. 2012;94(4):1166–72.

60. Fortner JG, Lincer RM. Hepatic resection in the elderly. Ann Surg. 1990;211(2):141–5.

61. Fong Y, Blumgart LH, Fortner JG, Brennan MF. Pancreatic or liver resection for malignancy is safe and effective for the elderly. Ann Surg. 1995;222(4):426–34. discussion 434–427.

62. Escarce JJ, Shea JA, Chen W, Qian Z, Schwartz JS. Outcomes of open cholecystectomy in the elderly: a longitudinal analysis of 21,000 cases in the prelaparoscopic era. Surgery. 1995;117(2): 156–64.

63. Tsujitani S, Katano K, Oka A, Ikeguchi M, Maeta M, Kaibara N. Limited operation for gastric cancer in the elderly. Br J Surg. 1996;83(6):836–9.

64. Gretschel S, Estevez-Schwarz L, Hunerbein M, Schneider U, Schlag PM. Gastric cancer surgery in elderly patients. World J Surg. 2006;30(8):1468–74.

65. Okada M, Koike T, Higashiyama M, Yamato Y, Kodama K, Tsubota N. Radical sublobar resection for small-sized non-small cell lung cancer: a multicenter study. J Thorac Cardiovasc Surg. 2006;132(4):769–75.

66. Mery CM, Pappas AN, Bueno R, et al. Similar long-term survival of elderly patients with non-small cell lung cancer treated with lobectomy or wedge resection within the surveillance, epidemiology, and end results database. Chest. 2005;128(1):237–45.

67. Barbas AS, Turley RS, Ceppa EP, et al. Comparison of outcomes and the use of multimodality therapy in young and elderly people undergoing surgical resection of pancreatic cancer. J Am Geriatr Soc. 2012;60(2):344–50.

68. Lawrence VA, Hazuda HP, Cornell JE, et al. Functional independence after major abdominal surgery in the elderly. J Am Coll Surg. 2004;199(5):762–72.

69. Seymour DG, Vaz FG. A prospective study of elderly general surgical patients: II. Post-operative complications. Age Ageing. 1989;18(5):316–26.

70. Dzankic S, Pastor D, Gonzalez C, Leung JM. The prevalence and predictive value of abnormal preoperative laboratory tests in elderly surgical patients. Anesth Analg. 2001;93(2):301–308, 302nd contents page.

71. Vaporciyan AA, Merriman KW, Ece F, et al. Incidence of major pulmonary morbidity after pneumonectomy: association with timing of smoking cessation. Ann Thorac Surg. 2002;73(2):420–5. discussion 425–426.

72. Mizushima Y, Noto H, Sugiyama S, et al. Survival and prognosis after pneumonectomy for lung cancer in the elderly. Ann Thorac Surg. 1997;64(1):193–8.

73. Reilly JJ. Preparing for pulmonary resection: preoperative evaluation of patients. Chest. 1997;112(4 Suppl):206S–8.

74. Goldhaber SZ, Tapson VF. A prospective registry of 5,451 patients with ultrasound-confirmed deep vein thrombosis. Am J Cardiol. 2004;93(2):259–62.

75. Jacobs LG. Prophylactic anticoagulation for venous thromboembolic disease in geriatric patients. J Am Geriatr Soc. 2003; 51(10):1472–8.

76. Berlauk JF, Abrams JH, Gilmour IJ, O'Connor SR, Knighton DR, Cerra FB. Preoperative optimization of cardiovascular hemodynamics improves outcome in peripheral vascular surgery. A prospective, randomized clinical trial. Ann Surg. 1991;214(3):289–97. discussion 298–289.

77. Bender JS, Smith-Meek MA, Jones CE. Routine pulmonary artery catheterization does not reduce morbidity and mortality of elective vascular surgery: results of a prospective, randomized trial. Ann Surg. 1997;226(3):229–36. discussion 236–227.

78. Ziegler DW, Wright JG, Choban PS, Flancbaum L. A prospective randomized trial of preoperative "optimization" of cardiac function in patients undergoing elective peripheral vascular surgery. Surgery. 1997;122(3):584–92.

79. Leppo JA. Preoperative cardiac risk assessment for noncardiac surgery. Am J Cardiol. 1995;75(11):42D–51.

80. Biagini E, Elhendy A, Schinkel AF, et al. Long-term prediction of mortality in elderly persons by dobutamine stress echocardiography. J Gerontol A Biol Sci Med Sci. 2005;60(10):1333–8.

81. Snowden CP, Prentis J, Jacques B, et al. Cardiorespiratory fitness predicts mortality and hospital length of stay after major elective surgery in older people. Ann Surg. 2013;257(6):999–1004.

82. Brunelli A, Pompili C, Berardi R, et al. Performance at preoperative stair-climbing test is associated with prognosis after pulmonary

83. Pollock M, Roa J, Benditt J, Celli B. Estimation of ventilatory reserve by stair climbing. A study in patients with chronic airflow obstruction. Chest. 1993;104(5):1378–83.

84. Brunelli A, Refai M, Xiume F, et al. Performance at symptom-limited stair-climbing test is associated with increased cardiopulmonary complications, mortality, and costs after major lung resection. Ann Thorac Surg. 2008;86(1):240–7. discussion 247–248.

85. Win T, Jackson A, Groves AM, Sharples LD, Charman SC, Laroche CM. Comparison of shuttle walk with measured peak oxygen consumption in patients with operable lung cancer. Thorax. 2006;61(1):57–60.

86. Simonsick EM, Fan E, Fleg JL. Estimating cardiorespiratory fitness in well-functioning older adults: treadmill validation of the long distance corridor walk. J Am Geriatr Soc. 2006;54(1): 127–32.

87. Robinson TN, Wu DS, Sauaia A, et al. Slower walking speed forecasts increased postoperative morbidity and 1-year mortality across surgical specialties. Ann Surg. 2013;258(4):582–8; discussion 588–590.

88. Afilalo J, Eisenberg MJ, Morin JF, et al. Gait speed as an incremental predictor of mortality and major morbidity in elderly patients undergoing cardiac surgery. J Am Coll Cardiol. 2010;56(20):1668–76.

89. Weinstein H, Bates AT, Spaltro BE, Thaler HT, Steingart RM. Influence of preoperative exercise capacity on length of stay after thoracic cancer surgery. Ann Thorac Surg. 2007;84(1): 197–202.

90. Audisio RA, Pope D, Ramesh HS, et al. Shall we operate? Preoperative assessment in elderly cancer patients (PACE) can help. A SIOG surgical task force prospective study. Crit Rev Oncol Hematol. 2008;65(2):156–63.

91. Internullo E, Moons J, Nafteux P, et al. Outcome after esophagectomy for cancer of the esophagus and GEJ in patients aged over 75 years. Eur J Cardiothorac Surg. 2008;33(6):1096–104.

92. Katlic MR. The Holy Grail of geriatric surgery. Ann Surg. 2013;257(6):1005–6.

93. Iwamoto K, Ichiyama S, Shimokata K, Nakashima N. Postoperative pneumonia in elderly patients: incidence and mortality in comparison with younger patients. Intern Med. 1993;32(4):274–7.

94. Kwon AH, Matsui Y. Laparoscopic cholecystectomy in patients aged 80 years and over. World J Surg. 2006;30(7):1204–10.

95. Landau O, Kott I, Deutsch AA, Stelman E, Reiss R. Multifactorial analysis of septic bile and septic complications in biliary surgery. World J Surg. 1992;16(5):962–4. discussion 964–965.

96. Meijer WS, Schmitz PI, Jeekel J. Meta-analysis of randomized, controlled clinical trials of antibiotic prophylaxis in biliary tract surgery. Br J Surg. 1990;77(3):283–90.

97. Watters JM, Clancey SM, Moulton SB, Briere KM, Zhu JM. Impaired recovery of strength in older patients after major abdominal surgery. Ann Surg. 1993;218(3):380–90. discussion 390–383.

98. Kudsk KA, Tolley EA, DeWitt RC, et al. Preoperative albumin and surgical site identify surgical risk for major postoperative complications. JPEN J Parenter Enteral Nutr. 2003;27(1):1–9.

99. Souba WW. Nutritional support. N Engl J Med. 1997;336(1): 41–8.

100. Bittner R, Butters M, Ulrich M, Uppenbrink S, Beger HG. Total gastrectomy. Updated operative mortality and long-term survival with particular reference to patients older than 70 years of age. Ann Surg. 1996;224(1):37–42.

101. Myrdal G, Gustafsson G, Lambe M, Horte LG, Stahle E. Outcome after lung cancer surgery. Factors predicting early mortality and major morbidity. Eur J Cardiothorac Surg. 2001;20(4):694–9.

102. Allen MS, Darling GE, Pechet TT, et al. Morbidity and mortality of major pulmonary resections in patients with early-stage lung cancer: initial results of the randomized, prospective ACOSOG Z0030 trial. Ann Thorac Surg. 2006;81(3):1013–9. discussion 1019–1020.

103. Cerfolio RJ, Bryant AS. Survival and outcomes of pulmonary resection for non-small cell lung cancer in the elderly: a nested case–control study. Ann Thorac Surg. 2006;82(2):424–9. discussion 429–430.

104. Coyle KA, Smith 3rd RB, Salam AA, Dodson TF, Chaikof EL, Lumsden AB. Carotid endarterectomy in the octogenarian. Ann Vasc Surg. 1994;8(5):417–20.

105. Maehara Y, Oshiro T, Oiwa H, et al. Gastric carcinoma in patients over 70 years of age. Br J Surg. 1995;82(1):102–5.

106. Jougon JB, Ballester M, Duffy J, et al. Esophagectomy for cancer in the patient aged 70 years and older. Ann Thorac Surg. 1997;63(5):1423–7.

107. de Perrot M, Licker M, Reymond MA, Robert J, Spiliopoulos A. Influence of age on operative mortality and long-term survival after lung resection for bronchogenic carcinoma. Eur Respir J. 1999;14(2):419–22.

108. Okada M, Nishio W, Sakamoto T, Harada H, Uchino K, Tsubota N. Long-term survival and prognostic factors of five-year survivors with complete resection of non-small cell lung carcinoma. J Thorac Cardiovasc Surg. 2003;126(2):558–62.

109. Thomas P, Sielezenff I, Rajni J, Giridicilli R, Fuentes P. Is lung cancer resection justified in patients aged over 70 years? Eur J Cardiothorac Surg. 1993;7:246–51.

110. Turrentine FE, Wang H, Simpson VB, Jones RS. Surgical risk factors, morbidity, and mortality in elderly patients. J Am Coll Surg. 2006;203(6):865–77.

111. Keller SM, Markovitz LJ, Wilder JR, Aufses Jr AH. Emergency and elective surgery in patients over age 70. Am Surg. 1987;53(11):636–40.

112. Bingener J, Richards ML, Schwesinger WH, Strodel WE, Sirinek KR. Laparoscopic cholecystectomy for elderly patients: gold standard for golden years? Arch Surg. 2003;138(5):531–5. discussion 535–536.

113. Tambyraja AL, Kumar S, Nixon SJ. Outcome of laparoscopic cholecystectomy in patients 80 years and older. World J Surg. 2004;28(8):745–8.

114. Tsai TP, Chaux A, Matloff JM, et al. Ten-year experience of cardiac surgery in patients aged 80 years and over. Ann Thorac Surg. 1994;58(2):445–50. discussion 450–441.

115. Tseng EE, Lee CA, Cameron DE, et al. Aortic valve replacement in the elderly. Risk factors and long-term results. Ann Surg. 1997;225(6):793–802. discussion 802–794.

116. Bender JS, Magnuson TH, Zenilman ME, et al. Outcome following colon surgery in the octaganarian. Am Surg. 1996;62(4):276–9.

117. Spivak H, Maele DV, Friedman I, Nussbaum M. Colorectal surgery in octogenarians. J Am Coll Surg. 1996;183(1):46–50.

118. Sisto D, Hoffman D, Frater RW. Isolated coronary artery bypass grafting in one hundred octogenarian patients. J Thorac Cardiovasc Surg. 1993;106(5):940–2.

119. Logeais Y, Langanay T, Roussin R, et al. Surgery for aortic stenosis in elderly patients. A study of surgical risk and predictive factors. Circulation. 1994;90(6):2891–8.

120. Maurice-Williams RS, Kitchen ND. Intracranial tumours in the elderly: the effect of age on the outcome of first time surgery for meningiomas. Br J Neurosurg. 1992;6(2):131–7.

121. Tan KY, Chen CM, Ng C, Tan SM, Tay KH. Which octogenarians do poorly after major open abdominal surgery in our Asian population? World J Surg. 2006;30(4):547–52.

122. Adam DJ, Craig SR, Sang CT, Cameron EW, Walker WS. Esophagectomy for carcinoma in the octogenarian. Ann Thorac Surg. 1996;61(1):190–4.

123. Mathisen DJ, Grillo HC, Wilkins Jr EW, Moncure AC, Hilgenberg AD. Transthoracic esophagectomy: a safe approach to carcinoma of the esophagus. Ann Thorac Surg. 1988;45(2):137–43.

124. Bandoh T, Isoyama T, Toyoshima H. Total gastrectomy for gastric cancer in the elderly. Surgery. 1991;109(2):136–42.

125. Katz NM, Chase GA. Risks of cardiac operations for elderly patients: reduction of the age factor. Ann Thorac Surg. 1997;63(5):1309–14.

126. Bernstein EF, Dilley RB, Randolph 3rd HF. The improving long-term outlook for patients over 70 years of age with abdominal aortic aneurysms. Ann Surg. 1988;207(3):318–22.

127. Lo CY, van Heerden JA, Grant CS, Soreide JA, Warner MA, Ilstrup DM. Adrenal surgery in the elderly: too risky? World J Surg. 1996;20(3):368–73. discussion 374.

128. Giannice R, Foti E, Poerio A, Marana E, Mancuso S, Scambia G. Perioperative morbidity and mortality in elderly gynecological oncological patients (>/= 70 Years) by the American Society of Anesthesiologists physical status classes. Ann Surg Oncol. 2004;11(2):219–25.

129. Henry L, Halpin L, Hunt S, Holmes SD, Ad N. Patient disposition and long-term outcomes after valve surgery in octogenarians. Ann Thorac Surg. 2012;94(3):744–50.

130. http://www.ssa.gov/OACT/STATS/table4c6.html. Period life table, 2009. Actuarial Publications, Statistical Tables [Accessed Feb 25, 2014].

131. Minino AM, Heron MP, Smith BL. Deaths: preliminary data for 2004. Natl Vital Stat Rep. 2006;54(19):1–49.

132. Nugent WC, Edney MT, Hammerness PG, Dain BJ, Maurer LH, Rigas JR. Non-small cell lung cancer at the extremes of age: impact on diagnosis and treatment. Ann Thorac Surg. 1997;63(1):193–7.

133. Beckett P, Callister M, Tata LJ, et al. Clinical management of older people with non-small cell lung cancer in England. Thorax. 2012;67(9):836–9.

134. Riaz SP, Linklater KM, Page R, Peake MD, Moller H, Luchtenborg M. Recent trends in resection rates among non-small cell lung cancer patients in England. Thorax. 2012;67(9):811–4.

135. Kuo CW, Chen YM, Chao JY, Tsai CM, Perng RP. Non-small cell lung cancer in very young and very old patients. Chest. 2000;117(2):354–7.

136. Fruh M, Rolland E, Pignon JP, et al. Pooled analysis of the effect of age on adjuvant cisplatin-based chemotherapy for completely resected non-small-cell lung cancer. J Clin Oncol. 2008;26(21):3573–81.

137. Cress RD, O'Malley CD, Leiserowitz GS, Campleman SL. Patterns of chemotherapy use for women with ovarian cancer: a population-based study. J Clin Oncol. 2003;21(8):1530–5.

138. Moore DH. Ovarian cancer in the elderly patient. Oncol (Huntingt). 1994;8(12):21–5; discussion 25, 29–30.

139. Edmonson JH, Su J, Krook JE. Treatment of ovarian cancer in elderly women. Mayo Clinic-North Central Cancer Treatment Group studies. Cancer. 1993;71(2 Suppl):615–7.

140. Singletary SE, Shallenberger R, Guinee VF. Breast cancer in the elderly. Ann Surg. 1993;218(5):667–71.

141. Wanebo HJ, Cole B, Chung M, et al. Is surgical management compromised in elderly patients with breast cancer? Ann Surg. 1997;225(5):579–86. discussion 586–579.

142. Swanson RS, Sawicka J, Wood WC. Treatment of carcinoma of the breast in the older geriatric patient. Surg Gynecol Obstet. 1991;173(6):465–9.

143. van Dalsen AD, de Vries JE. Treatment of breast cancer in elderly patients. J Surg Oncol. 1995;60(2):80–2.

144. Guadagnoli E, Shapiro C, Gurwitz JH, et al. Age-related patterns of care: evidence against ageism in the treatment of early-stage breast cancer. J Clin Oncol. 1997;15(6):2338–44.

145. Hebert-Croteau N, Brisson J, Latreille J, Blanchette C, Deschenes L. Compliance with consensus recommendations for

the treatment of early stage breast carcinoma in elderly women. Cancer. 1999;85(5):1104–13.

146. Hurria A, Hurria A, Zuckerman E, et al. A prospective, longitudinal study of the functional status and quality of life of older patients with breast cancer receiving adjuvant chemotherapy. J Am Geriatr Soc. 2006;54(7):1119–24.

147. Silliman RA, Ganz PA. Adjuvant chemotherapy use and outcomes in older women with breast cancer: what have we learned? J Clin Oncol. 2006;24(18):2697–9.

148. Bilimoria KY, Stewart AK, Palis BE, Bentrem DJ, Talamonti MS, Ko CY. Adequacy and importance of lymph node evaluation for colon cancer in the elderly. J Am Coll Surg. 2008;206(2):247–54.

149. Chalmers RT, Stonebridge PA, John TG, Murie JA. Abdominal aortic aneurysm in the elderly. Br J Surg. 1993;80(9):1122–3.

150. Blanche C, Matloff JM, Denton TA, et al. Cardiac operations in patients 90 years of age and older. Ann Thorac Surg. 1997;63(6):1685–90.

151. Pierard S, Seldrum S, de Meester C, et al. Incidence, determinants, and prognostic impact of operative refusal or denial in octogenarians with severe aortic stenosis. Ann Thorac Surg. 2011;91(4):1107–12.

152. Riall TS, Sheffield KM, Kuo YF, Townsend CM, Jr., Goodwin JS. Resection benefits older adults with locoregional pancreatic cancer despite greater short-term morbidity and mortality. J Am Geriatr Soc. 2011;59(4):647–54.

153. Owonikoko TK, Ragin CC, Belani CP, et al. Lung cancer in elderly patients: an analysis of the surveillance, epidemiology, and end results database. J Clin Oncol. 2007;25(35):5570–7.

154. Kiran RP, Attaluri V, Hammel J, Church J. A novel nomogram accurately quantifies the risk of mortality in elderly patients undergoing colorectal surgery. Ann Surg. 2013;257(5):905–8.

155. Koppert LB, Lemmens VE, Coebergh JW, et al. Impact of age and co-morbidity on surgical resection rate and survival in patients with oesophageal and gastric cancer. Br J Surg. 2012;99(12):1693–700.

156. Finlayson E, Fan Z, Birkmeyer JD. Outcomes in octogenarians undergoing high-risk cancer operation: a national study. J Am Coll Surg. 2007;205(6):729–34.

157. Moskovitz AH, Rizk NP, Venkatraman E, et al. Mortality increases for octogenarians undergoing esophagogastrectomy for esophageal cancer. Ann Thorac Surg. 2006;82(6):2031–6. discussion 2036.

158. Ngaage DL, Cowen ME, Griffin S, Guvendik L, Cale AR. Early neurological complications after coronary artery bypass grafting and valve surgery in octogenarians. Eur J Cardiothorac Surg. 2008;33(4):653–9.

159. Leo F, Scanagatta P, Baglio P, et al. The risk of pneumonectomy over the age of 70. A case–control study. Eur J Cardiothorac Surg. 2007;31(5):780–2.

160. Lee JD, Bonaros N, Hong PT, et al. Factors influencing hospital length of stay after robotic totally endoscopic coronary artery bypass grafting. Ann Thorac Surg. 2013;95(3):813–8.

161. Barnett SD, Halpin LS, Speir AM, et al. Postoperative complications among octogenarians after cardiovascular surgery. Ann Thorac Surg. 2003;76(3):726–31.

162. Jarvinen O, Huhtala H, Laurikka J, Tarkka MR. Higher age predicts adverse outcome and readmission after coronary artery bypass grafting. World J Surg. 2003;27(12):1317–22.

163. Lightner AM, Glasgow RE, Jordan TH, et al. Pancreatic resection in the elderly. J Am Coll Surg. 2004;198(5):697–706.

164. Sosa JA, Mehta PJ, Wang TS, Boudourakis L, Roman SA. A population-based study of outcomes from thyroidectomy in aging Americans: at what cost? J Am Coll Surg. 2008;206(3):1097–105.

165. Mamoun NF, Xu M, Sessler DI, Sabik JF, Bashour CA. Propensity matched comparison of outcomes in older and younger patients after coronary artery bypass graft surgery. Ann Thorac Surg. 2008;85(6):1974–9.

166. Fraioli B, Pastore FS, Signoretti S, De Caro GM, Giuffre R. The surgical treatment of pituitary adenomas in the eighth decade. Surg Neurol. 1999;51(3):261–6. discussion 266–267.

167. Derks W, De Leeuw JR, Hordijk GJ, Winnubst JA. Elderly patients with head and neck cancer: short-term effects of surgical treatment on quality of life. Clin Otolaryngol. 2003;28(5):399–405.

168. Uruno T, Miyauchi A, Shimizu K, et al. Favorable surgical results in 433 elderly patients with papillary thyroid cancer. World J Surg. 2005;29(11):1497–501. discussion 1502–1493.

169. Salameh JR, Myers JL, Mukherjee D. Carotid endarterectomy in elderly patients: low complication rate with overnight stay. Arch Surg. 2002;137(11):1284–7. discussion 1288.

170. Durward QJ, Ragnarsson TS, Reeder RF, Case JL, Hughes CA. Carotid endarterectomy in nonagenarians. Arch Surg. 2005;140(7):625–8. discussion 628.

171. Beauford RB, Goldstein DJ, Sardari FF, et al. Multivessel off-pump revascularization in octogenarians: early and midterm outcomes. Ann Thorac Surg. 2003;76(1):12–7. discussion 17.

172. Chiappini B, Camurri N, Loforte A, Di Marco L, Di Bartolomeo R, Marinelli G. Outcome after aortic valve replacement in octogenarians. Ann Thorac Surg. 2004;78(1):85–9.

173. Collart F, Feier H, Kerbaul F, et al. Valvular surgery in octogenarians: operative risks factors, evaluation of Euroscore and long term results. Eur J Cardiothorac Surg. 2005;27(2):276–80.

174. Ferguson Jr TB, Hammill BG, Peterson ED, DeLong ER, Grover FL. A decade of change–risk profiles and outcomes for isolated coronary artery bypass grafting procedures, 1990–1999: a report from the STS National Database Committee and the Duke Clinical Research Institute. Society of Thoracic Surgeons. Ann Thorac Surg. 2002;73(2):480–9. discussion 489–490.

175. Huber CH, Goeber V, Berdat P, Carrel T, Eckstein F. Benefits of cardiac surgery in octogenarians–a postoperative quality of life assessment. Eur J Cardiothorac Surg. 2007;31(6):1099–105.

176. Rice DC, Correa AM, Vaporciyan AA, et al. Preoperative chemoradiotherapy prior to esophagectomy in elderly patients is not associated with increased morbidity. Ann Thorac Surg. 2005;79(2):391–7; discussion 391–397.

177. Ruol A, Portale G, Zaninotto G, et al. Results of esophagectomy for esophageal cancer in elderly patients: age has little influence on outcome and survival. J Thorac Cardiovasc Surg. 2007;133(5):1186–92.

178. Ruol A, Portale G, Castoro C, et al. Effects of neoadjuvant therapy on perioperative morbidity in elderly patients undergoing esophagectomy for esophageal cancer. Ann Surg Oncol. 2007;14(11):3243–50.

179. Poon RT, Law SY, Chu KM, Branicki FJ, Wong J. Esophagectomy for carcinoma of the esophagus in the elderly: results of current surgical management. Ann Surg. 1998;227(3):357–64.

180. Kunisaki C, Akiyama H, Nomura M, et al. Comparison of surgical outcomes of gastric cancer in elderly and middle-aged patients. Am J Surg. 2006;191(2):216–24.

181. Avital S, Kashtan H, Hadad R, Werbin N. Survival of colorectal carcinoma in the elderly. A prospective study of colorectal carcinoma and a five-year follow-up. Dis Colon Rectum. 1997;40(5):523–9.

182. Barrier A, Ferro L, Houry S, Lacaine F, Huguier M. Rectal cancer surgery in patients more than 80 years of age. Am J Surg. 2003;185(1):54–7.

183. Law WL, Choi HK, Ho JW, Lee YM, Seto CL. Outcomes of surgery for mid and distal rectal cancer in the elderly. World J Surg. 2006;30(4):598–604.

184. Aldrighetti L, Arru M, Caterini R, et al. Impact of advanced age on the outcome of liver resection. World J Surg. 2003;27(10):1149–54.

185. Cescon M, Grazi GL, Del Gaudio M, et al. Outcome of right hepatectomies in patients older than 70 years. Arch Surg. 2003;138(5):547–52.

186. Ferrero A, Vigano L, Polastri R, et al. Hepatectomy as treatment of choice for hepatocellular carcinoma in elderly cirrhotic patients. World J Surg. 2005;29(9):1101–5.

187. Menon KV, Al-Mukhtar A, Aldouri A, Prasad RK, Lodge PA, Toogood GJ. Outcomes after major hepatectomy in elderly patients. J Am Coll Surg. 2006;203(5):677–83.

188. Sohn TA, Yeo CJ, Cameron JL, et al. Should pancreaticoduodenectomy be performed in octogenarians? J Gastrointest Surg. 1998;2(3):207–16.

189. Petrowsky H, Clavien PA. Should we deny surgery for malignant hepato-pancreatico-biliary tumors to elderly patients? World J Surg. 2005;29(9):1093–100.

190. Geisler JP, Geisler HE. Radical hysterectomy in patients 65 years of age and older. Gynecol Oncol. 1994;53(2):208–11.

191. Anderson JG, Wixson RL, Tsai D, Stulberg SD, Chang RW. Functional outcome and patient satisfaction in total knee patients over the age of 75. J Arthroplasty. 1996;11(7):831–40.

192. Wurtz LD, Feinberg JR, Capello WN, Meldrum R, Kay PJ. Elective primary total hip arthroplasty in octogenarians. J Gerontol A Biol Sci Med Sci. 2003;58(5):M468–71.

193. Hamel MB, Toth M, Legedza A, Rosen MP. Joint replacement surgery in elderly patients with severe osteoarthritis of the hip or knee: decision making, postoperative recovery, and clinical outcomes. Arch Intern Med. 2008;168(13):1430–40.

194. Malata CM, Cooter RD, Batchelor AG, Simpson KH, Browning FS, Kay SP. Microvascular free-tissue transfers in elderly patients: the leeds experience. Plast Reconstr Surg. 1996;98(7):1234–41.

195. George TJ, Kilic A, Beaty CA, Conte JV, Mandal K, Shah AS. Septuagenarians bridged to heart transplantation with a ventricular assist device have outcomes similar to younger patients. Ann Thorac Surg. 2013;95(4):1251–60; discussion 1260–1251.

196. Morgan JA, John R, Weinberg AD, et al. Long-term results of cardiac transplantation in patients 65 years of age and older: a comparative analysis. Ann Thorac Surg. 2003;76(6):1982–7.

197. Goldstein DJ, Bello R, Shin JJ, et al. Outcomes of cardiac transplantation in septuagenarians. J Heart Lung Transplant. 2012;31(7):679–85.

198. Mahidhara R, Bastani S, Ross DJ, et al. Lung transplantation in older patients? J Thorac Cardiovasc Surg. 2008;135(2):412–20.

199. Minor ME, Ellozy S, Carroccio A, et al. Endovascular aortic aneurysm repair in the octogenarian: is it worthwhile? Arch Surg. 2004;139(3):308–14.

200. St Peter SD, Craft RO, Tiede JL, Swain JM. Impact of advanced age on weight loss and health benefits after laparoscopic gastric bypass. Arch Surg. 2005;140(2):165–8.

201. Chautard J, Alves A, Zalinski S, Bretagnol F, Valleur P, Panis Y. Laparoscopic colorectal surgery in elderly patients: a matched case–control study in 178 patients. J Am Coll Surg. 2008;206(2):255–60.

202. Gianetta E, de Cian F, Cuneo S, et al. Hernia repair in elderly patients. Br J Surg. 1997;84(7):983–5.

203. Amemiya T, Oda K, Ando M, et al. Activities of daily living and quality of life of elderly patients after elective surgery for gastric and colorectal cancers. Ann Surg. 2007;246(2):222–8.

204. Zierer A, Melby SJ, Lubahn JG, Sicard GA, Damiano Jr RJ, Moon MR. Elective surgery for thoracic aortic aneurysms: late functional status and quality of life. Ann Thorac Surg. 2006; 82(2):573–8.

205. de Vincentiis C, Kunkl AB, Trimarchi S, et al. Aortic valve replacement in octogenarians: is biologic valve the unique solution? Ann Thorac Surg. 2008;85(4):1296–301.

206. Vicchio M, Della Corte A, De Santo LS, et al. Tissue versus mechanical prostheses: quality of life in octogenarians. Ann Thorac Surg. 2008;85(4):1290–5.

207. Dunlop WE, Rosenblood L, Lawrason L, Birdsall L, Rusnak CH. Effects of age and severity of illness on outcome and length of stay in geriatric surgical patients. Am J Surg. 1993;165(5): 577–80.

208. Akoh JA, Mathew AM, Chalmers JW, Finlayson A, Auld GD. Audit of major gastrointestinal surgery in patients aged 80 years or over. J R Coll Surg Edinb. 1994;39(4):208–13.

209. Battafarano RJ, Piccirillo JF, Meyers BF, et al. Impact of comorbidity on survival after surgical resection in patients with stage I non-small cell lung cancer. J Thorac Cardiovasc Surg. 2002; 123(2):280–7.

210. Mehta RH, Eagle KA, Coombs LP, et al. Influence of age on outcomes in patients undergoing mitral valve replacement. Ann Thorac Surg. 2002;74(5):1459–67.

211. Muravchick S. Anesthesia for the elderly. In: Miller RD, editor. Anesthesia. 5th ed. Philadelphia: Churchill Livingston; 2000. p. 2140–56.

212. Barzan L, Veronesi A, Caruso G, et al. Head and neck cancer and ageing: a retrospective study in 438 patients. J Laryngol Otol. 1990;104(8):634–40.

213. Gupta R, Kawashima T, Ryu M, Okada T, Cho A, Takayama W. Role of curative resection in octogenarians with malignancy. Am J Surg. 2004;188(3):282–7.

214. Martin 2nd RC, Jaques DP, Brennan MF, Karpeh M. Extended local resection for advanced gastric cancer: increased survival versus increased morbidity. Ann Surg. 2002;236(2):159–65.

215. Siegelmann-Danieli N, Khandelwal V, Wood GC, et al. Breast cancer in elderly women: outcome as affected by age, tumor features, comorbidities, and treatment approach. Clin Breast Cancer. 2006;7(1):59–66.

216. Levy B. Stereotype embodiment: a psychosocial approach to aging. Curr Dir Psychol Sci. 2009;18(6):332–6.

217. Tsilimparis N, Perez S, Dayama A, Ricotta 2nd JJ. Age-stratified results from 20,095 aortoiliac aneurysm repairs: should we approach octogenarians and nonagenarians differently? J Am Coll Surg. 2012;215(5):690–701.

Nutritional Considerations in Pelvic Medicine and Surgery

5

Arif R. Chaudry, Megan Kahn-Karen, and David A. Gordon

General Considerations

Nutrition and Metabolism is an area that, not surprisingly, is often at the forefront when it comes to a discussion regarding abdominal surgery or even abdominal processes in general. Interestingly, however, this is often *not* the case when it comes to the pelvis. Patients suffering with chronic pelvic disease or facing even the possibility of having to undergo surgery can be thrust into an array of pathophysiological challenges that could affect their nutritional status. Stone disease, inflammatory bladder disorders, urinary tract infection, nausea with hyperemesis, chronic pelvic pain, and anorexia may play devastating roles as comorbidities in patients who have to undergo even minor surgery. Moreover, catabolism and wound healing may be additional hurdles for patients after major operations. Poor nutritional status can compromise the function of many organ systems, including the heart, lungs, kidneys, and gastrointestinal (GI) tract. The effects of nutritional compromise will then often spill over into areas responsible for our "host defense mechanisms." Consequently, immune function and muscle strength may also be impaired, leaving these patients more vulnerable to infectious complications. Naturally, this may further lead to a "domino effect" that may impact wound healing, thus prolonging the patient's surgical recovery. All these factors may contribute to increased morbidity and a longer hospital stay, higher readmission rates, and markedly increased health care costs.

A.R. Chaudry
Department of Surgery, Sinai Hospital of Baltimore, Baltimore, MD, USA

M. Kahn-Karen
Department of Food and Nutrition, Sinai Hospital of Baltimore, Baltimore, MD, USA

D.A. Gordon (✉)
Division of Pelvic NeuroScience, Department of Surgery, Sinai Hospital of Baltimore, 2401 W. Belvedere Ave, Baltimore, MD 21215, USA
e-mail: dgordon@lifebridgehealth.org

Also, it is important to remember that even well-nourished patients can experience adverse outcomes if metabolic and nutrition issues are not adequately assessed or addressed. During periods of increased metabolic demand even mild delays in dealing with adequate nutritional and metabolic concerns can hamper a patient's convalescence, hospital course and worst of all, postoperative recovery. Interestingly, there is a "flip side" to all of this. It may seem surprising that the nutritional status does not always improve clinical outcomes. The inherent risks associated with artificial NS may outweigh the benefits in certain patient populations. Therefore, it is important to (1) identify early which patients may benefit from enteral nutrition (EN) or even worse, parenteral nutrition (PN) intervention, (2) provide the optimal combination of nutrients, and (3) closely monitor patient progress throughout the course of therapy. This type of protocol can reduce risks of adverse clinical outcomes.

Dietary Modifications for Calcium Oxalate Urolithiasis

Kidney stones are common occurrences in the general population all over the world. Some experts refer to this disorder as nephrolithiasis while others say urolithiasis. In actuality, these terms are not totally interchangeable. The term nephrolithiasis refers to a more global metabolic picture allowing for the formation, precipitation and passage of crystal agglomerates called calculi through the renal microtubules onto the renal papillae and then into the urinary tract. Urolithiasis, on the other hand, refers to calcifications that form in the urinary system, primarily in the renal pelvis as the calcifications of nephrolithiasis fall off of the renal papillae and into the capacious renal pelvis and then ureter. From there, they can migrate into the lower urinary tract, namely the bladder or urethra. Urinary tract stone disease has been documented historically as far back as the Egyptian mummies. As much as 10 % of the US population will develop a kidney stone in their lifetime. Upper urinary tract stones (kidney, upper ureter) are more common in the USA than in the rest of the world. Researchers attribute the incidence of nephrolithiasis in the USA to dietary preferences. Not surprisingly, there are many different types of stones from a metabolic perspective. Of course some regions are more predisposed to certain types of stones rather than others. Nevertheless, the etiology of these dysfunctional metabolic processes is multifactorial and uniquely associated with dietary lifestyle habits or practices. Proper management of calculi that occur along the urinary tract includes investigation into causative factors in an effort to prevent recurrences. Urinary calculi or stones is the most common cause of acute ureteral obstruction. Approximately 1 in 1000 adults in the USA are hospitalized annually for treatment of urinary tract stones, resulting in medical costs of approximately $2 billion/year.

Any factor that reduces urinary flow or causes obstruction, which results in urinary stasis or reduces urine volume through dehydration and inadequate fluid intake, increases the risk of developing kidney stones. Low urinary flow is the most common abnormality, and most important factor to correct with kidney stones. It is important for health practitioners to concentrate on interventions for correcting low urinary volume in an effort to prevent recurrent stone disease. Consequently, increasing free water intake or increasing the baseline state of hydration of the individual is the single most important therapeutic intervention that can be done.

Increasing urine volume can reduce supersaturation, and is widely known to help prevent stone formation. Recommendations for urinary output vary, but there is general agreement that it should exceed 2 l/day, while some even encourage urinary outputs in excess of 3 l/day. A key point is that the dilution of urine is necessary "24/7," or all day, every day. A patient who voids the recommended 2 l a day between the hours of 8 am and 10 pm, but only 300 ml during the remaining 10 h of the day will have saturated urine overnight, with the possibility of precipitation and aggregation during the sleeping hours. Patients must accept the necessity of getting up at least twice at night to urinate, and should consume more water each time they rise to void. When patients who suffer with stone disease ask how they should increase their state of hydration, the simple answer is that water is best. In the USA, the most common metabolic dysfunction allows for the formation of calcium oxalate urolithiasis. For those with excessive urinary oxalates, tea products should be eliminated because teas are high-oxalate beverages. The Nurses' Health Study (NHS) showed that the type of foods consumed proved relevant for stone formers. Not surprisingly, when the "at risk" patients increased their dietary consumption of oxalates their incidence of stone formation increased. Conversely, intake of liquids that inhibited ADH (antidiuretic hormone) such as caffeine or beer allowed for an increased diuresis and decreased the incidence of calcium oxalate urolithiasis. Although calcium intake was previously considered a culprit, current evidence indicates that urinary oxalate is the most important determinant of calcium oxalate crystallization. Individuals who tend to form stones of this type experience a significant increase in urinary oxalate excretion with even small increases in oxalate intake, whereas persons who do not form these stones do not experience a similar increase in urinary oxalate excretion with increased oxalate intake.[7] Patients should be advised to avoid high-oxalate foods, such as rhubarb, spinach, strawberries, chocolate (especially dark), wheat bran, nuts, beets, and tea. Alternatively, certain food preparation methods may be used to reduce oxalate content. Boiling, for example, reduces soluble oxalate content by 30–87 %, compared with steaming, which achieves a 5–53 % reduction.

Limit dietary intake in foods high in oxalate. By avoiding foods very high in oxalate, you may reduce the oxalate in your urine. A list of high oxalate foods include:

- Protein Foods (soy and otherwise)
- Grains
- Carmel colored beverages such as colas
- Caffeine containing beverages such as coffee or teas.
- Fruits (plums, strawberries, blackberries, and Blueberries)
- Vegetables (beets, greens, carrots, cauliflower, and rhubarb)
- Nuts (including peanut butter)
- Tofu grits

Though only a minority percentage of urinary oxalates come from dietary sources. Dietary reduction of oxalate should be advised for calcium oxalate stone formers. It has been suggested that because there is much less oxalate in the urine than calcium in the urine, urinary oxalate concentration is much more critical to the formation of calcium oxalate crystals than is the urinary calcium concentration. Therefore, reducing urine oxalates will have a more powerful effect on stone formation than can reduction of urine calcium. Patients with calcium oxalate stones, particularly those with documented hyperoxaluria, should avoid foods high in oxalates. Vitamin C is a precursor to endogenous production of oxalates, so some clinicians recommend avoiding mega-doses of vitamin C. Understanding the importance of modulating dietary intake of oxalate in patients who suffer with calcium oxalate urolithiasis, it is still important to remember that there are other metabolic manipulations which can be added to any therapeutic regimen to help decrease the tubular precipitation of calcium oxalate crystals. These would include (1) decreasing sodium intake, (2) decreasing protein intake, and (3) decreasing percentage of body fat and decreasing total body weight.

Because sodium competes with calcium for reabsorption in the renal tubules, excess sodium intake and consequent excretion result in loss of calcium in the urine. High-sodium diets are associated with greater calcium excretion in the urine. Metabolic studies in patients who are placed on high sodium diets reveal exceptionally high levels of urine calcium over 24 h. Patients may often deny salt intake, feeling that if they do not use the "salt shaker" that their diet is "low sodium." They quite likely are ignorant of hidden sodium sources in the diet. Sodium is a common preservative in canned and frozen foods, and is endemic in restaurant foods. Instruction on careful inspection of food labels and wise food choices helps patients identify and reduce sodium in their diets. Consultation with a registered dietician may help the patient achieve the specific goal of a sodium intake of 2000 mg or less per day.

Although it is emphasized to a lesser degree, some experts feels that Obesity and Body Mass Index is associated with an Increased Risk of Calcium Oxalate Urolithiasis. Although there is some evidence to support this, it has not been well proven clinically.

Interestingly is that this association is even more pronounced in women. Nevertheless, it must be remembered that the absolute value of weight loss with respect to stone formation in general has not been proven to a statistically significant standard.

Finally, it is important to remember that one does not necessarily have to wait to see a registered dietician or a physician to discuss dietary modification in stone disease. There are excellent educational resources on the Internet for patients seeking nutritional counseling. A great example is Nutrition Data. Here patients can search by category to view things like the standard sodium content, as well as additional information regarding vitamin and mineral content, calories, suggested healthier substitutes, and even the individual amino acid compositions of each protein. Under "Tools," patients can search within food categories like "dairy products" for choices highest in calcium and lowest in sodium. This site is complex and may be overwhelming to patients without good computer and Web skills, but is extraordinarily comprehensive.

Dietary Suggestions for Cystitis: Infectious, Inflammatory, & Interstitial

Cystitis is the inflammatory swelling of the bladder wall and is one of the dreaded eventualities of life as a female. However, in an effort to not be construed as sexist, it should be noted that, of course males are susceptible to cystitis but their attendant gross anatomy makes the initiation of this process much more challenging and much less likely. In any event, from a symptomatic perspective, cystitis translates as an unpleasant sensation deep in the anterior pelvis. The associated sensory phenomena of pain, pressure, and discomfort are quickly related to the urinary bladder with an even quicker desire by the patient for rapid eradication. This situation is most often implicated to some type of infectious agent, which incites a

physiologic response that kicks off a cascade of events bringing inflammatory cells and inflammatory mediators to the bladder wall to face off with the infecting microorganisms. Hence begins the microscopic "Battle Royale"! Fortunately for most females, the prescription for relief is simple and associated with beginning therapy which is targeted at the destruction of the microorganism. Most often, this means some type of antibiotic or antiviral agent. These agents work hand in hand with the host's natural inflammatory defense mechanisms to remove the infecting microorganism. Once successful eradication has been achieved, the host's natural physiologic response should "shut down" those inflammatory cascades and segue into the relief of her lower urinary tract symptoms. It is very important to note here that it is the "transmural inflammatory reaction" at the level of the bladder wall that is primarily implicated in the genesis and perpetuation of these painful lower urinary tract symptoms, NOT the infecting microorganism! So, what happens if the antibiotic or the antiviral agent successfully achieves eradication of the offending microorganism BUT the host's natural inflammatory response does NOT subside? What is the patient left with? If this situation exists, then the patient is left with an active inflammatory reaction within the substance of a swollen, tender, erythematous bladder wall and hence "persistence of painful urinary urgency" WITHOUT an active offending microorganism! For a long time, this was considered an "oxymoron," i.e. cystitis without infection. Nevertheless, essentially, what the patient is left with is a Noninfectious Inflammatory Cystitis. Perhaps, the most dreaded complication of all within this arena.

Interstitial Cystitis is a disease characterized by hypersensitivity of the bladder lining, even after resolution of the inflammation of the bladder wall. IC is largely diagnosed due to specific notable symptoms as there are currently no specific tests for the definitive diagnosis of the condition. In essence, it is a disease of exclusionary criteria as it is necessary to rule out conditions with similar symptoms. Approximately 90 % of IC patients are women, which may suggest a genetic link to this disease. The most common symptoms of IC, seen in over 60 % of patients, include urinary frequency, urinary urgency, and pelvic pain exacerbating by the filling or emptying of the bladder. Additional symptoms may include pelvic pain associated with menstrual cycle, constipation or irritable bowel syndrome, slow urinary stream, pain with sexual intercourse, depression, pain at the tip of the penis, the groin, or in the testicles in male patients. One of the most interesting aspects of this process is the symptomatic association with worsening lower urinary tract symptoms after GI processing and renal excretion of biochemical intake. Essentially, a very close dietary association, where flares of lower urinary tract pressure and pain are individually linked with specific foods or beverages. In fact, when it comes to a discussion of diet with respect to symptomatic clinical flares of dysfunctional abdominal or pelvic processes, there is not much else that expresses the intricate degree of predictability that IC possesses.

"To Eat or Not to Eat", the Big Question with IC

If every well-intentioned family or friend who encouraged my patients with almost any type of cystitis to take a few swigs of cranberry juice because they believed it was "good for all that ails you when it comes to the bladder," it seems that they are woefully wrong!! Furthermore, if they had to live with 2 min of bladder burning that one can develop after imbibing a "high acid" liquid, believe me, that type of advice would be altered. Research has confirmed that foods and beverages high in acid can worsen bladder symptoms. Something as simple as a daily cup of a citrus drink can provoke serious pain and discomfort. Dietary modification is a simple, affordable and often times, the MOST effective strategy for patients with cystitis.

In July 2007, formative research on IC and diet was published in The Journal of Urology, which listed the top trigger foods for IC. These foods were the same foods that patients had been talking about for 20 years, validating patients' experiences shared via Internet message boards and face-to-face support groups. Subsequently, in 2011, the American Urological Association published guidelines that specifically recommended diet modification as one of the first-line self-care therapies for newly diagnosed IC patients and RDs as the vehicles to deliver such therapy. Most importantly the best way to help these patients is to learn as much about the disease as possible.

Just how does diet affect IC symptoms? Much of that remains to be answered, but much of that research will come in time. The foundation of that initial research article on IC and diet is going to help pave the way for answers. Urologists, gynecologists, PAs, NPs, and most of all RDs should use is the previously mentioned list of trigger foods to potentially predict IC flares. That is, those foods most likely to produce problems for the majority of IC. When counseling new IC patients, Beyer suggests showing them this list and asking them to try eliminating as many of these foods as possible. Many patients often do very well with dietary modification alone.

Up to 90 % of patients with IC report insensitivities to various food items. The following foods have been known to exacerbate symptoms in those with IC:

- citrus fruits (oranges, grapefruits, lemons), apricots, apples, avocados, bananas, cantaloupes, cranberry, grapes, peaches, plums, and some berries
- tomatoes and tomato sauces
- coffee, tea, and various caffeinated beverages
- carbonated and alcoholic beverages
- spicy foods
- Vitamin C
- Artificial sweeteners

Dietary modifications play an instrumental role in managing the symptoms of Interstitial Cystitis. For the IC patient, trigger foods vary and elimination diets may be the first means of regulating symptoms. Keeping a food log and tracking foods consumed, trends, and associated symptoms is recommended in order to initially isolate foods or food groups that may elicit symptoms. If a specific food tends to cause an increase in symptoms, removing that food for 1–2 weeks will help to determine if that is one to be eliminated. Trial and error is often the best means of developing a specific diet in those with IC. Fluid intake can also play a vital role in the management of symptoms. Many IC patients limit fluid intake in the hopes of decreasing urinary urgency and frequency. However, limiting water intake specifically can actually concentrate the urine leading to worsened symptoms. Due to dietary restrictions, those with IC may benefit from a daily multivitamin as deficiencies may occur with the exclusion of specific food groups.

How to Begin an IC Diet

With respect to the treatment of Interstitial Cystitis most experts would agree that few things, if anything, are more important than diet. Having said that, what is often confounding about this whole thing, is the individuality that surrounds metabolic and dietary interventions with respect to IC. In fact, it is the individual variations between the baseline genetics of patients that frustrate physicians who deal with this disease. Just when you think that you have the "acid-base balance" associated with diet figured out for your practice, you run into a series of patients that seem to breakdown the protocol. Again, although this probably doesn't have to be stated out right, BUT, when diet is not well controlled, the patient's general state of well being is usually suboptimal. Suffice it to say that, diet is crucial to ultimately getting control of the pain component in Interstitial Cystitis.

Here it is important to note that this part of IC is where the "doctor-patient" relationship takes on its biggest role. In a certain way, it is this relationship that really defines how well patients do in the long run. Perhaps the key to this relationship is the ability for both the patient and the doctor to accept "joint responsibility" with respect to "outcomes." The physician can *NOT* be solely responsible for interventional therapy while letting the patient manage their own dietary and nutraceutical issues. This is a prescription for disaster! However, this is also the point where it is important for physicians who make the decision to commit to the treatment of these patients to build an infrastructure that will allow them to effectively manage these subtle, difficult but important components of a patient's treatment protocol. In this arena, being able to work with an RD who has an interest and experience can be a significant "value added" service that a practice can offer to a patient.

To begin to put together a diet for the IC patient who is becoming difficult to get under control with respect to pelvic pressure and pelvic pain, one must go back to the biochemical basics of metabolism and diet. Here the "Acid/Base Balance" becomes extremely important. It is that "charged species" such as the hydrogen ion (H+) in acidic foods as well as anions (negatively charged molecules) such as oxalate can cause electrophysiologic dysfunction of the more superficial layers of the bladder lining. Even worse is if these caustic ions are able to penetrate more deeply, they may even allow for depolarization of the underlying detrusor muscle. Consequently, working with a certified RD to create, as best as physiologically possible, an ionically neutral menu. At that point, the hope is that it will decrease the inflammatory cascade within the mucosal and submucosal lining, allowing the inflammatory process within the bladder to "calm itself." Not surprisingly, if one had to characterize this diet, the common verbal description often includes the word "bland." Although this word is somewhat nonspecific, the goal of this type of diet is to eradicate the ionically active particles in food that have a tendency to react and inflame the more superficial soft tissue of the lower urinary tract. Essentially, one can look at constructing this diet in two ways. The first is to imagine "wiping the slate clean" and incorporating those foods that have the potential to be less ionically active, or *to eliminate* those foods which seem to tend to cause irritation at the bladder level. Some people would consider this a type of Elimination Diet, which is not an uncommon technique in the world of Allergy and Immunology. The specifics of this technique are as follows.

The Elimination Technique for IC Dietary Modification

How about a dietary protocol to begin with boiled chicken, boiled potatoes, and oatmeal as the initiating ingredients. The key is to be plain, using no other additives. Salt is discouraged but if you have to use it, keep it to a minimum. To begin, only 3–4 very bland foodstuffs should be on the menu for the first 2–3 days, depending on how long you can stand it or how longs it takes your bladder to calm itself, whatever comes first. Referring to Helena de Jong in "Cooking with IC" which is a very popular and informative internet blog. These patients need a place to experiment in a creative fashion, in the world of food while following the IC diet. If one uses the "Cooking with IC" recommendations as a template, then your individual beginning IC Diet might start by picking 2–3 foods from the initiation column.

For the first 5 days, select 3–4 of these most plain basic foods from the column below. This should help to start to decrease the unbridled inflammatory response that is usually the perpetuating component with respect to pelvic pain in IC.

- Turkey
- Tuna
- Venison
- Lamb
- Rice
- potatoes well cooked with no skin
- Canned: Peaches, Cherries, Apricots, Nectarines, Plums, Prunes

Once you've made it through the first 5-day phase, then the patient can start adding food groups. You add as much of each food group as possible for 2 days. The fresh vegetables and fruit should be tested in the raw uncooked state if possible. Finally, if you already know that a food group bothers you, then there is no need to test that group.

1. *Dairy Products*—Milk and cheeses (exclude any colored cheeses that have food dyes)
2. *Cereals and Grains*—barley, corn oats, rye, wheat,
3. *Legume Pea Family*—peanuts, beans, (navy, lima, green), peas, tofu, bean sprouts.
4. *Meats*—beef, chicken, pork
5. Eggs
6. *Fruits* (1)—apple, strawberry, raspberry pears
7. *Vegetables* (high carbohydrate) potato, tomato, eggplant
8. *Fruits* (2)—fresh peaches, cherries apricots, nectarines, plums, prunes, almonds
9. *Miscellaneous*—lettuce, sesame seeds, sunflower seeds, carrots, celery, parsley, parsnip

In any event, when the patient gets to the point where you are adding food groups, it should be done with daily assessments and reassessments of "pain levels." Here the use of validated instruments may be helpful. In any event, if pelvic pain and pressure remain manageable, then a second foodstuff may be introduced. For instance, one may add sautéed white meat chicken. If it does not increase your pain level, you can consider it a success and move on to the next food. When you come upon a food that puts you in a flare, STOP TESTING foods until the flare is gone. Again, although this is a very time-consuming process, it is the best way to control the attendant inflammation that leads to clinically significant flares. If there is something that you notice immediately throws you into a flare reaction, here is what you should do. Take some powdered baking soda and mix 1/2 tablespoon with water. This should neutralize the upstart inflammatory response at the level of the bladder fairly quickly. Finally, remember, if part of our treatment strategy for IC is maintaining a metabolism that is as close to electrophysiologically neutral as possible, then diet takes on an extremely important role. Obviously, we have gone through the basics as well as what to do when emergent flares arise. However, the key to success is chronicity. So, to that end, it is always good to keep some calcium glycerol phosphate around, aka Prelief. It can be used on foods just prior to eating and is very effective in establishing neutrality. The recommended dose is two tablets or packets, depending on what is available in your area. However, do not be afraid to double this dose if need be. It is a great adjunct.

Nutritional Aspects in Surgery

Pelvic Surgery in the Nutritionally Compromised Patient

Malnutrition prior to surgery can negatively impact post-surgical acute care patients in relation to poor wound healing, increased length of stay, increased hospital care costs, muscle wasting, increased risk of both morbidity and mortality, hospital admissions. Nutrition screening can identify those at nutritional risk for operative complications. Malnutrition can be diagnosed using six specific criteria: insufficient or reduced energy intake, unintentional weight loss, changes in body composition including loss of muscled mass and/or loss of subcutaneous fat, localized or generalized fluid accumulation, and diminished functional status such as reduced hand grip strength. It is recommend that diagnoses are determined based on two or more of these characteristics.

Malnutrition in surgical patients probably occurs more commonly after surgery. There are many reasons for this, including changes in metabolic demands such as those seen with systemic infections, inadequate energy intake (related to poor appetite, changes in mental status, issues with chewing or swallowing), malabsorption related to pathological diseases of the gut, and increases in losses via emesis, fistulae, or diarrhea. Serum albumin can serve as an indicator as a barometer of current nutritional status only for many patients. However, the use of albumin and an indicator is much more effective when the patient is ambulatory and in pre-operative settings in which no other co-morbidities are present. In the acute-care setting, albumin should be assessed concurrently with pre-albumin and inflammatory markers such as C-reactive protein and white blood cell counts. Fluid shifts and vascular permeability can augment the concentration of serum proteins making them poor indicators of nutritional status.

Perioperative Nutritional Optimization

Optimizing nutritional status in patients at risk for malnutrition prior to surgical procedures can greatly impact post-surgical outcomes. One study found that a weight loss of less than 10 % in the 6 months prior to major abdominal surgeries lead to higher incidences of post-operative surgical complications when compared with those without weight loss prior to surgery.

In the "not so distant" past, the entire focus of more traditional programs for nutritional care in an operative setting was focused on GI rest. That is, it stressed resting the gastrointestinal tract before resumption of feeding. Now, however, a perioperative care program has become preferred. One such program is the Enhanced Recovery After Surgery protocol or ERAS. ERAS has been shown to reduce recovery time and length of stay by 2–3 days on average. In addition, this program may even reduce perioperative complications by 30–50 %. This care plan emphasizes optimization of nutritional status before, during, and following surgical procedures.

Pre-operative fasting is the older traditional protocols were due to concerns of pulmonary aspiration. This kind of situation actually places patients in a more catabolic state, which can attenuate suboptimal surgical outcomes and delay the healing process. Surgeons and anesthesiologists ensure gastric contents are less than 200 ml prior to surgery in order to avoid potentiating aspiration the potential for its attendant pneumonitis. However, a study by the Cochran Review demonstrated *NO* cases of aspiration when there is consumption of clear liquids even when they are offered to the patient up to 2 h prior to surgery. In fact, avoidance of excessive pre-operative fasting may lead to more positive outcomes in the post-surgical patient. That same Cochrane review also showed that solid meals can be safely consumed up to 6 h prior to surgery. This is NOT to say that this is the way it must be done in all cases now. However, it does suggest that strict adherence to the 8 h. time table may NOT be an absolute, and, although not completely clear, there may actually be benefits to some intake of clear liquids within that time frame.

Surgical intervention is known to cause alterations in metabolic demands. These metabolic alterations are usually up-regulatory in nature. In addition, there may be associated endocrine changes augmenting the entire process. For example, surgery can trigger insulin resistance and hyperglycemia in the post operative period. Durations are variable, but they can last up to 2–4 weeks. Obviously, the way that carbohydrates are processed is directly linked to changes in metabolism. Here the American Society of Parenteral and Enteral Nutrition (A.S.P.E.N.) has studied this relationship between metabolic changes, endocrine effects, and carbohydrate demands extensively. To that end, ASPEN has studies these relationships in detail and has shown that pre-operative carbohydrate-loading combined with epidural anesthesia is thought to decrease the stress hormones, epinephrine and cortisol. This in turn may decrease insulin resistance by 50 %. Consequently, ASPEN has set up protocols which have now been elevated to guideline status in this regard. Here, ASPEN has developed the following pre-operative carbohydrate protocol that has received much attention. Here, 800 ml of clear, carbohydrate-rich liquids given at midnight. This equates to about 100 g of pure carbohydrate by weight which translates to 400 kcal of energy. Subsequently, 400 ml of the same carbohydrate-rich formula is given 2 h prior to surgical intervention. ASPEN has shown that this simple protocol can decrease postoperative complication rates by almost 50%! Their rationale is that clear, carbohydrate-rich fluids pre-procedure stimulate an anabolic state leading to reduced glycogenolysis, which increases blood glucose control, and then stimulates the uptake of glucose by skeletal muscle cells. Sports drinks, which contain approximately 6–7% of carbohydrates may not provide a significant benefit in controlling post-surgical catabolism. Instead, what is necessary are fluids containing approximately 12% carbohydrate in the form of a complex sugar such as maltodextrin should be provided to limit osmolality and delays in gastric emptying.

After carbohydrates, protein metabolism has gleaned much interest by many groups as a modality to help improve surgical outcomes. High-protein foods or oral supplements prior to surgical procedures have been shown to improve surgical outcomes, especially in the malnourished preoperative population. In a study by Dock-Nascimento et al. preoperative fasting with maltodextrin and a glutamine-rich clear beverage 2 h prior to procedure led to less insulin resistance, a more favorable acute-phase response of Interleukin-6 and C-reactive protein, as well as reduced nitrogen losses when compared with the control. Another protein alternative known as whey protein contains essential amino acids including the branched chain amino acids and can be quickly digested and taken up by skeletal muscle cells to attenuate skeletal protein losses in stressful situations such as surgery and trauma.

When one divides the surgical experience into phases, there are three major categories. These are, respectively, the "Pre-Operative Phase," the "Operative Phase," and the "Post-Operative Phase." With respect to the "Post-Operative Phase," the most coveted position to have, is that of "Anabolism." The most desired post-operative anabolic state is achieved by trying to maximize all macronutrient needs. Unfortunately, a common scenario in the Post-Operative Phase is the patient with adequate protein provision despite inadequate energy intake. This scenario can attenuate muscle protein losses in the surgically stressed patient. ASPEN guidelines recommend 20–25% of energy intake, or 1.5–2.0 g/kg/day, from protein sources in the surgically stressed patient population. In the obese populations with a BMI greater than 30 2.0 g/kg of ideal body weight is recommended. Nitrogen Balance can be a useful clinical tool in assessing protein status in the acute care population. A 24-h urine collection following surgery can assist in determining current protein turnover and subsequent needs. By assessing urinary urea nitrogen concentrations, clinicians can estimate total protein needs based on total nitrogen intake and total nitrogen output related to nitrogen losses from skin, urine, stool, and body fluids provided there are no excess GI losses via tubes, drains, etc. As previously noted, albumin and pre-albumin should not be used to inflammation and fluid shifts and as such are confounders when it comes for benchmarks of protein intake.

Immuno-Nutrition is an emerging area when it comes to post-operative phase assessment. Essentially, Immuno-nutrition emphasizes the use of nutrients known to improve general cell biology and modulate inflammation. There are five nutrients that have been shown to have the most promise in this arena include amino acids (1) L-arginine and (2) glutamine, polyunsaturated long-chain fatty acids, specifically (3) (ω-3 PUFAs), and antioxidants such as (4) ascorbic acid and (5) selenium. Glutamine, the most abundant amino acid in the blood, is known for tissue protection, immune regulation preservation of glutathione and antioxidant capacity, and preservation of cellular metabolism following injury. L-Arginine is another essential amino acid recommended following surgery, trauma, and injury due to its role in T-lymphocyte function and nitric oxide production leading to improved microcirculation. ASPEN notes plasma arginine levels are noted to decrease by up to 50% for days to week following trauma or surgery. In the case of ω-3 PUFAs, an essential fatty acid that must be acquired from the diet, inflammation may be controlled through the formation of EPA and DHA which are further responsible for the formation of the 3-series prostaglandins and 5-series leukotrienes eicosanoids. EPA and DHA have been known to decrease arachidonic acid-derived inflammatory mediators. In addition, ω-3 PUFAs are incorporated into the phospholipid-rich membranes of immune cells such as macrophages, monocytes, and neutrophils influencing fluidity and the activity of membrane-bound proteins. Ascorbic acid, or Vitamin C, is a powerful antioxidant that interacts with superoxide, hydroxyl radicals, and singlet oxygen to prevent cellular damage. Selenium has also been noted to protect against oxidative injury. A study by Marik et al. found that immunonutrition significantly reduced the risk of acquired infections, wound complications, and length of stay in high risk-surgical patients compared to those on a controlled enteral diet. Together, these immunonutrients may positively affect post-surgical outcomes through immunomodulating and anti-inflammatory mechanisms.

Patients at high risk for nutritional deficiencies and malnutrition should receive oral, enteral, or parenteral nutritional support when deemed appropriate. When the gut is fully functional, oral nutrition is recommended prior to trialing nutrition support in order to prevent gut atrophy. In cases where nutritional needs are unable to be met orally, enteral nutrition is preferred over parenteral nutrition with the goal of preventing catabolism and stimulating anabolism.

Suggested Reading

1. Barbosa-Cesnik C, Brown MB, Buxton M, DeBusscher J, Foxman B. Cranberry juice fails to prevents recurrent urinary tract infection: results from a randomized placebo-controlled trial. Clin Infect Dis. 2011;52(1):23–30.
2. Bassaly R, Downes K, Hart S. Dietary consumption triggers in interstitial cystitis/bladder pain syndrome patients. Female Pelvic Med Reconstr Surg. 2011;17(1):36–9.
3. Borges Dock-Nascimento D, de Aguilar-Nascimento JE, Sepulveda Magalhaes Faria M, Caporossi C, Linetzky Waitzberg D. Evaluation of the effects of a preoperative 2-hour fast with maltodextrine and glutamine on insulin resistance, acute-phase response, nitrogen balance, and serum glutathione after laparoscopic cholecystectomy: a controlled randomized trial. JPEN J Parenter Enteral Nutr. 2012;36(1):43–52.
4. Evans DC, Martindale RG, Kiraly LN, Jones CM. Nutrition optimization prior to surgery. Nutr Clin Pract. 2014;29(1):10–21.
5. Fearon KC, Luff R. The nutritional management of surgical patients: enhanced recovery after surgery. Proc Nutr Soc. 2003;62:807–11.
6. Friedlander JI, Shorter B, Moldwin RM. Diet and its role in interstitial cystitis/bladder pain syndrome (IC/BPS) and comorbid conditions. BJU Int. 2012;109:1584–91.
7. Gillis C, Nguyen TH, Liberman AS, Carli F. Nutrition adequacy in enhanced recovery after surgery: a single academic center experience. Nutr Clin Pract. 2015;30(3):414–9.
8. Guay DR. Cranberry and urinary tract infections. Drugs. 2009;69(7):775–807.
9. Jepson RG, Williams G, Craig JC. Cranberries for preventing urinary tract infections. Cochrane Datab Syst Rev. 2012;17(10):CD001321.
10. Ljungqvist O. ERAS- enhanced recovery after surgery: moving evidence-based perioperative care to practice. J Parent Enteral Nutr. 20143;38 (5):559–66.
11. Marik PE, Zaloga GP. Immunonutrition in high-risk surgical patients: a systematic review and analysis of the literature. J Parenter Enteral Nutr. 2010;34(4):378–86.
12. Martindale RG, McClave SA, Taylor B, Lawson CM. Perioperative nutrition: what is the current landscape? J Parenter Enteral Nutr. 2013;37(1):5S–20.
13. Moldwin RM. The interstitial cystitis survival guide. Oakland: New Harbinger Publications; 2000.
14. Mueller CM, Kovacevich DS, McClave SA, Miller SJ, Baird Schwartz D. The A.S.P.E.N. adult nutrition support core curriculum. Am Soc Parent Enteral Nutr. 2012
15. Mueller C, Compher C, Ellen DM. A.S.P.E.N clinical guidelines. J Parenter Enteral Nutr. 2011;35(1):16–24.
16. Peres Pimenta G, de Aguilar-Nascimento JE. Prolonged preoperative fasting in elective surgical patients: why should we reduce it? Nutr Clin Pract. 2014;29(1):22–8.
17. Pogatschnik C, Steiger E. Review of preoperative carbohydrate loading. Nutr Clin Pract. 2015;30(5):660–4.
18. Raz R, Chazan B, Dan M. Cranberry juice and urinary tract infection. Clin Infect Dis. 2004;38(10):1413–9.
19. Ronald A. The etiology of urinary tract infection: traditional and emerging pathogens. Am J Med. 2002;113(1):14–9.
20. van Stijn MF, Korkic-Halilovic I, Bakker MS, van der Ploeg T, van Leeuwen PA, Houddijk AP. Preoperative nutrition status and postoperative outcome in elderly general surgery patients: a systematic review. J Parenter Enteral Nutr. 2013;37(1):37–43.
21. Wang C-H, Fang C-C, Chen N-C, Liu SS-H, Yu P-H, Wu T-Y, et al. Cranberry-containing products for prevention of urinary tract infections in susceptible populations. Arch Intern Med. 2012;172(13):988–96.
22. White J, Guenter P, Jensen G, Malone A, Schofield M. Consensus statement of the academy of nutrition and dietetics/American society for parenteral and enteral nutrition: characteristics recommended for the identification and documentation of adult malnutrition (undernutrition). J Acad Nutr Diet. 2012;112(5):730–8.

Microbiology of Virulence: Urinary Tract Infection Versus Colonization

6

Rupinder Singh, Ashrit Multani, and John Cmar

Introduction

There has been great controversy as to what differentiates infection of the urinary tract from mere colonization. The term colonization may be considered obsolete, or, it may be viewed as a clinical scenario on the same continuum as infection. The urinary tract is a sterile medium, and therefore, any presence of bacteria in the urine should be regarded as an infection, regardless of symptomatology. The requirement of delineation between asymptomatic and symptomatic bacteriuria occurs at the level of whether treatment is warranted or not. The additional presence of a catheter adds another level of complexity to the clinical equation. Catheter-associated urinary tract infections are the leading cause of secondary nosocomial bacteremia. An estimated 20 % of hospital-acquired bacteremias arise from the urinary tract, and the mortality associated with this condition is about 10 %. This chapter will seek to increase the understanding of the definitions, epidemiology, etiology (including risk factors and microbiology), pathogenesis, clinical presentation, diagnosis, treatment (including information on antimicrobial drug resistance), complications, and prevention of urinary tract infections.

Definitions

Urinary tract infection (UTI), in patients without a bladder catheter, is defined as the presence of symptomatology in combination with a positive urine culture, containing at least

R. Singh
Department of Geriatric Pelvic Medicine and Neurourology, Department of Internal Medicine, Sinai Hospital of Baltimore, Baltimore, MD 21215, USA

A. Multani • J. Cmar (✉)
Department of Medicine, Sinai Hospital of Baltimore, 2435 West Belvedere Ave, Hoffberger Bldg, Ste 56, Baltimore, MD 21215, USA
e-mail: jcmar@lifebridgehealth.org

10^5 colony-forming units (CFU) per milliliter with the isolation of fewer than two microorganisms.

Catheter-associated urinary tract infection (CAUTI) must contain at least 10^3 CFU/mL, with the urine sample being obtained with an aseptic technique.

Asymptomatic bacteriuria is defined as isolation of a specified quantitative count of bacteria in an appropriately collected urine specimen from an individual without symptoms or signs (e.g., the absence of fever greater than 38 °C, suprapubic tenderness or costovertebral angle pain or tenderness) of urinary tract infection [1].

For women, asymptomatic bacteriuria is defined as two consecutive clean-catch voided urine specimens with isolation of the same organism in quantitative counts of at least 10^5 CFU/mL [2].

For men, asymptomatic bacteriuria is defined as a single clean-catch voided urine specimen with one bacterial species isolated in counts of at least 10^5 CFU/mL in the absence of symptoms [2]. The presence of pyuria (at least 10 leukocytes/mm^3 of uncentrifuged urine) is insufficient for the diagnosis of bacteriuria [3].

Symptomatic catheter-related bacteriuria is defined as the presence of fever greater than 38 °C, suprapubic tenderness, costovertebral angle tenderness, or otherwise unexplained systemic symptoms (e.g., malaise, altered mental status, hypotension, metabolic acidosis, respiratory alkalosis, or a systemic inflammatory response syndrome), together with one of the following:

- Urine culture with greater than 10^5 CFU/mL irrespective of urinalysis
- Urine culture with greater than 10^3 CFU/mL with evidence of pyuria (urinalysis positive for leukocyte esterase and/or nitrite, microscopic pyuria or presence of microbes seen on the Gram stain of unspun urine) [4].

Patients who have had indwelling urinary catheters within the past 48 h (even if they are not in place at the time of infection) are considered to have catheter-associated UTI if they meet these definitions.

In asymptomatic catheterized men or women, bacteriuria is defined as a single catheterized specimen with isolation of a single organism in quantitative counts of at least 10^2 CFU/mL [2].

Infections of the urinary tract include cystitis (infection of the urinary bladder, or the lower urinary tract), pyelonephritis (infection of the kidney, or the upper urinary tract), or both. Prostatitis, inflammation of the prostate gland, is a separate but similar clinical entity that is beyond the scope of this chapter.

Emphysematous urinary tract infections are infections (cystitis, pyelitis, or pyelonephritis) of the lower or upper urinary tract associated with gas formation.

A urinary tract infection involving a healthy, ambulatory woman with no history suggestive of anatomical or functional urinary tract abnormality is termed as uncomplicated.

A urinary tract infection becomes complicated when it is associated with another underlying condition that increases the risk of treatment failure. These conditions include diabetes, pregnancy, symptoms for at least a week prior to seeking medical attention, hospital-acquired infection, urinary tract obstruction, presence of urinary tract hardware (e.g., indwelling urethral catheter, stent, nephrostomy tube, or urinary diversion), recent urinary tract instrumentation, functional or anatomical urinary tract abnormality, history of childhood urinary tract infection, or renal transplantation. In addition, any urinary tract infection in a male, by definition, is considered to be complicated because they are more likely to be associated with anatomic abnormalities (e.g., bladder outlet obstruction secondary to prostatic hypertrophy or recent instrumentation), and may require surgical intervention to prevent further complications.

Infection with a multidrug resistant organism is also considered complicated, although these patients are not at a higher risk of treatment failure so long as an appropriate antibiotic, based on susceptibility profiles, is used.

Acute complicated pyelonephritis is the progression of an upper urinary tract infection to emphysematous pyelonephritis, renal corticomedullary abscess, perinephric abscess, or papillary necrosis.

The distinction between reinfection and relapse is difficult to make and is arbitrarily defined. A recurrent infection is called a relapse if the infecting strain is the same as the prior infection, and the recurrence occurs within 2 weeks of treatment completion for the prior infection. A recurrent infection is called a reinfection if the infection recurs more than 2 weeks after treatment completion, regardless of the nature of the uropathogenic strain. If there is a documented sterile urine culture between the two infections, and the patient is off antibiotics, the recurrence is also called a reinfection.

Epidemiology

Urinary tract infections are the most common bacterial infection encountered in the ambulatory setting. They accounted for 8.6 million visits nationally in 2007, with 84% of those cases involving women. By age 32, half of women have had at least one urinary tract infection [5].

For sexually active young women, symptomatic UTI carries a high incidence. Increased risk is seen with recent sexual intercourse, recent spermicide use, and a personal history of UTI [6]. Cystitis also occurs in postmenopausal women [7]. Recurrent uncomplicated UTIs are seen even with anatomic and physiologic urinary tract normality. Acute pyelonephritis is less common than acute cystitis. Recurrent pyelonephritis in healthy women is uncommon. Infections with *Escherichia coli* (*E. coli*) in particular tend to recur within the first 6 months [8].

The prevalence of asymptomatic bacteriuria among healthy women tends to increase with age. It affects approximately 1% of schoolgirls and more than 20% among women over the age of 80 years. This also tends to correlate with sexual activity [9]. Greater prevalence is seen in premenopausal married women than nuns of the same age [10]. There is no significant difference between pregnant (2%) and nonpregnant (7%) women [11]. Asymptomatic bacteriuria generally has a transient (rarely lasting longer than a few weeks) in young healthy women.

Diabetic women have a three- to fourfold higher prevalence (8–15%), with a correlation seen between the duration and presence of long-term diabetic sequelae. Duration of diabetes more than 10 years has a relative risk of 2.6. Insulin use also appears to carry an increased risk with a relative risk of 3.7 [12].

In pregnancy, bacteriuria occurs in 2–7%, especially in multiparous women. This prevalence is similar to that seen in nonpregnant women. The organisms are also similar in species and virulence between pregnant and nonpregnant women [13]. Bacteriuria is commonly seen in the first month of pregnancy [14]. Acute cystitis occurs in 1–2% of pregnant women. There is a greater likelihood among pregnant women for bacteriuria to progress to pyelonephritis. Up to 30–40% of pregnant women with untreated asymptomatic bacteriuria will develop symptomatic UTI, including pyelonephritis. This risk is reduced by 70–80% if the bacteriuria is treated [15].

For young healthy adult men, the incidence of symptomatic UTI (5–8 UTIs per year per 10,000 young to middle-aged men) is much lower than that in women. Asymptomatic bacteriuria is rare among healthy young males [16]. The prevalence rises to 6–15% among men over the age of 75 years [17]. The presence of diabetes does not confer any additional risk of asymptomatic bacteriuria among males.

Candiduria is becoming increasingly common, with nosocomial UTIs due to Candida species being 22% between

1986 and 1989 to almost 40 % between 1992 and 1997 [18]. Many of these patients were asymptomatic; therefore, a distinction between infection versus colonization could not be delineated [19].

Indwelling bladder catheters confer a significant risk of bacteriuria. Patients develop bacteriuria at a rate of 3–10 % per day of catheterization [20]. The clinical significance of catheter-associated asymptomatic bacteriuria is not known. About 10–25 % of patients will be symptomatic [21].

Urinary tract infections encompass almost half of infectious complications of renal transplantation [22]. The incidence of UTI following transplantation has been reduced with improvements in surgical procedures, greater attention to rapid catheter removal, refinements in immunosuppressive therapy, and routine administration of antibiotic prophylaxis [23].

Etiology

Many different variables are responsible for the causation of urinary tract infections. Sexual intercourse, diaphragm-spermicide use, and a history of recurrent UTIs are strong and independent risk factors [6]. There is an increased risk for approximately 24 h post-coitus. Increased sexual intercourse frequency correspondingly increases risk of infection. Having a new sexual partner within the past year increases risk [24].

Spermicide-coated condom use increases risk, as does recent antimicrobial use, even if used for UTI treatment [25]. Antimicrobials (beta-lactams are more heavily implicated than trimethoprim-sulfamethoxazole) lead to an alteration of urogenital flora, especially Lactobacillus. A lack of Lactobacilli in the vaginal flora predisposes to UTI as these organisms competitively exclude uropathogens through epithelial adhesion. Lactobacilli also produce lactic acid which lowers the vaginal pH, creating an inhospitable environment for uropathogens. They also produce bacteriocins and surfactants, and are involved in H_2O_2 production, in combination with chloride and myeloperoxidase in the vagina. Lactobacilli loss can also be caused by menopause (leading to a loss of estrogen and increased vaginal pH) and bacterial vaginosis [26].

Another identified risk factor is having the first UTI before the age of 15 years. Despite widespread thought that bathroom hygiene and wiping habits are associated with increased risk for UTIs, there has been no data to support this claim [24].

The use insulin and longer diabetes duration (greater than 10 years) confer an increased risk. Diabetics do not exhibit a different microbial profile compared to non-diabetics [12]. Diabetes mellitus and urinary tract obstruction (mainly papillary necrosis and ureteral calculi) confer an increased risk for emphysematous UTIs [27].

Anatomical and urologic differences may also account for infections and recurrences. These include obstruction, stone formation, indwelling catheters, scarring, trauma, fistula formation, urinary incontinence, presence of a cystocele, post-void residual urine, a history of UTI before attaining menopause, and non-secretor status (discussed in Pathogenesis section) [28]. Neurogenic bladder carries an increased risk due to altered urodynamics and microtrauma from repeated intermittent catheterizations.

Specific risk factors identified for UTIs in men include insertive anal intercourse and lack of circumcision [29].

Risk factors for catheter-associated bacteriuria or UTI include female gender, diabetes mellitus, prolonged catheterization, bacterial colonization of the drainage bag, and errors in catheter care [30].

The microbes implicated in uncomplicated cystitis and pyelonephritis are mainly *Escherichia coli* (75–95 %), with occasional other Enterobacteriaceae (such as *Proteus mirabilis* and *Klebsiella pneumoniae*), and *Staphylococcus saprophyticus*. Other Gram-negative and Gram-positive organisms are rarely isolated in uncomplicated infections [31].

Complicated UTIs involve a larger microbial spectrum, including the aforementioned pathogens, along with Pseudomonas, Serratia, Providencia, Enterococci, Staphylococci, and fungi. Organisms leading to complicated infections are more prone to exhibit antimicrobial drug resistance patterns [32]. Risk factors for progression to complicated pyelonephritis include urinary tract obstruction, urologic dysfunction, antibiotic resistant pathogen(s), and diabetes (particularly for emphysematous pyelonephritis and papillary necrosis).

Emphysematous infections are usually due to *E. coli* or *Klebsiella pneumoniae* [27]. Candida is a rare cause [33].

If organisms such as Lactobacilli, Enterococci, Group B Streptococci, and coagulase-negative Staphylococci (excluding *Staphylococcus saprophyticus*) are isolated in otherwise healthy individuals, contamination of the urine specimen is a reasonable conclusion. However, if these cultures are seen in symptomatic women when found in voided midstream urine at high counts with pure growth, they can be considered pathogenic [5].

Funguria is common among hospitalized patients and is generally benign. Invasive kidney infection is unusual, but difficult to treat. Risk factors for funguria included urinary tract drainage devices, prior antibiotic use, diabetes, urinary tract pathology, and malignancy. Common fungal isolates in the urine are Candida species (predominantly *Candida albicans* and *Candida glabrata*). A variety of other fungi can rarely involve the kidney as a result of disseminated infection. These include Aspergillus, Fusarium, Trichosporon, Mucorales (Rhizopus, Mucor), Dematiaceous molds, *Cryptococcus neoformans*, *Histoplasma capsulatum*, Coccidioides, Blastomyces *dermatitidis*, *Paracoccidioides brasiliensis*, *Sporothrix schenckii*, and *Penicillium marneffei*.

Risk factors for UTI in transplant patients include the same risk factors that apply to the general population, in addition to additional factors related to the transplantation itself. Risk factors unrelated to transplantation include advanced age, female gender, reflux kidney disease prior to transplantation, and diabetes mellitus. Risk factors directly related to transplantation include deceased donor kidney, kidney–pancreas transplant, retransplantation, antithymocyte globulin administration, urinary bladder catheterization, allograft rejection and subsequent increased immunosuppression, and ureteral stent placement [22].

Renal transplant patients exhibit many differences in microbial patterns. In general, infections are caused by Gram-negative organisms, predominantly *E. coli*. The other Gram-negative uropathogens that have been isolated include *Pseudomonas aeruginosa*, *Enterobacter cloacae*, *Klebsiella pneumoniae*, *Klebsiella oxytoca*, *Serratia marcescens*, *Stenotrophomonas maltophilia*, *Citrobacter freundii*, *Proteus mirabilis*, *Achromobacter xylosoxidans*, *Acinetobacter baumannii*, and *Morganella morganii*. Because of the common practice of administering antibiotic prophylaxis among transplant recipients, these organisms tend to exhibit increased resistance patterns [34]. Fungal UTIs occur in 5–11 % of transplant recipients with UTI, with *Candida albicans* being the most common cause. Other species include *Candida tropicalis*, *Candida glabrata*, and *Candida krusei* [35].

Pathogenesis

The pathogenesis of urinary tract infections involves a complex balance and interaction between a variety of factors. The main factors implicated include host-related factors (such as innate factors, urinary tract abnormalities, and behavioral factors) and pathogen-related factors (such as virulence).

Humans have a built-in normal defense mechanism against urinary tract infections. The mechanical force of urine flow helps expel any existing organisms from the genitourinary system. Superficial umbrella cells in the bladder will exfoliate in response to bacteria binding to surface uroplakins (a type of membrane protein). Underlying cells will rapidly differentiate into superficial facet cells [36, 37].

There is also an innate immune response to urinary tract infections. There are antimicrobial peptides, such as beta-defensin 1 and cathelicidin LL-37, in urine that bind and disrupt bacterial membranes. Elements involved in host iron sequestration include lactoferrin, transferrin, and lipocalin-2. Tamm-Horsfall protein, or uromodulin, is responsible for binding and blocking bacterial fimbriae. Bladder and kidney cells are capable of upregulating cytokines and chemokines in response to bacteria, of which interleukin (IL) 8 appears to be a key factor by functioning as a neutrophil attractant. There are also a variety of Toll-like receptors (TLR) that recognize different patterns as part of the host response. TLR1 and TLR2 recognize lipopeptides, TLR4 recognizes fimbriae and lipopolysaccharides, and TLR5 recognizes flagellin. These Toll-like receptors upregulate NFkB that subsequently increases the production of IL-6 and IL-8 [36, 37].

Urinary tract infections in women generally originate with fecal flora that colonize the vaginal introitus. These organisms then ascend the urethra to enter the bladder. Alterations in the normal vaginal flora, especially a decrease in H_2O_2-producing lactobacilli, can predispose to introital colonization with *E. coli*. Pyelonephritis is a result of pathogen ascent to the kidneys through the ureters. Underlying host and microbial factors that lead to progression from cystitis to pyelonephritis are not well understood at this time. Pyelonephritis may be caused by seeding of the kidneys as a result from bacteremia or from bacteria present in the lymphatic system [26].

There is a predisposition for developing pyelonephritis in pregnancy. This may be related to pregnancy-related anatomic changes in the urinary tract, such as increased pressure on the bladder from the enlarging gravid uterus, and an increase in ureteral size due to smooth muscle relaxation. The immunosuppression of pregnancy may also play a role, including lower mucosal IL-6 levels and serum antibody responses to *E. coli* antigens [38].

Recurrences, in general, follow the same basic principles as sporadic infection. Recurrences due to the same bacterial strain may be due to reinfection, with the source being a remnant uropathogen reservoir in the bladder epithelium from a prior infection. This may be related to intracellular bacterial communities and quiescent intracellular reservoirs [39]. There is evidence of clonal invasion of epithelial cells in biofilm structures. This allows the bacteria to evade host defenses. Antibiotics are not capable of penetrating these structures well. The majority of cystitis recurrences are reinfections. The initial pathogenic strain can persist in the fecal flora after being eliminated from the urinary tract. *E. coli* strains can be responsible for recurrent UTIs 1–3 years later, although most recurrences occur within the first 3 months [40].

Women with recurrent infections have an increased susceptibility to vaginal colonization with uropathogens. This is partially due to a greater tendency for uropathogenic coliforms to adhere to the uroepithelium in women with a history of recurrences when compared to women without recurrent infections [41]. Genetic determinants also play a role. The non-secretor and the P1 phenotypes have higher expression among females with recurrent UTI and recurrent pyelonephritis, respectively. Uroepithelial cells from women who are non-secretors of ABH blood group antigens have stronger adherence of uropathogenic *E. coli* when compared with cells from secretors [42]. The non-secretors also express unique glycolipid receptors that bind uropathogenic *E. coli*. The IL-8 receptor (IL8R or CXCR1) is another implicated genetic factor. IL-8 promotes neutrophil migration across infected uroepithelium [43].

Asymptomatic bacteriuria and symptomatic urinary tract infection are significantly less common in men when compared to women. This is because of inherent anatomical differences in men, namely the longer urethral length, drier periurethral environment (with subsequent less frequent bacterial colonization), and prostatic fluid's antibacterial properties.

The lack of symptoms with asymptomatic bacteriuria may be related to the specific pathogen, the host, or both. When comparing asymptomatic bacteriuria, cystitis, and pyelonephritis, the microbiology is similar. There may be some strains that exhibit subtle adaptations that promote pathogenesis. In order for symptomatic infection to occur, bacteria irreversibly attach to the urinary tract via fimbrial adhesins. Some strains with reduced fimbrial expression grow more rapidly, which then leads to asymptomatic bacteriuria [44]. The strains implicated in asymptomatic bacteriuria might be less virulent, and therefore, may not constitute true pathogens and are unlikely to progress to serious infection [45]. Because of this, it is postulated that colonization with "uroprotective" bacterial strains (especially strains of *E. coli*) may protect against infection from invasive uropathogens [46]. Host factors that may be implicated in asymptomatic bacteriuria may be related to lower levels of neutrophil Toll-like receptor 4 (TLR4) expression. TLR4 is responsible for the mucosal response to *E. coli*, and its inactivation can lead to a carrier state resembling asymptomatic bacteriuria [47].

Bacterial adhesion to mucosal or urothelial cells is an important determinant of bacterial virulence. Infection in the urinary tract is partly related to the bacteria's ability to adhere and colonize other locations (e.g., the gut, perineum, urethra, bladder, and kidneys) [48]. Adhesion is especially of interest when infections occurs in an anatomically normal urinary tract, but it also plays a significant role in recurrent cystitis and catheter-associated infections [49].

Uropathogenic Enterobacteriaceae are electronegative and too small to overcome repulsion by the net negative charge of epithelial cells. Therefore, bacterial adhesion cannot happen in the absence of fimbrial or other non-fimbrial surface adhesion systems, which have favorable electrical charge and promote adhesion via hydrophobicity [50].

Bacterial virulence does not appear to be related to antimicrobial drug resistance.

Virulence of uropathogenic *E. coli* appears to be related to several O-serotypes (O1, O2, O4, O6, O7, O16, O18, and O75) [51]. While they only comprise 28 % of normal fecal flora isolates, they are the culprit in 80 % of pyelonephritis cases, 60 % of cystitis cases, and 30 % of asymptomatic bacteriuria cases [52].

The presence of adhesins on the tip of bacterial fimbriae (also known as pili) and on the bacterial surface (non-fimbrial adhesins) is the most important factor in *E. coli* uropathogenicity. Most adhesins are lectins that recognize binding site conformations from oligosaccharide sequences on the epithelial cell surface [53].

Two major fimbrial adherence systems (PAP and SFA) have been identified in *E. coli* strains associated with urinary tract infections. The PAP adhesin is found on the tip of P fimbriae. The term P fimbriae relates to the PAP adhesin's ability to recognize the human digalactoside P blood group determinants on human erythrocytes and urothelial cells, that then facilitates increased adhesion. This plays an important role in host susceptibility to infection. Epithelial binding and invasion appears to be accomplished by Dr fimbriae [53].

Non-fimbrial adhesins include many different proteins, including AFA and the AT (autotransporter) family of trimeric proteins. Two of these latter proteins have structural similarity to the *E. coli* K12 antigen 43 (Ag43a), which promotes biofilm growth. Its expression is associated with long-term *E. coli* bladder colonization. UpaG is another non-fimbrial adhesin that binds to the epithelium, mediates cell aggregation, and relates to biofilm formation [54].

The frequency of PAP, SFA, and AFA operons is approximately 75 %, 25 %, and 10 %, respectively in pyelonephritis; 45, 20, and 12 % in cystitis; and 24, 27, and 0 % in asymptomatic bacteriuria [55]. Virtually all young females with a normal urinary tract and pyelonephritis have been found to have at least one adhesin system [56].

Because of the aforementioned findings, patients with UTI who are infected with non-uropathogenic (non-fimbrial) bacteria should undergo further investigations to detect a structural defect (e.g., intermittent reflux, neuromuscular bladder dysfunction, or bladder neck obstruction) leading to infection [56].

Apart from the presence of adhesins, bacterial fimbriae also appear to have other virulence properties that are responsible for development of infection, but these are not yet well defined. Other virulence factors include the presence of flagellae (which are responsible for motility), hemolysin production (which form pores in the epithelial cell membrane and lead to inflammation, damage, and hemorrhage), and aerobactin production (which is necessary for iron uptake in the iron-deficient urinary tract). CNF1 appears to play a role in adherence and invasion, and can stimulate bladder cell apoptosis [51].

Escherichia coli is capable of evading host defense mechanisms, as well. Its type 1 fimbriae make the siderophore enterobactin, which is neutralized by the host protein lipocalin-2. The bacteria can glycosylate enterobactin into salmochelin, which lipocalin-2 cannot recognize. *E. coli* can also synthesize factors that blunt cytokine responses and help resist free radicals. It can also produce immunosuppressants such as SisA and SisB [36, 37].

Escherichia coli may also have an effect on ureteral peristalsis. Multiple strains of *E. coli* were tested. Non-uropathogenic strains had no significant effect on ureteral motility. However, uropathogenic strains demonstrated some effect, from 9.47 to 96.7 % ureteral dysmotility over 8 h. This effect is postulated to be related to the FimH adhesin on the end of type 1 fimbriae [57].

Proteus mirabilis has its own armamentarium of virulence factors, including urease production, hemolysin production, IgA protease production, iron acquisition, flagellae, and fimbriae. Urease hydrolyzes urea to ammonia and carbon dioxide. Ammonia combines with hydrogen to form ammonium. This leads to urine alkalinization with the urine pH being frequently above 7.0 and can even reach as high as 9.0. The alkalinity promotes precipitation of phosphate, carbonate, and magnesium, which form struvite stones and then large staghorn calculi. These stones contain a mixture of proteinaceous matrix, leukocytes, struvite, and bacteria. Because the stone is Proteus-contaminated, it becomes a permanent source of bacteria. It also leads to urinary stasis, which then furthers bacterial multiplication, urinary alkalinization, and deposition of new struvite layers. Hemolysin in Proteus species works in a similar fashion to Escherichia species in that it leads to epithelial cell inflammation, damage, and hemorrhage. Another entity, Proteus toxic agglutinin, remains anchored on the bacterial surface and leads to bacterial auto-agglutination. This process is directly toxic to bladder and kidney cells [58].

Proteus mirabilis produces at least 4 fimbrial types that do not appear to be requisite for causing infection. At least 2 fimbrial systems may contribute to colonization, namely the MR/P fimbriae for bladder and kidney infection; and the PMF fimbriae for bladder infection. UCA fimbriae bind epithelial cells and can target a variety of surface receptors. ATF fimbriae is another structure that appears to be expressed optimally at room temperature, and may play a role in the organism's survival outside of the urinary tract. ZapA is a zinc metalloprotease that cleaves IgG, IgA, complement, and antimicrobial peptides [58].

A particular phenotype termed "swarm cell differentiation," characterized by the formation of very long flagellae, appears to facilitate ascent into the urinary tract [59].

Staphylococcus saprophyticus is a common cause of cystitis in young sexually active women. It rarely leads to pyelonephritis. This organism adheres strongly to the urothelium apparently because of a lactosamine residue [60].

Microorganisms have uptake and transport systems that steal essential metals from the host. The most important metals that have been identified are iron and zinc. Iron is critical for a variety of host processes. Zinc plays a key role in metalloprotease activity and piliation. The host sequesters these nutrients as a defense mechanism. However, bacteria are able to generate siderophores in order to harvest iron [36, 37].

The pathogenesis of funguria is not as well understood. Fungal multiplication is commonly found within the kidney, a phenomenon which does not appear to occur in any other organ. It is not known whether fungi preferentially localize in the kidney or are cleared from other organs more efficiently. The pathogenesis of fungal renal infection appear to be related to the attachment of fungi to endothelial surfaces and penetration into tissue. The presence of yeast in the capillary beds of the kidneys elicits an inflammatory response. The yeasts survive only if they are able to penetrate the capillary walls and invade the interstitium. Invasion is expedited by attachment of the fungi via adherence mechanisms to the capillary walls. Pseudohyphal and hyphal forms facilitate penetration through the capillary walls. Ascending infection of the kidneys appears to be related to vesicoureteral reflux of fungi from the bladder [61].

Catheter-associated urinary tract infections may be extraluminal or intraluminal. Extraluminal infections occur with bacterial entry into the bladder along the biofilm that forms around the catheter in the urethra. Intraluminal infections occur due to urinary stasis because of drainage failure, or due to drainage bag contamination with subsequent ascending infection. Extraluminal infections are more common than intraluminal [62].

The organisms that cause urinary tract infections in a hospital or nursing home are usually of different species and often have greater antibiotic resistance profiles when compared to pathogens seen in the general community. Ambulatory patients with indwelling catheters tend to acquire uropathogens similar to those seen in hospitalized patients. These organisms may lack some virulence factors that allow the usual uropathogen to adhere to uroepithelial cells, but they can still easily access the bladder via the catheter. Upper urinary tract infection is also an important consequence of CAUTIs [63].

Clinical Presentation

There is a crucial distinction to be made when evaluating a patient with bacteriuria—whether they are symptomatic or not. This distinction will serve to determine whether treatment is warranted. Many patients with bacteriuria will be asymptomatic, and may not always require antibiotic treatment. Symptomatic patients, on the other hand, will always require treatment. This will be further discussed later.

Patients with cystitis have dysuria, frequency, urgency, suprapubic pain/discomfort, and/or hematuria [64].

Patients with pyelonephritis may or may not complain of the symptoms associated with cystitis, in addition to fever, chills, flank pain, costovertebral angle tenderness, nausea, and/or vomiting. Symptoms may mimic pelvic inflammatory disease. On rare occasions, acute pyelonephritis may manifest as acute kidney injury, sepsis, multiple organ dysfunction syndrome (MODS), and/or shock [64].

Patients with emphysematous cystitis most commonly present with abdominal pain. Emphysematous pyelonephritis and emphysematous pyelitis are indistinguishable from severe acute pyelonephritis based on presentation. The symptoms may present suddenly or may evolve over 2–3 weeks.

Complicated pyelonephritis may present as weeks to months of malaise, fatigue, nausea, or abdominal pain.

Chronic pyelonephritis is an uncommon cause of chronic tubulointerstitial disease, usually associated with a chronically obstructing calculus or vesicoureteral reflux, in which patients again present with weeks to months of insidious non-specific symptoms.

Patients with indwelling catheters are rarely symptomatic. Even when faced with fever, urinary symptoms, and leukocytosis, it can be difficult to attribute these to an active UTI [21].

Funguria is a common occurrence in the presence of indwelling catheters. When asymptomatic, the presence of yeasts generally reflect colonization. Infected patients may have dysuria, frequency, and suprapubic discomfort. When present, symptoms of fungal kidney involvement may include flank pain, costovertebral angle tenderness, abdominal pain, and/or abdominal tenderness [65].

Symptoms of urinary tract infection in pregnancy are no different from the nonpregnant population.

Patients in the extremes of age may have subtle symptoms. Elderly patients with indwelling catheters often have atypical presentations of infection. The clues to the presence of infection may be the development of fever or otherwise unexplained systemic manifestations compatible with infection, such as altered mental status, delirium, fall in blood pressure, metabolic acidosis, tachypnea, and respiratory alkalosis. However, fever may not be present [21].

In renal transplant patients, urinary tract infection usually occurs within the first year after transplantation. Now, due to multiple factors (routine administration of prophylactic antibiotics, refinements in immunosuppression, improvements in surgical techniques, and greater attention to early catheter removal post-operatively), more patients are presenting with UTI after the first year of transplantation. Patients can present with either uncomplicated cystitis (without pyelonephritis of allograft or native kidney and without sepsis) or pyelonephritis involving either the native kidney or allograft. Symptoms are generally comparable to non-transplant patients [34]. Occasionally, patients may lack all clinical manifestations of UTI because of immunosuppression and denervation of the renal allograft [66].

Diagnosis

Clinical history is of the utmost importance in diagnosis of uncomplicated cystitis or pyelonephritis along with clinical manifestations mentioned above. The likelihood of cystitis is more than 50 % in a woman with any of the symptoms of urinary tract infection presented above (clinical manifestations section) but the probability of urinary tract infection is usually greater than 90 % in a woman presenting with dysuria and frequency in the absence of vaginal discharge or irritation [3, 64].

Physical examination is another important entity and should consist of evaluation for fever, costovertebral angle tenderness, and complete abdominal examination including signs of guarding and rigidity. Complete pelvic exam should also be considered in cases where vaginitis or urethritis is present. In addition, testing for pregnancy is crucial in women of child bearing age presenting with symptoms of urinary tract infection.

Further assessment with laboratory diagnostic testing includes urinalysis and urine culture with susceptibility information. Urinalysis with microscopy or dipstick is acceptable depending on inpatient versus outpatient setting and is a quick and cheap diagnostic tool complimenting urine culture. However, urinalysis without a urine culture is also considered adequate for diagnosing uncomplicated cystitis if clinical symptoms are indicative of urinary tract infection unless there is strong suspicion for antimicrobial resistance or other confounding features including indwelling catheters, anatomic abnormalities, history of renal transplant, and clinical signs/symptoms indicating complicated cystitis with pyelonephritis.

Routine imaging studies are not indicated for diagnosing acute uncomplicated cystitis but may be required in certain complicated cases, recurrent UTIs, and pyelonephritis.

The most important aspect of urinalysis is searching for pyuria when evaluating a patient for urinary tract infection. Lack of pyuria on urinalysis should strongly instigate the clinician to look for alternative diagnosis as pyuria is present in nearly all patients presenting with acute cystitis or pyelonephritis [67].

Evaluating an unspun midstream voided urine sample with a hemocytometer is the most precise technique of assessing for pyuria. A positive result is reported with ≥10 leukocytes/microL [3].

Presence of white blood cell casts in the urine is indicative of upper tract infection. Red blood cells are common in UTI setting but uncommon in urethritis or vaginitis and therefore are helpful to the clinician when making treatment decisions. Hematuria, on the other hand, is neither an indication for longer therapy nor is a predictor for more severe infection.

Commercially available dipsticks are used to detect the presence of leukocyte esterase which is an enzymatic product of leukocytes indicating pyuria. Dipsticks also detect for nitrite, a by-product of Enterobacteriaceae which convert urinary nitrate to nitrite.

Leukocyte esterase may also be used to look for >10 leukocytes per high power field which has sensitivity of 75–96 % and specificity of 94–98 % [68]. Furthermore, the presence of nitrite is appreciably sensitive and specific for detecting $\geq 10^5$ CFU of Enterobacteriaceae per mL of urine but it does not have acceptable sensitivity to detect for other organisms. Consequently, negative results should not be taken for granted [69]. Further caution should be used when interpreting positive nitrite results because false positive nitrite tests can result when compounds that can make urine red are involved, such as bladder analgesic phenazopyridine or ingestion of beats.

The dipstick exam is useful in assessing for UTI when positive for either leukocyte esterase or nitrite with sensitivity of 75 % and a specificity of 82 % [64]. However, positive or negative dipstick results cannot accurately rule in or rule out a UTI because the clinical history along with presenting signs and symptoms of an individual patient is always considered more reliable.

Obtaining a proper urine culture may also be required when evaluating a patient with suspected UTI as treatment with antibiotics is considered. This has been increasingly more important in the face of increasing prevalence of antimicrobial resistance amid uropathogens. It is also crucial to obtain a urine culture when dealing with a complicated UTI [70]. For instance, urine culture with susceptibility testing should be performed in all patients presenting with signs and symptoms of acute pyelonephritis [71]. Furthermore, a urine culture should be obtained for susceptibility data of uropathogens if a patient is suffering from recurrent UTIs or symptoms persist after completing a course of antibiotics. A voided midstream urine specimen should be obtained for best results.

Treatment and Resistance

Treatment guidelines presented in this section are intended for treating uncomplicated acute cystitis and pyelonephritis. Complicated cystitis and pyelonephritis therapy guidelines are not covered in this chapter as they are beyond the scope of this text.

Treatment of UTI is based on the severity of the infection. A key decision point in selecting an appropriate antibiotic regimen is whether a cystitis or pyelonephritis is present. Antibiotic selection for treatment of acute cystitis further depends on certain key factors that include resistance profiles of uropathogens, efficacy of selected antimicrobial agent along with its side effect profile, drug availability, and cost [72].

Some of the commonly suggested antimicrobial agents for the treatment of acute cystitis are as follows:

Nitrofurantoin: Nitrofurantoin monohydrate/macrocrystals with suggested dose of 100 mg twice daily has reported efficacy rate of 90–95 % when used for 5–7 days orally according to randomized trials [73].

Special consideration: Nitrofurantoin is contraindicated in patients with creatinine clearance of <60 mL/min.

Trimethoprim-sulfamethoxazole (TMP-SMX): TMP-SMX with suggested dose of 160/800 mg (one double strength tablet) twice daily has reported efficacy rate of 86–100 % when used for 3–7 days orally according to randomized trials [74]. TMP-SMX should be dose adjusted at 50 % of recommended dose for patients with creatinine clearance of 15–30 mL/min.

Special consideration: Trimethoprim-sulfamethoxazole is contraindicated in patients with creatinine clearance of less than 15 mL/min.

Fosfomycin: Fosfomycin trometamol has reported efficacy rate of 91 % when given 3 g as a single dose according to one randomized trial [75]. However, it is considered inferior in efficacy when compared to other first-line agents suggested for treatment of acute cystitis [76].

Pivmecillinam: Pivmecillinam with suggested dose of 400 mg twice daily has reported efficacy of 55–82 % when given for 3–7 days orally according to randomized trials [77]. Evidently, it has lower clinical efficacy when compared to the other agents mentioned above. Pivmecillinam is currently not available in the USA.

Pyelonephritis is a more severe infection compared to cystitis and therefore requires special attention and selection of broader-spectrum antimicrobial agents. Definitive treatment of pyelonephritis is generally based on susceptibility profiles of causative microbes. However, empiric choice of antimicrobial agents is again based on the severity of illness. One important decision point in treating pyelonephritis is whether to initiate inpatient treatment (which generally requires intravenous antibiotics) or if outpatient treatment with oral antibiotics is adequate.

Outpatient management of pyelonephritis is deemed appropriate for patients who have mild to moderate illness (with mild symptoms and low grade fever) that can be treated with oral antibiotic and oral hydration [78].

Oral fluoroquinolones are the cornerstone of outpatient empiric therapy for patients with acute uncomplicated pyelonephritis. There has been ongoing concern for increasing resistance of uropathogens to currently available fluoroquinolones but clinical efficacy remains high when these antibiotics are used in accordance with susceptibility profiles [79].

For outpatient empiric treatment of pyelonephritis, the commonly suggested oral fluoroquinolones are ciprofloxacin and levofloxacin. For example, 500 mg of ciprofloxacin orally twice daily for 7 days or 1000 mg of extended release oral ciprofloxacin for 7 days are suggested regimens.

Alternatively, 750 mg of oral levofloxacin for 5–7 days is also acceptable.

Of note, fluoroquinolones are contraindicated in pregnancy. Therefore, when fluoroquinolones are used for treatment or prophylaxis in women in the reproductive age group, an effective contraception should be advised. Other serious side effects of fluoroquinolones include prolonged QTc interval in patients with certain cardiac conditions and risk of tendon rupture.

Albeit, final selection of oral antibiotic is then based on susceptibility profiles of the infection causing organisms and side effect profiles of antimicrobial agents selected.

On the contrary, inpatient management is mandatory for patients with pyelonephritis who present with more severe illness demonstrating high fever, hemodynamic instability, and inability to take adequate oral hydration or medications due to marked nausea/vomiting, excessive pain, and pregnancy. Empiric intravenous antibiotic therapy should be initiated promptly which is then tailored as susceptibility data becomes available. Commonly suggested intravenous antibiotics include fluoroquinolones, aminoglycosides, extended-spectrum cephalosporins, extended-spectrum penicillins, as well as carbapenems depending on the severity of the infection, other complicating factors, and prevalence of local resistance [5].

Moreover, when extended-spectrum beta-lactamase (ESBL) producing microbes are involved, intravenous carbapenems should be the choice for antibiotics [80].

Hospitalized patients receiving intravenous antibiotics should be monitored closely and should be switched to appropriate oral agents when significant clinical improvement is evident and patients are able to tolerate oral hydration as well as medications [81].

Most of the discussion on diagnosis and treatment so far has been devoted to urinary tract infections in women because asymptomatic bacteriuria and symptomatic urinary tract infections are much less common in men due to longer urethral length, relatively dry periurethral environment leading to lower frequency of colonization around the urethra and antibacterial properties of prostatic fluid [82].

Traditionally, all urinary tract infections in men between the age of 15 and 50 have been deemed complicated because most UTIs occur in infants and the elderly that have urologic anomalies, such as bladder outlet obstruction, or men with neurogenic bladders leading to altered urinary dynamics and microtrauma from intermittent catheterization, and urologic procedures. Nevertheless, clinical diagnosis and treatment of uncomplicated cystitis and pyelonephritis in men with normal urinary systems is comparable to diagnosis and treatment in women for all practical purposes.

There are some special circumstances where screening for and treating asymptomatic bacteriuria in men between the ages of 15 and 50 may be justified as well. These special considerations include transurethral resection of the prostate or other urologic procedures that put the patient at risk of bacteremia with instrumentation causing mucosal bleeding which can lead to sepsis and septic shock [2, 29].

Men with recurrent cystitis additionally warrant special consideration and evaluation for prostatitis with focus on physical examination and may require digital rectal examination for further management. In addition, the possibility of urethritis should be considered in young sexually active men presenting with UTI symptoms.

Imaging studies are also not routinely needed for diagnosing uncomplicated acute cystitis and pyelonephritis in men but may be helpful in certain circumstances.

Finally, growing uropathogen resistance can present a considerable challenge when selecting antimicrobial agents. Microbial resistance patterns vary significantly depending on geographic location and this is mostly true for *E. coli*. For instance, multiple studies show that resistance rates are higher amongst medial centers in the USA when compared to Canadian medical centers [83]. Resistance rates as high as greater than 20 % have been reported in many regions for trimethoprim (with or without sulfamethoxazole). Resistance for fluoroquinolones has been reported close to 10 % in most parts of North America [84]. Furthermore, ciprofloxacin resistance rates have been reported to have increased from 3 to 17 % between the years of 2000 and 2010 [79]. First and second generation oral cephalosporins are reported to have less than 10 % resistance. Nitrofurantoin is reported to have good in vitro activity in all regions generally [85]. Based on this reported data, the agents with least resistance may be used for empiric therapy in uncomplicated urinary infections caused by *E. coli*.

Complications

Recurrent uncomplicated urinary tract infections are relatively common in otherwise young, healthy woman even with normal anatomical and physiological urinary tracts. There have been no reported long-term complications including renal disease, permanent urinary tract injury, or other sequela leading to long-term health problems from recurrent UTIs in absence of anatomic or functional abnormalities of the urinary tract.

Patients presenting with complicated (please refer to the definitions section above for definition of complicated UTI) urinary tract infections leading to pyelonephritis can have a number of dire complications that require a special attention. Acute complicated pyelonephritis for instance can lead to sepsis, multi-organ system failure, shock, and acute renal failure. Moreover, progression of acute complicated pyelonephritis can lead to such complications as renal corticomedullary abscess, perinephric abscess, emphysematous pyelonephritis, or papillary necrosis. Some important risk factors for more advanced disease with progression to complicated pyelonephritis include urinary tract obstruction, urinary dysfunction, infection with multi-drug resistance uropathogens, and diabetes. Diabetes alone is a significant risk factor particularly for emphysematous pyelonephritis and papillary necrosis. Patients presenting with complicated acute pyelonephritis associated symptoms therefore should alert a clinician to diagnose and treat this potentially life threatening condition with a sense of urgency.

Prevention

Recurrent UTIs in women could present a significant burden and increase the risk of developing antibiotic resistance.

A number of behavioral interventions have been suggested that may be helpful in preventing recurrent UTIs in women. However, many of these behavioral interventions have not been sufficiently studied and tested clinically. Clinicians and patients arguably hold strong biases about the usefulness of these behavioral interventions and therefore it is important to consider them as tools of preventing UTIs that may help in limiting the use of antibiotics.

For instance, use of spermicides (especially coupled with diaphragms) in sexually active woman has been suggested to increase the risk of recurrent UTIs. These women should be counseled on the association between UTIs and use of spermicides during sexual intercourse. Avoiding the usage of spermicide consisting *products* is expected to reduce the risk of recurrent UTIs.

Another popular behavioral intervention often suggested is an early postcoital voiding and generous fluid intake to increase the frequency of micturition.

Furthermore, decreasing the frequency of sexual intercourse or complete abstinence are also commonly suggested strategies for preventing recurrent UTIs but may not be very practical.

Cranberry juice has also been widely used by patients for prevention of recurrent UTIs. A few laboratory studies have suggested that cranberry juice may inhibit adherence of urinary tract microbes to uroepithelial cells [85]. However, most clinical studies reported on clinical efficacy of cranberry juice have been suboptimal and limited (due to lack of power or other design limitations) [86]. Routine use of cranberry juice is not recommended clinically. Additionally, cranberry juice may also put patients at risk of unwanted gastrointestinal side effects such as gastroesophageal reflux as demonstrated by some studies [87].

Prophylactic antibiotics are a reasonable option in patients with recurrent UTIs who do not wish to undergo behavioral interventions such as changing their mode of contraception or other behavioral modifications. Antibiotic prophylaxis should be considered especially in patients who suffer two or more symptomatic recurrent UTIs within 6 months and/or three or more within 12 months period [88]. Antibiotic prophylaxis in patients with these characteristics has been proven to be an effective way of preventing recurrent UTIs [89]. Nevertheless, due to the concern for increasing antibacterial resistance, prophylactic antibiotics should be used conservatively. They should be reserved for patients exhibiting discomfort and more serious UTIs.

Conclusion/Summary

Urinary tract infection is defined as a combination of symptoms and positive urine culture containing at minimal 10^5 colony forming units per milliliter of urine with isolation of less than two microorganisms in a patient without a bladder catheter.

On the other hand, catheter-associated urinary tract infection must contain at least 10^3 CFU/mL, with the urine sample obtained by an aseptic technique.

Asymptomatic bacteriuria is defined as isolation of a significant count of bacteria in an appropriately collected urine specimen from a patient without any signs or symptoms of UTI.

Urinary tract infection is considered complicated when it is associated with other conditions that increase the risk of treatment failure. Such conditions include diabetes, pregnancy, symptoms lasting 1 week or longer prior to starting medical treatment, hospital-acquired infections, urinary tract obstruction, presence of hardware, recent instrumentation, functional or anatomical abnormality, history of childhood UTIs, and renal transplantation.

The prevalence of asymptomatic bacteriuria among healthy women tends to increase with age. Symptomatic UTIs are more prevalent in sexually active young women. Prevalence of UTIs is three-to-fourfold higher in diabetic women.

Asymptomatic bacteriuria is rare among young healthy men, and the incidence of symptomatic UTIs is much lower than that in women.

Pyelonephritis is a more serious infection than cystitis as it includes the upper urinary tract infection involving the kidney(s).

Some of the strong independent etiologic risk factors for UTIs include history of recurrent UTIs, receptive sexual intercourse, and diaphragm-spermicide use. Other risk factors include, having first UTI before the age of 15, diabetes, anatomical or functional urinary tract abnormalities, indwelling urinary catheters, and recent instrumentation.

Among uropathogens, *E. coli* is the most commonly implicated uropathogen responsible for majority of UTIs. Severity of infections depends on variety of host factors, virulence, and antibiotic resistance properties of uropathogens.

Patients with symptomatic cystitis could present with a variety of symptoms including dysuria, increased urinary frequency, urgency, suprapubic pain/discomfort, and hematuria.

Patients with pyelonephritis on the contrary may or may not present with symptoms commonly associated with cystitis but may exhibit fever, chills, flank pain, costovertebral angle tenderness, nausea, and/or vomiting.

Clinical history is immensely important in diagnosis of uncomplicated cystitis or pyelonephritis. Laboratory studies with urinalysis and urine culture also provide valuable information in diagnosis and treatment of UTIs. Routine imaging studies are not indicated for diagnosing acute uncomplicated cystitis but may be required in certain complicated cases and pyelonephritis.

Treatment of UTI is based on the severity of the infection. Appropriate antibiotic regimen is selected based on whether it is cystitis or pyelonephritis.

Treatment of acute cystitis further depends on resistance profiles of uropathogens, efficacy of selected antimicrobial agent along with its side effect profile, drug availability, and cost. Treatment of pyelonephritis generally requires inpatient therapy with intravenous antibiotics.

Growing antibiotic resistance among uropathogens presents a special challenge when selecting antimicrobial agents.

Behavioral interventions may be helpful in reducing the risk of recurrent UTIs but may not be very practical and more studies are needed to prove their clinical efficacy.

Prophylactic antibiotics may be a reasonable option in patients with recurrent UTIs that do not wish to undergo behavioral interventions but because of concern for increasing antibacterial resistance, prophylactic antibiotics should be used conservatively.

References

1. www.cdc.gov/nhsn/pdfs/pscManual/7pscCAUTIcurrent.pdf. Accessed 04 Jan 2010.
2. Nicolle LE, Bradley S, Colgan R, Rice JC, Schaeffer A, Hooton TM. Infectious Diseases Society of America guidelines for the diagnosis and treatment of asymptomatic bacteriuria in adults. Clin Infect Dis. 2005;40(5):643.
3. Stamm WE. Measurement of pyuria and its relation to bacteriuria. Am J Med. 1983;75(1B):53.
4. Hooton TM, Bradley SF, Cardenas DD, Colgan R, Geerlings SE, Rice JC, Saint S, Schaeffer AJ, Tambayh PA, Tenke P, Nicolle LE, Infectious Diseases Society of America. Diagnosis, prevention, and treatment of catheter-associated urinary tract infection in adults: 2009 International Clinical Practice Guidelines from the Infectious Diseases Society of America. Clin Infect Dis. 2010;50(5):625.
5. Hooton TM. Clinical practice. Uncomplicated urinary tract infection. N Engl J Med. 2012;366(11):1028–37. doi:10.1056/NEJMcp1104429.
6. Hooton TM, Scholes D, Hughes JP, Winter C, Roberts PL, Stapleton AE, Stergachis A, Stamm WE. A prospective study of risk factors for symptomatic urinary tract infection in young women. N Engl J Med. 1996;335(7):468.
7. Jackson SL, Boyko EJ, Scholes D, Abraham L, Gupta K, Fihn SD. Predictors of urinary tract infection after menopause: a prospective study. Am J Med. 2004;117(12):903.
8. Foxman B, Gillespie B, Koopman J, Zhang L, Palin K, Tallman P, Marsh JV, Spear S, Sobel JD, Marty MJ, Marrs CF. Risk factors for second urinary tract infection among college women. Am J Epidemiol. 2000;151(12):1194.
9. Hooton TM, Scholes D, Stapleton AE, Roberts PL, Winter C, Gupta K, Samadpour M, Stamm WE. A prospective study of asymptomatic bacteriuria in sexually active young women. N Engl J Med. 2000;343(14):992.
10. Kunin CM, McCormack RC. An epidemiologic study of bacteriuria and blood pressure among nuns and working women. N Engl J Med. 1968;278(12):635.
11. Nicolle LE. Asymptomatic bacteriuria: when to screen and when to treat. Infect Dis Clin North Am. 2003;17(2):367.
12. Boyko EJ, Fihn SD, Scholes D, Abraham L, Monsey B. Risk of urinary tract infection and asymptomatic bacteriuria among diabetic and nondiabetic postmenopausal women. Am J Epidemiol. 2005;161(6):557.
13. Stenqvist K, Sandberg T, Lidin-Janson G, Orskov F, Orskov I, Svanborg-Edén C. Virulence factors of Escherichia coli in urinary isolates from pregnant women. J Infect Dis. 1987;156(6):870.
14. Kaitz AL. Urinary concentrating ability in pregnant women with asymptomatic bacteriuria. J Clin Invest. 1961;40:1331.
15. Smaill F, Vazquez JC. Antibiotics for asymptomatic bacteriuria in pregnancy. Cochrane Database Syst Rev. 2007;18, CD000490.
16. Lipsky BA. Urinary tract infections in men. Epidemiology, pathophysiology, diagnosis, and treatment. Ann Intern Med. 1989;110(2):138.
17. Boscia JA, Kobasa WD, Knight RA, Abrutyn E, Levison ME, Kaye D. Epidemiology of bacteriuria in an elderly ambulatory population. Am J Med. 1986;80(2):208.
18. Sobel JD, Fisher JF, Kauffman CA, Newman CA. Candida urinary tract infections--epidemiology. Clin Infect Dis. 2011;52 Suppl 6:S433.
19. Richards MJ, Edwards JR, Culver DH, Gaynes RP. Nosocomial infections in medical intensive care units in the United States. National Nosocomial Infections Surveillance System. Crit Care Med. 1999;27(5):887.
20. Haley RW, Hooton TM, Culver DH, Stanley RC, Emori TG, Hardison CD, Quade D, Shachtman RH, Schaberg DR, Shah BV, Schatz GD. Nosocomial infections in U.S. hospitals, 1975–1976: estimated frequency by selected characteristics of patients. Am J Med. 1981;70(4):947.
21. Tambyah PA, Maki DG. Catheter-associated urinary tract infection is rarely symptomatic: a prospective study of 1,497 catheterized patients. Arch Intern Med. 2000;160(5):678.
22. Alangaden GJ, Thyagarajan R, Gruber SA, Morawski K, Garnick J, El-Amm JM, West MS, Sillix DH, Chandrasekar PH, Haririan A. Infectious complications after kidney transplantation: current epidemiology and associated risk factors. Clin Transplant. 2006;20(4):401.
23. de Souza RM, Olsburgh J. Urinary tract infection in the renal transplant patient. Nat Clin Pract Nephrol. 2008;4(5):252.
24. Scholes D, Hooton TM, Roberts PL, Stapleton AE, Gupta K, Stamm WE. Risk factors for recurrent urinary tract infection in young women. J Infect Dis. 2000;182(4):1177.
25. Fihn SD, Boyko EJ, Normand EH, Chen CL, Grafton JR, Hunt M, Yarbro P, Scholes D, Stergachis A. Association between use of spermicide-coated condoms and Escherichia coli urinary tract infection in young women. Am J Epidemiol. 1996;144(5):512.
26. Gupta K, Stamm WE. Pathogenesis and management of recurrent urinary tract infections in women. World J Urol. 1999;17(6):415.
27. Huang JJ, Tseng CC. Emphysematous pyelonephritis: clinicoradiological classification, management, prognosis, and pathogenesis. Arch Intern Med. 2000;160(6):797.

28. Raz R, Gennesin Y, Wasser J, Stoler Z, Rosenfeld S, Rottensterich E, Stamm WE. Recurrent urinary tract infections in postmenopausal women. Clin Infect Dis. 2000;30(1):152.

29. Hooton TM, Stamm WE. Diagnosis and treatment of uncomplicated urinary tract infection. Infect Dis Clin North Am. 1997;11(3):551.

30. Platt R, Polk BF, Murdock B, Rosner B. Risk factors for nosocomial urinary tract infection. Am J Epidemiol. 1986;124(6):977.

31. Echols RM, Tosiello RL, Haverstock DC, Tice AD. Demographic, clinical, and treatment parameters influencing the outcome of acute cystitis. Clin Infect Dis. 1999;29(1):113.

32. Warren JW. Catheter-associated urinary tract infections. Infect Dis Clin North Am. 1987;1(4):823.

33. Hildebrand TS, Nibbe L, Frei U, Schindler R. Bilateral emphysematous pyelonephritis caused by Candida infection. Am J Kidney Dis. 1999;33(2), E10.

34. Valera B, Gentil MA, Cabello V, Fijo J, Cordero E, Cisneros JM. Epidemiology of urinary infections in renal transplant recipients. Transplant Proc. 2006;38(8):2414.

35. Krcmery S, Dubrava M, Krcmery Jr V. Fungal urinary tract infections in patients at risk. Int J Antimicrob Agents. 1999;11(3–4):289–91.

36. Nielubowicz GR, Mobley HL. Host-pathogen interactions in urinary tract infection. Nat Rev Urol. 2010;7:430–41.

37. Stapleton AE. Infect Dis Clin Nor Am. 2013. doi:10.1016/j.idc.2013.10.006.

38. Sweet RL. Bacteriuria and pyelonephritis during pregnancy. Semin Perinatol. 1977;1(1):25.

39. Russo TA, Stapleton A, Wenderoth S, Hooton TM, Stamm WE. Chromosomal restriction fragment length polymorphism analysis of Escherichia coli strains causing recurrent urinary tract infections in young women. J Infect Dis. 1995;172(2):440.

40. Stamm WE, McKevitt M, Roberts PL, White NJ. Natural history of recurrent urinary tract infections in women. Rev Infect Dis. 1991;13(1):77.

41. Schaeffer AJ, Jones JM, Falkowski WS, Duncan JL, Chmiel JS, Plotkin BJ. Variable adherence of uropathogenic Escherichia coli to epithelial cells from women with recurrent urinary tract infection. J Urol. 1982;128(6):1227.

42. Sheinfeld J, Schaeffer AJ, Cordon-Cardo C, Rogatko A, Fair WR. Association of the Lewis blood-group phenotype with recurrent urinary tract infections in women. N Engl J Med. 1989;320(12):773.

43. Godaly G, Proudfoot AE, Offord RE, Svanborg C, Agace WW. Role of epithelial interleukin-8 (IL-8) and neutrophil IL-8 receptor A in Escherichia coli-induced transuroepithelial neutrophil migration. Infect Immun. 1997;65(8):3451.

44. Roos V, Nielsen EM, Klemm P. Asymptomatic bacteriuria Escherichia coli strains: adhesins, growth and competition. FEMS Microbiol Lett. 2006;262(1):22.

45. Roos V, Schembri MA, Ulett GC, Klemm P. Asymptomatic bacteriuria Escherichia coli strain 83972 carries mutations in the foc locus and is unable to express F1C fimbriae. Microbiology. 2006;152(Pt 6):1799.

46. Klemm P, Hancock V, Schembri MA. Mellowing out: adaptation to commensalism by Escherichia coli asymptomatic bacteriuria strain 83972. Infect Immun. 2007;75(8):3688.

47. Fischer H, Yamamoto M, Akira S, Beutler B, Svanborg C. Mechanism of pathogen-specific TLR4 activation in the mucosa: fimbriae, recognition receptors and adaptor protein selection. Eur J Immunol. 2006;36(2):267.

48. Mulvey MA. Adhesion and entry of uropathogenic Escherichia coli. Cell Microbiol. 2002;4(5):257.

49. Reid G, van der Mei HC, Tieszer C, Busscher HJ. Uropathogenic Escherichia coli adhere to urinary catheters without using fimbriae. FEMS Immunol Med Microbiol. 1996;16(3–4):159.

50. Oelschlaeger TA, Dobrindt U, Hacker J. Virulence factors of uropathogens. Curr Opin Urol. 2002;12(1):33.

51. Johnson JR. Virulence factors in Escherichia coli urinary tract infection. Clin Microbiol Rev. 1991;4(1):80.

52. Johnson JR, Roberts PL, Stamm WE. P fimbriae and other virulence factors in Escherichia coli urosepsis: association with patients' characteristics. J Infect Dis. 1987;156(1):225.

53. Servin AL. Pathogenesis of Afa/Dr diffusely adhering Escherichia coli. Clin Microbiol Rev. 2005;18(2):264.

54. Valle J, Mabbett AN, Ulett GC, Toledo-Arana A, Wecker K, Totsika M, Schembri MA, Ghigo JM, Beloin C. UpaG, a new member of the trimeric autotransporter family of adhesins in uropathogenic Escherichia coli. J Bacteriol. 2008;190(12):4147.

55. Le Bouguénec C, Lalioui L, du Merle L, Jouve M, Courcoux P, Bouzari S, Selvarangan R, Nowicki BJ, Germani Y, Andremont A, Gounon P, Garcia MI. Characterization of AfaE adhesins produced by extraintestinal and intestinal human Escherichia coli isolates: PCR assays for detection of Afa adhesins that do or do not recognize Dr blood group antigens. J Clin Microbiol. 2001;39(5):1738.

56. Meyrier A, Condamin MC, Fernet M, Labigne-Roussel A, Simon P, Callard P, Rainfray M, Soilleux M, Groc A. Frequency of development of early cortical scarring in acute primary pyelonephritis. Kidney Int. 1989;35(2):696.

57. Floyd RV, et al. Escherichia coli-mediated impairment of ureteric contractility is uropathogenic E. coli specific. J Infect Dis. 2012;206(10):1589–96.

58. Schulz WA. Uropathogenic bacteria leave a mark. Lab Invest. 2011;91(6):816–8.

59. Mobley HL, Island MD, Massad G. Virulence determinants of uropathogenic Escherichia coli and Proteus mirabilis. Kidney Int Suppl. 1994;47:S129.

60. Latham RH, Running K, Stamm WE. Urinary tract infections in young adult women caused by Staphylococcus saprophyticus. JAMA. 1983;250(22):3063.

61. Barnes JL, Osgood RW, Lee JC, King RD, Stein JH. Host-parasite interactions in the pathogenesis of experimental renal candidiasis. Lab Invest. 1983;49(4):460.

62. Nickel JC, Costerton JW, McLean RJ, Olson M. Bacterial biofilms: influence on the pathogenesis, diagnosis and treatment of urinary tract infections. J Antimicrob Chemother. 1994;33(Suppl A):31.

63. Schaberg DR, Haley RW, Highsmith AK, Anderson RL, McGowan Jr JE. Nosocomial bacteriuria: a prospective study of case clustering and antimicrobial resistance. Ann Intern Med. 1980;93(3):420.

64. Bent S, Nallamothu BK, Simel DL, Fihn SD, Saint S. Does this woman have an acute uncomplicated urinary tract infection? JAMA. 2002;287(20):2701.

65. Lehner T. Systemic candidiasis and renal involvement. Lancet. 1964;1(7348):1414.

66. Ramsey DE, Finch WT, Birtch AG. Urinary tract infections in kidney transplant recipients. Arch Surg. 1979;114(9):1022–5.

67. Wilson ML, Gaido L. Laboratory diagnosis of urinary tract infections in adult patients. Clin Infect Dis. 2004;38:1150.

68. Pappas PG. Laboratory in the diagnosis and management of urinary tract infections. Med Clin North Am. 1991;75:313.

69. Eisenstadt J, Washington JA. Diagnostic microbiology for bacteria and yeasts causing urinary tract infections. In: Mobley HL, Warren JW, editors. UTIs: Molecular pathogenesis and clinical management. Washington: ASM Press; 1996. p. 29.

70. Warren JW, Abrutyn E, Hebel JR, et al. Guidelines for antimicrobial treatment of uncomplicated acute bacterial cystitis and acute pyelonephritis in women. Infectious Diseases Society of America (IDSA). Clin Infect Dis. 1999;29:745.

71. Gupta K, Hooton TM, Stamm WE. Increasing antimicrobial resistance and the management of uncomplicated community-acquired urinary tract infections. Ann Intern Med. 2001;135:41.

72. Gupta K, Hooton TM, Naber KG, et al. International clinical practice guidelines for the treatment of acute uncomplicated cystitis and pyelonephritis in women: a 2010 update by the Infectious Diseases Society of America and the European Society for Microbiology and Infectious Diseases. Clin Infect Dis. 2011; 52:e103.

73. McKinnell JA, Stollenwerk NS, Jung CW, Miller LG. Nitrofurantoin compares favorably to recommended agents as empirical treatment of uncomplicated urinary tract infections in a decision and cost analysis. Mayo Clin Proc. 2011;86:480.

74. Arredondo-García JL, Figueroa-Damián R, Rosas A, et al. Comparison of short-term treatment regimen of ciprofloxacin versus long-term treatment regimens of trimethoprim/sulfamethoxazole or norfloxacin for uncomplicated lower urinary tract infections: a randomized, multicentre, open-label, prospective study. J Antimicrob Chemother. 2004;54:840.

75. Stein GE. Comparison of single-dose fosfomycin and a 7-day course of nitrofurantoin in female patients with uncomplicated urinary tract infection. Clin Ther. 1999;21:1864.

76. Fosfomycin for urinary tract infections. Med Lett Drugs Ther. 1997; 39:66.

77. Ferry SA, Holm SE, Stenlund H, et al. Clinical and bacteriological outcome of different doses and duration of pivmecillinam compared with placebo therapy of uncomplicated lower urinary tract infection in women: the LUTIW project. Scand J Prim Health Care. 2007;25:49.

78. Ward G, Jorden RC, Severance HW. Treatment of pyelonephritis in an observation unit. Ann Emerg Med. 1991;20:258.

79. Sanchez GV, Master RN, Karlowsky JA, Bordon JM. In vitro antimicrobial resistance of urinary Escherichia coli isolates among U.S. outpatients from 2000 to 2010. Antimicrob Agents Chemother. 2012;56:2181.

80. Pitout JD. Infections with extended-spectrum beta-lactamase-producing enterobacteriaceae: changing epidemiology and drug treatment choices. Drugs. 2010;70:313.

81. Mombelli G, Pezzoli R, Pinoja-Lutz G, et al. Oral vs intravenous ciprofloxacin in the initial empirical management of severe pyelonephritis or complicated urinary tract infections: a prospective randomized clinical trial. Arch Intern Med. 1999;159:53.

82. Krieger JN, Ross SO, Simonsen JM. Urinary tract infections in healthy university men. J Urol. 1993;149:1046.

83. Zhanel GG, Hisanaga TL, Laing NM, et al. Antibiotic resistance in Escherichia coli outpatient urinary isolates: final results from the North American Urinary Tract Infection Collaborative Alliance (NAUTICA). Int J Antimicrob Agents. 2006;27:468.

84. Swami SK, Liesinger JT, Shah N, et al. Incidence of antibiotic-resistant Escherichia coli bacteriuria according to age and location of onset: a population-based study from Olmsted County. Minnesota Mayo Clin Proc. 2012;87:753.

85. Sobota AE. Inhibition of bacterial adherence by cranberry juice: potential use for the treatment of urinary tract infections. J Urol. 1984;131:1013.

86. Avorn J, Monane M, Gurwitz JH, et al. Reduction of bacteriuria and pyuria after ingestion of cranberry juice. JAMA. 1994; 271:751.

87. Stapleton AE, Dziura J, Hooton TM, et al. Recurrent urinary tract infection and urinary Escherichia coli in women ingesting cranberry juice daily: a randomized controlled trial. Mayo Clin Proc. 2012;87:143.

88. Ronald AR, Conway B. An approach to urinary tract infections in ambulatory women. Curr Clin Top Infect Dis. 1988;9:76.

89. Stamm WE, Hooton TM. Management of urinary tract infections in adults. N Engl J Med. 1993;329:1328.

Chronic Catheter Associated Complications and Catheter-Associated Urinary Tract Infection

7

JoAnn Coleman

Urinary catheters are standard medical devices used in hospitals and long-term care (LTC) facilities. The most frequent complication associated with these devices is the development of nosocomial catheter-associated urinary tract infections (CAUTIs), accounting for almost 40 % of infections reported by acute care hospitals [1, 2].

CAUTI increases hospital cost and is associated with increased morbidity and mortality [2–4]. Each year, more than 13,000 deaths are associated with urinary tract infections (UTIs) [3, 4]. In 2007, the cost of treating CAUTIs was estimated at \$400 million per year [5]. Although the absolute cost of each CAUTI may not be overwhelming, the frequency of episodes over a year greatly increases their significance [6].

In addition to the health and financial burden of CAUTI, there are additional patient safety concerns associated with urinary catheterization, such as patient discomfort, restriction of activity, delay in discharge, and the potential development of a reservoir of multidrug-resistant organisms that can spread to other patients [7, 8]. Indwelling catheter usage may also prolong hospital stay if the patient is unable to void normally after the catheter is removed near the time of a planned discharge [9].

The prevalence of indwelling urinary catheter use is 15–25 % in the acute care setting and 5–10 % in long-term care (LTC) facilities. Long-term indwelling urinary catheters are used most commonly in the elderly, in patients who are disabled or have debilitating neurological conditions such as a spinal cord injury. CAUTI in the LTC resident can lead to complications of cystitis, pyelonephritis, bacteremia, and septic shock. These complications associated with CAUTI can result in decline in resident function and mobility, acute care hospitalizations, and increased mortality [10, 11].

CAUTIs are considered by the Centers for Medicare and Medicaid Services (CMS) to represent a reasonably preventable complication of hospitalization and the first healthcare-associated infection (HAI) where no payment is provided to hospitals for CAUTI treatment-related costs [12]. Reduction of CAUTI is a reasonable goal but elimination may not be feasible, especially in patients who require long-term catheterization [5, 13].

The CMS rule change on nonreimbursement for CAUTI has fueled an increased focus on the prevention of CAUTI and an increased interest in distinguishing CAUTI from asymptomatic bacteriuria (ASB). The ability to distinguish symptomatic CAUTI from ASB currently relies on clinical symptoms (Table 7.1) and is not easily made even with the help of various guidelines [14]. The presence of bacteria in urine does not imply a UTI [15] and more than 90 % of cases of catheter-associated bacteriuria are symptom-free [16].

Asymptomatic Bacteriuria vs Symptomatic Urinary Tract Infection

Asymptomatic CAUTIs are common in hospitalized patients and catheterized LTC facility residents. There is 100 % ABS in LTC facility residents with chronic indwelling urinary catheters. They are associated with a low incidence of sequelae and morbidity, and in most patients resolve spontaneously on removal of the catheter. Despite consensus guidelines developed to help diagnose UTI, a single, evidence-based approach to distinguish symptomatic UTI from ASB does not exist. Routine screening and treatment for ASB are not recommended [17].

However, ASB comprises a reservoir of microorganisms in health care settings [18]. Urine cultures should only be obtained from patients with symptoms of UTI [19]. Overtreatment with antibiotics for suspected UTI remains a significant problem and leads to a variety of consequences including the development of multidrug-resistant organisms,

J. Coleman (✉)
Sinai Hospital, 2401 West Belvedere Avenue, Baltimore, MD 21215, USA
e-mail: jocolema@lifebridgehealth.org

© Springer Science+Business Media New York 2017
D.A. Gordon, M.R. Katlic (eds.), *Pelvic Floor Dysfunction and Pelvic Surgery in the Elderly*,
DOI 10.1007/978-1-4939-6554-0_7

Table 7.1 Comparison of CDC and IDSA definitions of asymptomatic bacteriuria and symptomatic catheter-related bacteriuria

Asymptomatic bacteriuria (ASB)	Symptomatic catheter-related bacteriuria (UTI)
CDC definition	
Absence of: Fever >38 °C Suprapubic tenderness or Costovertebral angle pain or tenderness Urine culture with >10^5 colony forming units (cfu)/mL of uropathogenic bacteria (CDC definition)	Presence of: Fever >38 °C Suprapubic tenderness Costovertebral angle tenderness or Unexplained systemic symptoms such as: Altered mental status Hypotension or Evidence of a systemic inflammatory response syndrome Along with one of the following: • Urine culture with >10^5 cfu/mL irrespective of urinalysis results • Urine culture with 10^3 cfu/mL with evidence of pyuria (dipstick positive for leukocyte esterase and/or nitrite, microscopic pyuria or presence of microbes seen on Gram stain of unspun urine)
IDSA definition	
Single catheterized specimen with isolation of a single organism in quantitative counts of ≥10^2 cfu/mL	Patients who are no longer catheterized but had indwelling urinary catheters within the past 48 h are also considered to have CAUTI if they meet these definitions

CDC Center for Disease Control;www.cdc.gov/nhsn/pdfs/pscManual/7pscCAUTIcurrent.pdf (Accessed on February 25, 2014)
IDSA Infectious Disease Society of America; Nicolle LE, Bradley S, Colgan R, et al. Infectious Diseases Society of America guidelines for the diagnosis and treatment of asymptomatic bacteriuria in adults. Clin Infect Dis 2005; 40:643

suprainfections, unnecessary costs [13, 19], and does not change chronic genitourinary symptoms or improve survival [20].

Patients with symptoms of a UTI, which include fever, chills, hematuria, suprapubic pain, are treated with antibiotics. Older adults may not exhibit the common UTI symptoms but may show a decline in mental state [21, 22]. A catheterized patient with symptoms or signs of a UTI and significant bacteriuria is diagnosed as having a CAUTI. Many patients are being diagnosed inappropriately with CAUTI, for which they receive treatment that is not recommended [13].

The prevalence of ASB in LTC residents can range from 25 to 50 %. Although the incidence of symptomatic UTI is lower, it still comprises a significant proportion of infections manifesting in LTC facilities and results in a large amount of antibiotic use [11]. In recent years, LTC facilities have admitted residents with higher acuity levels with concomitant increase in indwelling devices and parenteral antibiotics, further exposing a greater number of residents to multidrug-resistant bacteria [23].

In LTC residents with a urinary catheter, the most common occult infectious source of fever is the urinary tract. The combination of fever and worsening mental or functional status in such residents meets the criteria for a UTI. Particular care should be taken to rule out other causes of these symptoms. A symptomatic UTI requires the presence of symptoms along with significant bacteriuria. However, symptomatic UTI in a catheterized LTC resident should always be a diagnosis of exclusion in the absence of localizing urinary tract findings [24]. If a catheterized resident meets the criteria for infection at a site other than the urinary tract, then the clinical diagnosis is an infection at the other site [25]. Risk factors for ASB and symptomatic UTI are presented in Table 7.2.

Table 7.2 Risk factors for asymptomatic bacteriuria and symptomatic urinary tract infection

Asymptomatic bacteriuria	Symptomatic urinary tract infection
Disconnection of drainage system	Prolonged catheterization
Insertion by one who lacks lower professional training	Female sex
Placement of catheter outside of OR	Older age
Incontinence	Impaired immunity
Diabetes	
Meatal colonization	
Renal dysfunction	
Orthopedic/neurology services	

The exact relationship between ASB and UTI remains unclear. The distinction currently relies on clinical symptoms and is not easily made, even with the help of various guidelines [14]. Even though treatment of ASB is not recommended, it is plausible that preventing ASB will decrease the incidence of symptomatic infection in catheterized patients [26].

CAUTI Definitions

The definition of CAUTI is controversial. A number of societies vary in their current definitions and recommendations but all agree that symptoms are not reliable for the diagnosis of CAUTI.

In 2008 the Society for Healthcare Epidemiology of America (SHEA), the Infectious Diseases Society of America (IDSA) jointly published the *Compendium of Strategies to Prevent Healthcare-Associated Infections in Acute Care Hospitals*, including strategies to prevent CAUTI [26].

Table 7.3 Criteria for diagnosis of CAUTI form IDSA/SHEA, CDC, APIC

Organization	Definition
Infectious Diseases Society of America (IDSA) and the Society for Healthcare Epidemiology of America (SHEA) http://www.idsociety.org/uploadedFiles/IDSA/Guidelines-Patient_Care/PDF_Library/Comp%20UTI.pdf 2009 These guidelines are for acute care hospitals Emphasis is on enabling the clinician to detect a CAUTI in an individual patient. These guidelines make a distinction between CAUTI and ASB. Although ASB may be a precursor for CAUTI, the majority of ASBs do not progress to symptomatic infection. Routine screening for ASB is not recommended except in specific research and other settings	Catheter-associated urinary tract infection is defined by the presence of symptoms or signs compatible with a urinary tract infection (UTI) with no identifiable source of infection along with $\geq 10^5$ colony forming units (CFU)/mL of ≥ 1 bacterial species in a single catheter urine specimen or in a midstream voided urine specimen from a patient whose urethral, suprapubic, or condom catheter has been removed within the previous 48 h
Centers for Disease Control and Prevention (CDC)/National Healthcare Safety Network 2008 http://www.cdc.gov/nhsn/pdfs/pscManual/7pscCAUTIcurrent.pdf CDC definitions are intended for infection control surveillance purposes in any type of health care setting	A UTI where an indwelling urinary catheter was in place for >2 calendar days on the date of event, with day of device placement being Day 1, *and* an indwelling urinary catheter was in place on the date of event or the day before. If an indwelling urinary catheter was in place for >2 calendar days and then removed, the UTI criteria must be fully met on the day of discontinuation or the next day Classification of CAUTI falls into two groups: symptomatic urinary tract infection (SUTI) and asymptomatic bacteriuric urinary tract infection (ABUTI). CAUTI includes those infections in which a patient had an indwelling urinary catheter at the time or within 48 h before onset of the event NOTE: There is no <u>minimum</u> period of time that the catheter must be in place for the UTI to be considered catheter-associated
CAUTI in Long-term Care Facilities	Catheter-associated SUTIs events occur when a resident develops signs and symptoms localizing to the urinary tract while having an indwelling urinary catheter in place or removed within 2 calendar days prior to the date of event (where day of catheter removal=day 1) NOTE: An indwelling urinary catheter should be in place for a minimum of 2 calendar days before infection onset (where day of catheter insertion=day 1) in order for the SUTI to be catheter-associated One or more of the following: 1. Fever 2. Rigors 3. New onset hypotension with not alternate site of infection 4. New onset suprapubic pain or costovertebral angle pain or tenderness 5. Acute pain, swelling, or tenderness of the testes, epididymis, or prostate 6. Purulent drainage from around the catheter AND any of the following: If urinary catheter removed within last 2 calendar days: 1. A voided urine culture with $\geq 10^5$ CFU/ml of not more than 2 species of microorganisms 2. Positive culture with $\geq 10^2$ CFU/ml of any microorganisms from straight in/out catheter specimen If urinary catheter in place: 3. Positive culture with 10^5 CFU/ml of any microorganisms from indwelling catheter specimen
Association for Professionals in Infection Control and Epidemiology (APIC) An APIC 2008 Guide to the Elimination of Catheter-Associated Urinary Tract Infections (CAUTIs) http://www.apic.org/Resource_/EliminationGuideForm/c0790db8-2aca-4179-a7ae-676c27592de2/File/APIC-CAUTI-Guide.pdf These guidelines are for acute and long-term settings	Uses the CDC/NHSN definition for SUTI and ASB Includes the McGeer definitions for CAUTI in the LTC setting (see Table 7.4)

In 2010, the IDSA published *Diagnosis, Prevention, and Treatment of Catheter-Associated Urinary Tract Infection in Adults: 2009 International Clinical Practice Guidelines From the Infectious Diseases Society of America* [27]. Later that same year, the Healthcare Infection Control Practices Advisory Committee (HICPAC) at the Centers for Disease Control (CDC) published an updated *Guideline for Prevention of Catheter-Associated Urinary Tract Infections 2009* [4]. Table 7.3 provides the criteria for diagnosis of CAUTI from these societies.

Table 7.4 McGeer and Loeb clinical criteria for symptomatic UTI for residents in LTC facility with an indwelling catheter [24, 28, 29]

McGeer criteria to identify a urinary tract infection (UTI) with an indwelling urinary catheter	Loeb criteria for initiating empiric antibiotic therapy with an indwelling urinary catheter

Both criteria 1 and 2 must be present:
1. At least 1 of the following sign or symptom
  a. Fever, rigors, or new onset hypotension, with no alternate site of infection
  b. Either acute change in mental status or acute functional decline, with no alternate diagnosis and leukocytosis
  c. New onset suprapubic pain or costovertebral angle pain
  d. Purulent discharge from around the catheter or acute pain, swelling, or tenderness of the testes, epididymis, or prostate
2. Urinary catheter specimen culture with at least 10^5 cfu/mL of any organism(s) Urinary catheter specimens for culture should be collected following replacement of the catheter (if current catheter has been in place >14 days)
	At least one of the following must be present:
	1. Fever (>37.9 °C) or 1.5 °C above baseline temperature
	2. New costovertebral angle tenderness
	3. Rigors (shaking chills) with or without an identified cause
	4. New onset delirium

Recent catheter trauma, catheter obstruction, or new onset hematuria may be localizing signs that are consistent with UTI but not necessary for diagnosis Diagnosis of UTI can be made without localizing symptoms if a blood culture isolate is the same as the organism isolated from the urine and there is no alternate site of infection	

In the LTC setting, the McGeer [28] definition is often used to guide clinical diagnosis and management of UTIs. These criteria were updated in 2012 by Stone et al. [24] Consensus criteria from SHEA and APIC for antibiotic use in LTC facilities was adapted by Loeb and colleagues [29] in 2001 for the treatment of UTI (Table 7.4).

Risk Factors for CAUTI

The risk of acquiring a UTI depends on the method of catheterization, duration of catheter use, the quality of catheter care, and patient susceptibility. The relationship between the duration of catheterization and the development of a UTI is firmly established [30].

Lack of proper training in catheter insertion and maintenance by healthcare persons may be the first introduction of bacteria into the urinary tract initiating CAUTI. The hands of the person inserting the indwelling catheter may be the first source of contamination [31]. Lack of asepsis or sterile equipment contamination during insertion of an indwelling urinary catheter by any healthcare person may be the first introduction of bacteria into the urinary tract and initiation of CAUTI. Lack of proper maintenance of an indwelling urinary catheter may also introduce bacteria into the urinary tract. Placement of an inappropriate size of catheter may also cause complications related to CAUTI [25–27, 32].

A patient with an indwelling urinary catheter has a 5 % daily risk for development of a UTI [33]. An indwelling urethral catheter in place for over 30 days is considered to be a long-term, or chronic catheter in a patient, and the risk of bacteriuria reaches 100 % after 30 days of the indwelling

Table 7.5 Risk factors for development of catheter-associated urinary tract infections

Prolonged catheterization
Improper catheter insertion technique
Female gender
Older age
Compromised immune system
Comorbid conditions (e.g., diabetes, renal dysfunction)

catheter [34, 35]. The most frequent indications for a long-term indwelling catheter are urinary retention in men and incontinence management in women [36].

Lack of attention or inability to maintain a closed drainage system, obstructed urinary flow, or improper placement of the drainage bag may place a patient at risk for CAUTI. Any unnecessary manipulation or break in the closed drainage system predisposes a patient to CAUTI [25–27, 32].

There are host factors which make individuals more susceptible to CAUTI, including being female, older age, having diabetes mellitus, receiving immunosuppressive therapy, having a neurogenic bladder, and the setting in which catheterization occurs [37]. Table 7.5 lists risk factors for the development of CAUTI.

Individuals 65 years of age and older are at increased risk for unnecessary catheterization [38–40]. Older adults may have a higher risk of developing complications, particularly infection, as the increased use of indwelling urinary catheters has been traditionally used to manage bladder emptying in those with cognitive impairment, incontinence, and decreased function in carrying out activities of daily living [40, 41], or convenience [42].

In the LTC resident, risk factors for developing bacteriuria and UTI include age-related changes to the genitourinary tract, comorbid conditions resulting in neurogenic bladder, and instrumentation required to manage bladder voiding [42].

Guidelines for CAUTI

The goals for placement of indwelling urinary catheters are the appropriate use of catheters and the safest possible management during the period when they are in use [43]. Given the clinical and economic consequences of CAUTI, updated consensus guidelines and prevention strategies to prevent this common and costly hospital-acquired complication have been published.

In 2008 the Society for Healthcare Epidemiology of America (SHEA) and the Infectious Diseases Society of America (IDSA) jointly published the *Compendium of Strategies to Prevent Healthcare-Associated Infections in Acute Care Hospitals*, including strategies to prevent CAUTI [44]. The Association for Professionals in Infection Control and Epidemiology (APIC) published the *Guide to the Elimination of Catheter-Associated Urinary Tract Infections (CAUTIs). Developing and Applying Facility-Based Prevention Interventions in Acute and Long-Term Care Settings* [45].

In 2010, the IDSA published *Diagnosis, Prevention, and Treatment of Catheter-Associated Urinary Tract Infection in Adults: 2009 International Clinical Practice Guidelines from the Infectious Diseases Society of America* [27]. Later that same year, the Healthcare Infection Control Practices Advisory Committee (HICPAC) at the Centers for Disease Control and Prevention (CDC) published an updated *Guideline for Prevention of Catheter-Associated Urinary Tract Infections 2009* [4]. IDSA/SHEA and APIC also published a joint statement concerning infection control in LTC facilities that addresses CAUTI [26].

The guidelines are generally drawn from the same pool of evidence. But there is a paucity of evidence, particularly when trying to determine the best practices for management of CAUTI [14]. A summary of these guidelines are presented in Table 7.6.

Three recommendations were present in all of these CAUTI guidelines: catheterize only when necessary and only for as long as necessary, insert catheters using aseptic techniques and sterile equipment, and maintain a closed, sterile drainage system. The indications for use of catheters were also agreed upon: acute urinary retention or obstruction, perioperative applications in select procedures, and the frequent, accurate measurement of urine output in critically ill patients [4, 27, 44, 45].

Table 7.6 Summary of recommendations from published guidelines

Recommendations	CDC	IDSA	SHEA
Limitation of catheter use			
Evaluate necessity of catheterization	Y	Y	Y
Review ongoing need for catheter	Y	Y	Y
Evaluate alternative methods of drainage	Y	Y	Y
Catheter insertion and selection			
Use of aseptic technique/sterile equipment	Y	Y	Y
Use of barrier precautions for insertion	Y	U	Y
Use smallest bore catheter possible	Y	U	Y
Use of silver alloy catheters	ND	T	N
Use of antimicrobial-impregnated catheters	ND	Y	N
Use of hydrophilic catheters	ND	N	ND
Catheter maintenance			
Maintain closed drainage system	Y	Y	Y
Replace collecting system if break in asepsis occurs	Y	ND	U
Maintain drainage bag below level of bladder	Y	Y	Y
Avoid routine irrigation	Y	Y	Y
Diagnostics and antimicrobials			
Avoid routine urine cultures	Y	Y	Y
Avoid use of systemic antimicrobial prophylaxis	ND	Y	Y
Do not treat asymptomatic bacteriuria	ND	Y	Y
General measures			
Practice strict hygiene	Y	ND	Y
Train all persons in catheter insertion and maintenance	Y	Y	Y
Written protocols for catheter care	ND	Y	Y

CDC US Centers for Disease Control and Prevention, *IDSA* Infectious Diseases Society of America; *N* not recommended, *ND*, not discussed, *SHEA*, Society for Healthcare Epidemiology of America, *U* unresolved (vary according to clinical experience and patients factors), *Y* recommended
Modified from Tambyah, PA and Oon, J, Catheter-associated urinary tract infection. Curr Opin Infect Dis. 2012 25(4): 365–370

Three recommendations for assuring the implementation of best practices were consistent across guidelines for the prevention of CAUTIs: train all persons responsible for catheter insertion and maintenance, document the indications for use of each catheter, and provide feedback and outcome measures to clinical staff and administrators [4, 27, 44, 45].

The definition of CAUTI was not consistent across guidelines. All guidelines acknowledged that a CAUTI is often asymptomatic [16]. IDSA and CDC guidelines distinguished catheter-associated asymptomatic bacteriuria by the presence of urgency, pelvic pain, fever, or bacteremia. IDSA and CDC guidelines also provided a written definition of CAUTI using these distinguishing criteria. However, only the IDSA guidelines included separate recommendations for the prevention of symptomatic CAUTIs vs. asymptomatic bacteriuria [46].

Although the guidelines differ in the amount of detail provided and their focus of efforts to prevent CAUTI, there is consistency of recommendations. Different grading systems for quality of evidence and strength of recommendation make comparisons difficult and what the recommendations purport to prevent remains unclear [46]. With the exception of IDSA, these recommendations do not distinguish between the prevention of symptomatic CAUTI and the prevention of catheter-associated asymptomatic bacteriuria. For clinicians seeking to prevent CAUTI, the distinction is a moot point, because all symptomatic CAUTI begins as asymptomatic bacteriuria. For clinicians making treatment decisions, the distinction between CAUTI and bacteriuria is important [14]. Separate guidelines address the management of asymptomatic bacteriuria [47]. Finally, the primary purpose of the guidelines was to assist clinicians in making decisions regarding UTI [46].

Pathogenesis of CAUTI

An indwelling urinary catheter provides a portal of entry into the urinary tract and increases the risk for UTI by compromising urinary tract defenses. It mechanically irritates the urethral and bladder mucosa, impairing local defense mechanisms and providing an ideal surface for growth of a bacterial biofilm [47]. A biofilm is the aggregation of microorganisms that form a structure on solid surfaces [27].

Biofilms on an indwelling urinary catheter consist of complex structures that include bacteria, extracellular products, and a host of components deposited on to the surface of the catheter [15]. Microbes attach to the biofilm and begin secreting polysaccharides that form the architectural structure of the biofilm (Fig. 7.1) [48]. Biofilms on urinary catheters may be composed of gram-negative or gram-positive bacteria or yeasts. Biofilms are a survival strategy for these microorganisms, offering protection from both the body's defenses and antimicrobial agents [49].

Biofilms are both tenacious and resistant to antimicrobial agents, thus their importance in the pathogenesis of catheter-associated infection [48]. Biofilm bacteria are up to 1000-fold more resistant to antimicrobial agents compared to planktonic bacteria, their free-floating counterparts. Biofilm bacteria that form on indwelling urinary catheters exhibit distinct characteristics and are treated differently from infections not associated with biofilms. [25] Figure 7.2 depicts the five stages of biofilm development.

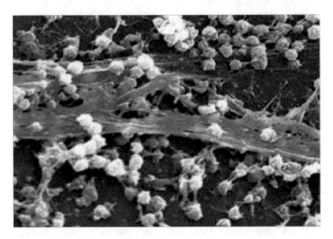

Fig. 7.1 Electron micrograph depicting round *Staphylococcus aureus* bacteria, with biofilm, the sticky-looking substance woven between the bacteria. *Source*: Donlan RM, Carr J, Public Health Image Library, Centers for Disease Control and Prevention; 2005

Fig. 7.2 Stages of biofilm development. This is a diagram of the five stages of biofilm development: initial attachment, irreversible attachment, maturation 1, maturation 2, and finally dispersal. Monroe D (2007) Looking for Chinks in the Armor of Bacterial Biofilms. PLoS Biol 5(11):e307. doi:10.1371/journal.pbio.0050307. © 2007 Don Monroe. This is an open-access article distributed under the terms of the Creative Commons Attribution License, which permits unrestricted use, distribution, and reproduction in any medium, provided the original author and source are credited

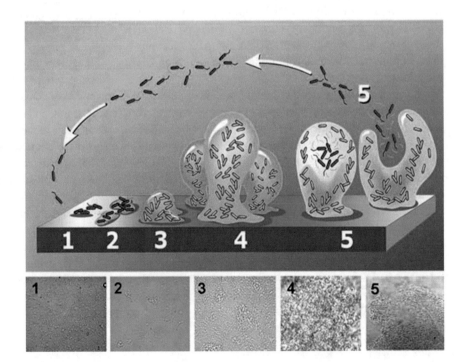

The catheterized urinary tract provides ideal conditions for the development of enormous biofilm populations. Catheterization allows for the formation of a biofilm between the catheter and the urethral mucosa. A urinary catheter interferes with normal host defenses and clearance of microbes from voiding and the bladder mucosa is diminished. Once a biofilm has developed on the external or internal surface of a urinary catheter, the only way to eliminate the risk of CAUTI is to remove the catheter [50]. The majority of CAUTI result from organisms ascending along the external surface of the catheter in a biofilm [51].

In a urinary catheter, the biofilm produces urease, which hydrolyzes urea in the patient's urine to ammonium hydroxide. The elevated pH can precipitate minerals in the biofilm that then encrust and block the lumen of the catheter [52, 53]. All types of catheters are vulnerable to encrustation by these biofilms, and clinical presentation strategies are needed, as bacteria growing in the biofilm are resistant to antibiotics and host defenses [50].

Most microorganisms that initiate CAUTI derive from the patient's own colonic and perineal flora (such as *Escherichia coli*) or from the hands of healthcare personnel during catheter insertion or manipulation of the collection system [31]. External contamination can occur by direct inoculation of the catheter tip from organisms on the external urethral meatus [31] and subsequent dragging of organisms along the full length of the urethra as the catheter is inserted fully into the bladder [54]. The tip is also the likely source of bacteria found on the inside of catheters that are carried downward by the flow of urine [54]. It has been hypothesized that perineal microorganisms, such as enterococci, staphylococci, and Candida species, ascend in the space between the catheter and the urethra [55] traveling by capillary action in the thin mucous film surrounding the catheter. Studies indicate that there are more bacteria on the external surface of the catheter than on the internal lumen. Bacteria from the outer surface of the catheter then colonize the bladder epithelium, contaminating the urine [54]. Common pathogens are presented in Table 7.7.

Table 7.7 Rank order of pathogens associated with catheter-associated urinary tract infections

1.	*Escherichia coli*
2.	*Pseudomonas aeruginosa*
3.	Klebsiella (pneumonia/oxytoca)
4.	*Candida albicans*
5.	*Enterococcus faecalis*
6.	Proteus spp.
7.	Enterococcus spp.
8.	Enterobacter spp.
9.	Other Candida spp.
10.	*Enterococcus faecium*

The usually sterile urinary tract can also become colonized in an ascending manner from the drainage bag or the catheter-bag junction, up through the lumen of the catheter. These routes are considered less likely than colonization from the flora of the distal urethra. Transport of a large quantity of contaminants from the inside of the catheter into the bladder may also occur by retrograde reflux of contaminated urine when the catheter or collection system is moved or manipulated [31].

On deflation of the retention balloon, crystalline debris from the biofilm can be shed into the bladder and initiate stone formation. The main complication is blockage in the urine through the catheter that results from the buildup of crystalline material on the internal surface. As a consequence, urine often leaks along the outside of the catheter and the patient becomes incontinent, resulting in the increased need for assistance and care. In addition, blockage of the catheter can lead to retention of urine in the bladder and vesicoureteric reflux of urine. If the blockage is not detected and if the catheter is not changed, patients can suffer episodes of pyelonephritis and septicemia [56, 57]. Internal bacterial ascension can also be introduced when opening the otherwise closed urinary drainage system. Microbes can ascend from the urine collection bag into the bladder via reflux (Fig. 7.3) [31].

Long-term indwelling catheters become colonized by extensive biofilms, which can lead to profound effects on the health of a patient [57]. Initially composed of single species, the biofilm on a long-term indwelling urinary catheter can also

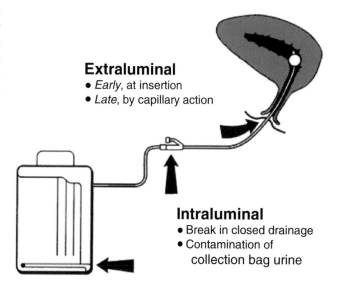

Extraluminal
- *Early*, at insertion
- *Late*, by capillary action

Intraluminal
- Break in closed drainage
- Contamination of collection bag urine

Fig. 7.3 Routes of entry of uropathogens to catheterized urinary tract. Maki DG, Tambyah PA. Engineering out the risk for infection with urinary catheters. Emerg Infect Dis. 2001 Mar-Apr; 7(2):342–7. © Maki DG, Tambyah PA 2001. This is an open-access article distributed under the terms of the Creative Commons Attribution License, which permits unrestricted use, distribution, and reproduction in any medium, provided the original author and source are credited

contain multiple species [48] with mixed-organism biofilms containing as many as 16 different strains of bacteria [54].

An ideal method for preventing biofilm formation on urinary catheters has not been developed. Future research needs to be aimed at identifying mechanisms for controlling biofilm formation and developing antimicrobial agents effective against bacteria in biofilms. [58].

Indications for a Chronic Indwelling Urinary Catheter

Many indwelling urinary catheters are used without clear indications, putting patients at unnecessary risk for complications [59]. Potentially serious complications associated with indwelling urethral catheters and the possible development of CAUTI warrant efforts to restrict the use of these devices by having clear indications for insertion and discontinuation [60]. Table 7.8 provides indications for an indwelling urinary catheter.

Complications of CAUTI

The most common complications of chronic indwelling catheters are bacteriuria, encrustation, and blockage [52]. Less common is the prevalence of bacteremia and renal disease. Risk factors for bacteriuria include female gender, older age, and long-term indwelling catheter use. Other complications include fever, acute pyelonephritis, urinary stones, chronic interstitial nephritis, renal failure, and even death [61, 62].

About half of the patients who have long-term catheterization will suffer the complication of catheter encrustation and blockage by bacterial biofilms at some time [52]. The welfare of many elderly and disabled patients is put at risk by the development of these complications, and considerable demands are made on the resources of the healthcare system to manage the complications [60]. Table 7.9 presents complications of indwelling urinary catheters in short-term and long-term catheterized persons.

Symptoms of CAUTI

Asymptomatic CAUTIs are common in hospitalized patients and catheterized long-term care residents. They are associated with a low incidence of sequelae and morbidity, and in most patients resolve spontaneously on removal of the catheter. However, ASB comprises a reservoir of microorganisms in healthcare settings [18]. Urine cultures should only be obtained from patients with symptoms of a urinary tract infection and, in the absence of signs and symptoms, may result in inappropriate treatment for ASB. Such unnecessary antimicrobial use may result in an increase in antimicrobial resistance and subject patients to otherwise avoidable adverse effects [19].

Urinary infection in residents with long-term indwelling catheters is usually asymptomatic. Despite this, the presence of a chronic indwelling catheter is associated with increased morbidity attributed to symptomatic urinary infection compared to bacteriuric LTC elderly residents without catheters. Symptomatic infection, when it occurs, usually manifests as fever, with or without bacteremia. Invasive infection frequently follows catheter obstruction or trauma to the genitourinary mucosa [63–65].

Patients with symptoms of a urinary tract infection, fever, chills, hematuria, suprapubic pain are treated with antibiotics [66]. Older adults may not exhibit the common urinary tract infection symptoms but instead show a decline in mental state [21]. Prophylactic antibiotics are not recommended

Table 7.9 Complications of catheterized patients

Short-term catheterization	Long-term catheterization
Fever	Fever
Acute pyelonephritis	Acute pyelonephritis
Bacteremia	Bacteremia
Death	Catheter encrustation and obstruction
	Urinary tract stones
	Local periurinary infections
	Chronic renal inflammation
	Chronic pyelonephritis
	Bladder cancer may develop over number of years

Table 7.8 Indications for an indwelling urinary catheter

Short-term indwelling catheterization	Long-term indwelling catheterization
Acute urinary retention/bladder outlet obstruction	Urinary retention with bladder outlet obstruction that cannot be managed by other methods
Need for accurate intake and output if critically ill	Urinary incontinence coexisting with urinary retention that cannot be managed by other methods
Perioperative use in selected surgical procedures	Delayed healing of a high-stage pressure ulcer owing to urinary incontinence
Urologic/other surgeries on contiguous structures of genitourinary tract	Palliative care setting where routine toileting is compromised by pain or immobility
Anticipated prolonged duration of surgery	
Operative patients with urinary incontinence	
Need for intraoperative hemodynamic monitoring	

with indwelling urinary catheterization as it leads to multidrug-resistant organisms [66].

If a CAUTI is suspected, the best practice is removal of the old catheter before obtaining a urine specimen in order to eliminate the confounding factor of possible catheter biofilm. If a patient suspected of having a CAUTI still requires urinary catheterization, the urine specimen should be obtained after replacing the old catheter [60].

The quality of the urine specimen for culture is important when determining if a true infection is present. Specimens collected from a newly inserted urine catheter are reliable, providing proper insertion technique was followed. Only specimens collected from a specifically designed sampling port or from the catheter directly should be submitted for analysis. A sample of urine should never be obtained from a drainage bag [60].

Prevention of CAUTI

There is a new enthusiasm for the prevention of CAUTI. Several strategies show promise for decreasing inappropriate insertion of urinary catheters and duration of catheterization, including a nurse-led multidisciplinary rounds in the hospital [67], computerized "stop orders" for urinary catheters, computer-based order entry for urinary catheters, nurse-generated reminders, and nurse empowerment to remove catheters [68].

Other prevention strategies fall under the headings of different types of catheters, different catheter materials, or alternatives to indwelling urinary catheters. At this time there is insufficient evidence to recommend the following potential alternatives to indwelling urinary catheters as a means to prevent CAUTI: antimicrobial catheters, intermittent catheterization, suprapubic catheters, and condom catheters [69–73].

The most effective means to prevent urinary infection is to avoid use of a chronic indwelling catheter. Continuing reassessment of the need for a chronic indwelling catheter should be part of the management of every resident with such a device. Approximately one half of residents with indwelling catheters transferred from an acute care facility can have the catheter removed at the LTC facility [74].

Long-term indwelling catheters seldom are indicated for management of incontinence in men. External collecting devices, such as condoms and leg bags, are an effective alternative for management, and their use is associated with lower morbidity from urinary infection [75]. For women, long-term indwelling catheters should be avoided as a means to manage incontinence. Routine toileting and use of diapers is preferred and usually effective [76].

Specific infection control practices to prevent CAUTI have been proposed. These include recommendations for catheter use, catheter insertion, closed drainage systems, irrigation of the catheter, maintenance of urinary flow, and indications for changing the catheter [32]. Policies and procedures should be reviewed and updated regularly. Educational strategies to make staff aware of issues relevant to the care of catheters also are necessary.

Routine urine specimens for culture are not useful in persons with chronic indwelling catheters as they will virtually always be bacteriuric. The only indications to obtain urine cultures from asymptomatic residents with chronic indwelling catheters would be during an outbreak investigation when the frequency of both asymptomatic and symptomatic infection in the facility may be important to determine, for a targeted screening program of limited duration with specific objectives, such as identification of the frequency of resistant organisms, or in an individual patient prior to an invasive genitourinary procedure. Otherwise, routine cultures of urine specimens from individuals with chronic indwelling catheters should be discouraged [66].

Pyuria, the presence of pus in the urine, is a universal accompaniment of infection in the presence of an indwelling urethral catheter. The presence of an indwelling catheter, by itself, can be irritating to the bladder and also cause pyuria, even without a positive culture [77]. The degree of pyuria does not correlate with symptomatic or asymptomatic infection, thus, pyuria is a nonspecific finding in the patient with a long-term indwelling catheter and does not assist in patient management. Routine urinalysis to identify the presence of pyuria also is discouraged [78].

Surveillance is recommended to identify the prevalence and duration of indwelling catheter use and the frequency of febrile morbidity and bacteremia attributed to the presence of an indwelling catheter. Surveillance for the presence of chronic indwelling catheters should include monitoring the proportion of individuals in an LTC facility with a catheter and explanation of the reasons for catheterization. Residents who could be considered for a trial without a catheter should be identified. Surveillance definitions for symptomatic infection in catheterized patients should be developed, including episodes of fever with and without localizing findings, bacteremia, and other catheter-associated complications, such as gross hematuria and obstruction. Problems in catheter care identified in surveillance for symptomatic episodes should be addressed systematically [26].

Because of the complications of long-term indwelling catheter usage, periodic assessment and voiding trials should be used to determine the continued need for a catheter. Interventions to be considered include closed versus open drainage systems, type of catheter, and size of catheter lumen. The closed-catheter system has helped to decrease bacteriuria. Silicone catheters and larger lumen size catheters are more resistant to encrustation than other catheter types and smaller lumen size catheters. Acidifying the urine without removing the urease-producing bacteria does not reduce encrustation. Removal of catheter blockage is preventive for renal disease. Evidence-based recommendations for managing indwelling urinary catheters include screening for risk factors and evaluating urinary white blood cell count for infection and assessment of the continued need for a catheter [79].

Antimicrobial agents are not indicated to prevent or treat bacteriuria in patients with indwelling urinary catheters, except for those with symptomatic infection, as it leads to antimicrobial resistance. Alternative devices such as condom catheters or suprapubic catheters may be preferable to the indwelling urethral catheter [80].

Constipation can exacerbate problems with indwelling urinary catheters and increase the risk of urinary tract infection caused by bladder instability or bladder outlet obstruction [81]. Hydration is especially important in catheterized patients as a way to prevent constipation, as is a bowel regimen consisting of high fiber diet and suppositories or minienemas if needed. Hydration is also important for internal flushing of the urinary tract. Wilde and Carrigan [82] reported that increased fluid intake reduced the incidence of urinary tract infection.

Patients with chronic indwelling urinary catheters and their reservoirs of bacteriuric organisms are sources of nosocomial outbreaks. Such outbreaks can be prevented and controlled with attention to catheter hygiene and prevention of patient-to-patient transmission on the hands of caregivers. While antimicrobial coated catheters may be used, current recommendations caution their use as a primary prevention strategy.

Recommendations

The most effective and consistent recommendation identified across guidelines is the removal of the catheter or avoidance of its use. Unfortunately, this recommendation is not always followed.

Reminder systems have been devised to assist in the prevention of CAUTI. Physical reminders consist of face-to-face encounters of staff nurses directly discussing with clinicians removal of the catheter. Paper-based reminders include the use of prewritten "stop orders" or protocols or stickers to encourage clinicians to insert catheters only when absolutely necessary or remove as soon as no longer indicated [67]. Virtual reminders involve the use of electronic devices to remind nurse and clinicians about catheter removal. Computerized automatic "stop orders" can be tied to computerized catheter orders or reminders can be sent via pagers [83].

The bundle design has been applied to urinary catheters. The concept of a "bundle" approach is the integrated and ide-

Table 7.10 Bladder Bundle

• Aseptic insertion and proper maintenance is paramount
• Bladder ultrasound may avoid indwelling catheterization
• Condom or intermittent catheterization in appropriate patients
• Do not use the indwelling catheter unless you must!
• Early removal of the catheter using reminders or stop orders appears warranted

ally synergistic effect of a group of straightforward, evidence-based practices. Currently, elements included in a CAUTI bundle are an appropriate clinical indication for use, aseptic insertion, hand hygiene, use of sterile lubricant, prompt removal, adequate catheter securement, as well as other less thoroughly researched interventions [84]. Table 7.10 presents simple elements of a bladder bundle. Clark et al. [85] also demonstrated that by bundling four easily implemented interventions resulted in a significant reduction in the CAUTI rate. This bundled intervention positively impacted patient safety and hospital costs. Whatever the number or types of interventions included, the bundle approach requires that all must be used as the benefit of a bundle results from the integrated and consistent use of its elements [84].

Although many recommendations are consistent across CAUTI prevention guidelines, the studies on which they are based are limited in number, size, and quantity [86]. In addition, most CAUTI prevention studies use bacteriuria as the outcome of interest, rather than more clinically relevant measures such as asymptomatic CAUTI or urosepsis [46].

Conclusion

As urinary catheters account for the majority of healthcare-associated UTIs, the most important interventions are directed at avoiding placement of urinary catheters and promoting early removal when appropriate. Education of all healthcare persons in the astute adherence to proper aseptic practices for catheter insertion, maintenance and the use of closed-catheter collection system for an indwelling urinary catheter is imperative for preventing CAUTI.

National quality and regulatory initiatives are closely aligned with the guidelines for preventing CAUTI. Research into preventing CAUTIs is needed to provide an increasing solid foundation of evidence to guide practice. The current interest in CAUTI is likely to lead to exciting advances in prevention and management of this healthcare-associated infection.

Key Points

• Urinary tract infections increase morbidity, length of stay, and increase healthcare delivery costs

- Catheter-associated urinary tract infection (CAUTI) is the most common health-care-associated infection in the USA and worldwide.
- Overuse of urinary catheters contributes to the frequency of urinary tract infections (UTIs)
- Differences in CAUTI definitions have led to confusion and misinterpretation of the actual numbers of CAUTI
- Risk assessment and surveillance systems must be established in order to identify areas of improvement in the prevention of CAUTI
- Prevention strategies must focus on clear indications for the insertion of a urine catheter, proper maintenance while in use, and early catheter removal
- A urine specimen with bacteriuria and pyuria in long-term care residents is not sufficient to confirm a diagnosis of clinically suspected urinary tract infection.
- Individuals with asymptomatic bacteriuria should not be prescribed antibiotics as this practice increases the risk of antimicrobial resistance and does not change chronic genitourinary symptoms or improve survival.
- Catheter-associated urinary tract infections in long-term care residents are challenging due to communication barriers, comorbidities, and the presence of chronic urinary symptoms

References

1. Edwards JR, Peterson KD, Andrus ML, Tolson JS, Goulding JS, Dudeck MA, Mincey RB, Pollock DA, Horan TC; NHSN Facilities. National Healthcare Safety Network (NHSN) Report, data summary for 2006, issued June 2007. Am J Infect Control. 2007; 35(5):290–301.
2. Klevens RM, Edward JR, Richards CL Jr, Horan TC, Gaynes RP, Pollock DA, Cardo DM. Estimating health care-associated infections and deaths in U.S. hospitals, 2002. Public Health Rep. 2007; 122(2):160–6.
3. Klevans RM, Edwards JR, Gaynes RP, National Nosocomial Infections Surveillance System. The impact of antimicrobial-resistant, health care-associated infections on mortality in the United States. Clin Infect Dis. 2008;47(7):927–30.
4. Gould CV, Umscheid CA, Agarwal RK, Kuntz G, Pegues DA; Healthcare Infection Control Practices Advisory Committee. Guideline for prevention of catheter-associated urinary tract infections 2009. Infect Control Hosp Epidemiol. 2010; 31(4):319–26.
5. Wald HL, Kramer AM. Nonpayment for harms resulting from medical care: catheter-associated urinary tract infections. JAMA. 2007;298(23):2782–4.
6. Nicolle LE. Catheter-acquired urinary tract infection: the once and future guidelines. Infect Control Hosp Epidemiol. 2010;31(4): 327–9.
7. Saint S, Lipsky BA, Baker PD, McDonald LL, Ossenkop K. Urinary catheters: what type do men and their nurses prefer? J Am Geriatr Soc. 1999;47(12):1453–7.
8. Saint S, Lipsky BA, Goold SD. Indwelling urinary catheters: a one-point restraint? Ann Intern Med. 2002;137(2):125–7.
9. Saint S, Olmsted RN, Fakih MG, Kowalski CP, Watson SR, Sales AE, Krein SL. Translating health care-associated urinary tract infection prevention research into practice via the bladder bundle. Jt Comm J Qual Patient Saf. 2009;35(9):449–55.
10. Benoit SR, Nsa W, Richards CL, Bratzler DW, Shefer AM, Steele LM, Jernigan JA. Factors associated with antimicrobial use in nursing homes: a multilevel model. J Am Geriatr Soc. 2008;56(11):2039–44.
11. Centers for Disease Control and Prevention (CDC). Urinary tract infection (UTI) event for long-term care facilities. [Internet] 2012 Aug 24. Available from: http://www.cdc.gov/nhsn/PDFs/LTC/LTCF-UTI-protocol_FINAL_8-24-2012.pdf.
12. Morgan DJ, Meddings J, Saint S, Lautenbach E, Shardell M, Anderson D, Milstone AM, Drees M, Pineles L, Safdar N, Bowling J, Henderson D, Yokoe D, Harris AD; SHEA Research Network. Does nonpayment for hospital-acquired catheter-associated urinary tract infections lead to overtesting and increased antimicrobial prescribing? Clin Infect Dis. 2012;55(7):932–9.
13. Saint S, Meddings JA, Calfee D, Kowalski CP, Krein SL. Catheter-associated urinary tract infection and the Medicare rule changes. Ann Intern Med. 2009;150(12):877–84.
14. Trautner BW. Management of catheter-associated urinary tract infection. Curr Opin Infect Dis. 2010;23(1):76–82.
15. Trautner BE, Darouiche RO. Role of biofilm in catheter-associated urinary tract infection. Am J Infect Control. 2004;32(3):117–83.
16. Tambyah PA, Maki DG. Catheter-associated urinary tract infection is rarely symptomatic: a prospective study of 1,497 catheterized patients. Arch Intern Med. 2000;160(5):678–82.
17. Rowe TA, Juthani-Mehta M. Diagnosis and management of urinary tract infection in older adults. Infect Dis Clin N Am. 2014;28(1):75–89.
18. Dalen DM, Zvonar RK, Jessamine PG. An evaluation of the management of asymptomatic catheter-associated bacteriuria and candiduria at The Ottawa Hospital. Can J Infect Dis Med Microbiol. 2005;16(3):166–70.
19. Colgan R, Nicolle LE, McGlone A, Hooton TM. Asymptomatic bacteriuria in adults. Am Fam Physician. 2006;74(6):985–90.
20. Rowe TA, Juthani-Mehta M. Urinary tract infection in older adults. Aging health. 2013;9(5). doi: 10.2217/ahe.13.28.
21. Midthun SJ. Criteria for urinary tract infection in the elderly: variables that challenge nursing assessment. Urol Nurs. 2004;24(3):157–62, 166–9, 186.
22. Genao L, Buhr G. Urinary tract infections in older adults residing in long-term care facilities. Ann Longterm Care. 2012;20(4):33–8.
23. Fleming A, Browne J, Byrne S. The effect of interventions to reduce potentially inappropriate antibiotic prescribing in long-term care facilities: a systematic review of randomized controlled trials. Drugs Aging. 2013;30(6):401–8.
24. Stone ND, Ashraf MS, Calder J, Crnich CJ, Crossley K, Drinks PJ, et al. Surveillance definitions of infections in long-term care facilities: revisiting the McGeer Criteria. Infect Control Hosp Epidemiol. 2012;33(10):965–77.
25. Vergidis P, Patel R. Novel approaches to the diagnosis, prevention, and treatment of medical device-associated infections. Infect Dis Clin North Am. 2012;26(1):173–86.
26. Smith PW, Bennett G, Bradley, Drinka P, Lautenbach E, Marx J, Mody L, Nicolle L, Stevenson K; Society for Healthcare Epidemiology of America (SHEA); Association for Professionals in Infection Control and Epidemiology (APIC). SHEA/APIC guideline: infection prevention and control in the long-term care facility. Am J Infect Control. 2008;36(7):504–35.
27. Hooton TM, Bradley SF, Cardenas DD, Colgan R, Geerlings SE, Rice JC, Saint S, Schaeffer AJ, Tambyah PA, Tenke P, Nicolle LE, Infectious Diseases of America. Diagnosis, prevention, and treatment of catheter-associated urinary tract infection in adults: 2009 International Clinical Practice Guidelines from the Infectious Diseases Society of America. Clin Infect Dis. 2010; 50(5):625–63.

28. Stone ND, Ashraf MS, Calder J, Crnich CJ, Crossley K, Drinks PJ, et al. Surveillance definitions of infections in long-term care facilities: revisiting the McGeer Criteria. Infect Control Hosp Epidemiol. 2012;33(10):965–77.

29. Loeb M, Bentley DW, Bradley S, Crossley K, Garibaldi R, Gantz N, McGeer A, Muder RR, Mylotte J, Nicolle LE, Nurse B, Paton S, Simon AE, Smith P, Strausbaugh L. Development of minimum criteria for the initiation of antibiotics in residents of long-term care facilities: results of a consensus conference. Infect Control Hosp Epidemiol. 2001;22(2):120–4.

30. Gray M, Newman DK, Einhorn CJ, Reid-Czarapata BJ. Expert review: best practices in managing the indwelling catheter. Perspectives 2006;1–11 (Special Edition).

31. Maki DG, Tambyah PA. Engineering out the risk of infection with urinary catheters. Emerg Infect Dis. 2001;7(2):342–7.

32. Tambyah PA, Oon J. Catheter-associated urinary tract infection. Curr Opin Infect Dis. 2012;25(4):365–70.

33. Tambyah PA, Knasinski V, Maki DG. The direct costs of nosocomial catheter-associated urinary tract infection in the era of managed care. Infect Control Hosp Epidemiol. 2002;23(1):27–31.

34. Warren JW. Catheter-associated urinary tract infections. Infect Dis Clin North Am. 1997;25(1):609–22.

35. Chenoweth CE, Saint S. Urinary tract infections. Infect Dis Clin North Am. 2011;25(1):103–15.

36. Newman DK. The indwelling urinary catheter: principles for best practice. J Wound Ostomy Continence Nurs. 2007;34(6):655–61.

37. Leone M, Albanese J, Garnier F, Sapin C, Barrau K, Bimar MC, Martin C. Risk factors for nosocomial catheter-associated urinary tract infection in a polyvalent intensive care unit. Intensive Care Med. 2003;29(7):1077–80.

38. Gokula RM, Smith MA, Hickner J. Emergency room staff education and use of a urinary catheter indication sheet improves appropriate use of foley catheters. Am J Infect Control. 2007;35(9):589–93.

39. Holyrod-Leduc JM, Sen S, Bertenthal D, Sands LP, Palmer RM, Kresevic DM, Covinsky KE, Landefeld SC. The relationship of indwelling urinary catheters to death, length of hospital stay, functional decline, and nursing home admission in hospitalized older medical patients. J Am Geriatr Soc. 2007;55(2):227–33.

40. Saint S. Clinical and economic consequences of nosocomial catheter-related bacteriuria. Am J Infect Control. 2000;28(1):68–75.

41. Hampton T. Urinary catheter use often "inappropriate" in hospitalized elderly patients. JAMA. 2006;295(24):2838.

42. Hazelett SE, Tsai M, Gareri M, Allen K. The association between indwelling urinary catheter use in the elderly and urinary tract infection in acute care. BMC Geriatr. 2006;6:15.

43. Hanchett M. Preventing CAUTI: a patient-centered approach. Prevention Strategist Autumn 2012;442–50.

44. Lo E, Nicolle L, Classen D, Arias KM, Podgorny K, Anderson DJ, Burnstin H, Calfee DP, Coffin SE, Dubberke ER, Fraser V, Gerding DN, Griffin FA, Gross P, Kaye KS, Klompas M, Marshall J, Mermel LA, Pegues DA, Perl TM, Saint S, Salgado CD, Weinstein RA, Wise R, Yokoe DS. Strategies to prevent catheter-associated urinary tract infections in acute care hospitals. Infect Control Hosp Epidemiol. 2008;29 Suppl 1:S41–50.

45. Association for Professionals in Infection Control and Epidemiology (APIC). Guide to the elimination of catheter-associated urinary tract infections (CAUTIs). Developing and applying facility-based prevention intervention in acute and long-term care settings. An APIC Guide [Internet]. 2008 [cited 2013 Dec 6]. Available from: http://www.apic.org/Resource_/EliminationGuideForm/c0790db8-2aca-4179-a7ae-676c27592de2/File/APIC-CAUTI-Guide.pdf.

46. Conway LJ, Pogorzelska M, Larson E, Stone PW. Adoption of policies to prevent catheter-associated urinary tract infections in United States intensive care units. Am J Infect Control. 2012;40(8):705–10.

47. Saye DE. Recurring and antimicrobial resistant infections: considering the potential role of biofilms in clinical practice. Ostomy Wound Manage. 2007;53(4):46–8, 50, 52.

48. Donlan RM. Biofilms and device-associated infections. Emerg Infect Dis. 2001;7(2):277–81.

49. Stickler DJ, Morgan SD. Observations on the development of crystalline bacterial biofilms that encrust and block Foley catheters. J Hosp Infect. 2008;69(4):350–60.

50. Stickler DJ. Bacterial biofilms in patients with indwelling urinary catheters. Nat Clin Pract Urol. 2008;5(11):598–608.

51. Tambyah PA. Catheter-associated urinary tract infections: diagnosis and prophylaxis. Int J Antimicrob Agents. 2004;24 Suppl 1:S44–8.

52. Stickler DJ, Feneley RC. The encrustation and blockage of long-term indwelling bladder catheters: a way forward in prevention and control. Spinal Cord. 2010;48(11):784–90.

53. Jacobsen SM, Shirtliff ME. Proteus mirabilis biofilms and catheter-associated urinary tract infections. Virulence. 2011;2(5):460–5.

54. Barford JM, Anson K, Hu Y, Coates AR. A model of catheter-associated urinary tract infection initiated by bacterial contamination of the catheter tip. BJU Int. 2008;102(1):67–74.

55. Drekonja DM, Johnson JR. Urinary tract infections. Prim Care. 2008;35(2):345–67.

56. Liedl B. Catheter-associated urinary tract infections. Curr Opin Urol. 2001;11(1):75–9.

57. Stickler DJ. Clinical complications of urinary catheters caused by crystalline biofilms: something needs to be done. J Intern Med. 2014. doi:10.1111/joim.12220.

58. Tenke P, Koves B, Nagy K, Hultgren SJ, Mendling W, Wullt B, Grabe M, Wagenlehner FM, Cek M, Pickard R, Botto H, Naber KG, Bjerklund Johansen TE. Update on biofilm infections in the urinary tract. World J Urol. 2012;30(1):51–7.

59. Gokula RR, Hickner JA, Smith MA. Inappropriate use of urinary catheters in elderly patients at a mid-western community teaching hospital. Am J Infect Control. 2004;32(4):196–9.

60. Bernard MS, Hunter KF, Moore KN. A review of strategies to decrease the duration of indwelling urethral catheters and potentially reduce the incidence of catheter-associated urinary tract infections. Urol Nurs. 2012;32(1):29–37.

61. Drinka PJ. Complications of chronic indwelling urinary catheters. J Am Med Dir Assoc. 2006;7(6):388–92.

62. Nicolle LE. Catheter-related urinary tract infection. Drugs Aging. 2005;22(8):627–39.

63. Warren JW, Damron D, Tenney JH, Hoopes JM, Deforge B, Muncie Jr HR. Fever, bacteremia, and death as complications of bacteriuria in women with long-term urethral catheters. J Infect Dis. 1987;155(6):1151–8.

64. Orr PH, Nicolle LE, Duckworth H, Brunka J, Kennedy J, Murray D, Harding GK. Febrile urinary infection in the institutionalized elderly. Am J Med. 1996;100(1):71–7.

65. Ouslander JG, Greengold B, Chen S. Complications of chronic indwelling urinary catheters among male nursing home patients: a prospective study. J Urol. 1987;138(5):1191–5.

66. Chenoweth CE, Gould CV, Saint S. Diagnosis, management, and prevention of catheter-associated urinary tract infections. Infect Dis Clin North Am. 2014;28(1):105–19.

67. Fakih MG, Dueweke C, Meisner S, Berriel-Cass D, Savoy-Moore R, Brach N, Rey J, DeSantis L, Saravolatz LD. Effect of nurse-led multidisciplinary rounds on reducing the unnecessary use of urinary catheterization in hospitalized patients. Infect Control Hosp Epidemiol. 2008;29(9):815–9.

68. Cornia PB, Lipsky BA. Commentary: indwelling urinary catheters in hospitalized patients: when in doubt, pull it out. Infect Control Hosp Epidemiol. 2008;29(9):820–2.

69. Neil-Weise BS, van den Broek PJ. Antibiotic policies for short-term catheter bladder drainage in adults. Cochrane Database Syst Rev. 2005;3, CD005428.

70. Niel-Weise BS, van den Broek PJ, da Silva EM, Silva LA. Urinary catheter policies for long-term bladder drainage. Cochrane Database Syst Rev. 2012;8, CD004201.

71. Moore KN, Fader M, Getliffe K. Long-term bladder management by intermittent catheterization in adults and children. Cochrane Database Syst Rev. 2007;4, CD006008.

72. Griffiths R, Fernandez R. Strategies for the removal of short-term indwelling urethral catheters in adults. Cochrane Database Syst Rev. 2007;2, CD004011.

73. Niel-Weise BS, van den Broek PJ. Urinary catheter policies for short-term bladder drainage in adults. Cochrane Database Syst Rev. 2005;3, CD004203.

74. Cools HJM, van der Meer JWM. Restriction of long-term indwelling urethral catheterization in the elderly. Br J Urol. 1986;58(6):683–8.

75. Hebel JR, Warren JW. The use of urethral, condom, and suprapubic catheters in aged nursing home patients. J Am Geriatr Soc. 1990;38(7):777–84.

76. Nicolle LE. The chronic indwelling catheter and urinary infection in long-term-care facility residents. Infect Control Hosp Epidemiol. 2001;22(5):316–21.

77. Tambyah PA, Maki DG. The relationship between pyuria and infection in patients with indwelling urinary catheters: a prospective study of 761 patients. Arch Intern Med. 2000;160(5):673–7.

78. Steward DK, Wood GL, Cohen RL, Smith JW, Machowiak PA. Failure of the urinalysis and quantitative urine culture in diagnosing symptomatic urinary tract infections in patients with long-term urinary catheters. Am J Infect Control. 1985;13(4):159–60.

79. Madigan E, Neff DF. Care of patients with long-term indwelling urinary catheters. Online J Issues Nurs. 2003;8(3):7.

80. Cravens DD, Zweig S. Urinary catheter management. Am Fam Physician. 2000;61(2):369376.

81. Vance J. Diagnosing and managing urinary tract infections: myths, mysteries and realities. Caring Ages. 2002;3(10):18–21.

82. Wilde MH, Carrigan MJ. A chart audit of factors related to urine flow and urinary tract infection. J Adv Nurs. 2003;43(3):254–62.

83. Cornia PB, Amory JK, Fraser S, Saint S, Lipsky BA. Computer-based order entry decreased duration of indwelling urinary catheterization in hospitalized patients. Am J Med. 2003;114(5):404–7.

84. Resar R, Griffin FA, Haraden C, Nolean TW. Using care bundles to improve health care quality. IHI Innovation Series white paper. Cambridge, MA: Institute for Healthcare Improvement; 2012. [Internet]. [cited 2013 Dec 6]; Available from: http://www.ihi.org/resources/Pages/IHIWhitePapers/UsingCareBundles.aspx.

85. Clark K, Tong D, Pan Y, Easley KA, Norrick B, Ko C, Wang A, Razavi B, Stein J. Reduction in catheter-associated urinary tract infections by bundling interventions. Int J Quality Health Care. 2013;25(1):43–9.

86. Conway LJ, Larson EL. Guidelines to prevent catheter-associated urinary tract infection: 1980 to 2010. Heart Lung. 2012;41(3):271–83.

Part II

Diagnosis of Pelvic Floor Disorders and Diagnostic Armamentarium

Physical Therapy Evaluation and Treatment of Pelvic Floor Dysfunction Including Hypertonic Pelvic Floor Dysfunction

Jennifer L. Ortiz

Abbreviations

CPP   Chronic pelvic pain
HPFD Hypertonic pelvic floor dysfunction
MTP   Myofascial trigger points
PFM   Pelvic floor muscles
PFPT Pelvic floor physical therapists

Introduction

On any given day, in any given urology, gastroenterology, or gynecology practice, a client will arrive at their appointment with previously undiagnosed hypertonic pelvic floor dysfunction (HPFD), also referred to as nonrelaxing pelvic floor dysfunction [1]. These clients will typically complain of a combination of symptoms which could include difficulty initiating flow of urine, altered micturition, slow urine stream, incomplete bladder emptying, frank urinary retention [2], incomplete bowel emptying, frequency, dyspareunia, pain with orgasm, constipation, chronic pelvic pain (CPP), and abdominal pain [1]. If the symptoms are acute, these clients are often first tested for urinary tract infection and/or yeast infection. If these tests are negative and the symptoms become chronic in nature, many times the physician will then order urodynamics testing, cystoscopy, colonoscopy, anorectal manometry as well as performing a traditional pelvic exam with speculum to rule out significant pathology. These are important diagnostics and they are often beneficial in determining the best overall treatment plan for these clients. However, too often, the pelvic floor, hip, and abdominal skeletal muscles are not examined or

even considered when diagnosing and treating these clients. As altered musculoskeletal health in the pelvic region can significantly affect the bladder and anorectal function [3], competency in the assessment and treatment of these muscles cannot be underrated. Pelvic floor physical therapists (PFPT) specialize in the assessment and treatment of the pelvic floor musculature (PFM) both externally and internally as well as the surrounding fascial, nervous, and skeletal tissue. This chapter will describe a PFPT evaluation and treatment of clients referred for pelvic floor dysfunction (PFD) of any kind. This chapter will also describe the typical findings and treatment of the client with HPFD. Ultimately, it is the goal of this chapter to encourage physicians who see clients with HPFD or any other type of PFD to give appropriate and early referrals to PFPT specialists for treatment as an important part of an interdisciplinary team [1].

The Importance of Communicating Empathy

When a PFPT first meets a client with symptoms typical to HPFD, often times these clients have either been referred by a physician with little experience in HPFD, especially as it relates to CPP, or the client has found out about physical therapy for the pelvic floor through a website or online support group. They are often apprehensive about physical therapy, thinking, "What could a physical therapist possibly do for me?" Many times these clients have seen multiple physicians prior to coming for treatment, many of whom have prescribed antifungals and antibiotics, even when the client tested negative for bacteria or yeast. These physicians have run every test they could think of, found no obvious sign of impairment or dysfunction and, while potentially important and very beneficial, their only recommendation is to suggest psychiatric treatment and evaluation as in their assessment there is no other clear etiology to explain these client's symptoms. The client often feels invalidated and misunderstood and they are near hopeless that there could be any

J.L. Ortiz (✉)
Her Physical Therapy, LLC, 10705 Charter Drive Ste 420, Columbia, MD 21044, USA
e-mail: jortizpt@yahoo.com

© Springer Science+Business Media New York 2017
D.A. Gordon, M.R. Katlic (eds.), *Pelvic Floor Dysfunction and Pelvic Surgery in the Elderly*,
DOI 10.1007/978-1-4939-6554-0_8

improvement of their symptoms. Many of these clients will have tried dietary changes, meditation, and other alternative interventions, which are often helpful to a small degree, but in no way entirely resolve their symptoms. As such an experienced PFPT may spend the first crucial moments of their initial consultation simply building trust with the client, often assuring the client that there are an array of treatments available to them, including but not limited to physical therapy. All clinicians who come into contact with these clients need to work to assure them that it is likely that their symptoms have a true physiological origin, even if their pain is now due in a large part to central sensitization [4, 5]. Furthermore, these PFPT need to educate their client that there are a growing network of specialists who are not only capable of treating their symptoms appropriately but who are also, what will become for these clients, an important part of an interdisciplinary team that the client will ultimately need to fully treat their PFD. This team includes gynecologists, urologists, physiatrists, psychiatrists, psychologists, neurourologists, neurologists as well as PFPT, all of whom have specialized in PFD, including HPFD and CPP.

A concerted effort needs to be made to provide comfort to these clients. Clients have reported that their level of comfort with their provider first influenced the likelihood that they would discuss concerns about sensitive issues and second, influenced whether or not they would trust in their provider's plan of care [6]. Clients with any type of PFD need to perceive compassion, as well as intelligence in their provider. It has been published that client perceived provider empathy significantly influences client satisfaction and compliance to treatment recommendations. This is in part because of the exchange of good information, the perceived expertise of the provider, the interpersonal trust established with the provider, and the perception of partnership with the provider [7]. Once the important step of establishing the trust and comfort of the client has taken place, the evaluation and treatment can continue far more successfully.

Medical History of the Client with PFD

As in any comprehensive medical consultation, a PFPT starts with a review of the client's past medical history. There are often important pieces of information gleaned from their past medical history that play a larger role than the client believes they would and so the client often fails to provide this information as they do not realize it is relevant. For example, a client may not mention any previous serious injuries. An experienced PFPT may ask a client, "Have you ever fallen and seriously hurt your tailbone?" Only then might the client recollect that they fell and hurt their coccyx so badly in high school that they could not sit normally for months. As a coccyx injury can cause many of the symptoms these

Table 8.1 Important considerations in the past medical history of clients with pelvic floor dysfunction

Multigravida	Ectopic pregnancy
Pelvic venous congestion syndrome	Traumatic vaginal birth
Cesarean section	Rectus diastasis
Hysterectomy	Oopherectomy
Irritable bowel syndrome	Coccygodynia
Sacral fracture	Hip dysplasia
Cerebral vascular accident	Multiple sclerosis
Uterine fibroids	Chronic constipation
Prostatitis	Groin strain
Inguinal hernia	Abdominal surgery
Competitive cyst	Competitive gymnast
Prolapsed pelvic organ	Sexually transmitted disease
Interstitial cystitis	Sexual or physical abuse
Frequent urinary tract infections	Frequent yeast infections
Primary dysmenorrhea	Adenomyosis

clients complain of and pain from this lesion may become recurrently symptomatic [8], that one question could have provided at least an important part of their etiology, helping to form their treatment plan. See Table 8.1 for other important pieces within the past medical history that can affect pelvic floor function.

A large percentage of the time, a skilled provider experienced in the treatment of PFD can make a preliminary diagnosis based on the history alone. The value of the history, of course, will depend on the provider's ability to elicit relevant information. All providers should do their best to remove any physical or otherwise client perceived barriers that stand between them and the client. The provider should move their chair closer to the client's, sit at equal height to the client when possible and maintain eye contact. In short, the provider should do all that can be done in the limited time the provider and the client have together, to place the provider and the client on equal footing. This helps to assure the client that the provider is completely focused on them during that time as well as helping to create an environment that will facilitate the exchange of useful information [7, 8].

A PFPT will ask many deeply personal questions about bowel, bladder, and sexual function and habits. As both the male and female client may perceive their penis or vagina to operate in isolation from their bowel and bladder, they will often wonder, why, if, for example, they came to a PFPT with the complaint of pain with intercourse, are they being asked about their bowel and bladder function. At this point the PFPT explains to the patient that the pelvic floor is a complex structure made up of muscles, ligaments, tendons, nerves, fascia, veins, arteries, mucosal tissue, and glands. Furthermore they will explain that the pelvic floor supports the urinary, fecal, sexual, and reproductive functions as well as the pelvic statics simultaneously [9]. If there is dysfunction or impairment in any one of these urological, gynecological, rectal or pelvic floor musculoskeletal systems, there will likely be impairment in another. Showing the patient a simple model or anatomical picture of the pelvic floor skeleton, muscles and nerves at this point in the evaluation is often helpful to better establish their understanding of their own pelvic floors.

The questions a PFPT asks in the subjective portion of the initial evaluation usually begin with bladder function and behavior. The client is asked how frequently do they urinate in the day and during the night? How much and what type of fluid do they consume? How long can they delay urination once they feel urge? How strong is their urge? Do they feel that their bladder empties completely and if not what strategies have they tried in order to accomplish more complete emptying (i.e., posturing, standing up and sitting down again, bearing down)? Do they have pain with full bladders or during urination? How much urine comes out when they do urinate intentionally (only a few drops of urine, or is it a small, medium, or large amount)? How fast or slow is their urine stream? Do they urinate at night and if so, how often? Do they leak urine and if so, how much and how often? Finally, how many incontinence pads do they wear in twenty-four hours and what size are they?

The Client with HPFD

The client with HPFD typically will report high frequency of urination, often urinating 10 to even 20 times or more during the day, and often this is regardless of whether or not they are consuming commonly recommended levels of daily water intake. Many dehydrate themselves, limiting fluid intake in an effort to make fewer trips to the restroom. Clients with HPFD will often describe needing to bear down or sit and wait patiently while trying to relax better in order to initiate their urine stream as well as to fully empty their bladders. They will many times describe a slow or hesitant urine stream that starts and stops frequently while urinating. In addition they will often report pain in the pelvic region with bladder filling and emptying, with occasional abdominal pain with bladder emptying. Finally, they will sometimes present with a varying degree of urge incontinence.

The line of questioning for any client then often turns to bowel function. The client is asked, how regular are their bowel movements? What is the typical consistency of the bowel movements and do they have to strain to initiate and/or complete the bowel movement? Do they take stool softeners, laxatives, or fiber supplements in order to accomplish a bowel movement on any kind of regular basis? Do they have anorectal or abdominal pain with the bowel movement? Do they have to change positions in order to evacuate their bowels? Do they have to brace manually with their hands on their perineum or, if female, in their vagina to evacuate their bowels? Do they leak feces and if so how much?

The Client with HPFD

The client with HPFD typically reports abdominal bloating, abdominal pain with bowel movement, anorectal pain with bowel movement, incomplete bowel emptying, straining to initiate and complete bowel movements as well as constipation.

The next category to be discussed with any client is sexual function. By this time in the evaluation, the provider has hopefully begun to earn their client's trust. Even if the client has come specifically to address their sexual function, it is still a difficult and deeply personal subject to discuss with anyone, much less a medical provider you have just met. The provider's confidence and comfort with the subject material, as well as the client's trust in the provider at this point in the evaluation are so important. The client's honesty and willingness to share details about their sexual function is vital to establishing a successful plan of care. As an example, a client was referred to our physical therapy practice by an obstetrician/gynecologist who had ruled out other pathology as a source of this client's pelvic pain.

The client initially only shared that she had severe pain with intercourse with her husband. Only after the client had developed confidence in the provider and only after the client had determined that the provider would be compassionate and nonjudgmental, did the client share that she did not have pain during intercourse with her lover like she did with her husband, despite the fact that her lover had a much larger penis. This allowed the physical therapist to determine, even before the physical and objective portion of the evaluation was performed, that this client would likely need counseling and psychological intervention more so than physical therapy. After the objective examination confirmed that the client's PFM had normal range of motion along with no other potential neuromuscular sources of pain, the client was educated on the complex relationship between her level of desire and its effect on her blood flow and glandular behavior in her vestibule and vagina. This knowledge helped to empower this client and convinced her to pursue psychology and counseling as her primary form of treatment. A 6-month follow-up by phone call confirmed that this was indeed the best course of action for this client. If the client had not felt comfortable enough to share that she had a lover and that intercourse was not painful with him, she may have had additional unnecessary and expensive medical testing or treatment, taken less effective medication and still not progressed towards her long-term goal of pain free intercourse with her husband.

When questioning about sexual function, first, if appropriate, it is important to determine the sexual orientation of the client, or at least the sexual practices of the client. Are they sexually active and if so, how many times in a month are they experiencing penetrative intercourse? If female or if a homosexual male, the client is asked if there is pain with penetration both at the entrance, middle and/or deep? Is there pain with movement of the penis or other sexual instrument, if utilized? Can the male patient achieve and maintain erection and can the female and/or male patient achieve orgasm? Is there pain with the orgasm if they can achieve it? Is there pain after penetrative intercourse or orgasm? Does the client have a history of penetrative or non-penetrative intercourse against their will? The relationship between sexual abuse and urinary tract symptoms, sexual abuse and gastrointestinal symptoms, or sexual abuse and sexual dysfunction has been well documented. One study published in 2009 in the Journal of Sexual Medicine found that patients with multiple pelvic floor complaints (micturition, defecation, and sexual function) related to pelvic floor dysfunction were more likely to have a history of sexual abuse than the patients with isolated complaints [10].

The Client with HPFD
The client with HPFD often reports insertional or deep dyspareunia often making intercourse intolerable as well as a pelvic and abdominal ache during and after intercourse and/ or orgasm.

Finally the PFPT will ask if the client has hip pain, middle or low back pain, sacroiliac pain and/or pubic bone pain? They will ask if the client has any radiating symptoms into their legs and if so, how severe is that pain? If the client reports any of these types and locations of pain, what activities or treatments have made that pain worse or better? Does the client participate in any type of exercise on a consistent basis and how intensely do they exercise when they do? Find out the occupation of the client and what if any physical requirements they have in their profession. Do not assume that if they have a desk job where they are seated much of the day that you do not need to be concerned about the physical demands of their job. Sedentary office workers with subacute, nonspecific low back pain have been found to have lower musculoskeletal fitness than healthy, age-matched controls, with the main difference found in endurance of the trunk muscles [10, 11]. This generalized decrease in musculoskeletal health can lead to orthopedic pain and dysfunction, including the pelvic and lumbar regions. Musculoskeletal pain and dysfunction throughout the pelvic and lumbar region commonly contribute to PFD [12]. In regard to questions about fitness, a patient's choice of exercise, especially if performed on a regular basis, can contribute to or even cause significant pelvic dysfunction. For example, a client who is a cyclist will experience prolonged perineal pressure as well as repeated and often vigorous hip flexion. Amongst other common physical injuries, cycling has also been known to cause pudendal nerve entrapment or inflammation [13] which can be a precursor to HPFD as well as other types of

PFD. Therefore if the client is a cyclist, again you may have stumbled upon a significant part of their etiology without performing a single objective test.

The Client with HPFD
Low back pain radiating to the thighs or groin unrelated to intercourse, as well as pelvic pain unrelated to intercourse are common in clients with HPFD [1].

Objective Measures

The role of the PFPT in the treatment of PFD for many years was widely debated.

Many felt that the treatments were unsubstantiated and therefore would not refer clients to physical therapy. In recent years these concerns have been laid to rest with multiple publications supporting the role of physical therapy in the treatment of PFD, including HPFD [14, 15]. The role of the PFPT is primarily in the assessment and treatment of the musculoskeletal system. Pelvic floor muscle dysfunction, such as myofascial trigger points (MTP) or palpable hypertonic PFM may be identified in as many as 85 % of clients suffering from urological, colorectal, and gynecological pelvic pain syndromes. In some clients, these MTP can be responsible for some, if not all, symptoms related to these syndromes [9]. Again, it cannot be emphasized enough that by the time the provider is ready to begin the objective portion of the evaluation, the client should have complete confidence in their provider's comfort and knowledge of their particular PFD. This confidence, along with the fact that the typical physical therapy pelvic floor initial evaluation is an hour in length, allowing the PFPT to go slowly and carefully through the objective portion of the evaluation, should make the client feel safe and secure throughout the examination. The PFPT occasionally finds that for reasons of time limitations or client comfort, an internal pelvic floor examination on the client during the initial visit is not possible or perhaps not indicated as the external dysfunction is so extensive. Many times the internal portion can be completed during a follow-up visit as again, a skilled provider can determine much about the patient from simply performing a comprehensive medical review and an external objective evaluation.

Featured and proposed at this point in the chapter is the Ortiz Stewart Pelvic Floor Dysfunction Physical Therapy Assessment and Treatment Algorithm (see Fig. 8.1). The authors of the OS Algorithm propose that it describes what a typical PFPT works through when evaluating and treating a client with PFD. The OS Algorithm is based on a compilation of research that when assembled gives a logical order to the objective evaluation and treatment of any client with

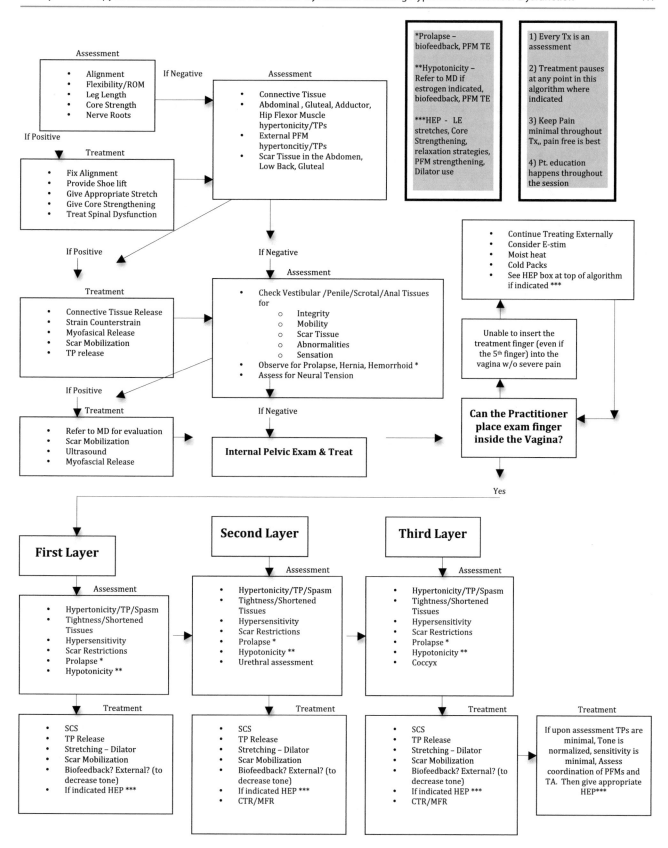

Fig. 8.1 The Ortiz Stewart Pelvic Floor Dysfunction Physical Therapy Assessment and Treatment Algorithm

PFD. We further propose that not only does the OS Algorithm potentially demonstrate what a more experienced PFPT would likely perform in any given treatment session but also that the OS Algorithm could be especially helpful in guiding the novice PFPT who has not yet established their own methodology. Further research needs to be conducted to determine if this algorithm is a truly successful guide to the PFPT. Clinically the author of this chapter and the coauthors of the OS Algorithm have had great success using this as a guide to assessment and treatment, however it must be remembered that each client and each physical therapist is entirely unique. Each situation may demand skipping forward in the OS Algorithm or staying put for a while without moving forward until indicated. Any other type of rigid checklist or formulaic approach would not be true to the fluid nature of PFPT. We will now review the various elements of the evaluation and treatment as described in the OS Algorithm (Fig. 8.1) and then mention what you would typically find while examining the client with HPFD.

Orthopedic Assessment

The objective evaluation begins with looking at the pelvic and lumbar alignment, the range of motion and flexibility of the hips and low back, assessing core strength and checking for leg length discrepancy. As already noted, dysfunction in any of those regions can contribute to HPFD as well as any other type of PFD, so the PFPT will need to determine what, if any, treatments will need to be performed to address any dysfunction in those regions [1, 12].

Most PFPT(s) will first check the flexibility and movement of the spine, hips, pelvis, knees and feet. This is often performed in standing first and can be observed and performed quickly. Some flexibility tests will be best performed in supine or prone and therefore are tested later in the evaluation if indicated (See Fig. 8.2). Once any loss of flexibility is assessed as well as any hinging or hypermobility of the spine is noted and documented, the PFPT will then perform any special tests indicated by the assessment of the client's range of motion (ROM) or movement dysfunction. Typically, hip and sacral dysfunction are diagnosed by standing and seated flexion tests as well as noting any asymmetry of the pelvic and sacral bony landmarks, which would indicate poor lumbopelvic alignment. A detailed write up of the numerous special tests, especially for the purpose of diagnosing hip and sacroiliac joint dysfunction are beyond the scope of this chapter, however please see the sources referenced in this chapter to read more about them [16, 17].

Lumbopelvic alignment is then assessed and treated by an experienced pelvic floor physical therapist, in any type of pelvic floor dysfunction. If the bony landmarks of the pelvis demonstrate that there is poor alignment, in theory one could

argue that the muscles attached to those bony landmarks will have an unequal length tension relationship, making it harder for the pelvic and hip musculature, pelvic floor musculature and lumbar musculature to function properly [18]. It has been shown that muscle tension in the pelvic floor muscles can cause pelvic misalignment, leading to pain and further dysfunction [19]. To check alignment, the client is observed first in standing, than in supine, and finally in the prone position. The PFPT will compare the position of the bilateral iliac crests, anterior superior iliac spines, posterior superior iliac spines, ischial tuberosities, gluteal folds, and greater trochanters as well as the pubic tubercles and the inferior lateral angles of the sacrum. Again, an experienced PFPT can compare these landmarks quickly and efficiently.

Next, the clinician needs to determine if there is any leg length discrepancy. Unfortunately this is diagnosed incorrectly too often, as it is either missed or, more commonly, given as a diagnosis when in reality the client does not have a true leg length discrepancy. Many times clients will report being given a shoe lift by a well-intentioned provider and the client will report that their symptoms are either unchanged or are worse than previous to the use of a heel lift. Once examined and treated they often are found to have what could be described as a functional leg length discrepancy and not a true leg length discrepancy [20, 21]. This means that with treatment, their leg length discrepancy "disappears," indicating that their shorter leg was not actually shortened but rather appeared so as the result of sacroiliac joint, hip, or pubic bone dysfunction. Leg length discrepancies whether true or functional lead to an unequal transmission of forces across the spine and pelvis during weight bearing activities which can lead to muscle dysfunction, joint impairment and ultimately to HPFD, and therefore need to be addressed. Some clinicians postulate that a leg length difference of three quarters of an inch or more is necessary to cause any significant dysfunction and therefore any client with this difference or greater could benefit from a shoe lift [22]; however, there are others that feel that differences as little as 4 mm are significant enough to warrant a shoe lift [23]. Finally the client needs to have their hip strength, sacroiliac joint stability and core strength and stability assessed including assessment for rectus diastasis. One of the most well-recognized methods to assess core strength and sacroiliac stability is the Asymmetrical Straight Leg Raise test (see Fig. 8.2). The supine active straight less raise (ASLR) test has been validated as a clinical test for measuring effective load transfer between the trunk and the lower limbs. When the lumbopelvic-hip region is functioning optimally, the leg should rise effortlessly from the table (effort can be graded from 0 to 5) and the pelvis should not move (flex, extend, laterally bend, or rotate) relative to the thorax or lower extremity. This requires proper activation of the muscles which stabilize the thorax, low back, and pelvis. There are several compensation strategies

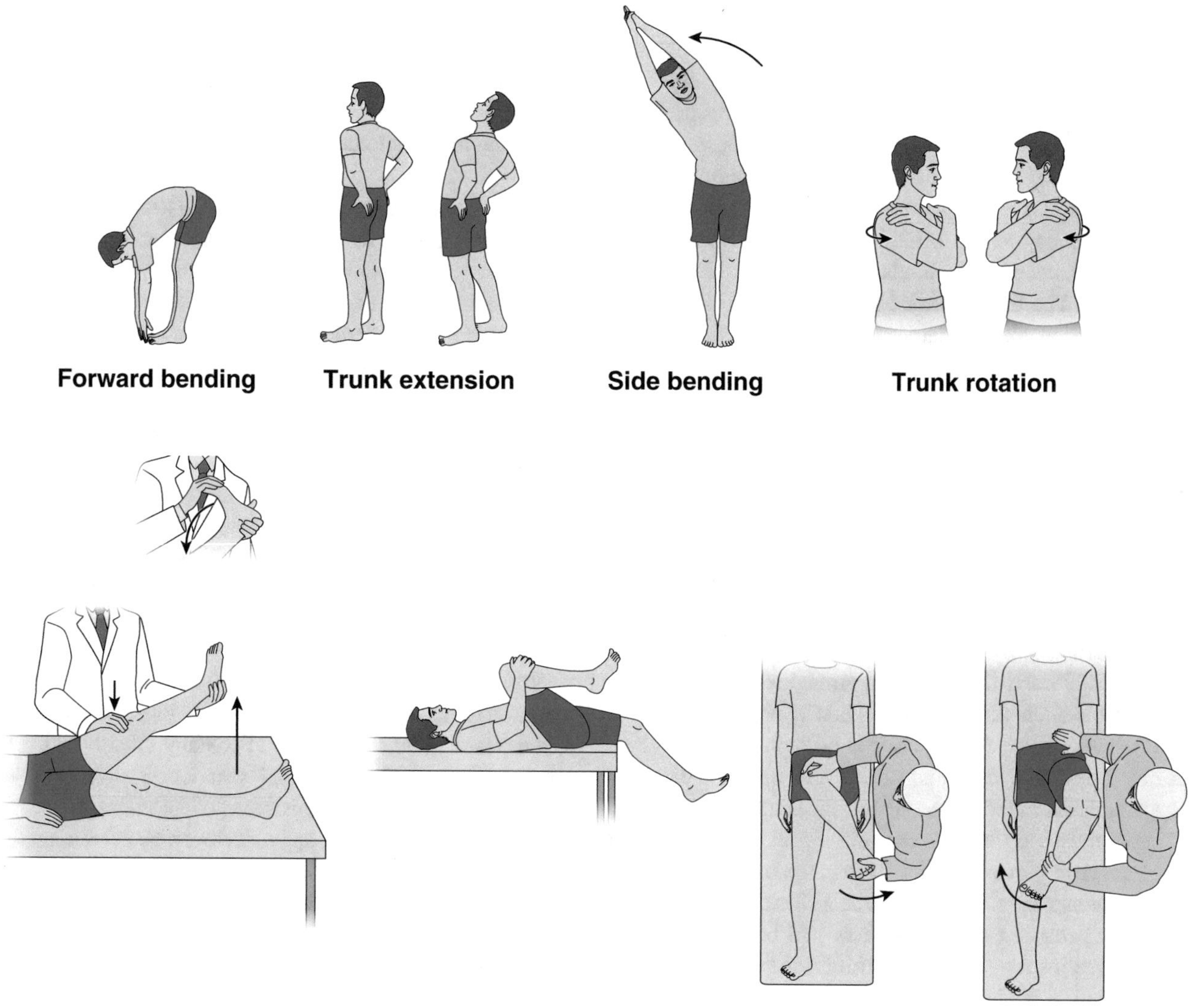

Forward bending   **Trunk extension**   **Side bending**   **Trunk rotation**

Straight leg raise   **Hip flexor tightness**   **Hip external and internal ROM**

Fig. 8.2 Common movement and flexibility testing performed in clients with pelvic floor disorders. *ROM* range of motion

when stabilization of the lumbopelvic region is lacking and the ASLR test can identify these strategies [24]. This test has been standardized and is well recognized to show instability in the SI joint [25]. Loss of core strength and sacroiliac stability can contribute to HPFD, general CPP and low back pain [26, 27]. The pelvic floor muscles can become hypertonic to compensate for the loss of integrity, as with a rectus diastasis, loss of stability and weakness of the core musculature as the pelvic floor muscles attempt to provide stability for the pelvis in ways those muscles were not intended to do so. As shown in the OS Algorithm (Fig. 8.1), there are times when a PFPT will treat a client who has no significant loss of range of motion or flexibility in their back and hips, no pelvic asymmetries, good core strength, no rectus diastasis and no leg length discrepancies, however this is the rare exception. Likely the client will present with a fair number of these

impairments. If this is the client's first assessment with the PFPT, you simply note the dysfunction or the lack thereof and continue on in the OS Algorithm (see Fig. 8.1) for further assessment. However if this is a treatment session, the clinician should treat and address these impairments first, as to neglect them would make further treatment of any type of PFD less effective [24]. Treatment would include correcting any lumbopelvic misalignment, giving customized core and hip strengthening where needed, giving stretches where there is significant tightness, providing extensive patient education and, only if indicated by a significant leg length discrepancy, a trial of a shoe lift. To correct alignment many physical therapy clinicians use Muscle Energy Technique (MET). A detailed description of this technique is outside the scope of this chapter, however, briefly, this technique is a common conservative treatment for pathology around the spine, particularly lumbopelvic pain. MET is considered a gentle manual therapy for restricted motion of the spine and extremities and is an active technique where the patient, and not the clinician, controls the corrective force. This treatment requires the patient to perform voluntary muscle contractions of varying intensity, in a precise direction, while the clinician applies a counterforce, allowing movement to occur. For many years, MET has been advocated to treat muscle imbalances of the lumbopelvic region such as pelvic asymmetry. The theory behind MET suggests that the technique is used to correct an asymmetry by targeting a contraction of the hamstring or the hip flexors on the painful side of the low back and moving the innominate in a corrected direction. It is worth noting, however, that evidence suggests that non-symptomatic individuals have also been shown to have pelvic asymmetries. Despite this, MET is frequently used by manual therapy clinicians as activating muscles in the region to assist with stimulating Type IIA mechanoreceptors and improving regional muscle function [18, 28, 29]. To date there are very few published prospective data to compare the efficacy of this treatment modality [26].

Clinical Pearl: Stretches and strengthening need to be given to the client judiciously, this is why physical therapists call it therapeutic exercise. There is no "cookie cutter" home exercise program where all clients can perform the same exact stretches in the same way nor the same exact strengthening exercises in the same way and expect the same benefit. The danger in providing a list of exercises in any textbook or on any website for that matter is that a client will perform the exercises because they believe they will be good for them when in reality, they can be harmful for the client. An example of this is a tendency by less experienced physical therapists and physicians to hand out pelvic floor contractions (also called Kegels) to clients with pelvic pain. If the client has hypotonic pelvic floor muscles with poor coordination and they need to strengthen their pelvic floor muscles, then this could be an appropriate exercise prescription assuming the client can perform the exercises correctly. However, many times clients with pelvic pain, especially clients with HPFD, have (as implied in the name) hypertonic pelvic floor muscles and their greatest need, at least initially, is to learn how to fully relax their pelvic floor musculature. If they try to perform pelvic floor muscle contractions, their tone could increase and their symptoms only worsen [1, 30]. That being said, therapeutic exercise including core strengthening and core and hip flexibility is often an important part of their rehabilitation and should not be neglected.

Soft Tissue Assessment and Treatment

One of the most important elements in the assessment and treatment of the client with HPFD or indeed any type of PFD is the soft tissue surrounding the pelvic region.

Specifically this includes assessment and treatment of the connective tissue, such as the skin and fascia around the pelvic, abdominal, lumbar, gluteal, and proximal thigh regions as well as the external skeletal muscle tissue for palpable hypertonicity, hypotonicity, and/or MTP(s).

Connective, Scar and Fascial Tissue Restriction

The PFPT evaluates the consistency and mobility of the various layers of the connective tissue. They will specifically assess and address the connective tissue in the abdominal wall, lower back, buttocks, vulva, and thigh by performing a specific technique that could be described as skin rolling. This technique can be quite painful, with the client who has the most restrictions experiencing the greatest amount of pain.

The Client with HPFD
Among with clients with HPFD, connective tissue abnormalities, such as connective tissue restrictions and trigger points, are common around the umbilicus, pubis, inguinal ligaments, lumbar region, and sacral regions [3].

While inspecting the connective tissue for restriction, it is common to find non-muscular trigger points in the skin, scar tissue, fascia, and ligaments [31]. Many clients with PFD present with previous surgical scar tissue sites or injury including perineal tears, episiotomy, laparoscopy, cesarean section, cholecystectomy, appendectomy, hysterectomy, and abdominoplasty. These MTP(s) in the connective tissue and scar tissue, which also cause radiating pain in the pelvic region, can be treated with Connective Tissue Release, a technique similar to skin rolling, elevating the tissue away from the skeletal muscle layer to release restriction [3].

Trigger Points and Hypertonicity in Skeletal Muscle

An MTP in a skeletal muscle is defined as a point of hyperirritability in a muscular taut band that is clinically associated with local twitch response and tenderness and/or referred pain upon manual examination [32]. Evidence suggests that the temporal profile of the spontaneous electrical activity at an MTP is similar to focal muscle fiber contraction and/or muscle cramp potentials, which contribute significantly to local tenderness and pain and motor dysfunction [33]. MTP(s) can create restriction, which can cause the tendon and ligaments attached to the muscle where they are located to over stretch, often causing pain in the associated joint or radiating elsewhere [34]. Studies have shown that abnormal conditions of the pelvic floor muscles and abdominal and pelvic region muscles are the probable etiologic site of men with genitourinary pain [35], women with vulvodynia [36], patients with interstitial cystitis [37], patients with abdominal pelvic pain syndrome [38], and HPFD [39].

Table 8.2 Muscle list

List of muscles to be assessed in examination of pelvic floor dysfunction as trigger points in these muscles have been shown to refer pain to the pelvic region, lower abdominal region, and perineal region:

- Adductor magnus
- Adductor longus
- Thoracolumbar paraspinal musculature
- Piriformis
- Gluteus magnus
- Gluteus minimus
- Gluteus medius
- Quadratus lumborum
- Iliacus
- Psoas major
- Obturator internus (often assessed internally)
- Tensor fascia lata (no direct referral to perineum or pelvic, however often found in clients with pelvic floor dysfunction

Table 8.3 List of muscles, ligaments, and bony landmarks assessed on the external pelvic floor

- Pubis symphysis
- Inferior pubic rami
- Ischial rami
- Sacrotuberous ligament
- Ischiocavernosus
- Bulbospongiosus
- Superficial transverse perineal
- Levator ani
- Perineal body
- Ischial tuberosity

It takes skill that is developed over time, as well as critical thinking and knowledge of anatomy to correctly palpate skeletal muscle tissue for hyper or hypotonicity, MTP(s), or restriction. Despite this, there is often good interrater reliability of palpation of MTP(s) and therefore it can be trusted as a good diagnostic tool [34, 40]. The PFPT will palpate the gluteal muscles, the hamstrings and low back muscles in prone. Then in supine, they will palpate the adductors, proximal quadriceps, the lateral hip musculature, hip flexors, and abdominal muscles. See Table 8.2 for a comprehensive list of muscles that should be assessed in any examination of a client with PFD. Then finally, when the patient is ready, they will evaluate the external pelvic floor musculature. Again, this typically takes gentle encouragement as many of the clients are apprehensive about this portion of the exam. The pressures used to examine the client need to be firm enough to ensure assessment of skeletal muscle; however, an effort should be made to stay within tolerable pain limits for the client. See Table 8.3 for a list of pelvic floor muscles and pelvic region bony landmarks assessed externally. If the client is not severely hypertonic and has little pain with palpation of the external pelvic floor, the PFPT may ask the client to perform a pelvic floor contraction to assess for and observe externally the client's coordination and more importantly their ability to relax after contraction. Many times however, the skilled PFPT will not assess the coordination of the client with HPFD symptoms prior to an internal assessment. With some clients, their external MTP(s) are so profound and their pelvic floor muscle hypertonicity so apparent, there is no indication for further assessment at that time. The client needs to have these MTP(s) and any other external soft tissue dysfunction treated before moving any further within the OS Algorithm (Fig. 8.1). As stated earlier, MTP(s) play a role in the vast majority of clients with PFD, especially in clients with CPP and HPFD [9]. Indeed, in some cases, it is possible for MTP(s) to be the only cause of pelvic pain.

Case Study
A 38-year-old woman gave a 14-year history of right lower quadrant pain, urinary retention, frequency, suprapubic pressure, and deep right-sided dyspareunia. These symptoms had arisen after a caesarian section that followed 2 days of traumatic labor. Her pelvic pain symptoms had been treated elsewhere with nine laparoscopic procedures for lysis of adhesions, a right oopherectomy, and total abdominal hysterectomy. When she presented to this clinic complaining of continued pain, external pelvic examination revealed myofascial trigger points of the right rectus abdominis muscles and a tender suprapubic scar. Internal pelvic examination disclosed myofascial trigger points of the right obturator internus, pubourethralis, and urinary sphincter. She was treated with internal myofascial release techniques (see below for a description of this technique), with eradicated the trigger points and hypertonus of the pelvic floor, and trigger point injections of 0.5% bupivacaine into the rectus abdominis trigger points and scar. She became completely asymptomatic after 12 treatments [41].

MTP being the sole source of pelvic pain is rarely seen in clinical practice. More commonly MTP(s) are just one component of a multilayered problem and usually present with connective tissue restriction, nerve inflammation, hormone irregularities, poor core, and pelvic floor skeletal muscle strength and flexibility and pelvic organ impairments such as overactive bladder, irritable bowel syndrome, and painful bladder syndrome (or interstitial cystitis). If the client presents with any of these external pelvic region impairments, they would be treated with connective tissue release (as described above), strain counterstrain, myofascial release, dry needling, manual scar mobilization (as described above), and manual trigger point release. A detailed description of these techniques is outside the scope of this chapter, however they are briefly described below:

Strain and Counterstrain

Strain and counterstrain (also called positional release therapy) is a manual soft tissue manipulation technique in which the practitioner locates and alleviates non-radiating tender points in the client's myofascial structures. The practitioner positions dysfunctional tissue at a point of balance in a direction opposite to the restrictive barrier. The position of ease, or the position in which the client no longer has pain to touch at the tender point, is held for ninety seconds, after which the patient is gently returned to the original position where the tender point is rechecked. The theory is that Strain counterstrain works to inhibit hyperactivity of the spasm reflex, allowing the muscle to relax by improving oxygenation and eliminating pain. To date, there is little data to support this technique, however, it is the author's experience that clients with allodynia in their vulvar and vaginal tissues respond very well to this technique.

Myofascial Release

Myofascial release is a soft tissue therapy for the treatment of skeletal muscle immobility and pain. It is theorized that this type of manual therapy relaxes hypertonic muscles, improves blood flow, increases lymphatic circulation, and stimulates stretch reflexes in the muscles. Many practitioners use the myofascial release technique developed by John Barnes. His method emphasizes light contact with the fascia, slowly stretching the fascia until reaching a barrier/restriction, maintaining this light pressure for 3–5 min and then feeling for a motion and softening of the tissue.

Dry Needling

Dry needling is a skilled intervention that uses a thin filiform needle to penetrate the skin and stimulate underlying myofascial trigger points, muscular, and connective tissues for the management of neuromusculoskeletal pain and movement impairments. Dry needling is a technique used to treat dysfunctions in skeletal muscle, fascia, and connective tissue and diminish persistent peripheral nociceptive input, and reduce or restore impairments of body structure and function leading to improved activity and participation [42].

Soft Tissue Mobilization

Soft tissue mobilization is defined as the hands-on mobilization of soft tissues, i.e. muscle and associated connective tissues that support it, and the tendons and ligaments. Soft tissue mobilization is theorized to produce improved neural ability, decreased muscle hypertonicity, increased muscle blood flow, improve lymphatic flow, and improved overall circulation in the area treated. A trained physical therapist localizes the source of pain or movement restriction through skilled, layer-by-layer assessment. They will look for soft tissue restrictions that could decrease motion and cause pain for the client. Once these areas of restriction are found, the trained therapist will use a variety of techniques to clear these restrictions, they are better prepared for therapeutic exercise.

Manual Trigger Point Release or Ischemic Compression

There are different manual techniques used to perform manual trigger points. The more common approaches are deep pressure and/or ischemic compression. Practitioners use their hands and fingers to find the trigger point, which is felt as a "speed bump" or knot in the tissue and then release it by applying deep pressure and/or ischemic compression. Many times, they will use their elbows or other various tools to apply pressure, to save their hands as the pressure needed is often so firm, they cannot maintain that force throughout the session, much less throughout the day. Fascia surrounding these trigger points should also be treated with therapeutic exercise, myofascial release or soft tissue mobilization to elongate and resolve strain patterns, otherwise muscles and connective tissue will simply be returned to positions where trigger points are likely to re-develop. See also references [9, 34–43] for more information both on the effectiveness of these treatments as well as further description of these treatments. If these treatments are not effective for the client in a timely manner, then a referral to a physician who can perform trigger point injections to the pelvic floor muscles and the surrounding pelvic and abdominal region musculature, using an anesthetic such as benzocaine or novocaine, using an anti-inflammatory or injection of botulinum toxin is indicated.

The Client with HPFD

A typical client with HPFD as well as CPP will present with muscle guarding. The guarding presents as muscles that have contracted tightly, for a prolonged period of time around a painful area. This guarding, unfortunately, restricts blood flow, leads to hypertonic muscles and MTP(s), causing more pain and guarding, leading to a vicious cycle. However hypertonic muscles or MTP(s) develop in the pelvic region, they often stick around well after the original cause of pain has cleared. See Table 8.4 for different ways pelvic region hypertonicity or MTP(s) can develop.

An easy analogy to demonstrate how trigger points and hypertonicity can develop: When you hold a fist tightly for a longer period of time, as in while holding several heavy bags of groceries in your hand as you carry them to your home from your car, and then you go to set the grocery bags down, many times your fist will not automatically relax. It stays very tense and perhaps only after some time has passed and you have shaken it out, does it finally relax back to baseline tension. In the same way, when you hold your pelvic floor muscles tight, sometimes not just for a few minutes but even for days or months because of pelvic pain, urinary urgency or heightened psychological stress, it is very difficult to get your pelvic floor muscles to relax and return to what their baseline is. Just as the hand would have pain if you kept holding the fist, the pelvic floor muscles have pain from being held or contracted, whether consciously or unconsciously.

Assessment of Vulvar Tissues and Prolapse

Again, in the rarest of patients, you will not find any of the previously described impairments. But whether you find these external impairments or not, the next objective assessment on the female client is to assess the vulva thoroughly.

Table 8.4 Different ways that pelvic region hypertonicity or MTPs can develop

- After receiving vaginal ultrasound
- Chronic or acute strain with defecation
- Fall on tailbone, back, pelvis, or hip
- Sexual abuse
- Physical abuse
- Urinary incontinence
- Fecal incontinence
- Urinary urgency and/or frequency
- Urinary tract infection (frequent or as few as one)
- Yeast infection
- Dyspareunia
- Cycling
- Vigorous high impact exercise
- Vaginal childbirth
- Episiotomy

See Table 8.5 for anatomical landmarks assessed and what a physical therapist looks for. On the male patient the PFPT will need to examine the penile and scrotal tissue and on both sexes they may need to examine the tissue around the anus. Again, this is obviously one of the more sensitive portions of the assessment. Many female and male clients are very hesitant to open their legs for this portion of the exam. The pressures on these delicate tissues should be kept well within tolerable limits. The provider should talk their way through the examination so the client knows what is being assessed and so that there are no surprises. PFPT(s) will often assess at this time for sensation, both allodynia and decreased sensation. A common test is the cotton swab test (Table 8.6). If indicated by observing upon examination scarring or restriction in the vulvar or scrotal tissues, a PFPT may perform scar tissue mobilization or myofascial release on these tissues. More often, if significant impairment is observed, the client is referred to a physician for further evaluation and treatment. At this point in the exam, the physical therapist can also perform reflex testing, if indicated, such as the anal wink test. The anal wink test is evoked by firmly stroking the perianal skin with a Q-tip®. The absence of an anal wink reflex suggests a defect in either sensory or motor nerves or in the central pathways that mediate this reflex [44]. A positive finding would indicate that the client could benefit from a referral to a neurologist or neurourologist for further testing. If indicated, at this point in the exam the PFPT will often assess for adverse neural tension [3], observe for profound prolapse or significant hemorrhoid sensitivity. A detailed description of techniques to release adverse neural tension, diagnose severity of prolapse, or assess hemorrhoid sensitivity is outside the scope of this chapter, however if the reader wishes for more information on these treatments or tests, please see the references provided at the end of the chapter [3, 40, 45, 46]. Again, the skilled PFPT would treat as

Table 8.5 Anatomical landmarks and what dysfunction a physical therapist will look for in these tissues

Mons pubis	Swelling, discoloration, thickening, unilateral hyper- or hypotrophy
Labia majora	Loss of anatomy, swelling, discoloration, thickening, unilateral hyper- or hypotrophy, redness, whiteness, loss of hair, lesions
Labia minora	Loss of anatomy, swelling, redness, thickening, whiteness, rigidity, micro tearing
Hart's line	Loss of appearance of a change in tissue between the vulva and the vagina, thickening, atrophy
Vestibule	Thinning of the tissue, thickening of the tissue, whiteness, redness, lesions
Bulbs of the vestibule	Swollen, atrophy
Great vestibular glands (Bartholin's glands)	Swollen, atrophy
Lesser vestibular glands	Swollen, atrophy
Paraurethral glands (Skene's glands)	Swollen, atrophy
Prepuce	Swollen, adhered to clitoris, thickened
Clitoris	Swollen, atrophied
Perineal body	Scarring, rigidity, redness, atrophy
Posterior fourchette	Scarring, rigidity, redness, atrophy
Anus	Hemorrhoids, redness, lesions, tearing

Table 8.6 Common swab test (Q-tip® test)

The test is used to assess for pain locations on the vulva. Each time the patient is touched by the Q-tip®, one method has the practitioner ask the patient if there is pain and if there is pain, is it mild, moderate, or severe. Another advises that if there is pain, the patient can rate the pain on a scale of 1–10:
1. Begin by touching the inner thigh
2. Touch the labia majora
3. Touch the clitoris/clitoral hood
4. Touch lateral to Hart's line, then just medial to Hart's line
5. Touch the vestibule at 1 and 11 o'clock (adjacent to the urethra at Skene's glands ostia)
6. Touch the vestibule at 4 and 8 o'clock (at the Bartholin's glands ostia)
7. Touch the vestibule at 6 o'clock
If there is pain in the 4–8 o'clock region indicates hypertonic pelvic floor dysfunction. If there is pain at the 1 and 11 o'clock region indicates intrinsic problem of the mucosa of the vestibule

indicated and if there are significant findings that demonstrate a potential need for surgery, they would refer the client to the appropriate physician for further evaluation.

The Internal Pelvic Floor Assessment and Treatment

Now the time has come in the evaluation and/or treatment session to assess and if indicated, treat the client internally. For a PFPT, as shown on the OS Algorithm, the first thing to determine is, can the client tolerate any internal assessment? There are female clients that cannot tolerate the placement of the tip of the fifth finger of the provider inside the vagina, much less the index finger. These clients are so allodynic that just contacting the opening of the vagina with light pressure causes severe pain. If this is the case, it is our clinic's practice to continue to treat the client externally, using, if indicated, external manual therapy as described above, core strengthening where indicated and hip stretches where indicated. After a few weeks of treatment, when there are fewer external impairments, the physical therapist can attempt internal assessment and treatment again as with improved external tissue health there is often an improvement in the client's tolerance of internal treatment. If the client does not develop tolerance of internal assessment and treatment over a relatively short amount of time, the PFPT may first try external transcutaneous electrical stimulation during internal treatment as it is theorized that analgesia is caused mainly by cutaneous afferent activation [47]. The electrical stimulation pads can be placed around the lateral borders of the sacrum, or in the pubic bone region and this has demonstrated to decrease vaginal allodynia in many of our clients. Also some clients are helped with cold packs or moist heat or relaxation exercises with deep diaphragmatic breathing for autonomic

Table 8.7 Internal pelvic floor muscles assessed and their corresponding layer in the pelvic floor

First layer (urogenital triangle)
• Superficial transverse perineal muscle
• Bulbospongiosus muscles (male)
• Bulbocavernosus muscle (female and male)
• Ischiocavernosus muscle (female and male)
Second layer (urogenital diaphragm)
• Sphincter urethra
• Urethrovaginal sphincter
• Compressor urethra
• Deep transverse perineal
Third layer (levator ani group and pelvic diaphragm)
• Pubococcygeus
• Puborectalis
• Iliococcygeus
• Coccygeus (ischiococcygeus)
• Piriformis
• Obturator internus

quieting. If these efforts are not successful, the PFPT will typically refer the client to their physician for consideration of topical analgesic that could be prescribed to allow tolerance of internal treatment as well for consideration of a muscle relaxant suppository to allow greater tolerance of internal treatment and therefore encourage a speedier progress towards long-term goals. Once the client can tolerate internal assessment, the PFPT assesses each muscle within each internal muscle layer, in a very systematic way. The muscles are assessed for pain and trigger point as well as muscle shortening with hyper or hypotonicity. See Table 8.7 for a list of internal pelvic floor muscles assessed and their layer in the pelvic floor. It is important to decrease the internal hypertonicity and palpable MTP(s) as well as to lengthen each shortened pelvic floor muscle to within a normal length. For example, MTP(s) in the obturator internus muscle, palpable in the third layer of the pelvic floor, can refer pain and irritability to the urethra and vagina [42]. The client with MTP(s) in their obturator internus would perceive their issue to be primarily in the bladder as they often experience burning and urgency there. These clients are often surprised when they are negative for urinary tract infection and could not know that their symptoms had a muscular origin. They are even more surprised when release of the MTP(s) in this muscle decreases their bladder symptoms. As described of external MTP(s) earlier in this chapter, internal MTP(s) as well as hypertonicity in the pelvic floor muscles can significantly affect sexual, bowel, and bladder function [9]. In fact the physiology and neurophysiology of the lower urinary tract and anorectum depends so highly on the proper function of the pelvic floor musculature, their shortness or weakness can have far greater implications for several physiological functions then, for example, muscle weakness in an extremity [3]. Any muscle affected by MTP(s) is shortened, tends to contract weakly and relaxes slowly [3]. The levator ani muscle group affected by MTP(s) will be held shortened and will potentially have decreased ability to limit the bladder from contracting during bladder filling; urinary urgency and frequency can result [39]. When the often fatigued and MTP filled levator ani is called upon to relax to allow voiding or defecation, relaxation can be delayed and urinary voiding dysfunction and/or constipation can result [3]. The PFPT at this time also assesses the internal mucosal tissue for scar tissue restrictions, tightness, thinning and hypersensitivity. Finally the PFPT will assess the pelvic organs for prolapse and hypersensitivity.

The Client with HPFD

The client with HPFD typically presents with moderately to severely hypertonic pelvic floor musculature, shortened and apparently weak pelvic floor muscles with multiple trigger points throughout the various pelvic floor muscle layers. The client tends to have moderate to severe tenderness even with movement of the assessment finger internally. The client with HPFD often is unable to relax the pelvic floor muscles upon verbal request to do so. Often they cannot demonstrate a normal bulge when asked to bear down. This contributes significantly to their complaints of difficulty initiating flow of urine, altered micturition, slow urine stream, incomplete bladder emptying, frank urinary retention [2], incomplete bowel emptying, frequency, dyspareunia, pain with orgasm, constipation, CPP and abdominal pain.

Treatment of the internal pelvic floor by a PFPT will include many of the same techniques and treatments used externally. With each treatment, every effort should be made to cause as little pain internally as possible. These treatments include internal pelvic floor muscle strain counterstrain, internal manual trigger point release, internal scar mobilization, internal pelvic floor muscle biofeedback, home exercises, self-treatment programs, internal connective tissue release, internal myofascial release and pelvic floor muscle stretching. There are very few studies supporting the use of strain counterstrain in general and especially its use intravaginal or intrarectal. However, the PFPT(s) in our practice find this technique to be highly effective as it releases the internal MTP(s) in a pain free way. Extensive research needs to be performed to confirm this treatment's efficacy in the pelvic floor rehabilitation setting. Stretching internally occurs both manually while in session with the PFPT using one to two treatment fingers as well as part of a home exercise program for the client to perform, usually involving a dilator [48]. Again, it is important that both while in session and at home, the stretching feel like stretching and that it not be painful. If painful stretching were effective, the client could have simply had frequent and severely painful inter-

course, often the reason they came to physical therapy in the first place, as this would be a form of stretching and therefore they could have avoided physical therapy treatment entirely. Painful stretching, like severely painful intercourse, causes the same muscle guarding, trigger point formation and downward spiral that you want your client to avoid and so careful education is given to the client to keep the dilator use pain free.

Once the internal pelvic floor tone is normalized and there is little pain to palpation, and once the client is near normal range of motion as demonstrated by their tolerance of the larger sized dilators, an assessment of their pelvic floor muscle coordination, strength and their ability to contract and relax volitionally is indicated and should be incorporated at this point. A detailed description of strain counterstrain (used externally or internally), trigger point release (used internally), internal scar tissue mobilization, pelvic floor biofeedback (used internally or externally to assess and train the client's pelvic floor muscles), typical home exercises given to the client with PFD and HPFD, internal connective tissue release, internal myofascial release and pelvic floor stretching protocol is outside the scope of this chapter, however there are also references provided at the end of the chapter if the reader wishes for more information both on the effectiveness and further description of these treatments [11, 22, 23, 49–53].

Conclusion

The musculoskeletal system is a significant factor in forming the diagnosis and treatment plan for clients with PFD, especially HPFD. Pelvic floor physical therapists are specifically trained in the assessment and treatment of the muscles and other soft tissues in the pelvic floor and surrounding area. As such, they should be considered an important part of a multidisciplinary team in the treatment of clients with pelvic floor dysfunction.

References

1. Faubian SS, Shuster LT, Bharucha AE. Recognition and management of the nonrelaxing pelvic floor dysfunction. Mayo Clin Proc. 2012;87(2):187–93.
2. Butrick CW. Discordant urination and defecation as symptoms of pelvic floor dysfunction. In: Butrick CW, editor. Pelvic pain. Diagnosis and management. Philadelphia: Lippincott, Williams and Wilkins; 2000.
3. FitzGerald MP, Kotarinos ÆR. Rehabilitation of the short pelvic floor. I: Background and patient evaluation. Int Urogynecol J Pelvic Floor Dysfunct. 2003;14:261–8.
4. McMahon SB, Jones NG. Plasticity of pain signaling: role of neurotrophic factors exemplified by acid induced pain. J Neurobiol. 2004;61(1):72–87.
5. Nazif O, Teichman JM, Gebhart GF, et al. Neural upregulation in interstitial cystitis. Urology. 2007;69(4 Suppl):24–33.

6. Pandhi N, Bowers B, Chen FP. A comfortable relationship: a patient derived dimension of ongoing care. Fam Med. 2007;39(4):266–73.

7. Saltini A, Del Piccolo L. Patient centered interviews in general practice. Recenti Prog Med. 2000;91(1):38–42.

8. Kaushal R, Bhanot A, Luthra S, Gupta PN, Sharma RB. Intrapartum coccygeal fracture, a cause for postpartum coccydynia: a case report. J Surg Orthop Adv. 2005;14(3):136–7.

9. Moldwin RM, Fariello JY. Myofascial trigger points of the pelvic floor: associations with urological pain syndromes and treatment strategies including injection therapy. Curr Urol Rep. 2013; 14(5):409–17.

10. Beck JJ, Elsevier HW, Pelger RC, Putter H, Voorhamvan der Zalm PJ. Multiple pelvic floor complaints are correlated with sexual abuse history. J Sex Med. 2009;6(1):193–8.

11. Del Pozo-Cruz B, Gusi N, Adusar JC, Del Pozo-Cruz J, Parraca JA, Hernandez-Mocholi M. Musculoskeletal fitness and health related quality of life characteristics among sedentary office workers affected by subacute, nonspecific low back pain: a cross sectional study. Physiotherapy. 2013;99(3):194–200.

12. Rosenbaum TY. Musculoskeletal pain and sexual function in women. J Sex Med. 2010;7(2 Pt 1):645–53.

13. Sacco E, Totaro A, Marangi F, Pinto F, Racioppi M, Gulino G, Volpe A, Gardi M, Bassi PF. Prostatitis syndromes and sporting activities. Urologia. 2010;77(2):126–38.

14. Burgio KL. Update on behavioral and physical therapies for incontinence and overactive bladder: the role of pelvic floor muscle training. Curr Urol Rep. 2013;14(5):457–64.

15. Rosenbaum TY, Owens A. The role of pelvic floor physical therapy in the treatment of pelvic and genital painrelated sexual dysfunction (CME). J Sex Med. 2008;5(3):513–23.

16. Laslett M. Evidence based diagnosis and treatment of the painful sacroiliac joint. J Man Manip Ther. 2008;16(3):142–52.

17. Freburger JK, Riddle DL. Using published evidence to guide the examination of the sacroiliac joint region. Phys Ther. 2001;81(5): 1135–43.

18. Selkow NM, Grindstaff TL, Cross KM, Pugh K, Hertel J, Saliba S. Short term effect of muscle energy technique on pain in individuals with non specific lumbopelvic pain: a pilot study. J Man Manip Ther. 2009;17(1):E14–8.

19. Bendová P, Růzicka P, Peterová V, Fricová M, Springrová I. MRI based registration of pelvic alignment affected by altered pelvic floor muscle characteristics. Clin Biomech (Bristol, Avon). 2007;22(9):980–7.

20. Knutson GA. Anatomic and functional leg length inequality: a review and recommendation for clinical decisionmaking. Part I, anatomic leg length inequality: prevalence, magnitude, effects and clinical significance. Chiropr Osteopat. 2005;13:11.

21. Coopersteina R, Lewb M. The relationship between pelvic torsion and anatomical leg length inequality: a review of the literature. J Chiropr Med. 2009;8(3):107–18.

22. Gurney B. Leg length discrepancy. Gait Posture. 2002;15(2): 195–206.

23. Martens MA, Backaert M, Vermaut G, Mulier JC. Chronic leg pain in athletes due to a recurrent compartment syndrome. Am J Sports Med. 1984;12(2):148–51.

24. Lee D, editor. The pelvic girdle, an approach to the examination and treatment of the lumbopelvichip region. 4th ed. Toronto: Elsevier; 2004.

25. Mens JM, Vleeming A, Snijders CJ, Koes BW, Stam HJ. Reliability and validity of the active straight leg raise test in posterior pelvic pain since pregnancy. Spine (Phila Pa 1976). 2001;26(10): 1167–71.

26. Dreyfuss P, Dreyer SJ, Cole A, Mayo K. Sacroiliac joint pain. J Am Acad Orthop Surg. 2004;12(4):255–65.

27. Hodges PW, Moseley GL. Pain and motor control of the lumbopelvic region: effect and possible mechanisms. J Electromyogr Kinesiol. 2003;13(4):361–70.

28. Ballantyne F, Fryer G, McLaughlin P. The effect of muscle energy technique on ham string extensibility: the mechanism of altered flexibility. J Osteopath Med. 2003;6:59–63.

29. Goodridge JP. Muscle energy technique: definition, explanation, methods of procedure. J Am Osteopath Assoc. 1981;81(4): 249–54.

30. FitzGerald MP, Kotarinos ÆR. Rehabilitation of the short pelvic floor II: treatment of the patient with the short pelvic floor. Int Urogynecol J Pelvic Floor Dysfunct. 2003;14(4):269–75; discussion 275.

31. Mense S, Simons DG. Muscle pain. Understanding its nature, diagnosis and treatment. Philadelphia: Lippincott, Williams and Wilkins; 2000.

32. Simons DG, Travell JG, Simons LS (eds). Myofascial pain and dysfunction: the trigger point manual, vol. 1. The upper half of body. Elsevier; 1983.

33. Ge HY, Arendt-Nielsen L. Latent myofascial trigger points. Curr Pain Headache Rep. 2011;15(5):386–92.

34. Bron C, Franssen J, Wensing M, Oostendorp RA. Interrater reliability of palpation of myofascial trigger points in three shoulder muscles. J Man Manip Ther. 2007;15(4):203–15.

35. Zermann DH, Ishigooka M, Doggweiler R, Schmidt RA. Neuro-urological insights into the etiology of genitourinary pain in men. J Urol. 1999;161:903–8.

36. McKay E, Kaufman RH, Doctor U, Berkova Z, Glazer H, Redko V. Treating vulvar vestibulitis with electromyographic biofeedback of pelvic floor musculature. J Reprod Med. 2001;46:337–42.

37. Lilius HG, Oravisto KJ, Valtonen EJ. Origin of pain in interstitial cystitis. Scand J Urol Nephrol. 1973;7:150–2.

38. Ling FW, Slocumb JC. User of trigger point injections in chronic pelvic pain. Obstet Gynecol Clin North Am. 1993;20:809–15.

39. Wesselman U, Burnett AL, Heinburg LJ. The urogenital and rectal pain syndromes. Pain. 1997;73:269–94.

40. Barbero M, Bertoli P, Cescon C, Macmillan F, Coutts F, Gatti R. Intrarater reliability of an experienced physiotherapist in locating myofascial trigger points in upper trapezius muscle. J Man Manip Ther. 2012;20(4):171–7.

41. Weiss JM. Pelvic floor myofascial trigger points: manual therapy for interstitial cystitis and the urgency frequency syndrome. J Urol. 2001;166(6):2226–31.

42. Travell JG, Simons DG. Myofascial pain and dysfunction: the trigger point manual, volume 2. Elsevier; 1989.

43. Davidson CJ, Ganion LR, Gehlsen GM, Verhoestra B, Roepke JE, Sevier TL. Rat tendon morphologic and functional changes resulting from soft tissue mobilization. Med Sci Sports Exerc. 1997; 29(3):313–9.

44. McFarlane MJ. The Rectal Examination. In: Clinical methods: the history, physical, and laboratory examinations. 3rd ed. Boston: Butterworth; 1990.

45. Lorenzo Rivero S. Hemorrhoids: diagnosis and current management. Am Surg. 2009;75(8):635–42.

46. Persu C, Chapple CR, Cauni V, Gutue S, Geavlete P. Pelvic organ prolapse quantification system (POPQ) a new era in pelvic prolapse staging. J Med Life. 2011;4(1):75–81.

47. Radhakrishnan R, Sluka KA. Deep tissue afferents, but not cutaneous afferents, mediate transcutaneous electrical nerve stimulation–induced antihyperalgesia. J Pain. 2005;6(10):673–80.

48. Fisher KA. Management of dyspareunia and associated levator ani muscle overactivity. Phys Ther. 2007;87(7):935–41.

49. Haddow G, Watts R, Robertson J. Effectiveness of a pelvic floor muscle exercise program on urinary incontinence following childbirth. Int J Evid Based Healthc. 2005;3(5):103–46.

50. Hodges PW. Changes in motor planning of feedforward postural responses of the trunk muscles in low back pain. Exp Brain Res. 2001;141(2):261–6.

51. Lewis C, Khan A, Souvlis T, Sterling M. A randomised controlled study examining the short term effects of Strain Counterstrain treat-

ment on quantitative sensory measures at digitally tender points in the low back. Man Ther. 2010;15(6):536–41.

52. Lewis C, Flynn TW. The use of Strain Counterstrain in the treatment of patients with low back pain. J Man Manip Ther. 2001; 9(2):92–8.

53. Abraham K, Scheufele L. Physical therapist management of patients with chronic pelvic pain. 2008, Section On Women's Health, APTA, Home Study Module. http://www.women-shealthapta.org/education/home-study-modules/.

Suggested Reading

Arab AM, Abdollahi I, Joghataei MT, Golafshani Z, Kazemnejad A. Interand intraexaminer reliability of single and composites of selected motion palpation and pain provocation tests for sacroiliac joint. Man Ther. 2009;14(2):213–21.

Baldry P, Y MB, Inanici F. Myofascial pain and fibromyalgia syndromes: a clinical guide to diagnosis and management. Elsevier Health Sciences; 2001. p. 36.

Barnes JF. Myofascial release: the search for excellence. Rehabilitation Services; 1990

Collins CK. Physical therapy management of complex regional pain syndrome I in a 14 year old patient using strain counterstrain: a case report. J Man Manip Ther. 2007;15(1):25–41.

Dardzinski JA, Ostrov BE, Hamann LS. Myofascial pain unresponsive to standard treatment. Successful use of a strain and counterstrain technique with physical therapy. J Clin Rheumatol. 2000;6:169–74.

DiGiovanna E, Schiowitz S, Dowling DJ. (2005) [1991]. Myofascial (soft tissue) techniques. In: An osteopathic approach to diagnosis and treatment, 3rd ed. Philadelphia: Lippincott Williams & Wilkins; 2005. p. 80–2.

Fernández De las Peñas C, Arendt-Nielsen L, Gerwin RD. Tension type and cervicogenic headache: pathophysiology, diagnosis, and management. Jones & Bartlett Learning; 2009. p. 250.

FitzGerald MP, Anderson RU, Potts J, Payne CK, Peters KM, Clemens JQ, Kotarinos R, Fraser L, Cosby A, Fortman C, Neville C, Badillo S, Odabachian L, Sanfield A, O'Dougherty B, HallePodell R, Cen L, Chuai S, Landis JR, Mickelberg K, Barrell T, Kusek JW, Nyberg LM; Urological Pelvic Pain Collaborative Research Network. Randomized multicenter feasibility trial of myofascial physical therapy for the treatment of urological chronic pelvic pain syndromes. J Urol. 2009;182(2):570–80.

Furlan AD, van Tulder MW, Cherkin DC, et al. Acupuncture and dry needling for low back pain. Cochrane Database Syst Rev. 2005; (1):CD001351.

Glossary of Osteopathic Terminology. American Association of Colleges of Osteopathic Medicine. April 2009. p. 28. Retrieved 25 August 2012.

Hay-Smith J, Mørkved S, Fairbrother KA, Herbison GP. Pelvic floor muscle training for prevention and treatment of urinary and faecal incontinence in antenatal and postnatal women. Cochrane Database Syst Rev. 2008;(4):CD007471.

Hunter G. Specific soft tissue mobilization in the management of soft tissue dysfunction. Man Ther. 1998;3(1):211.

Kotarinos RK. Pelvic floor physical therapy in urogynecologic disorders. Curr Womens Health Rep. 2003;3(4):33–49.

Laslett M, Aprill CN, McDonald B, Young SB. Diagnosis of sacroiliac joint pain: validity of individual provocation tests and composites of tests. Man Ther. 2005;10(3):207–18.

Lewis C, Souvlis T, Sterling M. Strain Counterstrain therapy combined with exercise is not more effective than exercise alone on pain and disability in people with acute low back pain: a randomised trial. J Physiother. 2011;57(2):91–8.

Lewit K. The needle effect in the relief of myofascial pain. Pain. 1979;6(1):83–90.

Betsch M, Wild M, Große B, Rapp W, Horstmann T. The effect of simulating leg length inequality on spinal posture and pelvic position: a dynamic rasterstereographic analysis. Eur Spine J. 2012;21(4): 691–7.

Nagrale AV, Glynn P, Joshi A, Ramteke G. The efficacy of an integrated neuromuscular inhibition technique on upper trapezius trigger points in subjects with nonspecific neck pain: a randomized controlled trial. J Man Manip Ther. 2010;18(1):37–43.

Reissing ED, Armstrong HL, Allen C. Pelvic floor physical therapy for lifelong vaginismus: a retrospective chart review and study. J Sex Marital Ther. 2013;39(4):306–20.

Wong CK. Strain Counterstrain: current concepts and clinical evidence. Man Ther. 2012;17(1):28.

Wong CK, Shauer C. Reliability, validity and effectiveness of Strain Counterstrain techniques. J Man Manip Ther. 2004;12(2):107–12.

Wong CK, Schauer Alvarez C. Effect of Strain Counterstrain on pain and strength in hip musculature. J Man Manip Ther. 2004; 12(4):215–23.

Multichannel Urodynamic Testing

9

Mikel Gray and Jessica Jackson

Introduction

The term urodynamics was introduced by David M. Davis [1]. The International Continence Society defines urodynamics as a set of tests used to measure urinary tract function and dysfunction [2]. Multichannel urodynamic testing refers to a set of tests that are typically performed together in order to provide a comprehensive evaluation of lower urinary tract function; the most commonly performed procedures are prestudy uroflowmetry, followed by filling cystometry with urethral pressure studies in selected cases, and voiding pressure flow study (Table 9.1) [3–6].

Uroflowmetry

Uroflowmetry may be performed immediately prior to multichannel urodynamic testing or as a stand-alone study. The patient is asked to arrive for testing with a moderate to strong desire to urinate and allowed to void promptly upon arrival. When combined with a multichannel urodynamic study or endoscopy, uroflowmetry should be completed prior to catheterization because urethral instrumentation has been shown to lower the maximum flow rate [7]. Urinary flow may be measured via one of several transducers; one measures weight changes as urine is collected in a beaker, and a second uses a spinning disc device that measures flow as it passes across the disc and alters the spin rate [3].

Urinary flow is determined by two factors: the velocity of urine flow as it exits the bladder vesicle and the cross sectional area of the urethra [8]. The velocity of urinary flow is primarily created by a detrusor contraction, although it may be augmented by abdominal straining [9]. Urethral caliber also influences urinary flow; a urethra with a larger diameter allows a higher flow rate, while a narrower urethral lumen restricts the maximum flow rate. The female urethra has a wider lumen than a male urethra and therefore, women tend to have a higher maximum urinary flow rate than men. In the normal urethra, flow is determined by its narrowest region (sometimes referred to as the flow determinant zone); this zone is found in the middle third of the female urethra and the membranous urethra in the male where the urethra traverses the rhabdosphincter. The flow determinant zone is shifted to the level of blockage in patients with bladder outlet obstruction. Because of the interaction between these factors, variability in either detrusor contraction strength or urethral diameter influences maximum and average urinary flow rate. In order to accurately identify the cause of an abnormal flow pattern simultaneous measurement of detrusor contraction pressure and urinary flow is needed.

A variety of potentially characteristic urinary flow patterns have been described, but we have found that a relatively simple classification schema based on three uroflow patterns is most useful for interpretation of the non-instrumented uroflowmetry [3, 10–12]. They are continuous (normal), prolonged, and interrupted/intermittent (Fig. 9.1) [3, 10–12]. The continuous flow pattern is characterized by a bell grade curve that tends to be slightly skewed to the left. The prolonged flow pattern is characterized by a lower maximum and average flow rate. The interrupted/intermittent flow pattern starts and stops at least once before voiding ends; the maximum flow rate may be comparable to values seen in the continuous flow pattern, but the average flow will be less than 50 % of the maximum flow rate.

Maximum and average flow rates vary among healthy women and men rendering it impossible to identify a single value describing a normal flow in an adult male or female. Limited evidence from studies in aging men undergoing prostatectomy for benign prostatic enlargement and adult women undergoing midurethral sling surgery suggests that a Qmax >15 ml/s is a reasonable cut point for distinguishing a

M. Gray (✉) • J. Jackson
Department of Urology, University of Virginia,
P.O. Box 800422, Charlottesville, VA 22908, USA
e-mail: mg5k@virginia.edu

© Springer Science+Business Media New York 2017
D.A. Gordon, M.R. Katlic (eds.), *Pelvic Floor Dysfunction and Pelvic Surgery in the Elderly*,
DOI 10.1007/978-1-4939-6554-0_9

Table 9.1 Typical components of a multichannel urodynamic study

Procedure	Brief description	Main parameters measured	Goals of study
Assessment of bladder filling/storage			
Filling cystometrogram (CMG)	Graphic representation of flow versus intravesical volume. Three pressures are routinely measured during the filling CMG: intravesical pressure (Pves), abdominal pressure (Pabd), and detrusor pressure (Pdet)	Cystometric capacity Bladder wall compliance Competence of the urethral sphincter mechanism Sensations of bladder filling Detrusor response to bladder filling	Evaluation of disorders related to bladder storage function including: small or large bladder capacity, low bladder wall compliance, stress incontinence with urethral incompetence of the sphincter mechanism, increased or reduced sensations of bladder filling, and detrusor response to bladder filling
Urethral pressure studies	Graphic representation of urethral pressure (Pura) Urethral pressure profile (UPP) measures maximum urethral closure pressure when the bladder is filled with 50–200 ml Cough-stress UPP measures competence of urethral closure in response to coughing	Urethral pressure measured in cm H_2O Maximum urethral closure pressure is a subtraction of the maximum urethral pressure from Pves	Evaluation of urethral sphincter competence
Assessment of bladder evacuation			
Prestudy uroflowmetry	Graphic representation of urinary flow (Q) as urine is collected in beaker placed over von Garrlet's flowmeter or when urine passes through spinning disc uroflowmeter	Maximum flow rate (Qmax): maximum flow sustained for 1 s or longer Average flow rate (Qave): mean flow rate calculated as voided volume divided by voiding time Voided volume: measured in ml Residual volume: measured by catheterization or bladder ultrasound	Characterized flow pattern, voided volume, and residual volumes Enables identification of abnormal flow patterns but does not indicate cause of voiding problems May be used for assessment of quality of voiding pressure flow study (voiding pressure flow study should reproduce flow pattern of non-instrumented prestudy uroflow study)
Voiding pressure flow study	Graphic representation of uroflowmetry, Pabd, Pves, and Pdet pressures with or without sphincter EMG	Uroflow with Qmax, Qave, voided volume Voiding pressures Pves, Pabd and Pdet Sphincter EMG may be recorded A second post void residual volume is measured immediately following the voiding pressure flow study	Evaluation of bladder evaluation including urinary flow, detrusor contraction strength, urethral resistance, and sphincter response to micturition when sphincter EMG is measured
Sphincter electromyography (EMG)	Graphic assessment of the electrical activity of pelvic floor muscles during bladder filling and storage; EMG is typically measured via transcutaneous patches that detect electrical signals from the pelvic floor muscles Alternatively, the electrical activity of motor units within the rhabdosphincter may be measured directly using EMG needle or the periurethral muscles may be directly measured via hooked wire electrodes	Summary activity measures gross motor movements of the pelvic floor muscles only Summary EMG may be displayed as a mirrored image; a wider tracing indicates greater EMG activity and a narrower image indicates lesser EMG activity Summary EMG activity may be measured via microvolts; normal resting tone is less than 5 microvolts; higher microvolts cause increased EMG activity Needle EMG allows assessment of individual motor units within the rhabdosphincter	During bladder filling/storage the EMG is assessed to determine pelvic floor muscle (PFM) response to voluntary pelvic floor muscle contraction (also called a Kegel contraction) Gently tapping the clitoris or squeezing the glans penis allows assessment of the bulbocavernosus reflex During bladder evacuation the EMG response to voiding is assessed, relaxation of the PFM causes quieting of the EMG tracing; paradoxical contraction of the pelvic floor EMG indicates dyssynergia (incoordination) of the striated sphincter and detrusor contraction or voluntary PFM contraction associated with voiding dysfunction

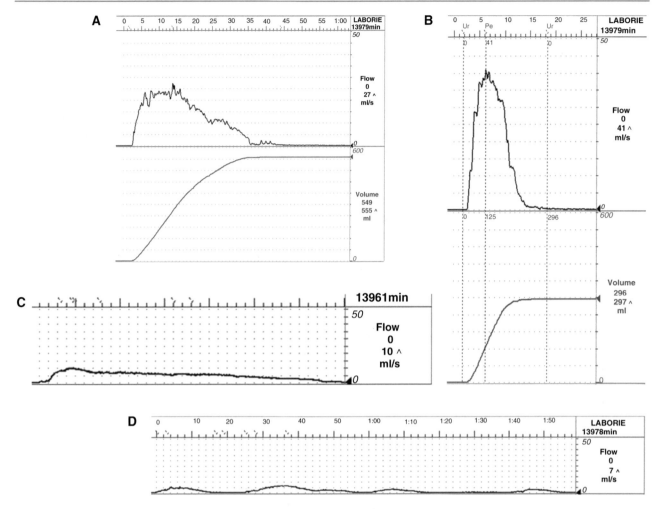

Fig. 9.1 Continuous flow pattern in an adult male (**a**), adult female (**b**), prolonged flow pattern in an adult male (**c**) and interrupted flow pattern in an adult female (**d**)

continuous from a prolonged flow pattern [12–14]. While it is tempting to associate a specific diagnosis to a particular flow pattern, such as bladder outlet obstruction with a prolonged flow pattern or underactive detrusor function augmented with abdominal straining with an interrupted/intermittent flow pattern, it is important to note that uroflowmetry alone cannot reliably distinguish the cause of an abnormal flow pattern. Instead, the uroflow results should be combined with a post void urine residual measurement and interpreted as indicating *either* underactive detrusor function or bladder outlet obstruction [15]. Differentiation of these conditions requires a voiding pressure flow study.

A post void residual measurement should be obtained immediately following the prestudy uroflow [3, 12]. When performed in the context of a multichannel urodynamic study, the residual is usually measured via catheterization. Nevertheless, estimation of the residual volume via ultrasound provides a less invasive alternative when uroflowmetry is performed as a stand-alone study [16, 17]. Similar to the maximum and mean flow rates, there is no absolute cut

point for a residual volume indicating the need for additional evaluation. In addition, residual volumes vary significantly among older adults, requiring repeat assessment to determine a consistent pattern of elevated residual urine volumes [18]. Nevertheless, clinical experience suggests that patients with consistently higher residual volumes (>200 ml) may benefit from a voiding pressure flow analysis to determine the cause of incomplete bladder emptying.

Filling Cystometrogram

The filling cystometrogram is a graphic representation of multiple pressures plotted against intravesical volume with or without pelvic floor muscle electromyography (EMG); the main goal of this study is to evaluate bladder storage and filling [19]. Multichannel filling cystometry typically involves measurement of 3 pressures. Intravesical pressure (Pves) is measured by placing a transducer into the urinary bladder. Pves is a reflection of both detrusor generated force and abdominal forces acting on the bladder wall. Abdominal pressure (Pabd) is measured by a tube placed in the rectal vault or vaginal vault. Pabd is a measurement of the abdominal forces acting on the pelvis including the lower urinary tract. A third pressure, detrusor pressure (Pdet) is a calculated pressure by subtracting abdominal pressure from intravesical catheter pressure (Pdet = Pves − Pabd) [3, 20].

Most urodynamic systems use one of three transducer technologies to measure pressure [21]. Water-charged systems measure pressure transmitted along a column of water established between the patient and a flexible membrane; the water-charged transducer is placed outside the body. A small reservoir of water (3–5 ml) within a specially designed tube is used to measure Pabd. Air-charge transducers are small balloons that are filled (charged) with 0.8 ml of air, which are then incorporated into a specially designed catheter or tube to measure pressure. Microtransducers are mounted directly onto a reusable catheter; the transducer comes into contact with the wall of the rectum or vaginal vault to measure pressure. A disposable system incorporating microtransducer technology has been designed but is not yet commercially available in the USA.

Evidence guiding selection of the optimal transducer type for urodynamic testing is sparse [21]. The International Continence Society (ICS) recommends use of water-charged transducers based on multiple factors including its relatively rapid response to rapid changes in pressures such as those created by a cough [8, 21]. The ICS nevertheless acknowledges limitations of water-charged transducers including artifact when the fluid filled lines connecting the patient to the transducer are jostled during testing. Air-charged transducers are gaining more widespread use in North American in particular. Both air-charged and microtransducers have strengths when compared to water-charged transducers including rapid setup and reduced sensitivity to artifact when jostled during urodynamic testing. Nevertheless, both technologies require placement of the transducer inside the patient's body, which is contributory to greater variability with establishing the reference level. The water-charged system, where the transducer remains outside the patient's body, enables more consistent placement at the recommended reference level. Both air-charged and water-charged transducers exhibit similar responses when measuring pressures during a voiding pressure flow study [22]. The ICS also notes that air-charge transducers tend to exhibit a diminished or delayed response to rapidly changing pressures such as those observed during a cough [21]. However, the magnitude of this difference and its clinical relevance has not been established.

Regardless of the type of transducer used to measure pressures during multichannel urodynamic testing, all transducers must be zeroed with respect to atmosphere and a proper reference level established to ensure high quality, reproducible measurements [2, 8, 23]. Zeroing with respect to atmosphere provides a consistent standard for pressure measurement in urodynamic testing and it is strongly preferred over more variability introduced when transducers are zeroed with respect to each patient. The reference level established by the International Continence Society is the superior margin of the symphysis pubis [2]. This level is easily established with water-charged transducers that can be situated parallel to the superior margin by visual inspection. The reference level is more difficult to establish with air-charged or microtransducer catheters; it may be established by performing a simple urethral pressure profile and placing the transducer several centimeters above the maximum urethral pressure measured. Alternatively, standard placement may be used; the catheters used for both systems are graduated in centimeters to make this process easier. Clinical experience suggests that catheter should be inserted approximately 12 cm in adult females and 20 cm in adult males. Once transducers are in place within the bladder pressure measurement is technically straightforward, as the bladder is a fluid filled chamber. Measurement of Pabd is more technically challenging since neither the rectal vault nor posterior vaginal vault is normally filled with a liquid medium. Hence there is a need for a specially designed tube with a small reservoir to measure pressure or a microtransducer system.

Sphincter electromyography (EMG) also may be monitored during filling cystometry. EMG information can be gathered through several methods. Transcutaneous (patch) electrodes or percutaneous needles can be placed on the perianal area. Alternatively hooked wire electrodes can be percutaneously inserted into the periurethral striated muscle [4]. Measurement of pelvic floor muscle activity provides an opportunity to evaluate how the pelvic floor responds to bladder filling/storage, the bulbocavernosus reflex, and provocative maneuvers such as coughing. The EMG allows the clinician to determine the patient's ability to identify, contract, and relax the pelvic floor muscles.

Filling cystometry is completed by filling the urinary bladder with sterile water, saline, or a radiographic contrast material [21, 23]. Supraphysiologic fill rates from 30 ml/min to as high as 100 ml/min may be used. However, slower fill rates (30–50 ml/min) are preferred since the small catheter size used for most urodynamic testing (5–7 French) limits the ability to fill the bladder at higher rates. In addition, higher rates have been shown to exert negative effects on urodynamic findings when compared to physiologic filling during ambulatory monitoring.

Data from the filling cystometrogram is used to answer five essential questions: (1) what is the cystometric capacity, (2) is bladder wall compliance normal or low, (3) is the urethral sphincter mechanism competent, (4) are sensations of bladder filling normal, reduced, or increased, and (5) what is the detrusor response to bladder filling [5]. The immediacy of each of these questions varies based on the clinical history of the patient and the lower urinary tract symptoms or disorders prompting urodynamic testing. Nevertheless, answering each ensures a comprehensive filling cystometrogram (Table 9.2).

Cystometric Capacity

The International Continence Society defines three types of bladder capacity: functional, cystometric, and anesthetic (often referred to as anatomic) [20]. Functional capacity is defined as the intravesical volume when an individual voluntarily elects to urinate; it varies considerably based on multiple factors such as social context and proximity to a toilet. A study of 300 healthy women found a mean voided volume of 204 ml and an average maximum voided volume of 330 ml over a 1 day data collection. Nevertheless, the range of voided volume varied widely from 90–1020 ml [24]. A similarly designed study in 284 healthy men found a median voided volume of 237 ml and a median maximum voided

volume of 382 ml [25]. In contrast to these values cystometric capacity tends to be higher in adults; it was 513 ml in a group of women without detrusor overactivity undergoing diagnostic urodynamic testing and 570–572 ml in a group of 30 healthy adult women undergoing sequential testing in a research setting [26, 27]. Cystometric capacity tends to be higher than functional bladder capacity because of the provocative nature of urodynamic testing. Patients are filled to a strong and persistent (imminent) desire to urinate, or until lower urinary tract symptoms such as urgency and urge incontinence are reproduced. This situation differs from the daily lives of patients with stress, urge or mixed urinary incontinence who tend to void at lower volumes in an attempt to prevent urinary leakage or involuntary voiding.

Whenever possible, cystometric capacity is calculated as voided volume plus residual volume. This technique is preferred over relying on the infused volume to determine capacity because of the renal contribution that occurs during provocative testing. A study of 186 adults undergoing

Table 9.2 Five questions for interpretation of the filling cystometrogram

Question	Normal range and cut point for clinically relevant abnormal finding	Effect of normal aging
(1) What is the cystometric capacity?	Normal range: 300–600 ml Cystometric capacity <300 ml often associated with detrusor overactivity, low bladder wall compliance, inflammation of the bladder wall Cystometric capacity >600 ml often associated with denervating disorders affecting lumbosacral spinal segments, metabolic disorders including diabetes mellitus and prolonged pattern of infrequent voiding	Functional bladder capacity does not decline with age [68]
(2) Is bladder wall compliance normal or low?	No absolute value for normal bladder wall compliance has been defined, whole bladder compliance values <10 ml/cm H_2O, sustained detrusor pressures $\geq$35 cm H_2O and detrusor leak point pressure $\geq$40 cm H_2O associate with urinary tract distress	No age related changes in bladder wall compliance have been observed [68]
(3) Is the urethral sphincter mechanism competent?	Any detectable abdominal leak point pressure (provoked by Valsalva maneuver or coughing) indicates urodynamic stress urinary incontinence; a negative pressure transmission ratio on cough-UPP indicates urodynamic stress UI A maximum urethral closure pressure <20 cm H_2O indicates intrinsic sphincter deficiency, an abdominal leak point pressure <60 cm H_2O assessed at 200 ml indicates intrinsic sphincter deficiency	Urethral sphincter incompetence (urodynamic stress UI) is not a component of normal aging Maximum urethral closure pressure declines with aging in healthy adult women [68]
(4) Are sensations of bladder filling normal reduced or increased?	First sensation of bladder filling, first desire to urinate and strong desire to urinate are found in healthy adult women subjected to urodynamic evaluation; they occur in a predictable order	Sensations of bladder filling diminish with age; the volume at which characteristic sensory thresholds increased 100 ml in a group of healthy women (mean age 55 years; range 22–90 years)
(5) What is the detrusor response to bladder filling?	No detrusor contractions during the filling cystometrogram is considered normal; some adults experience lower amplitude, phasic detrusor contractions that do not cause urgency or urge incontinence	Detrusor overactivity with urgency or incontinence is not a normal response of the aging bladder [68]

urodynamic testing found that all participants had higher voided plus residual volume than infused volumes; the mean renal contribution was 14 % above infused volume [28]. Nevertheless, infused volume must be used when voided volume cannot be measured in the neurologically impaired or older adult unable to sit safely on a toilet for a voiding pressure flow study.

Large cystometric capacity is often accompanied by reduced sensations of bladder filling with or without incomplete bladder emptying. A large cystometric capacity is seen in multiple conditions affecting older adults such as diabetes mellitus and denervating disorders affecting lumbosacral spinal segments such as cauda equina syndrome or spinal stenosis [29, 30]. While supporting evidence is sparse, clinical experience strongly suggests that a lifelong pattern of infrequent voiding also increases bladder size. Voluntary restriction of voiding, often related to working in an environment when voiding is restricted such as a factory floor, long haul trucking industry, or health care profession may lead to a chronic pattern of less frequent voiding and increased bladder capacity [31]. Smaller cystometric capacity has been linked to inflammation of the bladder wall, detrusor overactivity, and low bladder wall compliance [32–35].

Bladder Wall Compliance

Compliance of the bladder wall is a measure of the relationship between detrusor pressure (Pdet) and intravesical volume during bladder filling and before the occurrence of a voluntary or overactive detrusor contraction [36, 37]. In the healthy person, Pdet remains at a comparatively stable and low value because of its ability to accommodate increasing intravesical volumes via its viscoelastic properties and low detrusor muscle resting tone. Low bladder wall compliance is characterized by a steady rise in Pdet during the filling cystometrogram. Bladder wall compliance can be assessed in several ways: pattern recognition, identification of pressure specific bladder volumes, and calculation of whole bladder compliance. Pattern recognition is used to "screen" for low bladder compliance. If visual inspection of the Pdet tracing during filling cystometry reveals a nearly flat slope, compliance is deemed normal. In contrast, if a steeper slope is visualized, low bladder compliance is suspected and further analysis is performed (Fig. 9.2). Low bladder wall compliance must be distinguished from overactive detrusor contractions [6]. Detrusor overactivity is characterized by a rapid rise in pressure caused by contraction of smooth muscle in the bladder wall, followed by a peak pressure (amplitude) and comparatively rapid decline to baseline (Fig. 9.3).

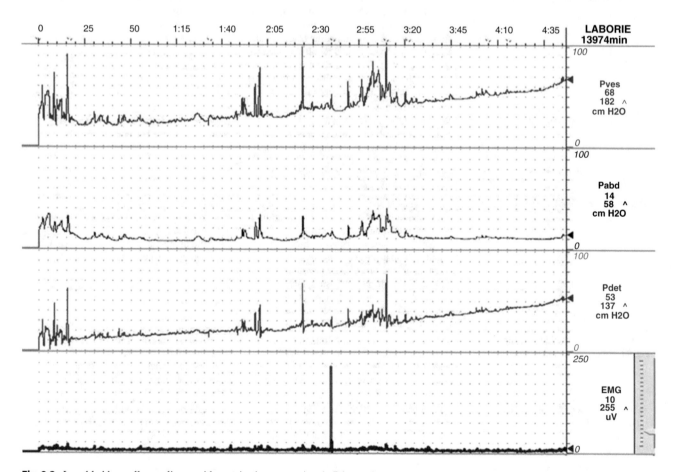

Fig. 9.2 Low bladder wall compliance with sustained pressure rises in Pdet tracing

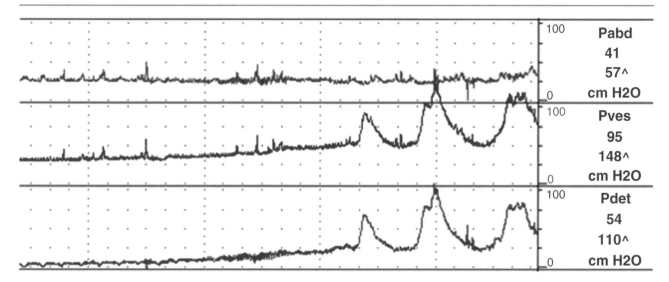

Fig. 9.3 Filling cystometrogram with low bladder wall compliance superimposed on phasic detrusor overactivity; note the rapid pressure rise of the overactive detrusor contractions as compared to the steady rise of Pdet characteristic of low bladder wall compliance

Identification of volume specific pressures is particularly relevant when determining the volume at which an individual can safely store urine; such knowledge is essential when determining the frequency of intermittent catheterization. One landmark study of bladder wall compliance evaluated 923 children with neurogenic bladders and 69 children with lower urinary tract complaints and normal urodynamic findings [38]. Children with normal urodynamic findings stored 95 % of intravesical volume at a Pdet <20 cm H_2O and 99 % at a Pdet <30 cm H_2O. Based on these findings, and observations of participants with lower bladder wall compliance, researchers concluded that a sustained Pdet ≤20 cm H_2O indicates normal bladder wall compliance. In contrast, a sustained Pdet of 21–30 cm H_2O indicates a low risk of urinary tract distress, and a sustained Pdet ≥35 cm H_2O indicates a high imminent risk of urinary tract distress (recurrent febrile urinary tract infections, vesicoureteral reflux, hydronephrosis, and/or compromised renal function). These findings are consistent with another landmark study of low bladder wall compliance in children with myelodysplasia. In this study a urodynamic outcome measure, the detrusor leak point pressure, was evaluated for its ability to predict urinary tract distress. The detrusor leak point pressure is the Pdet required for a low compliant bladder to overcome urethral closure and produce overflow urinary incontinence; study findings revealed that all subjects with a detrusor leak point pressures ≥40 cm H_2O had urinary tract distress [39].

Calculation of whole bladder compliance is a third alternative for measuring bladder wall compliance. It provides a single number designed to summarize the compliance curve during the entire filling storage phase of bladder function [6, 20, 37]. It is calculated using the formula: Compliance = infused volume/ΔPdet. Compliance is expressed as ml per cm H_2O;

infused volume is the volume of fluid instilled at cystometric capacity, and ΔPdet is the difference in detrusor pressure at cystometric capacity immediately prior to the onset of a voluntary or overactive detrusor contraction minus Pdet at the beginning of filling. A cut point of ≤10 cm H_2O is used to identify clinically relevant low bladder wall compliance [6, 37]. Values indicating normal bladder wall compliance are less well defined; 40 ml/cm H_2O was identified as normal compliance in a group of adult women [6, 39, 40]. However, clinical experience overwhelmingly suggests that many patients have much higher values.

Low bladder wall compliance is clinically relevant because of its deleterious effects on urinary tract function [6, 38–41]. Low bladder wall compliance has been associated with diminished blood flow and histologic changes in the bladder wall [42]. It has also been associated with urinary tract distress, manifested as recurring febrile urinary tract infections, vesicoureteral reflux, hydronephrosis, and impaired renal function [6, 38, 39, 41, 43]. In the older adult, low bladder wall compliance is associated with neurological disorders such as spinal cord injury, multiple sclerosis, cauda equina syndrome, tethered spinal cord, and non-neurologic conditions including tuberculous cystitis, pelvic radiation, long-term interstitial cystitis, and chronic bladder outlet obstruction due to prostatic enlargement [35, 43–47].

Urethral Sphincter Competence

Stress urinary incontinence (UI) can be defined as a symptom, physical sign noted during physical assessment, or a medical diagnosis. The International Continence Society defines urodynamic stress UI as a urodynamic observation; it occurs when abdominal forces exceed urethral closure forces resulting in urinary leakage [20]. Urodynamic evaluation of urethral sphincter competence addresses two questions: (1) does this patient have urodynamic stress UI, and (2) does this patient have intrinsic sphincter deficiency (sometimes referred to as urethral sphincter incompetence or deficiency) [48]. Two urodynamic techniques are used to determine urethral sphincter competence: abdominal leak point pressure measurement and urethral pressure profilometry. The clinical relevance of the first question (does the patient have any stress UI) is apparent. The accurate identification of the type of incontinence is necessary since the surgical management of intrinsic sphincter deficiency differs from other forms of incontinence, and therefore may influence surgical outcomes [49].

The abdominal leak point pressure is defined as the magnitude of intravesical pressure required to overcome urethral closure and provoke urinary leakage in the absence of a detrusor contraction [20]. It should be measured in the upright (sitting or standing) position. The patient's bladder is filled to 200 ml, the fill is temporarily discontinued, and the patient is asked to perform Valsalva's maneuver with sufficient vigor to raise Pves at least 100 cm H_2O. The intravesical pressure at which leakage is observed is recorded and subtracted from the baseline

intravesical pressure (Fig. 9.4) [45]. Any measureable value indicates urodynamic stress UI; in addition, an abdominal leak point pressure <60 cm H_2O indicates intrinsic sphincter deficiency [49]. While this strategy will provoke urodynamic stress UI in many women and men, additional maneuvers are often required to detect urodynamic stress UI without intrinsic sphincter deficiency. Therefore, when straining does not produce urine loss, the patient is asked to cough while observing for urine loss. Because of the very rapid pressure changes provoked by a cough, it is not possible to determine the precise abdominal leak point pressure using this technique. Instead, the maximum pressure produced with the cough when leakage is observed is recorded and the event is labelled "cough leak point pressure." If urodynamic stress UI is not produced using either maneuver, cystometric filling is continued and these maneuvers are repeated every 150–200 ml until cystometric capacity is reached. If none of these maneuvers produces stress UI, the intravesical catheter may be removed and Pabd is used as a proxy for Pves; this technique has also been recommended for routine investigation of men with stress UI following radical prostatectomy [50]. Removal of the intravesical catheter is recommend because it has been found to "unmask" subtle cases of urodynamic stress UI when the intravesical tube is removed from the urethra.

Fig. 9.4 Abdominal leak point pressure measurement demonstrating urodynamic stress urinary incontinence

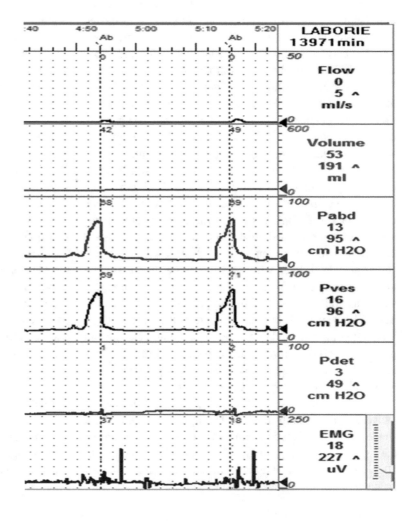

The presence of severe pelvic organ prolapse (Pelvic Organ Prolapse Quantification System Stages 3 and 4) may obscure urodynamic stress UI [51]. In this case, reduction of severe prolapse using a gauze vaginal pack, ring pessary, or other maneuver is recommended to detect urodynamic stress UI that may be revealed when pelvic organ prolapse is repaired surgically.

Urethral pressure profilometry may also be used to assess urethral sphincter competence [48]. Unlike the abdominal leak point pressure, urethral pressure profilometry relies on direct assessment of urethral pressure (Pura), ideally combined with simultaneous measurement of intravesical pressure (Pves) and urethral closure pressure (Pclo), a computer generated tracing calculated by subtracting Pves from Pura. The technique for measuring urethral pressure presents unique challenges to the urodynamic clinician because of the narrow lumen of the urethra during bladder filling/storage and absence of a fluid medium in the urethra required for accurate pressure measurement. When measuring urethral pressures with water-charged transducers the clinician must create a small pocket of water by slowly perfusing water through the pressure monitoring line as it is pulled through the urethra. Measurement of Pura by a microtransducer does not require infusion of water; instead the catheter may be pulled through the urethra and pressures are recorded as the transducer interacts with the urethral wall. However, this technique is prone to artifact when the comparatively stiff catheter interacts with the urethral wall resulting in variable pressure readings depending on the orientation of the catheter [52]. The air-charged catheter creates a fluid environment via the small air filled balloon incorporated into the catheter. This design enables the catheter to be pulled through the urethra without significant discomfort. Since pressure is measured in a small fluid filled chamber, the artifact created by the microtransducer is eliminated.

A urethral pressure profile (UPP) is obtained by filling the bladder with 50–200 ml and slowly pulling the catheter through the urethra [48, 53]. Multiple parameters may be measured with the UPP including maximum urethral pressure, maximum urethral closure pressure, total profile length, and functional profile length. However, only one of these parameters, maximum urethral closure pressure, has proved useful for diagnosis of intrinsic sphincter deficiency [54]. A maximum urethral closure pressure <20 cm H_2O indicates intrinsic sphincter deficiency. While the UPP is useful for evaluation of urethral closure pressures, it is not a dynamic study and does not directly diagnose stress UI. In addition no cutoff point has been determined for the maximum urethral closure pressure (or any other parameter measured during the UPP) that reliably differentiates women with stress UI from those with a competent urethral sphincter mechanism [55]. These limitations can be overcome by combining a traditional UPP with a cough-stress UPP. The Cough-stress UPP is completed by asking the patient to cough individually as the catheter is slowly pulled through the urethra while measuring Pura, Pves, and Pclo. Individuals with competent urethral sphincter mechanisms (no stress UI) will have a positive pressure transmission ratio (upward spike seen on the Pclo tracing) while those with stress UI will have a negative pressure transmission ratio (downward spike seen on the Pclo tracing) (Fig. 9.5).

The predictive power of these tests for detection of any stress UI was measured in 108 women undergoing multichannel urodynamic evaluation [56]. Abdominal leak point pressure testing was determined to be most likely to reproduce any stress UI. Nevertheless, the evidence supporting use of a UPP for diagnosing intrinsic sphincter deficiency is stronger than that supporting use of the abdominal leak point pressure [54]. We therefore recommend completing both investigations when completing urodynamic testing in contemplation of surgical management of stress UI in the older adult.

Sensations of Bladder Filling

Assessment of sensations of bladder filling is particularly difficult in the context of multichannel urodynamic testing [57]. The presence of pressure monitoring lines in the bladder and rectal or posterior vaginal vault almost certainly alter sensations of bladder filling. This effect is further intensified by the clinical setting (the urodynamic suite) which bears little resemblance to the relative privacy of most toilets. Three sensations are commonly identified during the filling cystometrogram, the first sensation of bladder filling, first desire to void, and strong desire to void [58, 59]. The first sensation of the bladder is described as initial awareness of bladder filling, the first desire to void is characterized by a desire to urinate at the next convenient moment, and a strong desire is defined as a strong and persistent desire to urinate at the earliest possible time. These characteristic sensations have been shown to occur in a predictable sequence when filling cystometry is performed in healthy volunteers [59].

In addition to identifying these characteristic sensations of bladder filling, the urodynamic clinician should assess the patient for urgency and pain. Urgency is defined as a sudden and strong desire to urinate that cannot be deferred [20]. It is the main lower urinary tract symptom associated with overactive bladder syndrome. Urgency differs from physiologic "strong desire to void" in several important ways: (1) it is sudden and difficult to defer, (2) it may occur at any bladder volume and tends to occur at lower volumes ultimately reducing cystometric and functional bladder capacity, (3) it is associated with detrusor overactivity on urodynamic testing, (4) it is often associated with urge incontinence [60, 61].

Evaluation of lower urinary tract pain is also challenging; painful bladder syndrome is often misdiagnosed as chronic pelvic pain, vulvodynia, endometriosis, or overactive bladder [62]. While urodynamic testing plays a limited role in the

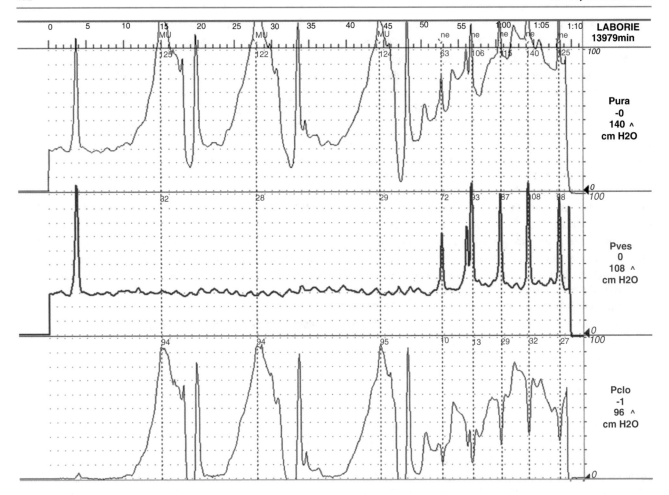

Fig. 9.5 Urethral pressure profile (UPP) demonstrating three maximum urethral closure pressure measurements varying from 94 to 95 cm H_2O and cough-stress UPP with negative pressure transmission ratios indicating urodynamic stress urinary incontinence

diagnosis of painful bladder syndrome, we have found that differentiation of urgency associated with fear of urinary leakage or incontinence from urgency associated with pain induced by bladder filling clinically relevant. A study of 214 patients found that that women with painful bladder syndrome/interstitial cystitis reported first sensation, first desire, and strong desire occurred at low volumes and were strongly associated with increased pain [32]. Nevertheless, this study did not associate pain with the symptom of urgency or with occurrences of detrusor overactivity. Further research is needed to establish the optimal approach for assessing the relationship between lower urinary tract pain to urinary urgency and detrusor overactivity in patients with chronic pelvic pain.

The ICS nomenclature committee has established multiple categories for summarizing sensations of bladder filling based on multichannel urodynamic testing [20]. Normal sensations of bladder filling are defined as awareness of the three characteristic sensory threshold events, first sensation to urinate, first desire to urinate, and strong desire to urinate. The term increased sensations of bladder filling is defined as an early and persistent desire to void (presumably sensations occurring at lower volumes). The description does not account for

the patient who described a first sensation and first desire to void at a higher intravesical volume with urgency with or without urge incontinence. The term reduced sensations of bladder filling is defined as awareness of bladder filling but absence of a specific desire to urinate. The term absent sensations is described as no reported sensations of bladder filling. A newer term, non-specific sensations of bladder filling, is defined as absence of specific bladder sensations; this person instead reports "abdominal fullness, vegetative symptoms or spasticity." The vagueness of these categories of sensory reports reflects our limited understanding of the sensory function of the urinary bladder and lower urinary tract.

Detrusor Response to Bladder Filling

In the healthy adult, the detrusor remains in a relaxed state resulting in the characteristic flat line Pdet tracing seen on urodynamic testing. Detrusor overactivity is a urodynamic observation characterized by an involuntary detrusor contraction that occurs during the filling cystometrogram [20]. Detrusor overactivity causes urgency and/or urge incontinence characteristic of overactive bladder syndrome. The ICS nomenclature committee defines two types of detrusor overactivity, phasic and terminal. Phasic detrusor overactivity occurs as the bladder is filled and before permission to void is granted; it may cause urgency and urinary leakage but it occurs and subsides allowing additional filling until cystometric capacity is reached. In contrast, terminal detrusor overactivity is characterized by a single detrusor contraction that occurs before permission to void is granted; it terminates bladder filling and causes involuntary voiding.

Detrusor overactivity may also be categorized based on its underlying cause [20]. Urodynamic testing alone cannot differentiate neurogenic from idiopathic detrusor overactivity. Neurogenic detrusor overactivity occurs in a patient with an established diagnosis of a neurologic disorder or lesion affecting the central nervous system. Prevalent disorders of the brain associated with neurogenic detrusor overactivity in the older adult include Alzheimer's dementia, stroke, or Parkinson's disease. Persons with neurogenic detrusor overactivity on urodynamic testing usually experience associated symptoms of urgency and urge incontinence [63, 64]. Spinal cord disorders associated with neurogenic detrusor overactivity include spinal cord injury, disc problems, spinal cord tethering, and stenosis. Persons with spinal cord lesions or disorders may also experience reduced or absent sensations of bladder filling and detrusor-striated sphincter dyssynergia. These bladder conditions may lead to incomplete bladder emptying and related complications such as recurring urinary tract infections. Multiple sclerosis is a special case because the denervating lesions occur in multiple levels of the central nervous system resulting in a variety of urodynamic findings, including neurogenic detrusor overactivity; some persons will experience urgency and urge

incontinence, while others may experience reduced or absent sensations of bladder filling, detrusor-striated sphincter dyssynergia, and incontinence without sensory awareness [64].

Voiding Pressure Flow Study

The voiding pressure flow study (VPFS) combines uroflowmetry with the pressures measured during the filling cystometrogram. It is considered the gold standard for evaluation of normal versus abnormal voiding caused by underactive detrusor function, bladder outlet obstruction, or a combination of these conditions [65, 66]. The VPFS is typically completed following the filling CMG. Patients with a normal detrusor response to bladder filling are asked to urinate when they perceive an imminent desire to void. Terminal detrusor overactivity causing bladder evaluation may be analyzed as a voiding pressure flow study only when the patient is given permission to void at the onset of the detrusor contraction; this maneuver is essential because it enables the patients and clinician to separate bladder storage from the voiding phase of a multichannel urodynamic evaluation [66]. An alternative to this approach when terminal detrusor overactivity occurs is to fill the bladder again to a lower volume and ask the patient to void voluntarily. Analysis of the VPFS focuses on three components: the urinary flow pattern, detrusor contraction strength, and urethral resistance. A synthesis of these components enables the clinician to differentiate a normal study from incomplete bladder evacuation caused by bladder outlet obstruction, underactive detrusor function, or a combination of these factors (Table 9.3).

Table 9.3 Elements of the voiding pressure flow study (VPFS)

Component of the VPFS	Normal range and cut point for clinically relevant abnormal findings	Effects of normal aging
Urinary flow pattern	Continuous flow pattern with Qmax >15 ml/s and Qave 50 % of Qmax is considered normal Lower residual volumes is considered normal; there is no absolute cut point for clinically relevant residual volume (consistent residual volumes >200 ml may indicate need for further evaluation) Qmax ≤15 ml/s is a cut point for distinguishing normal from prolonged or interrupted flow pattern	Q max declines significantly with aging in healthy adult women and men [66, 68] Residual volumes remained low in a group of 85 healthy women with and without detrusor overactivity, median residual volume 12 ml (IQR 0–14 ml) [68]
Detrusor contractility	Normal values have not been well defined; they vary according to age and gender Women tend to void with lower Pdet@Qmax than men	Detrusor contraction strength declines with aging [68]
Urethral Resistance	Values <20 on the ICS obstruction nomogram indicate no obstruction on women and men Values >40 on the ICS obstruction nomogram indicate higher magnitude obstruction in men Values >30 on the ICS obstruction nomogram indicated higher magnitude obstruction in women	Precise effect not well studied, urethral resistance tends to decline with aging in women and increase with aging in men
Pelvic floor muscle EMG response to voiding	Reflexive relaxation of the pelvic floor muscles and striated sphincter leads to reduction in EMG activity	No known effects of aging on EMG response

Pelvic floor muscle EMG is often measured during the VPFS. In the healthy adult, the striated sphincter and pelvic floor muscles reflexively relax during micturition, which is reflected in a reduction in EMG activity seen on the VPFS tracing [67]. In contrast, patients with detrusor-striated sphincter dyssynergia (discoordination between detrusor muscle and striated sphincter contractions seen in neurological lesions or disorders affecting spinal segments below the pontine micturition center and above the sacral micturition center) have increased EMG activity, usually accompanied by an interrupted flow pattern.

The events that characterize a normal voiding pressure flow study include relaxation of the pelvic floor muscles seen on EMG that occurs several seconds before onset of a detrusor contraction. Urinary flow begins when Pdet overcomes urethral resistance; this event is labelled urethral opening pressure. Flow continues until the detrusor contraction begins

to fade; at some point during this process urinary flow stops and Pdet gradually declines until it returns to baseline [65, 66]. Some patients will experience a detrusor contraction after the bladder has emptied; the detrusor after-contraction presents as a strong and rapid rise in detrusor pressure occurring after bladder evacuation. The clinical relevance of the detrusor after-contraction is unknown (Fig. 9.6) [68, 69].

Visual Inspection of the Voiding Pressure Flow Study

Identification of the urinary flow pattern is based on the same categorization schema used to interpret a prestudy or stand-alone uroflow study. A continuous flow pattern in the healthy adult resembles a bell shaped curve that tends to be skewed slightly to the left; Qmax should be ≥15 ml/s in men and often

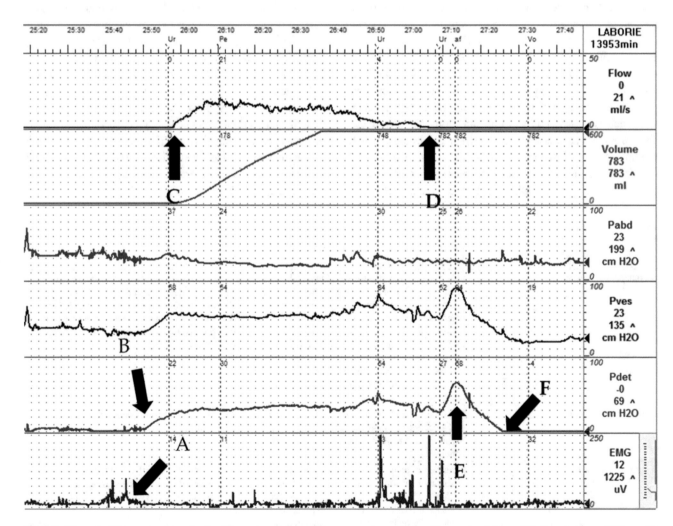

Fig. 9.6 Characteristic events of a normal voiding pressure flow study. (A) Relaxation of striated sphincter with reduction in pelvic floor EMG activity. (B) Onset of detrusor contraction, (C) Urethral opening pressure is reached with onset of flow. (D) Termination of Flow. (E) Detrusor after-detrusor contraction occurs after bladder evacuation. (F) Detrusor pressure returns to baseline

higher in women and Qave should be 50 % of Qmax. A prolonged flow pattern remains continuous (without interruption) but its Qmax is <15 ml/s. An interrupted (intermittent) urinary flow pattern starts and stops more than once during micturition; Qmax may be >15 ml/s but Qave will be <50 % of the maximum flow rate. However, unlike this screening study, analysis of the flow pattern during the VPFS is combined with evaluation of the detrusor contractility and urethral resistance in order to determine the cause of an abnormal flow pattern.

Urodynamic evaluation of detrusor contractility begins with assessment of the amplitude and duration of the Pdet tracing during voiding. Ultimately, this assessment is combined with analysis of the flow pattern and urethral resistance. Because of the invasive nature of the VPFS, few studies have been completed in otherwise healthy adult women and men. A study of 24 healthy women revealed an average maximum detrusor voiding pressures (Pdet@Qmax) of 29 cm H_2O in women aged 22–39 years, a mean Pdet@Qmax of 26 cm H_2O in women aged 45–53 years of age and a mean Pdet@Qmax of 24 cm H_2O in women aged 55–80 years [70]. A study of 33 healthy adult men aged 18–44 years of age revealed a mean Pdet@Qmax of 53 cm H_2O [71]. Because of variability in urethral resistance in adult women and men of varying ages, no single cut point for a Pdet@Qmax indicating bladder outlet

obstruction or underactive detrusor function has been determined; instead, detrusor contractility must be evaluated in the context of flow pattern and urethral resistance.

Urodynamic evaluation of urethral resistance is based on a comparison of urinary flow and detrusor pressure. These relationships can be assessed qualitatively by inspection of the urinary flow and Pdet at maximum or minimum flow, or it can be quantitatively evaluated via a voiding pressure nomogram. Adult women have a shorter and straighter urethral course than do adult men. As a result, they tend to urinate with a higher Qmax and lower Pdet@Qmax than do men [70]. Adult men have a more torturous urethral course that passes through the prostate, as a result they tend to void with a lower Qmax and higher Pdet@Qmax [71]. This difference is more apparent in aging men who experience benign prostatic enlargement and increased urethral resistance versus aging women who experience a reduction in urethral resistance measured on a UPP [72, 73].

Bladder outlet obstruction is diagnosed on the VPFS when urethral resistance is increased due to an anatomic or functional increase in urethral resistance; this event causes a rise in detrusor contraction pressures as the lower urinary tract attempts to maintain urinary flow and ensure complete bladder evacuation (Fig. 9.7). Functional bladder outlet obstruction

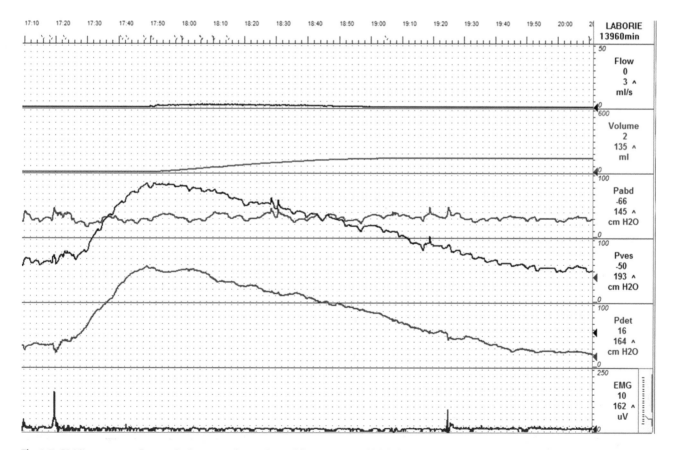

Fig. 9.7 Voiding pressure flow study demonstrating prolonged flow pattern and high detrusor contraction pressure characteristic of bladder outlet obstruction. Sphincter EMG response to voiding is normal; obstruction in this 78-year-old male was caused by benign prostatic enlargement

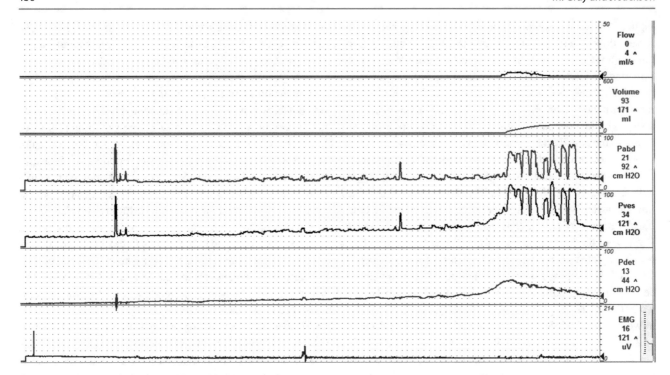

Fig. 9.8 Voiding pressure flow study demonstrating prolonged flow pattern and low detrusor contraction pressure characteristic of underactive detrusor function in a 67-year-old male with spinal stenosis. He attempts to augment bladder emptying with abdominal straining noted in intravesical and abdominal pressure tracings

associated with detrusor-striated sphincter dyssynergia may be diagnosed when pelvic floor EMG is monitored during the VPFS; it is more likely to produce an interrupted/intermittent urinary stream as the striated sphincter and periurethral muscles contract and relax in an uncoordinated manner during micturition. Underactive detrusor function is characterized by a prolonged flow pattern combined with a lower detrusor contraction pressures (Fig. 9.8).

A number of pressure flow nomograms have been developed that provide a more quantitative analysis of urethral resistance and detrusor contractility. The most widely used in urodynamic testing are the ICS nomogram and the linear passive urethral resistance relationship (linPURR) nomogram [74]. The ICS nomogram measures urethral resistance by comparing Qmax and Pdet@Qmax; the resulting ICS obstruction number (also referred to as the urethral resistance algorithm, URA) is used to describe the magnitude of obstruction; values <20 indicate no clinically relevant obstruction, values from 20 to 40 indicate equivocal (lower magnitude) obstruction and values >40 indicate higher magnitude obstruction [75]. Values from this nomogram have been extrapolated for clinical use in women; a single cut point of 20 was used to differentiate clinically relevant bladder outlet obstruction from normal urethral resistance in women [76]. The linPURR nomogram compares Pdet at minimum flow to evaluate urethral resistance; it divides obstruction into seven grades

(0–VI) [75]. This nomogram also allows assessment of detrusor contractility, which is divided into six categories ranging from very weak to strong. Similar to the ICS nomogram, it was developed and validated in a group of older men with obstruction related to benign prostatic enlargement. It has not been adapted for use in adult or aging women. An ICS composite nomogram has been developed that merges the ICS obstruction nomogram (describe above) and the ICS bladder contractility nomogram; this composite nomogram allows categorization of patients into nine zones reflecting the complex relationship of bladder outlet obstruction and detrusor contractility [77, 78].

Multichannel Urodynamic Testing in the Aged Adult: Case Examples

The American Urological Association (AUA) and Society for Urodynamics and Female Urology (SUFU) have generated a clinical practice guideline for urodynamic testing in adults [79]. Several principles are particularly useful when considering indications for multichannel urodynamic testing in adults. The following cases review scenarios where multichannel urodynamic testing provided clinically useful information in the evaluation of an elderly patient with complex lower urinary tract dysfunction.

Case 1: Multichannel Urodynamic Testing in a 75-Year-Old Female with Mixed Urinary Incontinence Symptoms

Mrs. A is a 75-year-old woman who complains of mixed urinary incontinence, along with weak urinary steam and feeling of incomplete bladder emptying. She also complains of constipation and a bulging sensation of the vaginal area. Recent pelvic examination reveals severe vaginal wall prolapse (Pelvic Organ Prolapse Quantification System Stage 4), defined as eversion of the vaginal wall ≥2 cm. Multichannel urodynamic testing was performed in contemplation of surgical repair of pelvic organ prolapse and stress urinary incontinence. Filling cystometry revealed a cystometric capacity of 428 ml, and normal bladder wall compliance (whole bladder compliance: 75 ml/cm H_2O). No stress UI was observed when provoked at 200 ml; a vaginal pack was inserted to reduce her cystocele; she then experienced stress UI with an abdominal leak point pressure of 64–68 cm H_2O (Fig. 9.9). Urethral pressure profilometry shows maximum urethral closure pressures of 22–24 cm H_2O; cough-stress UPP showed negative pressure transmission ratio indicating stress UI. Sensations of bladder filling were normal and no detrusor overactivity was observed on urodynamic testing. Voiding pressure flow study was completed after vaginal pack had been removed; it revealed prolonged flow pattern with Qmax of 12 ml/s and Qave of 5 ml/s and her Pdet@Qmax was high at 84 cm H_2O. In this case, urodynamic testing revealed urodynamic stress UI that was apparent only after her vaginal wall prolapse had been reduced. No evidence of urge incontinence (increased sensations of bladder filling with or without detrusor overactivity). Voiding pressure flow study was consistent with bladder outlet obstruction probably attributable to her cystocele.

The AUA/SUFU guideline task force noted that urodynamic testing is not indicated for routine evaluation of all adults with stress or urge incontinence [79]. However, testing is recommended for selected patents with mixed urinary incontinence when considering invasive, potentially morbid, or irreversible treatments. Testing was ordered for Mrs. A because she desired surgical repair of her vaginal prolapse. Guideline statements recommend filling cystometry to identify detrusor overactivity or low bladder wall compliance, along with assessment of urethral function. Filling cystometry revealed normal bladder wall compliance, normal sensations

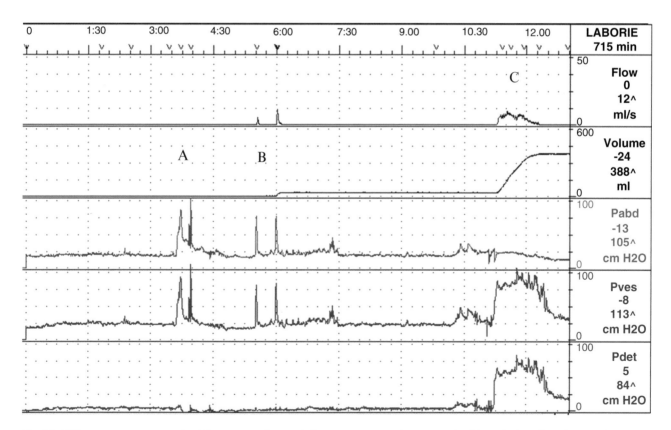

Fig. 9.9 Filling cystometrogram and voiding pressure flow study in a 75-year-old female with mixed urinary incontinence symptoms and pelvic organ prolapse. (A) No leakage when abdominal leak point pressure measured without reduction of vaginal wall prolapse. (B) Urodynamic stress urinary incontinence when abdominal leak point pressure testing repeated with vaginal wall prolapse reduced. (C) Voiding pressure flow study showing prolonged flow pattern and elevated detrusor contraction pressure indicating bladder outlet obstruction associated with severe vaginal wall prolapse

of bladder filling and no detrusor overactivity. Urethral function was evaluated via urethral pressure profilometry and abdominal leak point testing; both demonstrated urodynamic stress UI but neither found evidence of intrinsic sphincter deficiency. Mrs. A underwent anterior repair and sacrocolpopexy for pelvic organ prolapse and placement of a suburethral sling for her stress UI. She reported resolution of stress UI and improvement in the force of her urinary stream.

Case 2: Urodynamic Testing in a 90-Year-Old Male with Urinary Retention Requiring Twice Daily Intermittent Catheterization Despite Transurethral Prostate Photovaporization 7 Years Ago

Mr. B is a 90-year-old gentleman with urinary retention requiring intermittent catheterization twice daily. He underwent transurethral resection of prostate using photovaporization 7

years prior to referral for urodynamic testing. Mr. B initially noted marked improvement in the force of his urinary stream and reduction of nocturia from 5 to 3 episodes per night. He reports increasing difficulty urinating over the past year and was found to have a 560 ml residual 1 month ago prompting initiation of intermittent catheterization twice daily (morning and before sleep) and urodynamic evaluation for possible repeat transurethral prostate resection. In addition to his difficulty emptying his bladder, Mr. B reports urgency and urge incontinence requiring absorptive briefs when away from his home. Multichannel urodynamic testing demonstrated a cystometric capacity of 407 ml and normal bladder compliance (whole bladder compliance was 129 ml/cm H_2O) (Fig. 9.10). Terminal detrusor overactivity occurred at a volume of 388 ml. He was given permission to urinate which revealed prolonged flow pattern with Qmax 6 ml/s and a Qave of 2 ml/s. His voided volume was 88 ml and his residual volume was 319 ml. Detrusor pressure at maximum flow was 15 cm H_2O and the

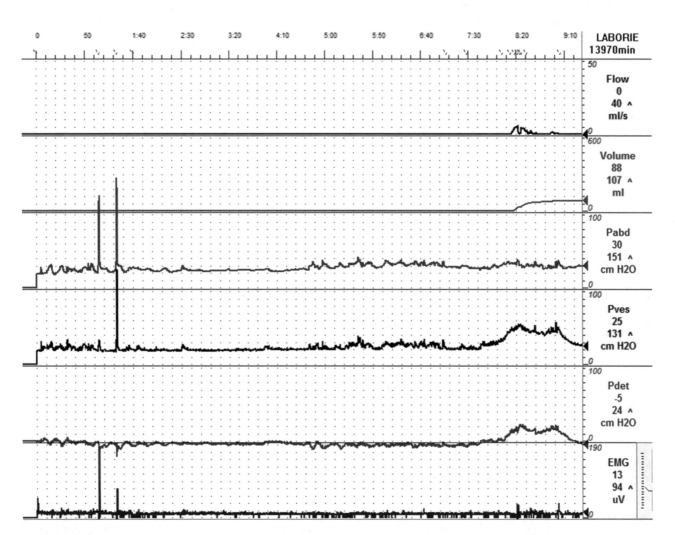

Fig. 9.10 Filling cystometrogram and voiding pressure flow study in a 90-year-old male with urinary retention managed by intermittent catheterization twice daily and urge incontinence. Voiding pressure flow study shows underactive detrusor contraction without bladder outlet obstruction

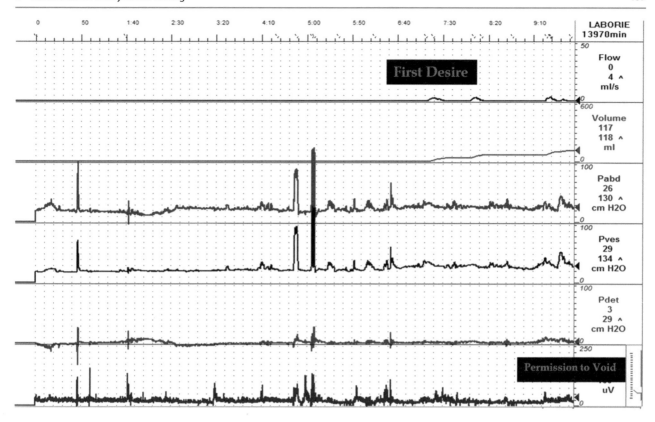

Fig. 9.11 Filling cystometrogram in an 89-year-old female with detrusor hyperreflexia with impaired contractile function

ICS obstruction nomogram revealed a URA of 12, indicating no clinically relevant bladder outlet obstruction.

The AUA/SUFU guidelines recommend VPFS to determine bladder outlet obstruction in men with lower urinary tract symptoms when invasive, potentially morbid, or irreversible treatment is considered. In this case, Mr. B was found to have no evidence of obstruction; instead, his incomplete bladder emptying was related to underactive detrusor function and repeat transurethral prostate resection was deemed inappropriate in the absence of obstruction. Catheterization frequency was increased to 4 times daily which reduced the frequency of daytime voiding and urge incontinence episodes.

Case 3: Detrusor Overactivity Combined with Underactive Detrusor Function (Impaired Contractility) in an 89-Year-Old Female

Mrs. D is an 89-year-old female with mild Alzheimer's disease who is brought in by her husband and daughter, who are her caretakers. They are for concerned for worsening urinary incontinence requiring use of adult briefs and recurring urinary tract infections. The patient has been hospitalized several times due to episodes of worsening confusion during UTIs. The patient is ambulatory with minimal assistance. Her medication list is only significant for donepezil. Multichannel urodynamic testing was performed to distinguish the cause of her incontinence and how this may relate to her recurrent infections. As seen in Fig. 9.11, cystometric capacity was 118 ml with a normal compliance. She has reduced sensation of bladder filling. During filling phase she had two low amplitude detrusor contractions with associated urgency and small volume urge incontinence. With permission to void her Pdet was 10 cm H_2O at a Qmax of 4 ml/s, indicating poor contractility. Her post void residual was 150 ml. This patient shows a common finding in elderly patients, detrusor hyperreflexia with impaired contractile function (DHIC). This condition is hypothesized to represent an advanced form of overactive bladder in which the detrusor has deteriorated over time resulting in an underactive bladder [80, 81]. Patients with DHIC in prospective observational study have been shown to have higher rates of urinary retention and recurrent cystitis than those with detrusor overactivity and preserved contractility [82].

Key Points

- Urodynamics is a set of tests used to measure lower urinary tract function and dysfunction; the most commonly employed tests are uroflowmetry, filling cystometrogram, voiding pressure flow study, and post void residual measurement.
- The prestudy uroflowmetry is a screening test; it is used to differentiate a normal (continuous) from abnormal (prolonged or interrupted) flow pattern but it cannot be used to determine the underlying cause of abnormal results.
- The filling cystometrogram is used to evaluate bladder filling/storage; however, normal cystometric capacity is usually higher than functional bladder capacity because it is intended to reproduce bothersome lower urinary tract symptoms.
- Urethral sphincter competence can be assessed by abdominal leak point pressure measurements; any detectable abdominal leak point indicates urodynamic stress urinary incontinence and if >60 cm H_2O, also indicates intrinsic sphincter deficiency.
- Detrusor overactivity is the occurrence of any detrusor contractions during the filling cystometrogram; this urodynamic finding is strongly associated with urgency and urge incontinence characteristic of overactive bladder dysfunction.
- Analysis of the voiding pressure flow study enables differentiation of normal micturition from abnormal flow with or without incomplete bladder emptying associated with underactive detrusor function or bladder outlet obstruction.
- Age related changes measured in healthy women include reduced sensations of bladder filling, reduced detrusor contraction strength, and reduced urethral closure pressures in women.
- Reduced bladder capacity is not seen in healthy older adults; it does occur in adults who also have detrusor overactivity.
- Multichannel urodynamics is useful for measurement of lower urinary tract dysfunction when considering invasive or potentially irreversible interventions.

References

1. Davis DM. The hydrodynamics of the upper urinary tract (urodynamics). Ann Surg. 1954;140(6):839–49.
2. Abrams P, Blaivas JG, Stanton SL, Andersen JT. The standardisation of terminology of lower urinary tract function. The International Continence Society Committee on Standardisation of Terminology. Scand J Urol Nephrol Suppl. 1988;114:5–19.
3. Gray M. Traces: making sense of urodynamics testing–part 2: uroflowmetry. Urol Nurs. 2010;30(6):321–6.
4. Gray M. Traces: making sense of urodynamics testing–part 3: electromyography of the pelvic floor muscles. Urol Nurs. 2011;31(1):31–8.
5. Gray M. Traces: making sense of urodynamics testing–part 5: evaluation of bladder filling/storage functions. Urol Nurs. 2011;31(3):149–53.
6. Gray M. Traces: making sense of urodynamics testing–part 6: evaluation of bladder filling/storage: bladder wall compliance and the detrusor leak point pressure. Urol Nurs. 2011;31(4):215–21. 235.
7. Issa MM, Chun T, Thwaites D, Bouet R, Hall J, Miller LE, et al. The effect of urethral instrumentation on uroflowmetry. BJU Int. 2003;92(4):426–8.
8. Schäfer W, Abrams P, Liao L, Mattiasson A, Pesce F, Spangberg A, et al. Good urodynamic practices: uroflowmetry, filling cystometry, and pressure-flow studies. Neurourol Urodyn. 2002;21(3):261–74.
9. Meffan PJ, Nacey JN, Delahunt B. Effect of abdominal straining on urinary flow rate in normal males. Br J Urol. 1991;67(2):134–9.
10. Kelly CE, Krane RJ. Current concepts and controversies in urodynamics. Curr Urol Rep. 2000;1(3):217–26.
11. Van de Beek C, Stoevelaar HJ, McDonnell J, Nijs HG, Casparie AF, Janknegt RA. Interpretation of uroflowmetry curves by urologists. J Urol. 1997;157(1):164–8.
12. Jarvis TR, Chan L, Tse V. Practical uroflowmetry. BJU Int. 2012;110(Suppl):28–9.
13. Jensen KM, Jørgensen JB, Mogensen P. Urodynamics in prostatism. I. Prognostic value of uroflowmetry. Scand J Urol Nephrol. 1988;22(2):109–17.
14. Wheeler TL, Richter HE, Greer WJ, Bowling CB, Redden DT, Varner RE. Predictors of success with postoperative voiding trials after a mid urethral sling procedure. J Urol. 2008;179(2):600–4.
15. Chancellor MB, Hanno PM, Malkowicz SB WA. Clinical manual of urology. 3rd ed. New York: McGraw-Hill; 2007, p. 448–50.
16. Coombes GM, Millard RJ. The accuracy of portable ultrasound scanning in the measurement of residual urine volume. J Urol. 1994;152(6 Pt 1):2083–5.
17. Byun SS, Kim HH, Lee E, Paick J-S, Kamg W, Oh S-J. Accuracy of bladder volume determinations by ultrasonography: are they accurate over entire bladder volume range? Urology. 2003;62(4):656–60.
18. Griffiths DJ, Harrison G, Moore K, McCracken P. Variability of post-void residual urine volume in the elderly. Urol Res. 1996;24(1):23–6.
19. Homma Y, Batista J, Bauer S, Griffiths D, Hilton P, KRAMER G, et al. Urodynamics. p. 317–72. Available from: http://www.ics.org/publications/ici_2/chapters/chap07.pdf.
20. Abrams P, Cardozo L, Fall M, Griffiths D, Rosier P, Ulmsten U, et al. The standardisation of terminology of lower urinary tract function: report from the Standardisation Sub-committee of the International Continence Society. Neurourol Urodyn. 2002;21(2):167–78.
21. Gammie A, Clarkson B, Constantinou C, Damaser M, Drinnan M, Geleijnse G, et al. International Continence Society guidelines on urodynamic equipment performance. Neurourol Urodyn. 2014;33(4):370–9.
22. McKinney TB, Babin E, Shah N, McKinney C, Glowack J. (2015) Comparison of water and air-charged transducer catheters during voiding pressure studies. Lecture presented at Tokyo, Japan; International Continence Society.
23. Klevmark B. Volume threshold for micturition. Influence of filling rate on sensory and motor bladder function. Scand J Urol Nephrol Suppl. 2002;(210):6–10.
24. Fitzgerald MP, Stablein U, Brubaker L. Urinary habits among asymptomatic women. Am J Obstet Gynecol. 2002;187(5):1384–8.
25. Latini JM, Mueller E, Lux MM, Fitzgerald MP, Kreder KJ. Voiding frequency in a sample of asymptomatic American men. J Urol. 2004;172(3):980–4.
26. Harris RL, Cundiff GW, Theofrastous JP, Bump RC. Bladder compliance in neurologically intact women. Neurourol Urodyn. 1996;15(5):483–8.
27. Brostrom S, Jennum P, Lose G. Short-term reproducibility of cystometry and pressure-flow micturition studies in healthy women. Neurourol Urodyn. 2002;21(5):457–60.

28. Heesakkers JPFA, Vandoninck V, van Balken MR, Bemelmans BLH. Bladder filling by autologous urine production during cystometry: a urodynamic pitfall! Neurourol Urodyn. 2003;22(3): 243–5.
29. Yuan Z, Tang Z, He C, Tang W. Diabetic cystopathy: a review. J Diabetes. 2015;7(4):442–7.
30. Srikandarajah N, Boissaud-Cooke MA, Clark S, Wilby MJ. Does early surgical decompression in cauda equina syndrome improve bladder outcome? Spine (Phila Pa 1976). 2015;40(8):580–3.
31. Palmer MH, Athanasopoulos A, Lee K-S, Takeda M, Wyndaele J-J. Sociocultural and environmental influences on bladder health. Int J Clin Pract. 2012;66(12):1132–8.
32. Kuo Y-C, Kuo H-C. The urodynamic characteristics and prognostic factors of patients with interstitial cystitis/bladder pain syndrome. Int J Clin Pract. 2013;67(9):863–9.
33. Nigro DA, Wein AJ, Foy M, Parsons CL, Williams M, Nyberg LM, et al. Associations among cystoscopic and urodynamic findings for women enrolled in the Interstitial Cystitis Data Base (ICDB) Study. Urology. 1997;49(5A Suppl):86–92.
34. Chen Y-C, Kuo H-C. Clinical and video urodynamic characteristics of adult women with dysfunctional voiding. J Formos Med Assoc. 2014;113(3):161–5.
35. Madersbacher S, Pycha A, Klingler CH, Mian C, Djavan B, Stulnig T, et al. Interrelationships of bladder compliance with age, detrusor instability, and obstruction in elderly men with lower urinary tract symptoms. Neurourol Urodyn. 1999;18(1):3–15.
36. Griffiths D. Urodynamics: the mechanics and hydrodynamics of the lower urinary tract. 2nd ed. Rotterdam: International Continence Society; 2014. p. 139–48.
37. Blaivas J, Chancellor M, Weiss J, Verhaaren M. Atlas of Urodynamics. 2nd ed. Victoria: Blackwell; p. 56–68.
38. Houle AM, Gilmour RF, Churchill BM, Gaumond M, Bissonnette B. What volume can a child normally store in the bladder at a safe pressure? J Urol. 1993;149(3):561–4.
39. McGuire EJ, Woodside JR, Borden TA, Weiss RM. Prognostic value of urodynamic testing in myelodysplastic patients. J Urol. 1981;126(2):205–9.
40. Gilmour RF, Churchill BM, Steckler RE, Houle AM, Khoury AE, McLorie GA. A new technique for dynamic analysis of bladder compliance. J Urol. 1993;150(4):1200–3.
41. Peterson A, Webster G. Urodynamic and videourodynamic evaluation of voiding dysfunction. In: Wein AJ, Kavoussi LR, Novick AC, Partin AW, Peters CA, editors. Campbell-Walsh urology. 9th ed. Philadelphia: Elsevier; p. 1986–2010.
42. Kershen RT, Azadzoi KM, Siroky MB. Blood flow, pressure and compliance in the male human bladder. J Urol. 2002;168(1):121–5.
43. Cho S-Y, Yi J-S, Oh S-J. The clinical significance of poor bladder compliance. Neurourol Urodyn. 2009;28(8):1010–4.
44. Shin JC, Park C, Kim HJ, Lee IY. Significance of low compliance bladder in cauda equina injury. Spinal Cord. 2002;40(12):650–5.
45. Kim SH, Kim TB, Kim SW, Oh S-J. Urodynamic findings of the painful bladder syndrome/interstitial cystitis: a comparison with idiopathic overactive bladder. J Urol. 2009;181(6):2550–4.
46. de Figueiredo AA, Lucon AM, Srougi M. Bladder augmentation for the treatment of chronic tuberculous cystitis. Clinical and urodynamic evaluation of 25 patients after long term follow-up. Neurourol Urodyn. 2006;25(5):433–40.
47. Viart L, Elalouf V, Petit J, Al Khedr A, Kristkowiak P, Saint F. [Prognostics factors of renal failure in multiple sclerosis]. Progrès en Urol J l'Association Fr d'urologie la Société Fr d'urologie. 2012;22(16):1026–32.
48. Gray M. Traces: making sense of urodynamics testing–part 7: evaluation of bladder filling/storage: evaluation of urethral sphincter incompetence and stress urinary incontinence. Urol Nurs. 2011;31(5):267–77, 289.
49. Smith AL, Ferlise VJ, Wein AJ, Ramchandani P, Rovner ES. Effect of A 7-F transurethral catheter on abdominal leak point pressure measurement in men with post-prostatectomy incontinence. Urology. 2011;77(5):1188–93.
50. Griffiths D. The pressure within a collapsed tube, with special reference to urethral pressure. Phys Med Biol. 1985;30(9):951–63.
51. Heesakkers JPFA, Vriesema JLJ. The role of urodynamics in the treatment of lower urinary tract symptoms in women. Curr Opin Urol. 2005;15(4):215–21.
52. Brown M, Wickham JE. The urethral pressure profile. Br J Urol. 1969;41(2):211–7.
53. Shah SM, Gaunay GS. Treatment options for intrinsic sphincter deficiency. Nat Rev Urol. 2012;9(11):638–51.
54. McGuire EJ, Cespedes RD, O'Connell HE. Leak-point pressures. Urol Clin North Am. 1996;23(2):253–62.
55. Betson LH, Siddiqui G, Bhatia NN. Intrinsic urethral sphincteric deficiency: critical analysis of various diagnostic modalities. Curr Opin Obstet Gynecol. 2003;15(5):411–7.
56. Gray M. Traces: making sense of urodynamics testing–part 8: evaluating sensations of bladder filling. Urol Nurs. 2011;31(6):369–74.
57. De Wachter SG, Heeringa R, van Koeveringe GA, Gillespie JI. On the nature of bladder sensation: the concept of sensory modulation. Neurourol Urodyn. 2011;30(7):1220–6.
58. Wyndaele JJ. The normal pattern of perception of bladder filling during cystometry studied in 38 young healthy volunteers. J Urol. 1998;160(2):479–81.
59. Wyndaele JJ, De Wachter S. Cystometrical sensory data from a normal population: comparison of two groups of young healthy volunteers examined with 5 years interval. Eur Urol. 2002;42(1):34–8.
60. Homma Y. OAB symptoms: assessment and discriminator for etiopathology. Curr Opin Urol. 2014;24(4):345–51.
61. Abrams P, Chapple CR, Jünemann K-P, Sharpe S. Urinary urgency: a review of its assessment as the key symptom of the overactive bladder syndrome. World J Urol. 2012;30(3):385–92.
62. Parsons CL. Diagnosing the bladder as the source of pelvic pain: successful treatment for adults and children. Pain Manag. 2014;4(4):293–301.
63. Haab F. Chapter 1: The conditions of neurogenic detrusor overactivity and overactive bladder. Neurourol Urodyn. 2014;33 Suppl 3:S2–5.
64. Ruffion A, Castro-Diaz D, Patel H, Khalaf K, Onyenwenyi A, Globe D, et al. Systematic review of the epidemiology of urinary incontinence and detrusor overactivity among patients with neurogenic overactive bladder. Neuroepidemiology. 2013;41(3–4):146–55.
65. Gray M. Traces: making sense of urodynamics testing – part 10: evaluation of micturition via the voiding pressure-flow study. Urol Nurs. 2012;32(2):71–8.
66. Rosier PFWM, Kirschner-Hermanns R, Svihra J, Homma Y, Wein AJ. ICS teaching module: analysis of voiding, pressure flow analysis (basic module). Neurourol Urodyn. 2016;35(1):36–8.
67. Gray M. Traces : making sense of urodynamics testing – part 3 : electromyography of the pelvic floor muscles. Urol Nurs. 2011;31(1):31–9.
68. Valentini FA, Marti BG, Robain G, Nelson PP. Detrusor aftercontraction: a new insight. Int Braz J Urol. 2015;41(3):527–34.
69. Rodrigues P, Hering F, Campagnari JC. Urodynamic aftercontraction waves: a large observational study in an adult female population and correlation with bladder and ureter emptying functions in women. Urol Int. 2014;93(4):431–6.
70. Pfisterer MH-D, Griffiths DJ, Rosenberg L, Schaefer W, Resnick NM. Parameters of bladder function in pre-, peri-, and postmenopausal continent women without detrusor overactivity. Neurourol Urodyn. 2007;26(3):356–61.
71. Rosario DJ, Woo HH, Chapple CR. Definition of normality of pressure-flow parameters based on observations in asymptomatic men. Neurourol Urodyn. 2008;27(5):388–94.

72. Sekido N. Bladder contractility and urethral resistance relation: what does a pressure flow study tell us? Int J Urol. 2012;19(3):216–28.

73. Pfisterer MH-D, Griffiths DJ, Schaefer W, Resnick NM. The effect of age on lower urinary tract function: a study in women. J Am Geriatr Soc. 2006;54(3):405–12.

74. Gray M. Traces: making sense of urodynamics testing–part 11: quantitative analysis of micturition via the voiding pressure flow study: pressure-flow nomograms. Urol Nurs. 2012;32(3):159–65. 147.

75. Schafer W. Current opinion in urology. 1992. p. 252–6. Available from: http://journals.lww.com/co-urology/Abstract/1992/08000/Urodynamics_of_micturition_.4.aspx.

76. Chassagne S, Bernier PA, Haab F, Roehrborn CG, Reisch JS, Zimmern PE. Proposed cutoff values to define bladder outlet obstruction in women. Urology. 1998;51(3):408–11.

77. Nitti VW. Pressure flow urodynamic studies: the gold standard for diagnosing bladder outlet obstruction. Rev Urol. 2005;7 Suppl 6:S14–21.

78. Abrams P. Bladder outlet obstruction index, bladder contractility index and bladder voiding efficiency: three simple indices to define bladder voiding function. BJU Int. 1999;84(1):14–5.

79. Winters J, Dmochowski R, Goldman H, Herndon C, Kobashi K, Kraus S. Adult urodnamics: AUA/SuFU guideline. 2012. Available from: https://www.auanet.org/common/pdf/education/clinical-guidance/Adult-Urodynamics.pdf.

80. Chancellor MB. The overactive bladder progression to underactive bladder hypothesis. Int Urol Nephrol. 2014;46 Suppl 1:S23–7.

81. Resnick NM, Yalla SV. Detrusor hyperactivity with impaired contractile function. An unrecognized but common cause of incontinence in elderly patients. JAMA. 1987;257(22):3076–81.

82. Stav K, Shilo Y, Zisman A, Lindner A, Leibovici D. Comparison of lower urinary tract symptoms between women with detrusor overactivity and impaired contractility, and detrusor overactivity and preserved contractility. J Urol. 2013;189(6):2175–8.

Anorectal Manometry

Askin Erdogan, Siegfried W.B. Yu, and Satish S.C. Rao

Introduction

Since Gower's first studies junction in 1877, physiologic testing using anorectal manometry (ARM) has been employed as a useful modality for assessing the physiologic and pathophysiologic characteristics of the anorectum [1]. Pelvic floor disorders involving the anorectum are among the conditions that can be evaluated with this modality. They affect up to a quarter of US women, with hysterectomy and multiparity having a strong causal association [2]. Constipation and fecal incontinence (FI) are common problems that involve the pelvic floor, and have a higher prevalence in the elderly. The prevalence of constipation was found to be 25.8 % in a community dwelling elderly population [3], and as high as 71.5 % in nursing home residents with age over 60 years [4]. FI affects between 6 and 19 % of elderly individuals aged 65 years and older living in the community, and is a major reason for nursing home placement. Unlike in younger patients, men and women are equally affected [5, 6].

Systemic disease, sphincter integrity, bowel motility, stool consistency, evacuation efficiency, cognitive and emotional affects, all of which tend to affect pelvic floor function the elderly population. Dyssynergic defecation, slow-transit constipation (STC), and constipation predominant irritable bowel syndrome (IBS-C) are examples of three pathophysiologic types of constipation and likewise fecal impaction with overflow and fecal incontinence are common problems. Patients may present to various specialists for treatment of these problems, and without a sound understanding of the underlying pathophysiology and appropriate testing methods, both diagnosis and treatment can be delayed.

Anorectal manometry provides detailed information about anorectal sensory and motor function. This includes pressures of the rectum and anal sphincters at rest, squeeze and with straining, anal sphincter length, rectal sensation, rectal capacity and compliance, and assessment of anorectal reflexes. In this chapter, we will discuss how to perform and interpret ARM, and review its role in the diagnosis and management of constipation, primarily dyssynergic defecation, and FI in the elderly.

Methods of Performing Anorectal Manometry

There are various methods of performing ARM, however, they all generally consist of a system with a probe (pressure sensing device), amplifier/recorder which converts the pressure signals, a monitor which displays the signal recordings, and a computer for data analysis and data storage. Because the equipment and procedures vary at different institutions, it is important to be familiar with the characteristics at one's own center. Different methods include the closed balloon system, the water-perfused system, and the manometry catheter system, which includes both water-perfused, and solid-state catheters.

Water-Perfused Catheter System

The water-perfused catheter system consists of a thin plastic tube with a central channel that is connected to a pneumo-hydraulic pump. The catheter, with a diameter ranging 3.5–7 mm, has multiple side holes (4–8) placed 0.5–2 cm apart from each other. The tip of the catheter has a 4 cm balloon for inflation. The pump is set with a pressure of 10–15 psi and nitrogen gas is used to pump water out of reservoir [7, 8]. Water flows through the side holes at a rate of 0.1–0.5 ml/min. Water-perfused catheter systems do not

A. Erdogan • S.W.B. Yu • S.S.C. Rao (✉)
Division of Gastroenterology and Hepatology, Augusta University, 1120 15th Street, BBR 2538, Augusta, GA 30912, USA
e-mail: srao@augusta.edu

© Springer Science+Business Media New York 2017
D.A. Gordon, M.R. Katlic (eds.), *Pelvic Floor Dysfunction and Pelvic Surgery in the Elderly*,
DOI 10.1007/978-1-4939-6554-0_10

record true sphincter pressures, but indirect measurements of intraluminal pressure using resistance pressure to the water flowing out of the catheter which is picked up by the transducers. Depending on the equipment used, conventional manometry and radial tracings can be generated. Although it has the advantage of having low cost and simplicity, the water perfusion system does not allow for performing studies in the sitting position, and the studies may be affected by abnormal voluntary reflexes induced by the contact of perfused water with rectal mucosa. Although the use of smaller manometry catheters has better patient tolerance, and radial catheters have the ability to record longitudinal pressures in the anal canal, the artifacts created by water-perfused systems have been criticized for some time [9].

Solid State Manometry System

The microtransducer technique was introduced to simplify ARM, and decreases the presence of stretch artifacts, however the use of a single microtip measured only a very small area, with the disadvantage of being very fragile. The introduction of solid-state microtip manometry catheters has improved this, and because these catheters do not require water perfusion, they are easier to use, accurate, and reliable, with much less artifact. Increasingly popular and widespread in use, they come in a variety of configurations with available probe adapters, and can be easily used in the ambulatory setting, permitting evaluation of anorectal function in different positions. The solid state manometry system consists of a thin flexible probe which has microtransducers that sense and measure pressures directly. A 4 cm long latex balloon is tied to the probe, and 6 sensors are located radially at an angle of 90° from each other at 1, 2, 3, 4, 5, and 9 cm from the "0" reference point. The 1 cm sensor is always located posteriorly. The probe is connected to an A-D connector and the pressures detected by the sensors are transmitted through the connector, and displayed on the monitor after being amplified. Conventional manometry tracings are generated by this system. The primary limitations of the solid state manometry system are its fragility and cost.

High Resolution Anorectal Pressure Topography (HRAPT) OR High Resolution Anorectal Manometry (HRARM)

Another advance was the introduction of HRAPT/HRARM. The probe consists of 10–12 circumferentially oriented 2.5 mm long sensors located 0.5–1 cm apart that detect pressures directly. There are 1–2 sensors located inside the rectal balloon and 8–10 sensors located along the anal canal. The pressure detected by sensors may be affected by changes in temperature (thermal drift), which can be adjusted for by using thermal compensation [10]. This system can generate conventional manometry tracings, and also provides 2-dimensional high resolution colored topographic imaging, more detailed intraluminal pressure, thus providing greater anatomic detail, and has been found to correlate well with the water-perfused systems [11]. Although it is easier to interpret, its main disadvantage is that the probe is fragile and expensive.

3-D High-Definition Anorectal Manometry

A further development is 3-D high-definition anorectal manometry (HDAM), a novel, solid state manometric system that can provide additional information about structural anorectal problems including excessive perineal descent, rectal prolapse, rectal intussusception, and anal sphincter defects. This system consists of a probe that has 256 solid-state microtransducers arranged in 16 rows, each row consisting of 16 circumferentially located sensors. The sensors are located 4 mm apart, however the software linearly interpolates the space between sensors and provides measurements at 1-mm spacing with minimal error. The probe is 10.75 mm in diameter, and has a central channel which facilitates inflation of a 3.3 cm long balloon that is attached to the probe. The balloon is made up of non-latex clear thermoplastic elastomer with a 400 ml capacity. The probe must be calibrated prior to use to correct for pressure drift. The advantage of HDAM is that it provides conventional as well as 2-dimensional high resolution images and 3-dimensional high resolution images in sagittal and cross-sectional planes, thereby providing a better understanding of anorectal function, anatomical structure, and sphincter defects. The disadvantage of the probe is that it is more expensive and fragile, and more rigid and bulky than HRAPT.

Performing Anorectal Manometry

Usually a bowel preparation is not required prior to performing ARM. The patient is asked to empty his/her bowel. Before ARM is performed, a digital rectal exam (DRE) should be performed, and in case there is significant stool in the rectum, an enema may be administered, and the test performed 2 h later. The DRE has the advantage of being a simple, bedside, physical examination maneuver that provides

At Rest

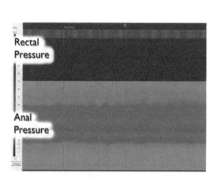

Squeeze

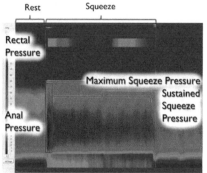

Bearing Down

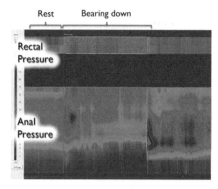

Fig. 10.1 Baseline manometric assessments. Typical anorectal manometry findings at rest, and while squeeze and bearing down. Rest: Resting profile shows high pressure zone of 67.2 mmHg corresponding with internal anal sphincter tone. Squeeze: Significant increase in anal sphincter pressure that has two components; max, mean squeeze pressure and sustained squeeze pressure. Bearing down: There is increase in rectal pressure coinciding with a decrease (reduction) in anal sphincter pressure showing a normal bearing down response

useful information [12]. The test may be easier to perform in the left lateral position. Details of systematic DRE exam have been published recently [12].

Probe Placement

The probe is placed with the patient lying down in the left lateral position, knees bent to 90° with the distal sensor located posteriorly from the anal verge. The probe should be placed into position with the sphincter pressure zone centered on the monitor. Calibration and accurate position are important for accurate interpretation. ARM consists of several standard measurements and maneuvers that evaluate anorectal anatomy and physiology, and are reviewed below (Fig. 10.1).

Anal Sphincter Length

In the absence of a solid state manometry system, the sphincter length is best measured with the pull-through technique. The sphincter length is determined by the level at which pressure is at least 5 mmHg above the rectal pressure. The normal length ranges from 3 to 5 cm, and men have longer sphincter length than women [13, 14].

Anal Sphincter Resting Pressure

To assess baseline anal sphincter pressure that primarily reflects mainly the internal anal sphincter (IAS) function. After placing the probe, a 5 min run-in period should be allowed before starting the recording to allow the pressures

to return to basal levels. During this period an ultraslow wave activity that has a phasic pressure activity at 1–1.5 cycles min⁻¹ with amplitude ≥40 mmHg can be seen which should be considered when interpreting the resting pressure [15]. Using the stationary technique, after the probe is placed correctly, the maximum highest pressure at any point in anal canal is taken as the resting pressure. This is the preferred technique for resting pressure.

The difference between maximum anal sphincter pressure and the basal pressure recorded at any level of the anal canal is defined as the maximal anal sphincter resting pressure. Resting pressure predominantly reflects the IAS (80 %) and normal values range between 50 and 80 mmHg [13]. In a study of 21 nulliparous females, 18 multiparous females and 20 males, mean maximum resting anal sphincter pressures were significantly higher in nulliparous women than in multiparous women, however no difference was noted between nulliparous females and males (Fig. 10.1) [16].

Anal Squeeze Sphincter Pressure

The anal squeeze sphincter pressure measurement assesses the strength of the EAS during a voluntary squeeze. The patient is asked to continuously squeeze the anal sphincter as long as possible, and for at least 30 s, as if holding a bowel movement. This maneuver is performed twice, with a 1 min resting interval, and the best attempt is chosen for interpretation [15]. This pressure is mostly due to contraction of the EAS, but also includes the puborectalis muscle. Maximum anal sphincter squeeze pressure is defined as the difference between the highest anal sphincter pressure and the atmospheric baseline and is the maximum pressure recorded at any level of the anal canal. After the initial peak of maximum

Fig. 10.2 High resolution manometric patterns showing typical examples of the Abdominopelvic Reflex (Party Balloon/Cough Reflex), Rectoanal Inhibitory Reflex (RAIR), Rectoanal Contractile Reflex (RACR), and the Sensorimotor Response (SMR)

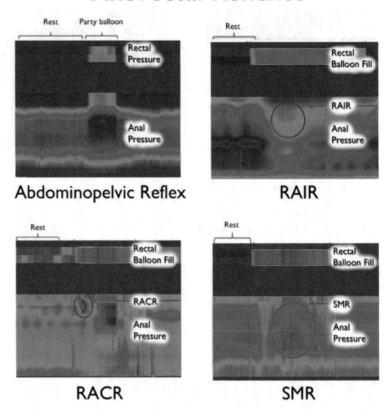

High Resolution Manometric Anorectal Reflexes

anal sphincter squeeze pressure, sustained squeeze pressure, which is important for continence, is defined as the pressure difference between the anal sphincter pressure and baseline pressure, which is sustained for at least 15 s at any level of the anal sphincter (Fig. 10.1).

Duration of Squeeze and Sustained Squeeze Krenor: The Total Period of Squeeze (Duration)

The period during which at least 50 % of the maximum squeeze pressure is maintained during the squeeze maneuver (Sustained squeeze), and is an important index of sphincter muscle fatigue. In a patient who cannot generate a good squeeze, the time difference between the onset of squeeze and the time to return to basal pressure is measured. The normal duration is between 25 and 31 s, however healthy people can squeeze up to 50 s [17]. Both maximum and sustained squeeze pressures are higher in men than in women, and nulliparous women have higher squeeze pressures than multiparous women (Fig. 10.1) [14, 16].

The Abdominopelvic Reflex (Party Balloon Test/Cough Test)

The abdominopelvic reflex maintains continence when there is a sudden increase in intra-abdominal pressure, by causing a reflex increase in both the intrarectal and anal sphincter pressure. This reflex arc is maintained by a local spinal reflex and is preserved in upper motor neuron lesions and impaired in cauda equina lesion or sacral plexus injury. To evaluate this reflex the patient is asked to blow into a party balloon for 10 s continuously, or to cough. This maneuver is performed twice after a 1 min interval. The maximum intrarectal pressure is the difference between the maximum rectal and basal rectal pressure. Similar to the measurement of squeeze pressures, the maximum intra-anal sphincter pressure during this reflex is the difference between the maximum and basal anal sphincter pressure. The findings of this reflex test must be interpreted with the findings of a voluntary anal sphincter squeeze. In lower motor neuron lesions, both this reflex and voluntary squeeze are absent. In upper motor neuron lesions, this reflex is present, but voluntary squeeze is absent (Fig. 10.2) [14].

Table 10.1 Anorectal manometry formulas

Formula	Definition	Useful for
Percentage of anal relaxation	$\dfrac{\text{Anal relaxation pressure}}{\text{Anal resting pressure}} \times 100$	Dyssynergic defecation
Defecation index (normal ≥ 1.2)	$\dfrac{\text{Maximum rectal pressure}}{\text{minimal residual pressure during bearing down}}$	Dyssynergic defecation
Percentage of saline retained	$\dfrac{\text{Volume of saline retained}}{\text{Volume of saline infused}} \times 100$	Fecal incontinence
Compliance	$\dfrac{dV}{dP} \; (\text{mL}/\text{mmHg})$	Rectal distensibility

Attempted Defecation (Bearing down maneuver)

Attempted defecation evaluates the rectal and anal canal pressure changes when bearing down (Valsalva maneuver), and characterizes the coordination of abdominal muscle contraction and rectal past effort along with anal canal relaxation. Simulated defecation should be performed both in the lying position and when sitting on a commode. The patient is initially asked to bear down as if having a bowel movement when lying on bed. This maneuver is performed twice after a 1 min interval. The residual anal pressure is the lowest pressure recorded at any level of the anal canal during attempted defecation. The percentage of anal relaxation (anal relaxation pressure/anal resting pressure × 100) and the defecation index (maximum rectal pressure/minimal residual pressure during bearing down) are 2 indices used to better understand anorectal function and problems related with attempted defecation. The normal defecation index is 1.2 (Table 10.1) [18].

In healthy subjects, the intrarectal pressure normally increases and anal sphincter pressure normally decreases during the bearing down maneuver. When this normal mechanism is impaired there is functional obstruction, also known as dyssynergic defecation, of which there are four different patterns (Fig. 10.3) [19]. Patients may have paradoxical anal contraction with normal propulsion (Type I), paradoxical anal contraction with impaired propulsion (Type II), impaired anal relaxation (<20 %) with adequate propulsion (Type III), and impaired anal relaxation with impaired propulsion (Type IV). When performed in the sitting position on a commode, the test simulates more physiologic conditions. The ARM probe is placed in the rectum and the intrarectal balloon is inflated with 60 ml of air to evoke the sensation of intrarectal fullness and simulate presence of stool. The patient is then asked to bear down as if having a bowel movement. During this maneuver the patient may expel the balloon. If not expelled, the balloon will be deflated and removed. Some healthy subjects may have a subclinical functional outlet obstruction that can be detected by this maneuver. This maneuver is also a useful parameter during biofeedback therapy.

Rectal Sensory Testing

Rectal sensory testing utilizes intrarectal balloon inflations to assess sensory thresholds in response to graduated balloon inflation. The rectal balloon is inflated in 10 ml increments until the patient describes a first sensation, and then by 30 ml increments until a maximum tolerable volume is reached (or up to a maximum volume of 320 ml). Each inflation is performed at a rate of 10 ml/s and maintained for 30 s. Between each inflation a rest period of 30 s is given. The sensory thresholds that are recorded include first sensation, constant sensation, desire to defecate, urge to defecate, and maximum tolerable volume (Table 10.2).

Normal sensation, rectal hyposensitivity, and rectal hypersensitivity can be elucidated by this test. Rectal hyposensitivity is defined as a higher than normal volume needed to elicit sensory thresholds with at least 2 out of 3 sensations (First sensation, desire to defecate, or urge to defecate) (2 standard deviations [SD] above normative data). Rectal hyposensitivity was found in 23 % of the patients with constipation and 10 % of patients with FI [20, 21]. Rectal hyposensitivity may also be found in patients with spinal cord injury, multiple sclerosis, and diabetes [22, 23]. Rectal hypersensitivity is defined as lower than normal volume needed to elicit sensory thresholds with at least 2 out of 3 sensations as noted above. This can be seen in patients with IBS and pelvic pain [17].

Rectal sensory abnormalities are important because they contribute to defecatory dysfunction, and can be corrected by sensory training and biofeedback therapy. Sensory results can be affected by the type of balloon used (elasticity, length, compliance, and shape), the distance of the rectal balloon from the anal verge, and the speed and technique of balloon inflation. Therefore, each motility laboratory must establish their own normative data with healthy subjects [24].

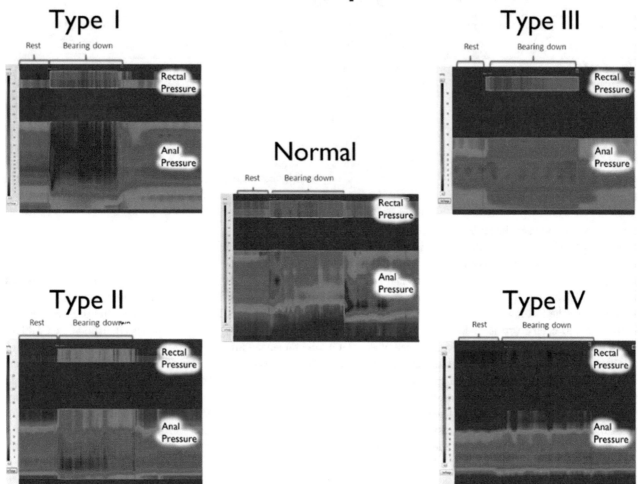

Fig. 10.3 High resolution manometric patterns showing typical examples of normal defecation pattern, type I, II, III, and IV dyssynergic defecation patterns. More recently additional subtypes for type 1 dyssynergia that include type 1P (Puborectalis), type 1A (Anal sphincter), type 1D (Diffuse), and similarly for type 2 dyssynergia (type II P, type II A and type II D) have been described

Table 10.2 Sensory thresholds in anorectal manometry

First sensation	A sensation of bloating, gas, or fullness which is transient[a]
Constant sensation	A sensation of gas which is constant and does not disappear through the inflation of balloon
Desire to defecate	A sensation which evokes the need to have a bowel movement and lasts >15 s[a]
Urge to defecate	An urgent sensation of desire to have a bowel movement (causing patient to rush to the bathroom)[a]
Maximum tolerable volume	The maximal volume that the patient can tolerate, often associated with severe urgency or pain

[a]Used in assessing for rectal hyposensitivity and rectal hypersensitivity

Rectal Compliance

Rectal compliance testing evaluates the distensibility and accommodation of the rectum by comparing pressure and volume changes. During graduated rectal balloon inflation, rectal pressure is recorded. Steady state rectal pressure for each inflation is assessed by subtracting the intraballoon pressure obtained in ambient air from the intrarectal pressure obtained during rectal distention. The intrarectal pressure increases as the rectum is inflated with an intrarectal balloon, then declines and reaches a steady state as a result of rectal accommodation to distention. Intrarectal volume and pressure responses to measured volumes are plotted on a graph and a compliance curve is obtained from the slope which represents the relationship between the change in intraballoon volume (dV) and the change in intrarectal pressure (dP) at the steady state (Table 10.1). The normal curve is nonlinear. The graph is useful to describe the volume–pressure relationships at various degrees of balloon inflation. Another option for assessing rectal compliance is a computerized balloon distending device, which uses a highly compliant balloon connected to a barostat [25, 26].

Rectoanal Inhibitory Reflex

The RAIR is a local enteric reflex mediated through the myenteric plexus, and is thought to facilitate anal sampling of rectal contents [27, 28]. As noted above, the intrarectal balloon is inflated with increasing amounts of air during the volumetric assessment. Balloon distention of the rectum produces a reflex relaxation of the IAS, and the lowest volume that evokes the RAIR is recorded. There are two components: a transient relaxation, then a sustained relaxation of the IAS that lasts throughout the period of rectal balloon distention. Cheeney et al. showed that relaxation increases until the balloon is filled with 71 ml, and then reaches a plateau [29]. This reflex is typically absent in patients with Hirschsprung's disease, which is typically diagnosed in earlier in life, not in the elderly (Fig. 10.2) [17, 30].

Sensorimotor Response

The SMR is an involuntary reflex contraction of the anal sphincter and puborectalis that occurs during rectal distention, and lasts 5–6 s. In healthy subjects, the lowest rectal distention volume required to elicit the SMR was 93 ± 26 ml, and it may be impaired in patients with rectal hyposensitivity [31]. This reflex is important for continence, is usually associated with desire the to defecate, and therefore to some extent is under voluntary control (Fig. 10.2) [32].

Rectoanal Contractile Response

The RACR is a reflex contraction of the EAS in response to distention of the rectum. This is a primordial reflex contraction that helps prevent accidental release of rectal contents, but disappears with continuous and increasing distention of the rectum (Fig. 10.2).

Balloon Expulsion Time

The Balloon Expulsion Time evaluates the patient's ability to expel an artificial stool (balloon) and is helpful in diagnosing dyssynergic defecation. This test is performed by placing a balloon 5 cm in length, which is fashioned from a condom or finger-cut, and attached to a short infusion line. The balloon is then soaked in water and placed in the rectum, and filled with 50 ml of warm water. The patient is asked to sit on a commode and expel the balloon in privacy. The patient is provided a stopwatch and instructed to start the timer when she/he starts, and stop the timer when the balloon is expelled. If the patient is not able to expel the balloon in 5 min, the examiner will remove the balloon manually. If the patient is not able to expel the balloon in 1 min, this is considered abnormal [14]. Although this test has a moderate to high specificity, negative, and positive predictive value (89 %, 64 %, and 97 % respectively) for the diagnosis of dyssynergic defecation [33], the sensitivity is as low as 40 % [34].

Complications of Anorectal Manometry

Great care needs to be taken when performing ARM. Rarely, colonic perforation has been reported in the literature as a complication of ARM [35, 36]. The probe must be gently inserted and removed in the rectum, and attention must be given to intrarectal balloon pressure during inflation. Any pain or discomfort that is reported by the patient should prompt caution, and a careful assessment regarding how to proceed. Special attention must be given to patients who are hyposensitive and/or postoperative.

Clinical Application of Anorectal Manometry in the Elderly

Descriptions of anatomic and physiologic data obtained from ARM in relation to aging have provided insights into age-related changes. Although gastrointestinal function is generally preserved with aging in healthy individuals, there is age-related neuronal loss, and changes in diet, mobility, comorbidity, polypharmacy, and prior trauma and surgeries

Table 10.3 Physiologic changes in the elderly

Structure	Proposed change	Pathophysiologic significance	Clinical problem
Number of HAPCs	Decreased	Decreased colonic propulsion	Constipation
Colonic transit time	Prolonged	Slow colon transit	Constipation
Internal anal sphincter	Thinning/atrophy	Weak sphincter	Fecal seepage/incontinence
External anal sphincter	Thinning/atrophy	Weak sphincter	Urgency/incontinence
Pudendal nerve function	Decreased	Impairment of colorectal sensorimotor function	Fecal seepage/incontinence
Rectal sensation	Decreased	Impairment of colorectal sensorimotor function	Fecal seepage/incontinence
Rectal Sensation	Decreased	Impaired reservoir function	Urgency/incontinence
Anal sphincter length	Decreased	Weak sphincter	Fecal seepage/urgency/incontinence
Rectal capacity	Decreased	Impaired reservoir function	Urgency/incontinence

Adapted from Yu, S.W. and S.S. Rao, *Anorectal physiology and pathophysiology in the elderly.* Clin Geriatr Med, 2014. **30**(1): p. 95–106 [37]

Table 10.4 Useful anorectal manometry data according to the underlying problem

Maneuver	Incontinence	Constipation
Resting pressure	Yes	Yes
Squeeze pressure/duration	Yes	Optional
Abdominopelvic reflex	Yes	No
Attempted defecation	Yes/No	Yes
Rectoanal inhibitory reflex	No	Yes
Rectal sensation	Yes	Yes
Rectal compliance	Optional	Optional
Simulated defecation	Yes/No	Yes

Adapted from Sun, W.M. and S.S. Rao, *Manometric assessment of anorectal function.* Gastroenterology clinics of North America, 2001. **30**(1): p. 15–32 [7]

that may predispose to impairment in function. In this regard, aging is associated with a variety of anatomic and physiologic changes that affect anorectal function, which include decreased colonic propulsion and slow transit, sphincter weakness, impaired sensorimotor function, and impaired reservoir function (Table 10.3) [37].

ARM provides an objective assessment of these changes in anorectal function that helps lead to the appropriate diagnosis and treatment of the underlying disorder. In one study, ARM provided new information in 88 % of evaluated patients, which led to appropriate changes in their management. Of those patients who were referred for FI, 53 % had low squeeze sphincter pressure, 36 % had impaired rectal sensation, and 50 % had pudendal neuropathy. Of those patients referred for constipation, 48 % were found to have Dyssynergic defecation, 58 % had impaired rectal sensation, and 43 % were successfully treated with biofeedback therapy [38]. In our increasingly comorbid and postsurgical elderly population with pelvic floor dysfunction, the benefit of ARM in providing diagnostic information that can effect specific management of these problems is clear. The useful ARM parameters for FI and constipation evaluation are similar, but are still dependent on the primary condition (Table 10.4).

Fecal Incontinence

Fecal continence is maintained with the help of several mechanisms, including normal IAS and EAS function, with the help of anal mucosal folds and the hemorrhoidal endovascular cushions. FI may result from deficits in IAS, EAS, or pelvic floor muscle function, the loss of endovascular cushions, impaired anorectal sensation, impaired rectal compliance/accommodation with aging, pelvic surgery, neuropathy related to pudendal, lumbosacral, and spinal cord lesions, or central nervous system deficits. Importantly, constipation can play an integral role in the development of FI, which can result from fecal impaction and subsequent overflow, IAS incompetence, decreased rectal or anal sensation, and from other structural pelvic floor or anorectal neuromuscular dysfunction caused by prior trauma from surgery or irradiation [39].

There are three clinical subtypes of FI, which include passive incontinence, urge incontinence, and fecal seepage. Although there is significant overlap between these subtypes, making a clinical distinction can help guide initial investigation and management (Table 10.3). A study by Deutekom et al. regarding these subtypes of incontinence, as reported by patients, showed that patients most often reported a combination of the different subtypes of FI (59 %), and their reported subtype did not correlate well with the underlying physiologic abnormalities ultimately identified with further testing—thus emphasizing the importance of physiologic testing such as ARM [40]. In the evaluation of FI, ARM can help describe the underlying sphincter, compliance, and sensory problems.

Patients with FI have been shown to have lower resting anal sphincter pressure and anal sphincter squeeze pressure [41]. Younger male and female subjects have been shown to have higher squeeze pressures than older subjects, [42, 43] which may predispose to FI in older individuals. Myogenic and neurogenic problems may be the underlying reason for the weaker squeeze pressures [17], which may be attributed to age-related changes in addition to the effects of comorbid disease. Aging was also found to be associated with lower anal resting pressures [43], although an earlier study performed in 18 healthy elderly and young adults did not show any effect of age on resting pressure [44], thus emphasizing the importance of disease in modulating the age-related predisposition to FI.

Rectal hyposensitivity, which can be diagnosed by volumetric rectal sensory testing during ARM, has been found in up to 10 % of patients with FI [20], and may also be found in patients with spinal cord injury, multiple sclerosis, and diabetes [22, 23]. Rectal hyposensitivity may contribute to FI through its association with constipation and subsequent overflow, impairment in reflexive or conscious anal sphincter contraction, and its association with pelvic floor weakness [21]. In one study of asymptomatic female patients, sensory testing was performed using a barostat, and volume thresholds were found to be similar, but pressure thresholds were found to be higher, although not significantly different, in older compared with younger females [43]. Rectal volumetric sensory assessments have not been found to be different between young and older healthy subjects [42]. The presence of disease comorbidities, which are more prevalent in older patients, again appears to be an important mitigating factor. The intrarectal volume needed to elicit the RAIR was not different in elderly patients compared younger patients, however elderly women required less volume than younger women [42]. Interestingly, in a study of the RAIR in patients with multiple sclerosis or spinal cord injury, FI correlated with a prolonged duration of RAIR [45], therefore prominence of and/or a lower threshold to elicit this reflex may be associated with FI.

The physiologic data obtained from ARM that helps in assessing FI includes decreased maximum resting pressure, low sustained squeeze pressure, and decreased squeeze duration. Testing of the abdominopelvic reflex with assessment of squeeze pressure can help differentiate patients with FI due to an upper (impaired squeeze alone and normal abdominopelvic reflex) or lower motor neuron lesion (impaired squeeze and abdominopelvic reflex) in the appropriate clinical scenario. Patients with FI as a group have been found to have lower compliance than continent patients [46], which may cause FI due to the effect of impaired rectal storage capacity. Attempted defecation on the commode also identifies patients with underlying dyssynergic defecation, which may underlie overflow FI. Saline continence testing also helps to characterize FI and can provide information regarding the severity of FI, and chance of successful biofeedback therapy [47]. Although is rarely used in clinical practice today.

Constipation

There are three major pathophysiological subtypes of constipation: STC, normal transit constipation which may include patients with IBS-C, and defecatory disorders, which includes patients with dyssynergic defecation. Age-related physiologic changes and neurodegenerative changes of the enteric nervous system, with increase in inhibitory neuron activity, may cause slow colonic transit, decreased colonic propulsion, and sensorimotor dysfunction [48]. Decrease in pelvic muscle strength and rectal hyposensitivity may contribute to dyssynergic defecation in aging patients [49].

Because symptoms alone are not able to clearly differentiate the subgroups of patients with dyssynergic defecation, ARM is a diagnostic tool of choice and plays a critical role in diagnosis, and is highly reproducible [50]. This is supported by the Rome III criteria for functional anorectal disorders, where ARM is a cornerstone in the diagnosis of functional defecation disorders, including dyssynergic defecation and inadequate defecatory propulsion [51].

The identification of dyssynergic defecation using physiologic data obtained from ARM does not differ in the elderly population, and important parameters include the intrarectal pressure, anal sphincter pressure including the percentage of relaxation, and the calculation of the defecation index. ARM has a positive yield for identifying dyssynergic defecation in a range between 20 and 75 %, and can also identify patients who will benefit from biofeedback therapy [52]. ARM not only detects dyssynergic defecation but also detects patients who have rectal hyposensitivity, which accompanies constipation in up to 50 % of patients [21, 53].

Biofeedback Therapy

Biofeedback therapy is the established treatment of choice for dyssynergic defecation and is effective in 71 % of patients, while only 8 % of patients with slow transit constipation benefit from biofeedback [38, 54]. One study showed that sensory training improved rectal sensation in 79 % of patients with rectal hyposensitivity [55]. For rectal hyposensitivity, the goal is to improve the thresholds for rectal sensory perception and to promote better awareness for stooling, which is important for both constipation and FI [56, 57]. Because intact physical and mental ability is important in effective biofeedback therapy, coexisting cognitive deficits such as dementia, and severe physical debility may be limitations to successful therapy in the elderly.

Conclusion

Pelvic floor disorders are common in the elderly. Although the pathophysiological changes of anorectal function are not fully understood in the elderly, ARM is a valuable diagnostic tool for understanding the physiologic and mechanistic changes in elderly patient with these disorders. Appropriate use of this diagnostic modality will guide management, and help to provide the much needed relief for patients who are suffering from anorectal disorders.

Acknowledgement Dr. SSC Rao was supported by NIH grant No. 2R01 KD57100-05A2.

References

1. Gowers W. The autonomic action of the sphincter ani. Proc R Soc Med (Lond). 1877;26:77–84.
2. Wu JM et al. Prevalence and trends of symptomatic pelvic floor disorders in U.S. Women. Obstet Gynecol. 2014;123(1):141–8.
3. Song HJ. Constipation in community-dwelling elders: prevalence and associated factors. J Wound Ostomy Continence Nurs. 2012; 39(6):640–5.
4. Fosnes GS, Lydersen S, Farup PG. Drugs and constipation in elderly in nursing homes: what is the relation? Gastroenterol Res Pract. 2012;2012:290231.
5. Goode PS et al. Prevalence and correlates of fecal incontinence in community-dwelling older adults. J Am Geriatr Soc. 2005;53(4): 629–35.
6. Santos-Eggimann B, Cirilli NC, Monachon JJ. Frequency and determinants of urgent requests to home care agencies for community-dwelling elderly. Home Health Care Serv Q. 2003; 22(1):39–53.
7. Sun WM, Rao SS. Manometric assessment of anorectal function. Gastroenterol Clin N Am. 2001;30(1):15–32.
8. Scott SM, Gladman MA. Manometric, sensorimotor, and neurophysiologic evaluation of anorectal function. Gastroenterol Clin N Am. 2008;37(3):511–38. vii.
9. Hancock BD. Measurement of anal pressure and motility. Gut. 1976;17(8):645–51.
10. Robertson EV et al. High-resolution esophageal manometry: addressing thermal drift of the manoscan system. Neurogastroenterol Motil. 2012;24(1):61–4. e11.
11. Jones MP, Post J, Crowell MD. High-resolution manometry in the evaluation of anorectal disorders: a simultaneous comparison with water-perfused manometry. Am J Gastroenterol. 2007;102(4): 850–5.
12. Tantiphlachiva K et al. Digital rectal examination is a useful tool for identifying patients with dyssynergia. Clin Gastroenterol Hepatol. 2010;8(11):955–60.
13. Fleshman JW. Anorectal motor physiology and pathophysiology. Surg Clin North Am. 1993;73(6):1245–65.
14. Rao SS et al. Manometric tests of anorectal function in healthy adults. Am J Gastroenterol. 1999;94(3):773–83.
15. Rao SS et al. Minimum standards of anorectal manometry. Neurogastroenterol Motil. 2002;14(5):553–9.
16. Cali RL et al. Normal variation in anorectal manometry. Dis Colon Rectum. 1992;35(12):1161–4.
17. Azpiroz F, Enck P, Whitehead WE. Anorectal functional testing: review of collective experience. Am J Gastroenterol. 2002;97(2): 232–40.
18. Patcharatrakul T, Gonlachanvit S. Outcome of biofeedback therapy in dyssynergic defecation patients with and without irritable bowel syndrome. J Clin Gastroenterol. 2011;45(7):593–8.
19. Rao SS. Dyssynergic defecation and biofeedback therapy. Gastroenterol Clin N Am. 2008;37(3):569–86. viii.
20. Gladman MA et al. Rectal hyposensitivity: prevalence and clinical impact in patients with intractable constipation and fecal incontinence. Dis Colon Rectum. 2003;46(2):238–46.
21. Burgell RE, Scott SM. Rectal hyposensitivity. J Neurogastroenterol Motil. 2012;18(4):373–84.
22. Caruana BJ et al. Anorectal sensory and motor function in neurogenic fecal incontinence. Comparison between multiple sclerosis and diabetes mellitus. Gastroenterology. 1991;100(2): 465–70.
23. Pannek J et al. Urodynamic and rectomanometric findings in patients with spinal cord injury. Neurourol Urodyn. 2001;20(1): 95–103.
24. Barnett JL, Hasler WL, Camilleri M. American Gastroenterological Association medical position statement on anorectal testing techniques. American Gastroenterological Association. Gastroenterology. 1999;116(3):732–60.
25. van der Schaar PJ, Lamers CB, Masclee AA. The role of the barostat in human research and clinical practice. Scand J Gastroenterol Suppl. 1999;230:52–63.
26. Kellow JE et al. Applied principles of neurogastroenterology: physiology/motility sensation. Gastroenterology. 2006;130(5): 1412–20.
27. Sangwan YP, Solla JA. Internal anal sphincter: advances and insights. Dis Colon Rectum. 1998;41(10):1297–311.
28. Duthie HL, Bennett RC. The relation of sensation in the anal canal to the functional anal sphincter: a possible factor in anal continence. Gut. 1963;4(2):179–82.
29. Cheeney G et al. Topographic and manometric characterization of the recto-anal inhibitory reflex. Neurogastroenterol Motil. 2012; 24(3):e147–54.
30. Noviello C et al. Role of anorectal manometry in children with severe constipation. Colorectal Dis. 2009;11(5):480–4.
31. De Ocampo S et al. Rectoanal sensorimotor response in humans during rectal distension. Dis Colon Rectum. 2007;50(10):1639–46.
32. Remes-Troche JM et al. Rectoanal reflexes and sensorimotor response in rectal hyposensitivity. Dis Colon Rectum. 2010;53(7): 1047–54.
33. Minguez M et al. Predictive value of the balloon expulsion test for excluding the diagnosis of pelvic floor dyssynergia in constipation. Gastroenterology. 2004;126(1):57–62.
34. Rao SS, Singh S. Clinical utility of colonic and anorectal manometry in chronic constipation. J Clin Gastroenterol. 2010;44(9): 597–609.
35. Park JS et al. Iatrogenic colorectal perforation induced by anorectal manometry: report of two cases after restorative proctectomy for distal rectal cancer. World J Gastroenterol. 2007; 13(45):6112–4.
36. Cho YB et al. Colonic perforation caused by anorectal manometry. Int J Colorectal Dis. 2008;23(2):219–20.
37. Yu SW, Rao SS. Anorectal physiology and pathophysiology in the elderly. Clin Geriatr Med. 2014;30(1):95–106.
38. Rao SS, Patel RS. How useful are manometric tests of anorectal function in the management of defecation disorders? Am J Gastroenterol. 1997;92(3):469–75.
39. Hall K. Effect of aging on gastrointestinal function. In: Ouslander JG, Halter JB, Tinetti ME, Studenski S, High KP, Asthana S, editors. Hazzard's geriatric medicine and gerontology. New York: McGraw Hill; 2009.
40. Deutekom M et al. Clinical presentation of fecal incontinence and anorectal function: what is the relationship? Am J Gastroenterol. 2007;102(2):351–61.

41. Rao SS. Diagnosis and management of fecal incontinence. American College of Gastroenterology Practice Parameters Committee. Am J Gastroenterol. 2004;99(8):1585–604.

42. Bannister JJ, Abouzekry L, Read NW. Effect of aging on anorectal function. Gut. 1987;28(3):353–7.

43. Fox JC et al. Effect of aging on anorectal and pelvic floor functions in females. Dis Colon Rectum. 2006;49(11):1726–35.

44. Loening-Baucke V, Anuras S. Effects of age and sex on anorectal manometry. Am J Gastroenterol. 1985;80(1):50–3.

45. Thiruppathy K et al. Morphological abnormalities of the recto-anal inhibitory reflex reflects symptom pattern in neurogenic bowel. Dig Dis Sci. 2012;57(7):1908–14.

46. Rasmussen OO. Fecal incontinence. Studies on physiology, pathophysiology and surgical treatment. Dan Med Bull. 2003; 50(3):262–82.

47. Ozturk R et al. Long-term outcome and objective changes of ano-rectal function after biofeedback therapy for faecal incontinence. Aliment Pharmacol Ther. 2004;20(6):667–74.

48. Rao SS et al. Evaluation of constipation in older adults: radioo-paque markers (ROMs) versus wireless motility capsule (WMC). Arch Gerontol Geriatr. 2012;55(2):289–94.

49. Bouras EP, Tangalos EG. Chronic constipation in the elderly. Gastroenterol Clin N Am. 2009;38(3):463–80.

50. Rao SS et al. Investigation of the utility of colorectal function tests and Rome II criteria in dyssynergic defecation (Anismus). Neuro-gastroenterol Motil. 2004;16(5):589–96.

51. Bharucha AE et al. Functional anorectal disorders. Gastroenterology. 2006;130(5):1510–8.

52. Rao SS, Ozturk R, Laine L. Clinical utility of diagnostic tests for constipation in adults: a systematic review. Am J Gastroenterol. 2005;100(7):1605–15.

53. Gladman MA et al. Clinical and physiological findings, and possi-ble aetiological factors of rectal hyposensitivity. Br J Surg. 2003;90(7):860–6.

54. Chiarioni G, Salandini L, Whitehead WE. Biofeedback benefits only patients with outlet dysfunction, not patients with isolated slow transit constipation. Gastroenterology. 2005;129(1):86–97.

55. Rao S, Erdogan A, Coss-Adame E, et al. Rectal hyposensitivity: randomized controlled trial of barostat vs. syringe-assisted sensory training. Gastroenterology. 2013;144 5 Suppl 1:S363.

56. Chiarioni G et al. Sensory retraining is key to biofeedback therapy for formed stool fecal incontinence. Am J Gastroenterol. 2002; 97(1):109–17.

57. Rao SS et al. Randomized controlled trial of biofeedback, sham feedback, and standard therapy for dyssynergic defecation. Clin Gastroenterol Hepatol. 2007;5(3):331–8.

Functional Anorectal Imaging: Radiologic Considerations and Clinical Implications

11

Ana Catarina A. Silva and Dean D.T. Maglinte

Introduction

"Functional" imaging of anorectal and pelvic floor dysfunction has assumed an important role in the diagnosis and management of these disorders. Defecation disorders and pelvic organ prolapse are common and affect up to 25 % of the population, mostly parous women [1, 2]. They cause significant morbidity, affect quality of life, and lead to psychological distress and work absenteeism. Functional/"dynamic" imaging has become increasingly central to the management of anorectal (AR) and pelvic floor dysfunction, the clinical treatment of which is often difficult [3, 4].

Pelvic floor anatomy is complex and DCP does not show the structural details pelvic floor magnetic resonance imaging (MRI) provides. Excellent reviews of anatomy, physiology, and functional diagnostic tests in pelvic floor imaging have recently been discussed by several authors [4–6] and will not be repeated. Technical advances allowing acquisition of dynamic rapid MR images with improved spatial resolution and soft tissue details in a single breath hold and multiplanar capability have made several authors state that MR should replace DCP because DCP utilizes radiation and does not show soft tissue details provided by MRI [7–22]. According to several reports, dynamic pelvic floor MRI not only shows anatomy but also diagnosis prolapses and can lead to a change in surgical therapy [5, 7, 10, 15, 18–20, 22–27]. However, the majority of these MRI studies do not include rectal evacuation (allowing for complete levator ani relaxation) or control for complete organ emptying. This limits the prolapses that can be seen.

A.C.A. Silva
Department of Radiology, Unidade Local de Saúde de Matosinhos, EPE, Ssenhora da Hora, Portugal

D.D.T Maglinte (✉)
Indiana University School of Medicine, IU Health – University Hospital, 550 N. University Blvd. UH 0279, Indianapolis, IN 46202-5253, USA
e-mail: dmaglint@iupui.edu

Predictions of hypothetical increase cancer incidence and deaths in patients exposed to radiation from data extrapolated from atomic bomb survivors [28–32], in addition to controversies relating to the clinical significance of DCP findings have added to the controversies between DCP and dynamic pelvic floor MRI. This chapter provides an update on the pros and cons between DCP and dynamic pelvic floor MRI, addresses interpretive controversies and their relevance to clinical management of these complex disorders.

Why Functional Voiding?

The term "pelvic floor" refers to the pelvic diaphragm (levator ani), the sphincter mechanism of the lower urinary tract, the upper and lower vaginal supports, and the internal and external anal sphincters. Understanding the levels and structure of pelvic floor supports, the restoration of which form the underlying basis for pelvic floor reconstructive surgery, is important for the diagnosis and staging of pelvic floor disorders [33]. Normal defecation involves an interaction between the colon and the rectum. The urge to defecate is initiated by rectal distention from high-amplitude propagating waves that move fecal contents into the rectum. The resulting distention relaxes the internal anal sphincter through the recto-anal inhibitory reflex in preparation for defecation. This allows for sampling to take place where the contents of the rectum come in contact with the sensory-rich areas below the dentate line to identify solids from liquids or gas. Evacuation, when desired, is then initiated by abdominal straining and voluntary pelvic floor relaxation. The anal canal opens and the rectum is squeezed from abdominal contraction. The rectum and about one-third of the left side of the colon will be emptied in normal physiologic defecation from continued mass colonic contractions and, most likely, some proximal rectal contractions [34]. The initiating movement for defecation is pelvic floor descent (PFD), which is defined as the descent of the AR junction from rest to maximum widening of the anal canal. The canal opens completely

© Springer Science+Business Media New York 2017
D.A. Gordon, M.R. Katlic (eds.), *Pelvic Floor Dysfunction and Pelvic Surgery in the Elderly*, DOI 10.1007/978-1-4939-6554-0_11

and in a second or so the rectum starts to empty. Emptying is rapid. When the patient stops straining, tone returns to the internal anal sphincter and levator ani so the anal canal closes and the AR angle becomes more acute; the pelvic floor and AR junction elevate to their normal resting position (the post-defecation reflex). Imaging studies do not invoke these physiological responses, and depend entirely on voluntary control of the pelvic floor and passive rectal emptying [35, 36]. The degree of rectal distention has bearing on functional imaging. Volumes of <300 mL may lower internal sphincter tone, but not increase intra-rectal pressure, whereas volumes of >300 mL may exceed rectal compliance and induce incontinence. Although rectal motor complexes might be activated by rectal distention, this does not seem to occur with volumes used in DCP. Rectal emptying is a passive phenomenon due to raised intra-abdominal pressure squeezing contrast out of the rectum.

The pelvic floor, unlike other skeletal muscles in the body, remains in a constant tone even during sleep. The only time this tone is interrupted is during defecation or urination; thus, actual evacuation must be part of the examination to show the full extent of pelvic organ prolapse (see Figs. 11.1 and 11.2) [3, 37, 38].

Association of Pelvic Compartment Defects with Defecatory Disorders

The frequency of associated pelvic abnormalities in patients presenting with AR disorders is high. In a study of patients with symptoms of defecatory disorders, DCP showed that 71 % had cystoceles, 65 % had a hypermobile bladder neck, and 35 % had vaginal vault prolapse of >50 % [37]. In another

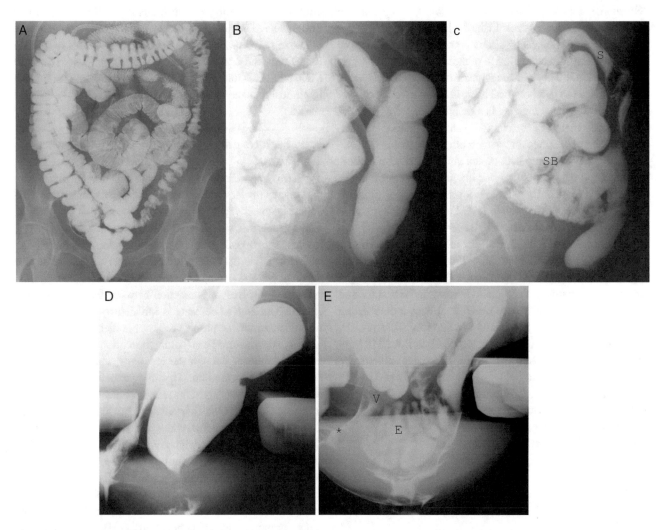

Fig. 11.1 A 39-year-old female patient with recurrent lower abdominal and pelvic pain with a prior history of endometriosis referred for enteroclysis prior to pelvic reconstructive surgery for possible small bowel obstruction. Recent DCP showed pelvic organ prolapse. (**a**) Overview of filled small bowel and colon following barium enteroclysis which did not show small bowel obstruction. (**b**) Lateral upright rest radiograph obtained following (**a**). No abnormality is seen. (**c**) Lateral radiograph obtained with patient straining. A small amount of rectal and sigmoid contrast was expelled but there is no evidence of pelvic organ prolapse. *S* sigmoid; *SB* small bowel. DCP was done on a locally made commode. (**d**) Rest radiograph of DCP done 1 week before the enteroclysis. Patient referred with a clinical history of constipation and dyspareunia, exclude anismus. The patient had prior hysterectomy. (**e**) Strain radiograph of DCP showing a Type C enterocele, recto-anal intussusception, Stage 1 posterior vaginal cuff prolapse and a Stage 1 rectocele. *PH; V, posterior vaginal cuff; E, enterocele

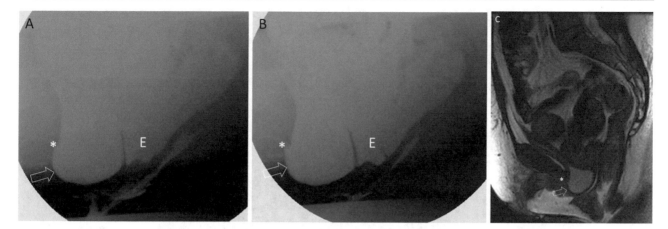

Fig. 11.2 Another patient a 52-year-old female had also with a clinical history of constipation and dyspareunia and prior hysterectomy. DPC examination during evacuation (**a, b**) shows a type B enterocele (E) that was missed at the dynamic MR examination that she had previously (**c**). Although vaginal opacification was not obtained, the persistent bladder catheter (*asterisks*) marks the bladder neck which in vivo is located at the same level as the hymen. An anterior vaginal wall prolapse due to cystocele is also present (*open arrow*) that is demonstrated at MR. (**d**)

This other 56-year-old patient with the same complaints of constipation and dyspareunia had an anterior vaginal wall prolapse due to a grade 2 cystocele (*arrow*) but she also showed at this phase (evacuation) a sigmoidocele (S) recognized by the barium paste inside and the filling defect that represents fecal material (*arrowhead*). This finding was missed at dynamic MR that the patient had previously. Also a grade 1 rectocele was present. *Asterisks* (bladder neck)

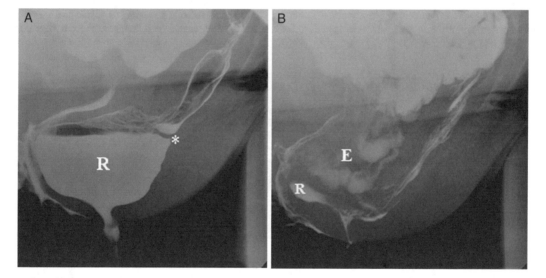

Fig. 11.3 DCP diagnosis of dyssynergic defecation. (**a**) 65-year-old multipara with prior hysterectomy referred for DCP because of chronic constipation and "pressure" on her vagina. Lateral radiograph with marked straining A at the end of defecation shows a large contrast retaining anterior rectocele (R) and retention of more than two thirds of

the rectal contents below the main fold (*asterisk*) consistent with anismus and (**b**) following vaginal digitations in the toilet show a Stage 2 enterocele (E) not shown in (**a**) because of undrained rectocele (R). The anterior rectocele is a combined distension and displacement type of rectocele; a Stage 2 posterior vaginal wall prolapse

report [39], 50 % of patients with urinary stress incontinence and 80 % of patients with uterovaginal prolapse had symptoms of obstructed defecation (prolonged rectal evacuation and need for digital assistance) (see Figs. 11.3, 11.4, 11.5, and 11.6). Thus, a global functional pelvic floor examination is needed in patients with defecatory disorders. The interrelationships of pelvic organ prolapse and the competition for space cannot be overemphasized [40]. Much of the uncertainty related to the value of DCP has been because of reports where the possibilities of functional defecatory disorders

have been ignored or where benefit has been evaluated in terms of outcome, an approach that inevitably includes assessment of any treatment [41, 42]. When a particular imaging technique is able to assist clinical understanding and management, it makes a relevant contribution in its assessment [43]. When this has been applied to investigation of DCP, the test has been found to be overwhelmingly valuable [44]. There is currently no prospective controlled study in which patient outcomes both with and without DCP or dynamic pelvic MRI have been evaluated [4].

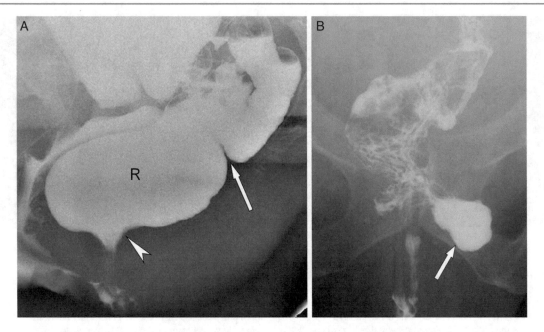

Fig. 11.4 Diagnosis of sigmoidocele and associated pelvic organ pro-lapses. A 57-year-old multipara with a history of a remote hysterectomy and more recently a urinary bladder suspension was referred for DCP because of worsening constipation and urinary incontinence. A Lateral rest radiograph following evacuation shows retention of almost all the rectal contrast below the main fold (*arrow*) consistent with dyssynergic defecation. R, rectum; arrow main fold; arrowhead posterior AR angle. B Lateral strain radiograph obtained following posterior vaginal wall digi-tations in the toilet shows a third-degree sigmoidocele (S), a displacement type anterior rectocele preventing the sigmoidocele from prolapsing fur-ther, a Stage 1 vaginal vault (V) prolapse and a Stage 2 recurrent cysto-cele (C). *Dashed line* PCL, *dashed dotted line* ischiococcygeal line

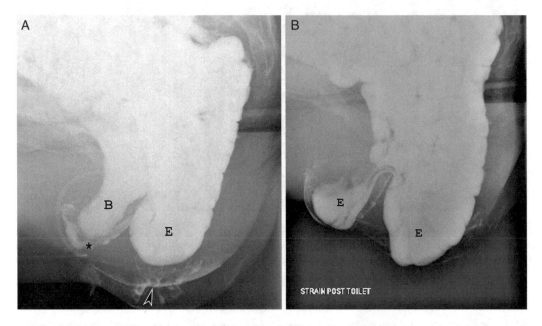

Fig. 11.5 Diagnosis of intra-vaginal enterocele. (**a**) 58-year-old patient referred for DCP because of excessive straining at defecation and sensation of incomplete emptying and urinary incontinence. A Lateral strain radio-graph obtained following the evacuation phase shows a Type C enterocele, Stage 2 cystocele and internal prolapse (*arrowhead*). *PH. (**b**) Lateral strain radiograph obtained following suction of urinary bladder through 8 F catheter and additional evacuation in the toilet shows an intra-vaginal enterocele (E) not shown in (**a**) because of a filled urinary bladder

Controversies in Pelvic Floor Imaging

"Functional imaging" of the pelvic floor is conducted in an arti-ficial surroundings that embarrass and inhibit the patient, and thus, the images do not represent physiologic defecation. In most MR protocols, the patient is imaged recumbent usually supine with legs extended rather than upright, a position in which patients are usually asymptomatic or less symptomatic. Having patient defecate supine in an artificial environment makes an embarrassing examination even less acceptable. Although some proponents of MRI imaging have stated that women do not mind

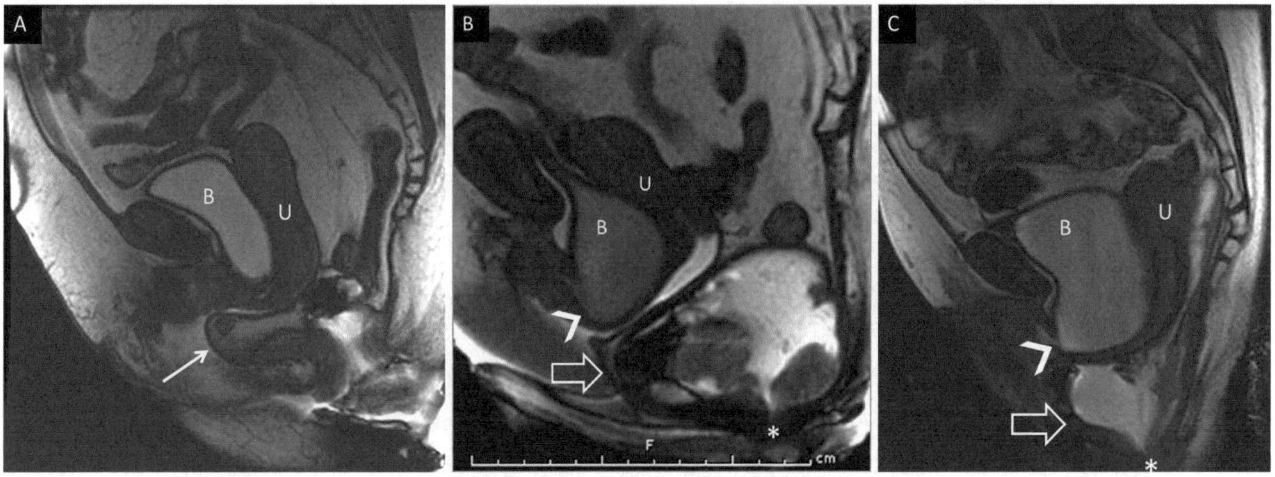

Fig. 11.6 Global characterization of pelvic floor by MR defecography of three different patients with the same major complaint of constipation. All three images were obtained at maximum strain post evacuation done in supine position. In all three cases the contrast resolution allows for a clear distinction between the pelvic compartments with easy identification of the bladder (B), uterus (U), vagina and rectum and also the plane of the hymen. In the first case (**a**) a grade 3 peritoneocele is pres-ent being recognized by its fat content (*arrow*). No other abnormalities were diagnosed in this patient. In the other two patients (**b, c**) an anterior vaginal wall prolapse due to grade 2 cystoceles (*arrowhead*) and posterior vaginal wall prolapses due to grade 2 rectocele (**b**) and grade 3 rectocele (**c**) (*open arrows*) without uterine prolapse are recognized. It was also present in both cases a fixed perineal descent. Note the abnormally low anorectal junction (*asterisks*)

defecating supine, we disagree with these statements and find this insensitive to patients concerns in our practice although we were the first to report that it could be done technically and did correlate with some DCP findings [45]. To be called functional, pelvic floor examinations should be done sitting in a commode similar to what patients do in life. This "functional position" provides the maximum stress to the pelvic floor, resulting in complete levator ani relaxation which is needed to diagnose defecation disorders and show maximum pelvic organ descent for accurate quantification of female organ prolapse that can only be inferred by physical examination [46–52].

Conclusions comparing supine and upright MRI studies demonstrate that sitting MR defecography is not superior to dynamic supine MRI for depiction of clinically relevant bladder descent and rectoceles [7]. These reflect limitations of the reports. The diagnosis of cystoceles and rectoceles is only part of the evaluation of pelvic floor abnormalities. In one report which showed greater degree of pelvic floor laxity on MRI in the sitting position it was concluded that it was not superior to standard supine MRI [53]. In another report [7], all intussusceptions were missed at supine MRI. AR descents of varying degrees and an enterocele, four small cystoceles and an anterior rectocele were also missed at supine MRI in the same report. No abnormalities seen at supine MRI were missed at upright MRI. However, all the missed findings at supine MRI were dismissed as not clinically relevant as there were no findings at physical examination.

The conclusion was that supine MRI is a valid alternative to upright MRI. Our own comparative study with DCP and dynamic pelvic MRI with patients defecating supine, both methods of examination done on the same patients underes-timated the extent of prolapse for sites other than rectoceles by approximately 15 % (see Figs. 11.2 and 11.7) [45]. The underestimates were caused by examining the patients in the supine position which has less gravitational influence than sitting as well as patients not completely relaxing the levator ani. As we gained more experience from our initial report of 10 patients, some patients have stated that their pelvic symptoms were only a problem when standing, sitting, or walking. Rectocele size is more influenced by rectal evacuation than by gravity. The limitations of physical examination have been recognized [36, 40, 46, 48, 54] even when done by experienced examiners [40, 46]; hence, the exclusion of abnormalities missed was not clinically relevant in the Bertschinger et al. [7] study because there were no physical examination findings should be questioned.

Physical examination does not allow for complete levator relaxation and therefore will miss more prolapses than defecography. In another report that showed MRI diagnosing more enteroceles than DCP and physical examination, both MRI and DCP were limited to a single-phase examination in which straining and evacuation of all opacified pelvic organs were performed at the same time. DCP did not involve the opacification of the small bowel in that report. These represent inferior techniques of performing these studies and will miss significant prolapse. In our current modification, diagnosis of peritoneoceles and enteroceles is done following emptying of the urinary bladder and rectum/rectoceles, hence recognition of a widened rectovaginal space is maximized for the diagnosis of peritoneoceles or enteroceles. Without complete emptying, these organs block descent of other organs. In addition, in patients with slow intestinal

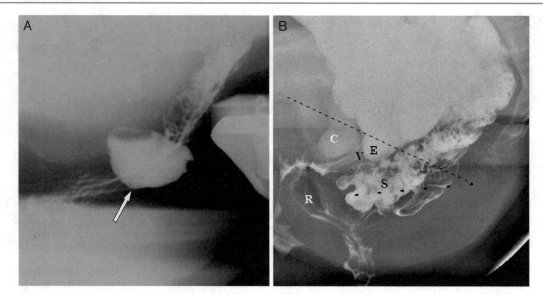

Fig. 11.7 Rectocele in a male. A 60-year-old male referred for proctography because of constipation; history of prior prostatectomy. (**a**) Lateral radiograph obtained shows a moderate size outpouching (*arrow*) retaining contrast. (**b**) Frontal radiograph obtained during straining shows a postero-lateral hernia retaining contrast medium (*arrow*)

transit, oral contrast may not have reached the small bowel. The contrast in the small bowel makes diagnosis of enteroceles more apparent because of the influence of gravity. In MRI studies done functionally sitting in a commode and defecation is part of the routine, the results will be comparable with DCP [15]. Conclusions and recommendations done with pelvic MRI supine even when done defecating do not consider the high reoperation rate in women who have undergone pelvic surgery [55]. Many pelvic floor surgeons believe that an attempt to correct all pelvic support defects, whether asymptomatic or not [56] should be done at one setting. If comprehensive repair is not done, coexisting asymptomatic support defects may become symptomatic within a relatively short time. The failure to recognize the full extent of pelvic organ prolapses pre-operatively based on physical examination done supine and the compartmental clinical approach to pelvic floor dysfunction (the "politics of the pelvic floor") may explain the high reoperation rate [57]. The reason women develop pelvic floor defects is likely multifactorial [58, 59] and the failure of surgical repair is not well understood. The relatively high rate of repeat surgery may reflect failure to recognize the full extent of prolapses pre-operatively if assessment is based predominantly on physical examination or incomplete methods of imaging where the levator ani is not fully relaxed. MRI done supine may be inadequate for recognition of AR disorders such as internal (intra-anal rectal intussusception) prolapse. These conditions are more reliably diagnosed when patients defecate during DCP or while seated in an open magnet [26, 36, 38, 50]. Currently, however, the relevance of DCP vs. dynamic pelvic floor MRI to patient outcomes has not been adequately addressed in a scientific manner.

The superior contrast resolution of MRI particularly in the anterior compartment requires [15] the use of endovaginal coil [5]. This is invasive and makes an embarrassing examination less acceptable to patients and will affect demonstration of prolapses because of space competition. The coil literally acts like a pessary, a device used to passively treat prolapse. In another report on patients with fecal incontinence, the results of MRI studies have led to a change of surgical therapy in 67 % of patients in whom some form of surgery was required to treat fecal incontinence [15]. It should be noted that the anal sphincters can be visualized with the body coil alone or with a phased-array or endoluminal coil [4, 60]. Examination with an endoluminal coil results in higher spatial resolution but a limited field of view. The spatial resolution provided by either a phased-array or a body coil is probably insufficient to aid in the diagnosis of sphincter abnormalities [61]. Rigid endoanal coils are preferred for optimal image quality and result in over-compression of adjacent structures. The use of T1-weighted sequence (e.g., fast spin-echo) with contrast medium increases cost, and their superiority over other sequences has not been established [4, 60]. The endopelvic fascia is not well visualized on conventional MRI; similar to DCP, defects or laxity is inferred indirectly through secondary findings [5]. An endovaginal coil [62] is needed to show these fascial condensations and their clinical significance as related to surgical repair may be irrelevant. Endoanal MRI is time-consuming compared to endoanal ultrasound (approximately 30 vs. 5 min) [61, 63]. In patients with anal incontinence, the findings at DCP can be used to recommend which appropriate imaging approach should be used. If incontinence is noted at rest in the pre-evacuation phase of the DCP, which suggest internal anal sphincter damage, endoanal ultrasound is recommended; if incontinence is noted when straining, endoanal MRI is recommended as it has been shown to be more accurate for the evaluation of the external anal sphincter than endoanal ultrasound [4, 15, 60]. Whether either of these changes surgical approach is not well studied. Putting together a separated anal sphincter which was damaged years earlier at childbirth may have little relevance on a 60-year-old patient. The neuromuscular function is probably of more significance and explains the relatively poor outcomes in anal sphincter repair in most long-term studies. The use of an open MRI system with patients defecating makes it "functional" similar to DCP [15]. With an open architecture magnet, however, one must contend with images of a lower signal-to-noise ratio and soft tissue resolution [5]. To make it a single non-invasive functional study to look at specific organ prolapse and direct visualization of the supporting structures specialized coils are needed to improve soft tissue resolution and visualize the pelvic supporting structures and fascial condensations. Specialized coils will make dynamic pelvic MRI more intrusive. Nonetheless even with the images obtained with current open MR systems, visualizing the soft tissue structures in obese patients to see reference points is better with MRI than DCP.

In our experience, patients who weigh >200 pounds and handicapped patients who cannot be seated safely in a stable position with the upright commode with DCP should undergo dynamic MRI done supine particularly if fecal incontinence is the clinical presentation. Placement of two markers aligned (pellets) on the inner lateral support of the DCP commode aids in visualizing the ischial tuberosities and ensures that measurements made (if the pubococcygeal line (PCL) is used) are midline with DCP. The volume and consistency of rectal pastes for DCP has undergone several modifications since the article of Mahieu et al. [64–66] and is standardized [33] in most DCP protocols. In MRI protocols, however, gels of varying amounts (from 60 to 120 mL) are used [10, 16, 19, 67]. The consistency and volume results in suboptimal straining particularly in the supine position that may mask the degree of pelvic organ prolapse and results in diminished conspicuity of visceral descent [67]. Some MR protocols using open MR system with appropriate contrast (potato starch consistency) have compared their protocol with MR using gel and have shown that the size and the degree of anterior rectocele evacuation and intussusception size are often underestimated when ultrasound gel is used for rectal enema [68]. In our modification of the DCP, prior to the administration of the rectal paste, high density low viscosity barium (50 mL Polibar, Bracco Diagnostics) is introduced followed by 50 mL of air from the same syringe. This improves rectal mucosal coating and diagnosis of rectal intussusceptions, entities that are important in the surgical management of AR disorders [69]. The vaginal paste allows us to delineate the vaginal fourchettes which are important anatomic landmarks in localizing the PH, the reference point used for the ICS POP-Q [70] which we have adopted to DCP for staging of prolapse [33]. A current problem with DCP is

that there is no commercially available commode for DCP examinations to our knowledge. A similar problem with MR is that only a few open magnet MRI systems are currently installed in radiology departments hence most dynamic pelvic MRI are done supine with extended legs. The DCP commode, however, can be constructed [71] (see Figs. 11.1 and 11.7). AR and pelvic floor dysfunction cause significant morbidity in women [1, 2, 33]. It appears to be an epidemic nobody talks about [33]; hopefully, a manufacturer will resolve this dilemma.

Although variable from country to country, important additional factors that should be considered are economics, logistics, and demonstrable clinical advantages of one method over the other. In our practice, pelvic MRI costs three to four times more than DCP. If the management consideration is based on diagnosis of prolapse, DCP is reliable, however, if visualizing the structural integrity of pelvic supportive tissues and endopelvic fascia is the relevant question to management, pelvic MRI with endoluminal coil to improve soft tissue resolution is the imaging of choice. Again, the disadvantage the coil has on displacing prolapse cannot be overemphasized if the examination was also done to evaluate pelvic organ prolapse. In most institutions in the USA the additional expense incurred with MRI compared with DCP and the relative lack of accessible time on an MR unit that is subject to heavy demand by other clinical specialties are important factors to consider. The logistics of performing a tailored examination (drainage of an undrained bladder and emptying of rectum or rectoceles) which will tamponade enteroceles or sigmoidoceles are important diagnostic considerations [41]. Another factor in our experience is the reluctance of many technologists to perform a longer, more complex examination. We were one of the earliest investigators who compared dynamic pelvic MRI done supine to DCP [46]. The attraction of a new technology and the lack of ionizing radiation in addition to economic considerations in private practice made us initially favor pelvic MRI done defecating supine in our prospective comparison of 10 patients, a number too limited to make appropriate recommendations. As we have gained more experience with the technology we have reverted back to DCP. Evacuation is pivotal for the evaluation of AR disorders and pelvic organ prolapse whether done with radiography or MR [33, 53] but making women defecate supine with extended legs without an open architecture magnet is not "functional" in our experience. Some patients in our practice have stated that they are not symptomatic in the supine position but perceive the pressure or bulging when they are sitting or upright. Our current DCP technique is faster than our prior technique [47]. Thus, when the relevant management question is on the anatomic/structural demonstration of the pelvic supporting tissues, a static-high definition MRI gives good soft tissue definition of the muscles and/or connective tissue tears that may alter management—information that can only be inferred with DCP [4, 61, 62, 64]. There is no controversy when soft tissue spatial resolution is the relevant consideration for management.

Imaging Pelvic Organ Prolapse Quantification/Grading

The radiology community has paid little attention to devising a grading or scoring system that has clinical correlates and understandable to clinicians who use the ICS POP-Q to stage pelvic organ prolapse [70]. Other clinical classification systems from colorectal surgeons for defecatory disorders [72, 73] have also not been addressed. With both DCP and "dynamic" pelvic MRI, grading of prolapses has been defined in reference to the PCL. In fact, there have been variable definitions in the literature where this line should be extended posteriorly from the inferior symphysis border. Most commonly, the line is described to extend from the inferior symphysis border to the sacrococcygeal junction [51]; others extend this line to the tip of the last horizontal sacrococcygeal joint [27], or the tip of the coccyx [66, 74, 75] while others join the inferior symphysis line to the coccygeal joint (joint not specified) [66, 74–76]. The PCL is considered to represent the approximate line of attachment of the pelvic floor muscles. In normal individuals, the levator plate is parallel to the PCL. Prolapse is inferred by imaging if a pelvic organ extends below the PCL. Two other reference lines, the H and M lines were introduced by Comiter et al. [10] to identify pelvic floor relaxation and prolapse. The H line measures the distance from the inferior symphysis pubic to the posterior AR junction in the midsagittal image and is indicative of the anteroposterior width of the levator hiatus. The M line is drawn perpendicular from the PCL to the most distal aspect of the H line and is indicative of the descent of the levator hiatus from the PCL. In that study, the H and M lines in normal women measured approximately 5 and 2 cm, respectively. These lines can also be drawn with the DCP but has not been adopted. Little is described in the literature quantifying the severity of prolapse using these reference lines. The ICS POP-Q has no correlates to the PCL and the H and M lines. These lines cannot be inferred clinically. The clinical ICS POP-Q uses the PH as the reference line [70]. This is because patients perceive the pressure/and or see a bulge when the prolapsing organ abuts or displaces the PH [77]. Singh and Berger [78] proposed a new method of grading with MRI using the same landmark as the clinical grading system. A new reference line, the midpubic line (MPL), corresponded to the PH in their cadaver study. Their early results showed good correlation with their clinical staging. More recent studies showed that the MPL has greater agreement with clinical staging than does the PCL. However, neither reference lines showed good agreement with clinical staging [79]. In a recent literature review [80], none of these reference lines showed clear superiority and this may relate to the fact that there is no complete levator ani relaxation during physical examination. The PCL, however, had the advantage of being the most widely used and is associated with high agreement for the evaluation of anterior and middle compartments.

The PCL as a reference point may have validity with colorectal surgeons [30–32, 80–83]. The agreement between methods of examination in the posterior compartment is lower for MRI. There is also high variability of pelvic MRI measurements among readers despite centralized training [80]. Interobserver agreement in the interpretation of DCP is reliable and reproducible [84]. In our experience using DCP, the use of the MPL will overstage prolapses [33]. Using the PCL will also overstage prolapses because it is higher than the MPL. This is because the PH in vivo is more anterior than the MPL in cadavers. It is at or slightly anterior to the anterior pubic line in patients in the sitting position. It is also variable from patient to patient and moves with straining—hence the lack of agreement between methods of staging and the high interobserver variability in measuring reference points with MRI. Anatomically, the external urethral meatus is at the same level as the PH in vivo; it is immediately posterior to the vaginal fourchettes. The vaginal fourchettes are seen on DCP as the most anterior segment of the vagina where the vaginal paste leaks out of the introitus inferiorly and superiorly. Because our current method of performing DCP, where a small urinary bladder catheter is left in place during the pre-evacuation and functional (evacuation) phases, determination of the PH in each patient is simplified (see Fig. 11.8). In our prior report, we determined the PH with an opaque marker (pellet) secured in the urethral meatus and localized it immediately posterior to the vaginal fourchettes [33] on DCPs. A line drawn crossing the posterior margin of the fourchettes parallel to the plane of the anterior cortex of the pubic bone determines the PH (see Fig. 11.9). In the DCP POP-Q, this plane is localized in the pre-evacuation or start of evacuation phases and the image selected which clearly shows it as it may be difficult to localize this plane precisely after defecation. The distance is marked from the anterior cortex of the pubic bone and a line parallel to the pubic bone is drawn in the rest and defecating/straining radiographs post-defecation and staging is measured from this line. Staging pelvic organ prolapse with DCP with similar reference point to the ICS POP-Q allows better communication between radiologists and surgeons. Our experience shows that this staging method is understood better by referring clinicians than using the PCL or the H or M lines. Pelvic organ prolapse staged with imaging studies done functionally will not correlate with physical examination (ICS POP-Q) findings since the levator ani is not maximally relaxed with the Valsalva maneuver in the supine position [84, 85]. This is why DCP and dynamic pelvic floor MRI in an open magnet with defecation in prior comparisons with physical examination have shown more abnormalities than the clinical examination [12, 47, 50, 52]. The imaging POP-Q is meant to complement the ICS POP-Q and not to compete with it [33]. The clinical POP-Q looks at different vaginal points whereas the imaging POP-Q is organ specific. DCP has proven value in patients with defecation disorders and

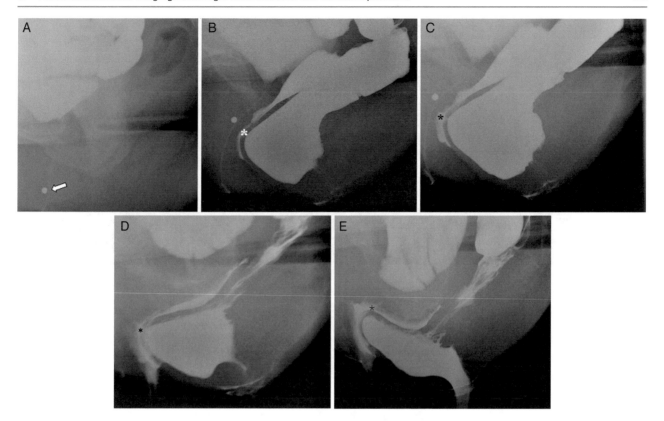

Fig. 11.8 Determination of the level of the PH with DCP, the reference point for staging pelvic organ prolapse. Lateral radiograph obtained (**a**) with the patient in the fluoroscopic table with a marker (*arrow*) secured at the level of the urethral meatus following contrast administration into the urinary bladder. Anatomically in vivo, the hymen is at the same level as the urethral meatus which is immediately posterior to the vagi-nal fourchettes (**b**) at rest following placement of vaginal and rectal contrast, (**c**) during straining, D at rest following defecation, and E during marked straining following defecation. Level of vaginal fourchettes is marked by *asterisk*. The leading edge of the anterior rectocele is anterior to the level of the PH, a stage 2 ICS posterior vaginal wall prolapse

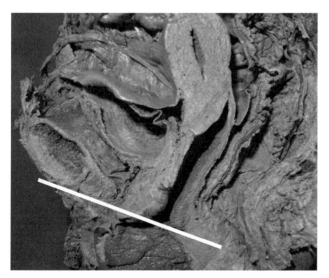

Fig. 11.9 Gross specimen showing the plane of the hymen. The *white line* is anterior to the anterior cortex of pubic bone crossing the vaginal fourchettes

in the diagnosis of associated prolapse in other compartments that may be clinically unrecognized [37]. Clinical examination enables the identification of only approximately 50 % of enteroceles but fares better in the recognition of rectoceles and cystoceles, an area where dynamic MRI is claimed to be superior to DCP [7]. The need for a small amount of contrast in the urinary bladder is poorly understood by radiologists who use the PCL as the reference point [86]. Although it appears that the extrinsic pressure by the urinary bladder on the anterior wall of the vagina can be discerned when using the PCL, it is not the leading edge of a cystocele relative to the PH. It cannot be accurately localized relative to the PH without contrast when using the DCP POP-Q. The presence of the catheter allows for faster drainage of urinary bladder especially those with urinary retention making the examination faster and ensuring that prolapses are not tamponade by an undrained bladder (see Fig. 11.5). Additionally, mobility of the bladder neck can be measured with the presence of the catheter and the contrast in the urinary bladder (see Fig. 11.10).

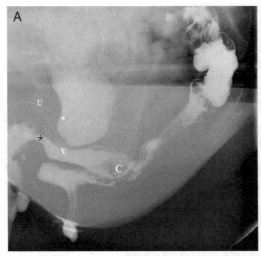
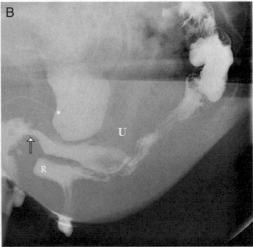

Fig. 11.10 Diagnosis of anterior vaginal wall prolapse. DCP performed of a 70-year-old patient who presented with a feeling of "something bulging" and urinary voiding dysfunction. (**a**) The axis of the urethra (U) is horizontal even at rest. Also note axis of the vagina (V) and Stage 1 uterine prolapse. C, cervix; U, urethra marked by catheter; *white asterisk* level of bladder neck; *black asterisk* PH. (**b**) Lateral strain radiograph shows displacement of the urethrovesical junction (*white asterisk*) by >1 cm from rest. The horizontal axis of the urethra and vagina is only minimally increased. A Stage 2 displacement anterior rectocele (R) is seen. The leading edge of the anterior rectocele (R) is at the same level as the PH (*arrow*) but measured from the anterior anal margin, the symptomatic rectocele would have been classified as small with conventional proctographic classification

The lesser sensitivity of clinical examination compared to functional imaging is almost certainly related to the patient's inability to relax the levator ani completely while performing the Valsalva maneuver. This should be understood to prevent further research trying to correlate imaging studies done functionally with clinical examinations. Vaginal topography staged with the ICS POP-Q clinically will not correlate with visceral position shown by the DCP [85]. The role of imaging in the management of AR and pelvic floor dysfunction is not completely understood. Our analysis of the literature relative to comparison of different imaging methods and the correlation of imaging with physical examination findings suggest that most comparisons are flawed as different landmarks and methods of examinations are used. Although the factors that lead to failure of surgical repair are not well understood and multifactorial, it appears that the limitations of physical examination in diagnosing all prolapses may lead to incomplete surgeries and may contribute to the high reoperation rate [56]. It is advisable to identify all areas of prolapse pre-operatively and plan accordingly as asymptomatic defects may become symptomatic within a relatively short time and all may require correction: ideally this is done at one surgical setting [87, 88]. Although incompetence of the internal and external anal sphincters can be predicted by history and by the rest and strain images obtained in the pre-evacuation sequence of a DCP [34] it cannot objectively demonstrate the structural defects that are shown with MRI using endoluminal coils [62, 89]. The role of DCP is in the diagnosis of commonly associated occult prolapses [37]. It remains the method of choice for patients who present with any symptom of the obstructed defecation syndrome [73].

Radiologists performing "functional" pelvic floor examinations should understand why it is relevant to use the PH as the reference point in staging pelvic organ prolapse [77]. Patients present to their physicians when they feel pressure or see the bulge suggesting laxity of pelvic support when the organs are close to or impinge on the hymen. Most prolapse is not truly symptomatic until it reaches the PH [77]. The use of the PH as a reference point, however, has limitations. It is a movable structure and measures vaginal points and not organ specific, hence the imaging POP-Q complements the clinical ICS POP-Q well. This is particularly true for posterior cul-de-sac prolapses and internal rectal prolapses. Additionally, AR symptoms do not correlate with the degree of posterior vaginal wall prolapse, nor does the presence of prolapse equate to abnormal physiologic test results. Bowel symptoms may result from primary AR abnormalities, which are demonstrated by functional studies [90]. In many cases, DCP is the only way these conditions may be reliably diagnosed.

Imaging Diagnosis, Limitations, and Clinical Relevance

Functional and Structural Disorders of Defecation

Differentiating functional from structural causes of obstructed defecation is difficult clinically. Constipation is a symptom, not a sign, and is based on the patient's perception. In the anorectum, most abnormalities are seen during and at the end of defecation. Rest and strain sequences without defecation as performed with some MR protocols are inadequate examinations. Evacuation while sitting on a commode in a position similar to that which precipitates the symptoms is logical. This is not achieved with supine MRI with patients legs extended and in protocols with rest and strain sequences only. DCP findings infer structural disorders by showing the maximum extent of intussusceptions or prolapses as well as demonstrate functional information in the diagnosis of defecation disorders. Dynamic pelvic floor MRI with the use of open architecture magnets achieves similar results with the exception of protocols that do not use fecal consistency rectal contrast and only uses ultrasound gel as rectal contrast. Intra-anal rectal intussusception (internal prolapse) may not be as apparent with MR since the mucosal folds are not well shown using sonographic gel. Determining the level of the ischial tuberosities in obese patients is difficult with DCP. Placing markers (pellets) on the lateral supports of the commode partially alleviates this problem and also helps determine the midline where prolapse severity is measured using a centimeter mid line marker. The DCP prolapse staging can be applied to dynamic pelvic MRI if the vaginal fourchettes can be identified. AR angle measurements have a wide variation or overlap of normality with abnormality [24, 66, 74, 91–93]; hence, its measurements do not appear to have relevance to management. Over emphasis on angle measurements has led some authors to question the clinical relevance of DCP [42]. Rectocele, rectal mucosal intussusceptions, rectal prolapse, solitary rectal ulcer syndrome (SRUS), descending perineum syndrome, enterocele, and sigmoidocele are common structural pelvic floor disorders that affect AR function.

Dyssynergic Defecation

This has been described in the literature with a plethora of other terms such as anismus, pelvic floor dyssynergy, paradoxical puborectalis contraction, non-relaxing puborectalis, pelvic outlet obstruction, and spastic pelvic floor syndrome. The term dyssynergic defecation has been recently recommended by several experts [8, 94]. This is not a clear-cut diagnosis. Historically, this has been diagnosed in patients with a history of prolonged straining during defecation if there is inappropriate puborectalis muscle contraction and if patients are unable to expel a balloon filled with 60 mL of water. It was initially assumed that this would be shown during defecography as a persistent indentation posteriorly, just above the AR junction. This finding has been poorly predictive of the diagnosis [36, 95]. In the study by Halligan et al., prolonged and/or incomplete evacuation of contrast material was shown to be far more sensitive and specific finding and was present in 83 % of patients and none of the control subjects. Rectal emptying

is a passive phenomenon, due to raised intra-abdominal pressure squeezing contrast out of the rectum. The combination of prolonged and incomplete evacuation gave a positive predictive value of 90 % compared with a physiologic diagnosis of anismus. A recent study has shown that normal electromyographic results or the ability to expel a 60-mL balloon does not exclude the presence of pelvic floor dyssynergy on defecography [96]. This adds further confusion as to which should be used to guide the recommendation for (and to then measure response) to biofeedback [97, 98]. The success of biofeedback treatments in these patients supports the value of making this diagnosis [61]. This is the importance of categorizing posterior compartment defects into functional and anatomic abnormalities which is reliably done with DCP [34]. In the past because puborectalis muscle dysfunction has been the main focus, a proctographic diagnosis of anismus was conventionally based on a prominent puborectalis muscle impression during voiding together with failure of the AR angle to open. There is little evidence that these findings are specific and simultaneous electromyographic and defecographic study has shown no correlation between muscular activity and AR junction configuration [96]. It is more appropriate to base a proctographic diagnosis on evacuation failure. Healthy subjects void rapidly and completely in contrast to patients with anismus whose evacuation is prolonged and incomplete, a difference that can be quantified by DCP [36]. This has not been done with pelvic MRI. Another study has shown that puborectalis morphology and AR angle measurements did not differentiate patients with anismus from asymptomatic controls but that prolonged and incomplete contrast medium voiding during proctography was highly specific [99] (see Fig. 11.3). The time taken to initiate anal canal opening and the rate of evacuation are more relevant than the final percentage of contrast evacuated because most patients will eventually fully empty their rectum if given enough time. Much of the uncertainty related to the benefits of DCP has been generated because of studies where the possibilities of functional diagnoses have been ignored, or where benefit has been evaluated in terms of outcome, an approach that inevitably includes assessment of any treatment [42, 43]. When this has been applied to evacuation proctography, the test has been overwhelmingly found to be valuable.

Rectocele

This refers to protrusion of the rectal wall, usually anterior towards the vagina. However, posterior rectocele may also occur as well as perineal rectocele. DCP and dynamic pelvic MRI can demonstrate rectocele, measure its size, and identify retention; however, its usefulness in clinical work-up has been limited. Eighty percent of asymptomatic controls may show small rectoceles [66, 91]. It is common in women after childbirth, particularly in patients with pelvic prolapse being present in 78–99 % [47, 100]. They may also be seen in obstructed defecation without prolapse and with dyssynergic defecation [101]. A depth of <2 cm is considered within normal limits [66] and may be considered large if >3.5 cm [102] with conventional DCP grading. If the depth and area of a rectocele are measured when filled and at the end of evacuation, retention of >10 % area defines barium trapping [103]. The size and trapping controversy is what makes grading with traditional radiology reference points limits its usefulness in management, hence clinical correlation is required [104]. As stated earlier, patients feel the pressure or the bulge when the leading edge is close to or beyond the PH hence grading rectoceles with the DCP POP-Q has relevance (see Fig. 11.10). Imaging measurements from the anterior anal margin may have limited the clinical usefulness of proctographic rectocele diagnosis. It may also make it better understood by referring clinicians if anterior rectoceles are categorized into distension rectocele (Type 1) and displacement rectocele (Type 2) with the imaging POP-Q staging since they have different anatomical, clinical, and therapeutic profiles (see Fig. 11.3) [105]. Clinical studies have shown that distension rectoceles are seen in patients with dyssynergic defecation and displacement rectoceles with excessive PFD or prolapse. Digitation provides convincing supporting evidence of the presence of a rectocele and is frequently seen when contrast trapping is present. Clinically, the only two symptoms to improve reliably with surgery are digitations and presence of the bulge. Small postero-lateral herniation of the rectum may result from levator ani damage during childbirth, and if >4 cm indicates an ischiorectal hernia [106]. Small anterior outpouchings may be seen after prostatectomy and have been reported in 17 % of men with obstructed defection (see Fig. 11.7) [106, 107].

Rectal Intussusceptions and the SRUS

Unlike children where rectal prolapse is secondary to an etiology such as malnutrition or cystic fibrosis, it is idiopathic in adults. There is a female preponderance with nulliparous and multiparous women almost equally affected although it is more common with generalized pelvic floor prolapse. Diagnosis is made clinically during forceful straining but defecography suggests that a significant proportion is missed on clinical examination [108]. Early studies with cineradiography have suggested that prolapse is initiated by an infolding of the rectal wall, which then intussuscepts into the anal canal and protrude beyond the anal verge to form an external prolapse [19]. Intussusceptions are classified as intra-rectal (rectorectal), intra-anal (internal prolapse), and extra-anal rectal intussusceptions (rectal prolapse). Rectorectal intussusception is diagnosed when the rectal mucosal folds intussuscepts but do not go below the level of

the upper recto-anal margin. It is diagnosed as internal prolapse if the rectal fold extends below the anal margin and rectal prolapse if it extends below the anal verge (see Fig. 11.11). Imaging protocols that do not show the folds may not be able to make these precise classifications unless it is extra-anal. The dynamic change in the anal canal width as the rectal fold enters is the most definite evidence of internal prolapse [109]. SRUS is almost always associated with either recto-anal or extra-anal intussusceptions. Mucosal ulceration is believed to result from forceful straining against an immobile or a non-relaxing pelvic floor together with trauma from digital manipulations as well as from ischemic necrosis of the intussuscepting rectal mucosa.

Patients usually present with rectal bleeding or pain, mucus discharge, straining and tenesmus, and a feeling of incomplete evacuation. About 55 % of patients present with constipation, 20–40 % with diarrhea, and 25 % are asymptomatic [110]. A quarter of these patients are misdiagnosed and treated as inflammatory bowel disease. The extent and direction of mucosal intussusceptions are reliably shown during the evacuation phase of a DCP. In one "dynamic" pelvic MRI study [7], all intussusceptions were missed at supine MR. The term "solitary rectal ulcer" is misleading because only erosion or erythema may be seen and more than one ulcer is often present [109]. The word "syndrome" was added because it was associated with other AR disorders and dysfunction of pelvic floor musculature (Fig. 11.11c) [111]. A clinical and defecographic diagnosis of rectal prolapse and the presence of SRUS in association with rectal intussusceptions are the best indicators for surgical correction [112]. Since constipation maybe the underlying mechanism for this disorder, surgery should only be performed in highly selected cases as the intussusceptions may merely be a secondary phenomenon [110]. Functional measurements of emptying are therefore important [95, 113].

Descending perineum syndrome and anterior mucosal prolapse

Parks and Hardcastle [114] linked chronic straining to PFD and anterior mucosal prolapse at proctoscopy when the patient strains. DCP can be used to suggest the diagnosis and measure the position of the pelvic floor at rest, when it is stressed by the weight of the abdominal contents in the sitting position, and on evacuation, when opening of the anal canal provides a clear end point. In younger patients, the pelvic floor is higher at rest, with greater descent at evacuation (dynamic perineal descent) of the AR junction. The converse applies to the elderly, with more descent at rest and less change at evacuation (fixed perineal descent) [115]. A low pelvic floor at rest is suggestive of muscle weakness and stretching of the elastic tissue of its fascial supports [116]. Perineal (AR) descent in this syndrome is defined as >3 cm

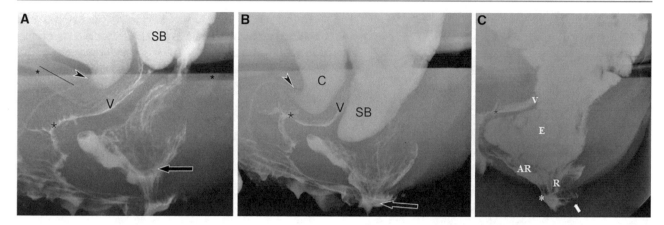

Fig. 11.11 Rectal intussusceptions. A 55-year-old nullipara with history of prior hysterectomy referred for DCP because of a sensation of vaginal pressure and constipation. (**a**) Lateral image obtained at rest following defecation shows near complete emptying of the rectum and an anterior rectocele. Note rectal intussusception into the proximal anal canal (*arrow*). *SB* small bowel; *V* vaginal vault; arrowhead urethrovesical junction; larger inferior asterisk PH (note clear delineation of both anterior and posterior vaginal fourchettes immediately anterior to asterisk), *small asterisks* in inferior symphysis margin (anterior) and tip of coccyx (posterior) indicates level of PCL. Straight line between anterior and posterior cortices of pubic bone indicates mid pubic line. (**b**) Lateral image during maximum straining at defecation shows a Type B enterocele (SB) prolapsing behind vaginal vault which was not seen at rest. Rectal intussusception is now noted to be below the anal verge (extra-anal). Also note Stage 2 cystocele displacing anterior vaginal wall inferiorly. A hypermobile bladder neck is also seen gauged by the degree of inferior displacement of the urethrovesical junction (*arrowhead*) from rest to strain (>10 mm). (**c**) Rectal prolapse and SRUS. Lateral radiograph of a 55-year-old patient referred for DCP because of rectal bleeding and severe pelvic pressure. Intussusception of the rectum (R) through the anal canal with a short segment seen below the anal verge (*arrow*). Associated Stage 1 vaginal cuff prolapse (V), Stage 2 (Type C) enterocele (E), and anterior rectocele (A) are seen. Global pelvic floor descent can be inferred by the marked increase distance from the AR junction (*asterisk*) to the level of the ischial tuberosities

or the AR junction is >3 cm below its normal position (at or above level of ischial tuberosities) at rest [66]. Imaging studies done supine or in the lateral position underestimate perineal descent which becomes maximal only at onset of defecation in the sitting position. The position of the pelvic floor is significantly higher at rest when the patient is in the left lateral position than when seating [7, 67, 117]. Excessive perineal descent at DCP may predict future anal incontinence [118].

Patients with the descending perineum syndrome present with tenesmus, pain, and sometimes bleeding. It was initially described as a proctologic diagnosis. The characteristics of anterior mucosal prolapse at DCP are variable. Inversion of the anterior rectal wall over the anal canal is a common finding with rectoceles [93] but should not enter the upper anal canal. Prolongation of the anterior rectal wall into the upper rectum without widening of the canal is suggestive of anterior mucosal prolapse (see Fig. 11.12). In one study [119], anterior rectocele and abnormal perineal descent were present in 70 % of women with anterior mucosal prolapse.

Enterocele, Sigmoidocele, and Peritoneocele

The incidence of enteroceles may have increased as a result of the widespread performance of prolapse or incontinence procedures that elevate the anterior vaginal wall exposing the poste-rior vaginal wall to increased intra-abdominal forces. This leads to enterocele formation and vaginal vault prolapse because damage occurs at the level of the vaginal apex. Enteroceles were seen in 64 % of patients who had undergone hysterectomy and in 27 % of those who had undergone cystopexy. Hysterectomy is not considered the risk factor for future prolapse unless the hysterectomy was performed for prolapse [87]. Urethropexy performed for incontinence pre-disposes to enterocele formation by lifting the anterior vaginal wall forward and opening up the cul-de-sac. Urethropexy has generally been replaced with the urethral sling procedure which is claimed not to increase the frequency of enterocele formation [87]. Enteroceles become evident only at the end of evacuation because of the space occupied by the distended rectum and urinary bladder. Repeated straining and making sure the urinary bladder is emptied after defecation are essential for the recognition of enteroceles. In one study [51], almost half (43 %) of enteroceles were seen only following evacuation and emptying of the urinary bladder emphasizing the importance of the post-evacuation/toilet phase of DCP. Evacuation should be as complete as possible because the unemptied rectum/rectocele and urinary bladder can prevent descent of an enterocele (see Fig. 11.3). Obtaining a post-toilet radiograph and emptying the urinary bladder with a catheter particularly those with urinary retention offers the best opportunity to diagnose enteroceles. Intra-vaginal enteroceles, unlike those that prolapse into the rectovaginal space, often compete with a cystocele; if the cystocele is not sufficiently drained, the

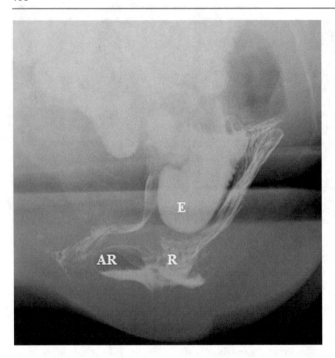

Fig. 11.12 Syndrome of the descending perineum and anterior mucosal prolapse. DCP performed on a 65-year-old patient because of tenesmus and symptoms of obstructed defecation. There is extension of the anterior rectal (R) wall into the anal canal without widening of the anal canal. Note Stage 2 anterior rectocele (A, displacement type) and a Stage 1 enterocele (E, type B)

presence of a coexisting enterocele may be overlooked or minimized (Fig. 11.5) [33, 37].

Enteroceles may be overdiagnosed owing to a lack of a clear definition of its diagnosis. A range from to 2 to 5 cm has been considered normal small bowel descent below vaginal apex [87]. Additionally, the vaginal apex moves. Enteroceles, sigmoidoceles, and peritoneoceles have been conventionally graded using the PCL but this may have little clinical significance. Controversy has existed as to whether enteroceles cause pressure on the rectum and obstruct rectal evacuation (the so-called defecation block). A prior report has suggested that it does [120] while a more recent study claimed that enteroceles do not obstruct rectal evacuation [121]. A more recent report has shown that enteroceles cause symptoms of obstructed defecation [73]. A clinical radiologic classification has been proposed by Morandi et al. [73]: Type A when the small bowel extends below the PCL during marked straining and returns back at rest without reaching or compressing the rectal ampulla, Type B when the enterocele descends below the PCL to extend through the rectovaginal space to compress the rectal ampulla at the end of evacuation, and Type C when the enterocele compressed the rectal ampulla at the beginning of defecation and moves towards the anal canal during defecation. This likely corresponds to the traditional radiologic grading using the PCL: minimal:<3 cm below PCL, moderate: 3–6 cm, and severe: >6 cm below PCL.

In that report, Type C was associated with symptoms of obstructed defecation, while Type B was associated frequently with abnormal perineal descent and anterior rectoceles. This classification using DCP appears relevant and merits further research. It appears that severe enteroceles produce symptoms of obstructed defecation. Rather than a linear measurement, volume of small bowel descending may be more relevant in the grading of enteroceles. Other symptoms typically associated with an enterocele are a sensation of pelvic pressure or dragging when standing or bearing down. The diagnosis of a previously undiagnosed enterocele may change the surgical approach from a transvaginal to a transabdominal route of entry. In many patients referred for DCP, this is an important information needed by the pelvic floor surgeon before surgery [87].

A sigmoidocele is a redundancy of the sigmoid colon that extends caudally into the cul-de-sac [72]. They are less common than are enteroceles and are found in approximately 5 % of proctograms [122]. This condition will be underdiagnosed at proctography if the sigmoid is not opacified but should be suspected on the basis of widening of the rectovaginal septum and air seen within fecal residue, hence the value of administering a small amount of gas following administration of high density barium mixture before administration of the feces consistency rectal paste. Lax presacral fixation of the rectosigmoid is seen by DCP and should be reported as it may be a risk factor for future development of a sigmoidocele. There is no agreed upon standard definition of a sigmoidocele. It has been defined as a sigmoid colon extending >4.5 cm below the PCL [122]. According to conventional radiologic classification this would constitute a moderate sigmoidocele. Sigmoidoceles are usually not detected at physical examination, even when large and are often associated with constipation [51, 72, 122]. The redundant sigmoid colon may compress the rectum and obstruct defecation. Stasis of solid debris in the redundant sigmoid gives rise to further discomfort and straining. A classification with clinical/surgical implications has been proposed by Jorge and Wexner [72] to provide a more objective approach to surgical treatment. The proposed classification was based on descent of the lowest portion of the sigmoid loop during marked straining at defecation relative to the PCL and the ischiococcygeal line (drawn from the ischial tuberosity to the tip of the coccyx).

Sigmoidoceles were classified as first degree when the intrapelvic loop of sigmoid abutted but did not descend below the PCL, second degree when the sigmoid loop descended below the PCL but remained above the ischiococcygeal line, and third degree when the sigmoid loop descended caudal to the ischiococcygeal line (see Fig. 11.4). The proposed classification yielded excellent correlation between the degree of sigmoidocele and clinical symptoms. All third-degree sigmoidoceles who underwent colonic resection reported symptomatic improvement [72]. There is only a minor difference of this classification from standard radiologic grading except for the addition of the ischiococcygeal line; it is simple and will be of value to colorectal surgeons to formulate an objective surgical approach.

Genital Prolapse

Uterine prolapse involves descent of the uterus into the vagina and often beyond the introitus. Vaginal vault prolapse involves descent of the apex of the vagina toward, through, or beyond the vaginal introitus after a previously performed total hysterectomy. Vaginal vault prolapse is almost always associated with prolapse of other pelvic organs, the most common of which is an enterocele. This reflects a loss of apical level support due to damage of the uterosacral–cardinal complex. Provided that adequate vaginal opacification is maintained at DCP, the location of the cervix and/or vaginal apex can be determined on DCP images. When there is partial or complete eversion, however, it may be difficult to determine the location of the vaginal apex. They are, however, clinically obvious. The direction of vaginal vault displacement is a valuable diagnostic adjunct. Although this is usually apparent from physical examination, what organ is behind that wall is not always evident. Anterior vaginal displacement is indicative of posterior vaginal wall prolapse, which traditionally is considered to be due to pressure from a rectocele. DCP, however, has shown that approximately one-third of patients with posterior colpoceles have an enterocele or a sigmoidocele [51]. Conversely, inferior/posterior displacement of the vaginal wall (anterior vaginal wall prolapse) is typically due to pressure from a cystocele, although in a minority of patients this finding may be due to an intra-vaginal enterocele [51]. These are usually underdiagnosed (Fig. 11.5). In either case, it represents loss of anterior vaginal wall support.

Cystocele

This is the result of a defect in the support of the anterior vaginal wall. The vaginal muscularis attaches laterally to the arcus tendineus pelvis and posteriorly to the cervix. Symptom caused by a cystocele may be minimal until it reaches the vaginal introitus; the most common symptoms are feeling of heaviness or "something bulging." Similar to other prolapses symptoms start to manifest clinically when the leading edge of the prolapsing organ abuts the PH. Large cystoceles may also lead to voiding dysfunction. Cystoceles are usually larger after rectal evacuation and are, therefore, optimally assessed by measuring the degree of displacement of the anterior vaginal wall during maximum straining after defecation. The presence of the 8 F catheter in our method of examination [33] also allows measurement of bladder neck mobility during maximum straining. This should be no >1 cm [27]. The urethral axis is normally <35 % of vertical (Fig. 11.10). Funneling (beaking) of the bladder neck at rest may suggest an incompetent urethral sphincter; however, it is a nonspecific sign and may also be seen in continent women [123]. In general, symptomatic cystoceles are

treated surgically with a variety of techniques. Some employ restorative measures such as paravaginal repair while others do a form of colpocleisis, anterior colporrhaphy.

What has been recognized more recently is the high degree of correlation between apical and anterior vaginal wall prolapse [124]. Surgeons have focused on the vaginal apex to correct anterior wall descent because of the strong association between the vaginal apex and the cystocele. An anti-incontinence procedure is frequently included because elevation of the bladder often unkinks the bladder neck and unmasks urinary incontinence.

Summary

The role of "functional" imaging of the pelvic floor is to complement deficiencies of physical examination. "Functional" imaging whether done with DCP or with dynamic pelvic MRI does not represent physiological defecation and is conducted in artificial surroundings that embarrass and inhibit the patient. Our analysis of the different controversies between DCP and dynamic pelvic MRI appears to reflect the authors preference. Most comparative studies use less rigorous gold standard such as physical examination whose shortcomings are well known. In several examinations, the authors did not compare both examinations on the same patients in the same position. When done functionally in an open magnet system, dynamic pelvic MRI images are of a lower signal-to-noise ratio and soft tissue resolution hence details of the pelvic supporting structures are not well defined. It has resulted in significant interobserver variations in determining reference points [5, 79]. Its improved soft tissue resolution with the use of appropriate endoluminal coil makes it difficult to use as a functional study to determine occult-associated pelvic organ prolapses as the coil itself blocks organ descent. It would be of benefit when all the limitations of functional pelvic floor MRI are overcome so more attention is given to improve the accuracy for subtle albeit important findings and not simply dismiss findings because of the lack of correlation with physical examination findings. DCP is a mature technology. Dynamic pelvic floor MRI is an evolving technology and its precise role in functional imaging of the pelvic floor still remains to be determined.

Conclusions reached by investigators on its use are conflicting. It has the potential to be a valid "functional" method for evaluating AR disorders and associated pelvic organ prolapse. Further developments and research on the use of functional MRI for defecatory disorders and pelvic organ prolapse can make it a valid alternative to DCP. It is likely that pelvic MR with increased soft tissue resolution with endoluminal coils will complement DCP where the need to see structural details of the pelvic supportive tissues and endopelvic fascia is required for surgical management. Their clinical significance as related to surgical repair has not been evaluated and may be irrelevant. Currently, both methods infer pelvic organ prolapses from different reference points most of which do not have physical examination correlates. The same argument applies to "functional" ultrasound examination which has the added disadvantage of requiring technical expertise not available in most practices.

DCP is time tested, well-established, and a widely available method. The ability of DCP to enable evaluation of function and infer anatomical structural integrity while the pelvic floor is being subjected to normal gravitational stress, similar to the daily maneuvers that precipitate patients symptoms makes this technique an important adjunct to physical examination. With current technical modifications to opacify all pelvic organs [92], it has evolved from a method to evaluate the anorectum for functional disorders (defecography) to its current status as a practical, "near functional" method for evaluating defecation disorders and associated pelvic organ prolapses with meaningful clinical information. "Functional" pelvic MRI has the potential to be an alternative or complementary examination. It has the technology required to demonstrate anatomical details of pelvic supporting structures including fascial condensations which are only inferred by DCP. The fascial defects seen by pelvic MRI, however, have not correlated with a change to surgical management in our practice. Currently, the evidence suggests that DCP is the "functional" examination for the diagnosis of AR and pelvic floor dysfunction [3, 33, 37]. Pelvic MR with endoluminal coils will complement DCP where the need to see anatomic details of pelvic supportive tissues are required for surgical management.

Key Points

Functional radiography provides the maximum stress to the pelvic floor resulting in levator ani relaxation accompanied by rectal emptying which is needed to diagnose defecatory disorders.

- This method provides organ-specific quantification of female pelvic organ prolapse, information that usually can only be inferred by means of physical examination.
- The ability of functional radiography to enable the evaluation of function and anatomy while the pelvic floor is being subjected to normal gravitational stress, similar to the daily maneuvers that have precipitated the symptoms, makes this method an important clinical adjunct to physical examination.
- Because there is only a limited amount of space in the pelvis, organs that do not empty after evacuation—which are difficult to recognize if unopacified—may prevent recognition of other prolapsed organs that are competing for this space.
- Dynamic cystocolpoproctography (DCP) is of value in patients with defecatory disorders, in patients with

symptoms or complaints that are not consistent with findings from physical examination, and in the diagnosis of associated prolapse in other compartments that may currently be asymptomatic.
- With the additional relevant diagnostic information DCP provides to the physical examination, the adoption of a radiologic method of staging prolapse with clinical correlates will enhance its role.

References

1. DeLancey JO. The hidden epidemic of pelvic floor dysfunction: achievable goals for improved prevention and treatment. Am J Obstet Gynecol. 2005;192(5):1488–95.
2. Sung VW, Hampton BS. Epidemiology of pelvic floor dysfunction. Obstet Gynecol Clin North Am. 2009;36(3):421–44.
3. Maglinte DD, Kelvin FM, Hale DS, Benson JT. Dynamic cystoproctography: a unifying diagnostic approach to pelvic floor and anorectal dysfunction. AJR Am J Roentgenol. 1997;169(3):759–67.
4. Stoker J, Halligan S, Bartram CI. Pelvic floor imaging. Radiology. 2001;218(3):621–41.
5. Law YM, Fielding JR. MRI of pelvic floor dysfunction: review. AJR Am J Roentgenol. 2008;191(6 Suppl):S45–53.
6. Barleben A, Mills S. Anorectal anatomy and physiology. Surg Clin N Am. 2010;90(1):1–15.
7. Bertschinger KM, Hetzer FH, Roos JE, et al. Dynamic MR imaging of the pelvic floor performed with patient sitting in an open-magnet unit versus with patient supine in a closed-magnet unit. Radiology. 2002;223(2):501–8.
8. Bharucha AE. Update of tests of colon and rectal structure and function. J Clin Gastroenterol. 2006;40(2):96–103.
9. Cappabianca S, Reginelli A, Iacobellis F, et al. Dynamic MRI defecography vs. entero-colpo-cysto-defecography in the evaluation of midline pelvic floor hernias in female pelvic floor disorders. Int J Colorectal Dis. 2011;26(9):1191–6.
10. Comiter CV, Vasavada SP, Barbaric ZL, Gousse AE, Raz S. Grading pelvic prolapse and pelvic floor relaxation using dynamic magnetic resonance imaging. Urology. 1999;54(3):454–7.
11. Eguare EI, Neary P, Crosbie J, et al. Dynamic magnetic resonance imaging of the pelvic floor in patients with idiopathic combined fecal and urinary incontinence. J Gastrointest Surg. 2004;8(1):73–82 (discussion 82).
12. El Sayed RF, El Mashed S, Farag A, Morsy MM, Abdel Azim MS. Pelvic floor dysfunction: assessment with combined analysis of static and dynamic MR imaging findings. Radiology. 2008;248(2):518–30.
13. Elshazly WG, El Nekady AA, Hassan H. Role of dynamic magnetic resonance imaging in management of obstructed defecation case series. Int J Surg. 2010;8(4):274–82.
14. Hecht EM, Lee VS, Tanpitukpongse TP, et al. MRI of pelvic floor dysfunction: dynamic true fast imaging with steadystate precession versus HASTE. AJR Am J Roentgenol. 2008;191(2):352–8.
15. Hetzer FH, Andreisek G, Tsagari C, Sahrbacher U, Weishaupt D. MR defecography in patients with fecal incontinence: imaging findings and their effect on surgical management. Radiology. 2006;240(2):449–57.
16. Hilfiker PR, Debatin JF, Schwizer W, et al. MR defecography: depiction of anorectal anatomy and pathology. J Comput Assist Tomogr. 1998;22(5):749–55.
17. Lamb GM, de Jode MG, Gould SW, et al. Upright dynamic MR defaecating proctography in an open configuration MR system. Br J Radiol. 2000;73(866):152–5.

18. Law PA, Danin JC, Lamb GM, et al. Dynamic imaging of the pelvic floor using an open-configuration magnetic resonance scanner. J Magn Reson Imaging. 2001;13(6):923–9.

19. Lienemann A, Fischer T. Functional imaging of the pelvic floor. Eur J Radiol. 2003;47(2):117–22.

20. Mortele KJ, Fairhurst J. Dynamic MR defecography of the posterior compartment: indications, techniques and MRI features. Eur J Radiol. 2007;61(3):462–72.

21. Rentsch M, Paetzel C, Lenhart M, et al. Dynamic magnetic resonance imaging defecography: a diagnostic alternative in the assessment of pelvic floor disorders in proctology. Dis Colon Rectum. 2001;44(7):999–1007.

22. Roos JE, Weishaupt D, Wildermuth S, et al. Experience of 4 years with open MR defecography: pictorial review of anorectal anatomy and disease. Radiographics. 2002;22(4):817–32.

23. Gousse AE, Barbaric ZL, Safir MH, et al. Dynamic half Fourier acquisition, single shot turbo spin-echo magnetic resonance imaging for evaluating the female pelvis. J Urol. 2000;164(5):1606–13.

24. Healy JC, Halligan S, Reznek RH, et al. Magnetic resonance imaging of the pelvic floor in patients with obstructed defaecation. Br J Surg. 1997;84(11):1555–8.

25. Gufler H, Laubenberger J, DeGregorio G, Dohnicht S, Langer M. Pelvic floor descent: dynamic MR imaging using a half- Fourier RARE sequence. J Magn Reson Imaging. 1999;9(3):378–83.

26. Schoenenberger AW, Debatin JF, Guldenschuh I, et al. Dynamic MR defecography with a superconducting, open-configuration MR system. Radiology. 1998;206(3):641–6.

27. Yang A, Mostwin JL, Rosenshein NB, Zerhouni EA. Pelvic floor descent in women: dynamic evaluation with fast MR imaging and cinematic display. Radiology. 1991;179(1):25–33.

28. Brenner D, Elliston C, Hall E, Berdon W. Estimated risks of radiation-induced fatal cancer from pediatric CT. AJR Am J Roentgenol. 2001;176(2):289–96.

29. Hall EJ, Brenner DJ. Cancer risks from diagnostic radiology. Br J Radiol. 2008;81(965):362–78.

30. Brenner DJ, Hall EJ. Computed tomography—an increasing source of radiation exposure. N Engl J Med. 2007;357(22):2277–84.

31. Brenner DJ, Hall EJ. Risk of cancer from diagnostic X-rays. Lancet. 2004;363(9427):2192 (author reply 2192–2193).

32. Brenner DJ, Hricak H. Radiation exposure from medical imaging: time to regulate? JAMA. 2010;304(2):208–9.

33. Maglinte DD, Bartram CI, Hale DA, et al. Functional imaging of the pelvic floor. Radiology. 2011;258(1):23–39.

34. Maglinte DD, Bartram C. Dynamic imaging of posterior compartment pelvic floor dysfunction by evacuation proctography: techniques, indications, results and limitations. Eur J Radiol. 2007;61(3):454–61.

35. Halligan S. Re: The benefits or otherwise of evacuation proctography (defecography). Abdom Imaging. 1995;20(3):280–1.

36. Halligan S, Malouf A, Bartram CI, et al. Predictive value of impaired evacuation at proctography in diagnosing anismus. AJR Am J Roentgenol. 2001;177(3):633–6.

37. Maglinte DD, Kelvin FM, Fitzgerald K, Hale DS, Benson JT. Association of compartment defects in pelvic floor dysfunction. AJR Am J Roentgenol. 1999;172(2):439–44.

38. Flusberg M, Sahni VA, Erturk SM, Mortele KJ. Dynamic MR defecography: assessment of the usefulness of the defecation phase. AJR Am J Roentgenol. 2011;196(4):W394–9.

39. Halligan S, Spence-Jones C, Kamm MA, Bartram CI. Dynamic cystoproctography and physiological testing in women with urinary stress incontinence and urogenital prolapse. Clin Radiol. 1996;51(11):785–90.

40. Kelvin FM, Maglinte DD. Dynamic cystoproctography of female pelvic floor defects and their interrelationships. AJR Am J Roentgenol. 1997;169(3):769–74.

41. Ott DJ, Donati DL, Kerr RM, Chen MY. Defecography: results in 55 patients and impact on clinical management. Abdom Imaging. 1994;19(4):349–54.

42. Hiltunen KM, Kolehmainen H, Matikainen M. Does defecography help in diagnosis and clinical decision-making in defecation disorders? Abdom Imaging. 1994;19(4):355–8.

43. Dixon A. Evidence based diagnostic radiology. Lancet. 1997;350:509–12.

44. Harvey CJ, Harvey CJ, Halligan S, et al. Evacuation proctography: a prospective study of diagnostic and therapeutic impact. Radiology. 1999;211:223–7.

45. Kelvin FM, Maglinte DD, Hale DS, Benson JT. Female pelvic organ prolapse: a comparison of triphasic dynamic MR imaging and triphasic fluoroscopic cystocolpoproctography. AJR Am J Roentgenol. 2000;174(1):81–8.

46. Kelvin FM, Maglinte DD, Hornback JA, Benson JT. Pelvic prolapse: assessment with evacuation proctography (defecography). Radiology. 1992;184(2):547–51.

47. Altringer WE, Saclarides TJ, Dominguez JM, Brubaker LT, Smith CS. Four-contrast defecography: pelvic "fluoroscopy". Dis Colon Rectum. 1995;38(7):695–9.

48. Brubaker L, Heit MH. Radiology of the pelvic floor. Clin Obstet Gynecol. 1993;36(4):952–9.

49. Hock D, Lombard R, Jehaes C, et al. Colpocystodefecography. Dis Colon Rectum. 1993;36(11):1015–21.

50. Kelvin FM, Hale DS, Maglinte DD, Patten BJ, Benson JT. Female pelvic organ prolapse: diagnostic contribution of dynamic cystoproctography and comparison with physical examination. AJR Am J Roentgenol. 1999;173(1):31–7.

51. Saclarides TJ, Brubaker LT, Altringer WE, Smith CS, Dominguez JM. Clarifying the technique of four-contrast defecography. Dis Colon Rectum. 1996;39(7):826.

52. Vanbeckevoort D, Van Hoe L, Oyen R, et al. Pelvic floor descent in females: comparative study of colpocystodefecography and dynamic fast MR imaging. J Magn Reson Imaging. 1999;9(3):373–7.

53. Fielding JR, Griffiths DJ, Versi E, et al. MR imaging of pelvic floor continence mechanisms in the supine and sitting positions. AJR Am J Roentgenol. 1998;171(6):1607–10.

54. Kelvin FM, Maglinte DD, Benson JT. Evacuation proctography (defecography): an aid to the investigation of pelvic floor disorders. Obstet Gynecol. 1994;83(2):307–14.

55. Olsen AL, Smith VJ, Bergstrom JO, Colling JC, Clark AL. Epidemiology of surgically managed pelvic organ prolapse and urinary incontinence. Obstet Gynecol. 1997;89(4):501–6.

56. Gill EJ, Hurt WG. Pathophysiology of pelvic organ prolapse. Obstet Gynecol Clin North Am. 1998;25(4):757–69.

57. Burnett LS, Buckley SL. Surgical failures in the management of pelvic floor relaxation. Curr Opin Obstet Gynecol. 1993;5(4):465–70.

58. Karasick S, Spettell CM. The role of parity and hysterectomy on the development of pelvic floor abnormalities revealed by defecography. AJR Am J Roentgenol. 1997;169(6):1555–8.

59. Karasick S, Spettell CM. Defecography: does parity play a role in the development of rectal prolapse? Eur Radiol. 1999;9(3):450–3.

60. Stoker J, Bartram CI, Halligan S. Imaging of the posterior pelvic floor. Eur Radiol. 2002;12(4):779–88.

61. Stoker J, Rociu E. Endoluminal MR imaging of anorecta l diseases. J Magn Reson Imaging. 1999;9(5):631–4.

62. Kim JK, Kim YJ, Choo MS, Cho KS. The urethra and its supporting structures in women with stress urinary incontinence: MR imaging using an endovaginal coil. Am J Roentgenol. 2003;180:1037–44.

63. Stoker J, Rociu E, Zwamborn AW, Schouten WR, Lameris JS. Endoluminal MR imaging of the rectum and anus: technique, applications, and pitfalls. Radiographics. 1999;19:383–98.

64. Mahieu P, Pringot J, Bodart P. Defecography: I. Description of a new procedure and results in normal patients. Gastrointest Radiol. 1984;9(3):247–51.

65. Ekberg O, Nylander G, Fork FT. Defecography. Radiology. 1985;155(1):45–8.

66. Shorvon PJ, McHugh S, Diamant NE, Somers S, Stevenson GW. Defecography in normal volunteers: results and implications. Gut. 1989;30(12):1737–49.

67. Fielding JR. Imaging of the female pelvis in the supine and upright position. J Magn Reson Imaging. 1996;88:750–6.

68. Solopova AE, Hetzer FH, Marincek B, Weishaupt D. MR defecography: prospective comparison of two rectal enema compositions. AJR Am J Roentgenol. 2008;190(2):W118–24.

69. Gagliardi G, Pescatori M, Altomare DF, et al. Results, outcome predictors, and complications after stapled transanal rectal resection for obstructed defecation. Dis Colon Rectum. 2008;51(2):186–95 (discussion 195).

70. Bump RC, Mattiasson A, Bo K, et al. The standardization of terminology of female pelvic organ prolapse and pelvic floor dysfunction. Am J Obstet Gynecol. 1996;175(1):10–7.

71. Bernier P, Stevenson GW, Shorvon PJ. Defecography commode. Radiology. 1988;155:891–2.

72. Jorge JM, Yang YK, Wexner SD. Incidence and clinical significance of sigmoidocele as determined by a new classification system. Dis Colon Rectum. 1994;37(11):1112–7.

73. Morandi C, Martellucci J, Talento P, Carriero A. Role of enterocele in the obstructed defecation syndrome (ODS): a new radiological point of view. Colorectal Dis. 2010;12:810–6.

74. Mahieu P, Pringot J, Bodart P. Defecography: II. Contribution to the diagnosis of defecation disorders. Gastrointest Radiol. 1984;9(3):253–61.

75. Bartolo DC, Roe AM, Virjee J, Mortensen NJ. Evacuation proctography in obstructed defaecation and rectal intussusception. Br J Surg. 1985;72:S111–6.

76. Healy JC, Halligan S, Reznek RH, et al. Dynamic MR imaging compared with evacuation proctography when evaluating anorectal configuration and pelvic floor movement. AJR Am J Roentgenol. 1997;169(3):775–9.

77. Barber MD, Brubaker L, Nygaard I, et al. Defining success after surgery for pelvic organ prolapse. Obstet Gynecol. 2009;114(3):600–9.

78. Singh K, Reid WM, Berger LA. Assessment and grading of pelvic organ prolapse by use of dynamic magnetic resonance imaging. Am J Obstet Gynecol. 2001;185(1):71–7.

79. Woodfield CA, Hampton BS, Sung V, Brody JM. Magnetic resonance imaging of pelvic organ prolapse: comparing pubococcygeal and midpubic lines with clinical staging. Int Urogynecol J Pelvic Floor Dysfunct. 2009;20(6):695–701.

80. Lockhart ME, Fielding JR, Richter HE, et al. Reproducibility of dynamic MR imaging pelvic measurements: a multi institutional study. Radiology. 2008;249(2):534–40.

81. Brenner DJ. Radiation risks potentially associated with low dose CT screening of adult smokers for lung cancer. Radiology. 2004;231(2):440–5.

82. Brenner DJ. It is time to retire the computed tomography dose index (CTDI) for CT quality assurance and dose optimization. For the proposition. Med Phys. 2006;33(5):1189–90.

83. Brenner DJ, Sachs RK. Estimating radiation-induced cancer risks at very low doses: rationale for using a linear nothreshold approach. Radiat Environ Biophys. 2006;44(4):253–6.

84. Pfeifer J, Oliveira L, Park UC, et al. Are interpretations of video defecographies reliable and reproducible? Int J Colorectal Dis. 1997;12:67–72.

85. Kenton K, Shott S, Brubaker L. Vaginal topography does not correlate well with visceral position in women with pelvic organ prolapse. Int Urogynecol J Pelvic Floor Dysfunct. 1997;8(6):336–9.

86. Altman D, Mellgren A, Kierkegaard J, et al. Diagnosis of cystocele—the correlation between clinical and radiological evaluation. Int Urogynecol J Pelvic Floor Dysfunct. 2004;15(1):3–9 (discussion 9).

87. Hale D. Clinical and surgical pelvic organ prolapse. In: Bartram CI, DeLancey JOL, editors. Medical radiology. Diagnostic and radiation oncology: pelvic floor disorders. 2nd ed. Heidelberg: Springer; 2008. pp. 165–86.

88. Benson T. Female pelvic floor disorders: investigation and management. New York: Norton; 1992.

89. Frudinger A, Bartram CI, Halligan S, Kamm M. Examination techniques for endosonography of the anal canal. Abdom Imaging. 1998;23(3):301–3.

90. da Silva GM, Gurland B, Sleemi A, Levy G. Posterior vaginal wall prolapse does not correlate with fecal symptoms or objective measures of anorectal function. Am J Obstet Gynecol. 2006;195(6):1742–47.

91. Felt-Bersma RJ, Luth WJ, Janssen JJ, Meuwissen SG. Defecography in patients with anorectal disorders. Which findings are clinically relevant? Dis Colon Rectum. 1990;33(4):277–84.

92. Ferrante SL, Perry RE, Schreiman JS, Cheng SC, Frick MP. The reproducibility of measuring the anorectal angle indefecography. Dis Colon Rectum. 1991;34(1):51–55. proctography: an investigation of rectal expulsion in 20 subjects without defecatory disturbance. Gastrointest Radiol 13(1):72–80.

93. Bartram CI, Turnbull G, Lennard-Jones JE. Evacuation proctography: an investigation of rectal expulsion in 20 subjects without defecatory disturbance. Gastrointest Radiol. 1988;13(1):72–80.

94. Bharucha AE, Wald A, Enck P, et al. Functional anorectal disorders. Gastroenterology. 2006;130:1510–8.

95. Halligan S, Bartram CI, Park HY, Kamm MA. Proctographic features of anismus. Radiology. 1995;197(3):679–82.

96. Bordeianou L, Savitt L, Dursun A. Measurements of pelvic floor dyssynergia: which test result matters? Dis Colon Rectum. 2011;54(1):60–5.

97. Rao SS. Advances in diagnostic assessment of fecal incontinence and dyssynergic defecation. Clin Gastroenterol Hepatol. 2010;8(11):910–9.

98. Rao SS, Go JT. Treating pelvic floor disorders of defecation: management or cure? Curr Gastroenterol Rep. 2009;11(4):278–87.

99. Halligan S, McGee S, Bartram CI. Quantification of evacuation proctography. Dis Colon Rectum. 1994;37:1151–4.

100. Kenton K, Shott S, Brubaker L. The anatomic and functional variability of rectoceles in women. Int Urogynecol J Pelvic Floor Dysfunct. 1999;10(2):96–9.

101. Mellgren A, Lopez A, Schultz I, Anzen B. Rectocele is associated with paradoxical anal sphincter reaction. Int J Colorectal Dis. 1998;13(1):13–6.

102. Siproudhis L, Ropert A, Lucas J, et al. Defecatory disorders, anorectal and pelvic floor dysfunction: a polygamy? Radiologic and manometric studies in 41 patients. Int J Colorectal Dis. 1992;7(2):102–7.

103. Halligan S, Bartram CI. Is barium trapping in rectoceles significant? Dis Colon Rectum. 1995;38(7):764–8.

104. Greenberg T, Kelvin FM, Maglinte DD. Barium trapping in rectoceles: are we trapped by the wrong definition? Abdom Imaging. 2001;26(6):587–90.

105. Pucciani F, Rottoli ML, Bologna A, et al. Anterior rectocele and anorectal dysfunction. Int J Colorectal Dis. 1996;11(1):1–9.

106. Grassi R, Pomerri F, Habib F, et al. Defecography study of outpouchings of the external wall of the rectum: posterior rectocele and ischio-rectal hernia. Radiol Med. 1995;90(1/2):44–8.

107. Chen HH, Iroatulam A, Alabaz O, et al. Associations of defecography and physiologic findings in male patients with rectocele. Tech Coloproctol. 2001;5(3):157–61.

108. Bremmer S, Ude'n R, Mellgren A. Defaeco-peritoneography in the diagnosis of rectal intussusception: a contribution for the discussion of causative mechanism. Acta Radiol. 1997;38(4):578–83.

109. Pomerri F, Zuliani M, Mazza C, Villarejo F, Scopece A. Defecographic measurements of rectal intussusception and prolapse in patients and in asymptomatic subjects. AJR Am J Roentgenol. 2001;176(3):641–5.

110. Felt-Bersma R, Tiersma ES, Cuesta M. Rectal prolapse, rectal intussusception, rectocele, solitary rectal ulcer syndrome, and enterocele. Gastroenterol Clin North Am. 2008;37:647–8.

111. Rutter KR, Riddell RH. The solitary ulcer syndrome of the rectum. Clin Gastroenterol. 1975;4(3):505–30.

112. Goei R. Anorectal function in patients with defecation disorders and asymptomatic subjects: evaluation with defecography. Radiology. 1990;174(1):121–3.

113. Halligan S, Nicholls RJ, Bartram CI. Evacuation proctography in patients with solitary rectal ulcer syndrome: anatomic abnormalities and frequency of impaired emptying and prolapse. AJR Am J Roentgenol. 1995;164:91–5.

114. Parks AG, Porter NH, Hardcastle J. The syndrome of the descending perineum. Proc R Soc Med. 1966;59(6):477–82.

115. Pinho M, Yoshioka K, Ortiz J, Oya M, Keighley MR. The effect of age on pelvic floor dynamics. Int J Colorectal Dis. 1990;5(4):207–8.

116. Bremmer S, Mellgren A, Holmstrom B, Lopez A, Uden R. Peritoneocele: visualization with defecography and peritoneography performed simultaneously. Radiology. 1997;202(2):373–7.

117. Jorge JM, Ger GC, Gonzalez L, Wexner SD. Patient position during cinedefecography: influence on perineal descent and other measurements. Dis Colon Rectum. 1994;37(9):927–31.

118. Berkelmans I, Heresbach D, Leroi AM, et al. Perineal descent at defecography in women with straining at stool: a lack of specificity or predictive value for future anal incontinence? Eur J Gastroenterol Hepatol. 1995;7(1):75–9.

119. Tsiaoussis J, Chrysos E, Glynos M, Vassilakis JS, Xynos E. Pathophysiology and treatment of the anterior rectal mucosal prolapse syndrome. Br J Surg. 1998;85(12):1699–702.

120. Wallden L. Defecation block in cases of deep rectogenital pouch. Acta Chir Scand. 1952;103(3):236–8.

121. Halligan S, Bartram C, Hall C, Wingate J. Enterocele revealed by simultaneous evacuation proctography and peritoneography: does "defecation block" exist? Am J Roentgenol. 1996;167(2):461–6.

122. Fenner DE. Diagnosis and assessment of sigmoidoceles. Am J Obstet Gynecol. 1996;175(6):1438–41 (discussion 1441–14 32).

123. Pannu HK, Kaufman HS, Cundiff GW, et al. Dynamic MR imaging of pelvic organ prolapse: spectrum of abnormalities. Radiographics. 2000;20(6):1567–82.

124. Rooney K, Kenton K, Mueller ER, FitzGerald MP, Brubaker L. Advanced anterior vaginal wall prolapse is highly correlated with apical prolapse. Am J Obstet Gynecol. 2006;195(6):1837–40.

Colonoscopy in Elderly Patients

Johannes Koch and Otto S. Lin

Introduction

Colonoscopy is currently the procedure of choice for evaluation of the whole colon in patients who present with lower gastrointestinal symptoms. In the USA, it is also the most effective and most commonly used modality for colorectal cancer (CRC) screening in asymptomatic individuals (with or without a family history), and for surveillance in patients at increased risk because of a personal history of adenomatous polyps, CRC, or inflammatory bowel disease. Finally, in appropriate circumstances it is a critical therapeutic procedure, allowing for biopsy of suspicious lesions, treatment of bleeding sources, placement of stents, and, most importantly, removal of colorectal adenomatous polyps, thereby preventing the potential occurrence of CRC [1].

Colonoscopy in Elderly Patients

Because the incidence of colorectal pathology and symptoms increase with age, a large proportion of diagnostic, screening, and surveillance colonoscopies are performed on "elderly" (defined for our purposes as those >65 years of age) and "very elderly" patients (>80 years). In the USA, the number of screening procedures in elderly patients has increased dramatically ever since Medicare began to cover screening colonoscopy in average-risk beneficiaries in 2001 [2]. However, performing colonoscopy in elderly patients poses a unique set of challenges. In the elderly, the risks and benefits of colonoscopy should be carefully assessed in light of lower life expectancy and the frequent presence of comorbidities, so as to ensure that the potential benefits outweigh the risks and morbidity. This chapter will discuss issues pertaining to the procedural yield, potential benefits, technical feasibility, complication risks, logistical difficulties and costs associated with performing colonoscopy in elderly and very elderly individuals.

Yield

The procedural yield is the percentage of patients who are found to have clinically significant findings (especially neoplasia) on colonoscopy. Generally, the yield of colonoscopy increases with age [3]. According to Surveillance Epidemiology End Results (SEER) registry data as of 2007, the incidence of CRC is 120 cases per 100,000 in persons aged 50–64 years of age, 186 per 100,000 in those 65–74, and 290.1 per 100,000 in those ≥75 [4]. It is well established that elderly patients have a higher prevalence of colorectal neoplasia [5, 6], as well as other pathology such as diverticulosis and hemorrhoids. As with younger patients, symptomatic elderly patients demonstrate a higher yield than those who are asymptomatic [7].

Numerous studies have confirmed a high yield for both screening and diagnostic colonoscopy in elderly patients (Table 12.1). The reported yield of colorectal neoplasia in symptomatic elderly patients has ranged from 3.7–12.7 % [8, 11, 14, 17]. In a study on 200 symptomatic octogenarians, 80 % had colonoscopic findings that explained their symptoms [18]. Controlled studies that compared the yield in patients of different ages have echoed these findings. In one study on 1353 elderly patients, the risk of CRC development was higher in patients >80 compared to those 70–74 years old [5]. In another study that included 915 symptomatic and screening patients, more advanced adenomas and invasive cancers were identified in 53 patients over the age of 80 than in younger controls [19]. Studies on European patients as well as minority

J. Koch • O.S. Lin (✉)
Digestive Disease Institute, Virginia Mason Medical Center, Seattle, WA, USA
e-mail: Otto.Lin@vmmc.org

© Springer Science+Business Media New York 2017
D.A. Gordon, M.R. Katlic (eds.), *Pelvic Floor Dysfunction and Pelvic Surgery in the Elderly*,
DOI 10.1007/978-1-4939-6554-0_12

Table 12.1 Yield of colonoscopy in studies with subgroups of symptomatic and/or screening/surveillance "elderly" patients

	N	Age (years)	Completion (%)	Cancers (%)	Adenomas/Polyps (%)
Bat et al. [8]	436	80+	63	14	29.8
Ure et al. [9]	354	70+	78	6	24
Sardinha et al. [10]	403	80+	94	4.5	–
Clarke et al. [11]	95	85+	–	12.7	–
Lagares-Garcia et al. [12]	103	80+	92.7	11.6	19.4
Arora and Singh [13]	110	80+	97[a]	20	–
Syn et al. [14]	225	80+	56	11	25
Yoong and Heymann [15]	316	85+	69	8.9	14.2
Karajeh et al. [16]	1000	65+	81.8	7.1	6[b]

[a]Adjusted for non-traversable stricture
[b]Large polyps ≥1 cm in size

groups in the USA have all reported similar results. A large study on 2000 English patients showed that compared with younger patients, those >65 years old had higher overall diagnostic yields (65 % versus 45 %) as well as CRC prevalence (7.1 % versus 1.3 %) [16], while another study on 1530 African American and Hispanic patients showed that the CRC yield was significantly higher in those over 65 than in younger counterparts (7.8 % versus 1.8 %) [20].

Complications and Adverse Events

One of the main concerns with performing colonoscopy on elderly patients is the potential for increased risk of complications. Adverse events are typically categorized as those occurring during or immediately after the procedure and those that have a delayed presentation. Cardiopulmonary complications are the most common peri-procedural adverse events. The level of sedation, presence of comorbidities, and procedure length and complexity all contribute to the risk and should be addressed to the extent known during preprocedural planning, especially for elective colonoscopies.

Although early, small studies suggested that colonoscopy in elderly patients did not result in more complications [21], more recent, larger, and better designed studies have shown convincingly that colonoscopy in the elderly is associated with more risk than in younger patients. As demonstrated by a recent meta-analysis, very elderly patients had a significantly higher rate of overall adverse events, gastrointestinal bleeding, and perforation (Table 12.2) [22]. Studies from Asia have also reported higher risks of cardiovascular complications despite the fact that elderly patients on average received lower doses of sedatives [23].

Nevertheless, when taken in context, the complication rate is still quite low even for patients over 85 years of age, and in most cases colonoscopy can be done safely with appropriate monitoring and precautions [24]. Furthermore, small studies

have shown that propofol sedation can also be used safely in very elderly patients [25]. The overall major complication rate in patients over 80 is low, between 0.2 % and 0.6 % [16, 17], although it increases with specific comorbid conditions [26]. Studies in minority patients (African Americans and Hispanics) [20], as well as from Asia [27], have confirmed that complication rates are low in elderly patients.

During the colonoscopy, the vital signs, oxygen saturation, and cardiac rhythm of all patients should be monitored continuously. Supplemental oxygen is often administered if patients are sedated. Increasingly, capnography is being used to identify early signs of respiratory depression. Conscious sedation is achieved by the use of a short-acting sedative with amnestic properties, such as intravenous midazolam or diazepam, and an opioid analgesic, such as fentanyl or meperidine. The use of deep sedation with propofol, typically administered by an anesthesia provider, is becoming more popular in the USA. However, gastroenterologist-administered propofol has also been shown to be safe in the elderly [28].

Up to one third of patients may have minor side effects after outpatient colonoscopy, most frequently bloating or abdominal cramps. Depending on their level of independence, elderly patients living alone may require additional post-procedure care. Post-procedure calls within 48 h by medical staff may be helpful.

Many elderly patients have implanted cardiac pacemakers or defibrillators. The use of monopolar electrocautery during snare polypectomy can cause pacemaker inhibition or false detection of cardiac arrhythmias [29]. Thus, these devices are generally inactivated during colonoscopy.

Colonoscopy Completion Rates

Complete colonoscopy requires cecal intubation or, for those who have had an ileocecectomy, reaching the ileocolonic anastomosis. In the USA, studies of all patients undergoing

Table 12.2 Complication risks based on data from meta-analysis by Day et al. [22]

Age group (years)	>65	>80
Cumulative adverse events	26.0ᵃ (25.0–27.0)	34.9ᵃ (31.9–38.0)
Perforation	1.0 % (0.9–1.5)	1.5 % (1.1–1.9)
Gastrointestinal bleeding	6.3 % (5.7–7.0)	2.4 % (1.1–4.6)
Cardiopulmonary complication	19.1 % (18.0–20.3)	28.9 % (26.2–31.8)
Mortality	1.0 % (0.7–2.2)	0.5 % (0.006–1.9)

ᵃPer 1000 colonoscopies

screening or surveillance colonoscopy report high completion rates above 95 % [30]. Studies on symptomatic patients (including those with non-traversable obstructing lesions) report completion rates of around 83 % [31].

Colonoscopy in the elderly is technically more challenging than in younger patients because of various factors, including more extensive colonic diverticulosis, higher incidence of tortuosity or post-surgical adhesions, and higher risk of complications [3]. Elderly patients are also less likely to tolerate large amounts of sedation, and have a higher probability of suffering inadequate bowel preparation [18, 32], both of which can preclude the possibility of complete colonoscopy.

A wide range of completion rates have been reported, including only 56 % (this included 8 obstructing lesions that could not be traversed) [14], 63 % (on the first attempt) or 89 % (second attempt) [8], 83.5 % [18], and as high as 88.1 % (for patients >73 years old) [32]. For patients over 65, the completion rate was quite respectable at 90.3 % in one study [20]. Overall, a meta-analysis showed that for elderly patients >65 years of age, the mean completion rate was 84 %, while for those >80, the completion rate was 84.7 % [22]. Many of the studies that directly compared completion rates between elderly patients and younger controls showed a significant difference in favor of the younger group [20, 33].

Bowel Preparation Issues

In a previous meta-analysis of 20 studies, suboptimal bowel preparation was documented in 18.8 % of patients >65 years of age, and in 12.1 % of those >80. As summarized in Fig. 12.1, elderly patients have a higher likelihood of poor bowel preparation due to slower colonic transit and higher incidence of obstipation [3, 36]. Inadequate bowel preparation was a big factor in many studies that demonstrated lower colonoscopy completion rates in older patients [18, 32]. The most commonly used bowel preparation regimen, 4 l of pegylated ethylene glycol, represents a substantial volume for ingestion in elderly patients, who are also more likely to have renal, cardiac, or hepatic conditions that make them ineligible for small volume alternative osmotic laxatives, such as sodium sulfate or sodium picosulfate. Moreover, frequent trips to the commode constitute a fall risk for the frail elderly patient with mobility issues.

Decision Analyses

Some decision analysis studies have addressed the costs, risks, and benefits of colonoscopy in elderly patients. The potential for screening-related complications was greater than estimated benefit in some population subgroups aged 70 years and older. At all ages and life expectancies, the potential reduction in mortality from screening outweighed the risk of colonoscopy-related death [37]. In another study, a patient with no familial risk factors with negative colonoscopy at age 50, 60, or 70 is less likely to benefit from additional screening colonoscopy compared to a 75-year-old individual with no antecedent screening. Furthermore, an individual in superb health at age 80 may benefit from colonoscopy whereas a patient with prior low risk adenomas but moderate to severe health impairment is unlikely to benefit from colonoscopy even at an age below 75. Investments in screening and polypectomy in younger persons may decrease CRC-related costs, including screening and surveillance, for healthcare payers for older Americans, including Medicare. While these savings could potentially be offset by future health costs for other diseases, screening may still be cost-effective [38].

Equipment and Logistical Issues

Colonoscopes and accessories are the same for elderly patients as their younger counterparts, although some endoscopists favor pediatric colonoscopes because the more flexible shaft can facilitate passage in the presence of tortuosity or diverticulosis. All patients undergoing sedation need an adult escort after the procedure, potentially posing a burden on some elderly individuals who live in social isolation.

Overview: Screening Colonoscopy in Elderly Patients

In the absence of additional risk factors such as family history, the prevailing consensus is to begin screening at age 50 and continue at intervals determined by the screening modality used, as well as any history of adenomatous polyps or cancer. Currently, all three US gastroenterology societies (American

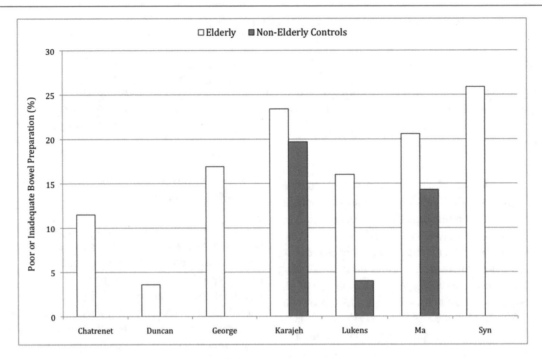

Fig. 12.1 Published studies reporting rates of poor or inadequate bowel preparation for colonoscopy in elderly patients and non-elderly controls: Chatrenet [18], Duncan [17], George [34], Karajeh [16], Lukens [35], Ma [23], and Syn [14]

Gastroenterological Association, American Society of Gastrointestinal Endoscopy, and American College of Gastroenterology), the American Cancer Society and the United States Preventive Services Task Force (USPSTF) have endorsed screening colonoscopy beginning at age 50 for average-risk patients, with subsequent intervals of every 10 years in the absence of any personal history of adenomas or family history of CRC [39–42]. However, the USPSTF is the only body to have formalized the recommendation to discontinue screening in low risk individuals at age 75 [42]. In a publication on colonoscopy created by the American Gastroenterological Association for the American College of Physicians "Choosing Wisely" Campaign, it is stated that "routine [colonoscopies] usually aren't needed after age 75."

There is concern that repeated screening into advanced age is associated with diminishing utility and increasing costs. Life expectancy in light of advanced age and comorbidities should be considered when considering screening in very elderly persons. Screening may not be warranted in asymptomatic patients for whom detecting and removing precancerous polyps would be unlikely to change their long term survival. Moreover, elderly patients who have been screened often incur frequent early repeat colonoscopies, leading to further risks, morbidity, and costs [43].

In a previous study using Declining Exponential Approximation of Life Expectancy (DEALE) analysis, we found that the prevalence of neoplasia was 13.8% in 50- to 54-year-old patients, 26.5% in the 75- to 79-year-old group, and 28.6% in the group aged 80 years or older. Despite higher prevalence of neoplasia in elderly patients, mean extension in life expectancy

was much lower in the group aged 80 years or older than in the 50- to 54-year-old group (0.13 versus 0.85 years). Even though prevalence of neoplasia increases with age, screening colonoscopy in very elderly persons (aged ≥ 80 years) results in only 15% of the expected gain in life expectancy in younger patients (Table 12.3) [44]. In a similar study, the survival of elderly patients undergoing colonoscopy was significantly lower than that for younger patients, with important screening implications [45]. Another decision analysis also showed that the benefits of screening were outweighed by screening-related complication risks in subgroups of patients over 75, especially if they were in poor health [37]. Surveys have shown that providers incorporate age and comorbidity in screening recommendations; however, their recommendations were often inconsistent with guidelines [46]. Other factors come into play when screening decisions are made; for example, elderly patients of low socioeconomic class were less likely to be screened for CRC regardless of insurance status [47].

Overview: Diagnostic Colonoscopy in Elderly Patients

Some conditions, such as constipation, incontinence, diverticulosis, and hemorrhoids, are more common with advancing age. CRC is much more common in symptomatic patients over 65 than in younger patients, with a risk ratio as high as 17 [34, 35, 48]. In all patients with colorectal symptoms, colonoscopy is usually the preferred diagnostic test for whole colon evaluation and has supplanted barium enemas and sigmoidoscopy. Direct

Table 12.3 Outcomes for 1244 individuals who underwent screening colonoscopy; classification is according to the most advanced lesion for each patient [44]

Age group (years)	N	Patients with advanced neoplasia (%)	Mean life expectancy (years)	Mean polyp lag time[a] (years)	Mean $LE_{extension}$ (years)	Adjusted mean $LE_{extension}$ (%)
50–54	1034	33[b] (3.2)	28.87	5.23	0.85	2.94
75–79	147	7 (4.7)	10.37	5.44	0.17	1.64
80+	63	9[c] (14)	7.59	3.58	0.13	1.71

$LE_{extension}$: Extension of life expectancy due to screening colonoscopy
Adjusted $LE_{extension}$ (%) = ($LE_{extension}$/LE) × 100
[a]These values are calculated only for patients with neoplastic findings, not the entire group
[b]Includes one patient with high-grade dysplasia and two patients with cancers
[c]Includes two patients with high-grade dysplastic polyps and one with cancer

visualization of the colonic mucosa can be extremely useful for diagnosis of colitis and confirmation of polyps or masses. Of course, colonoscopy also allows for histologic assessment through biopsies. Certainly any elderly patient without prior colonoscopy who presents with new colorectal symptoms should be offered diagnostic colonoscopy.

One of the most common colorectal symptoms leading to hospitalization is lower gastrointestinal bleeding. With advancing age there is an increased incidence of bleeding from diverticulosis, arteriovenous malformations, malignancy, ischemic colitis, radiation colitis, and ano-rectal lesions. When feasible, colonoscopy is the best diagnostic test and may offer therapeutic options. In elderly patients, completing a 4 l polyethylene glycol preparation can be difficult and time-consuming; it sometimes requires placement of a nasogastric tube. As an alternative diagnostic modality, the technetium red blood cell scan can localize active bleeding, while angiography is another diagnostic option, and like colonoscopy offers therapeutic possibilities.

Overview: Therapeutic Colonoscopy in Elderly Patients

Colonoscopy offers a variety of therapeutic options to control bleeding, remove polyps and small tumors, and relieve colonic obstructions caused by benign or malignant strictures; these maneuvers are especially useful in elderly patients because they may obviate the need for surgery.

For bleeding patients, endoscopic hemostasis can be achieved using injection of epinephrine, thermal or electrocoagulation, or deployment of clips. Polypectomy is performed in the same manner independent of age, i.e. small polyps are removed with cold snare polypectomy or biopsy forceps, larger polyps are removed with snare polypectomy with monopolar coagulation, and flat or sessile polyps are removed after saline submucosal injection, perhaps supplemented by argon plasma coagulation. With advancing age, large and flat polyps are more common. Benign colonic strictures may be

seen in patients with a surgical anastomosis, or in the presence of chronic ischemic colitis, inflammatory bowel disease, or diverticulitis. In such patients, endoscopic dilation can be attempted under fluoroscopic observation. Malignant strictures are at greater risk of perforation with dilation. In selected patients with colonic malignancy who are not surgical candidates or need preoperative decompression, permanent self-expanding stents can be placed across the obstruction.

Summary

Colonoscopy in very elderly patients (over 80 years of age) carries a greater risk of complications, adverse events, and morbidity than in younger patients, and is associated with lower completion rates and higher chance of poor bowel preparation. Although colonoscopic yield increases with age, several studies have suggested that the potential benefits are significantly decreased because of shorter life expectancy and greater prevalence of comorbidities. Thus, screening colonoscopy in very elderly patients should be performed only after careful consideration of potential benefits, risks, and patient preferences. Diagnostic and therapeutic colonoscopy are more likely to benefit even very elderly patients, and in most cases should be performed if indicated.

Key Points

- Diagnostic, screening, and surveillance colonoscopy are important tools in the care of elderly patients.
- Colonoscopic yield generally increases with age.
- Colonoscopy in very elderly patients carries a greater risk of complications, adverse events, and morbidity than in younger patients.
- Colonoscopy in very elderly patients is associated with lower completion rates and higher chance of poor bowel preparation.

- The potential benefits are also decreased because of shorter life expectancy and greater prevalence of comorbidities.
- Screening colonoscopy in very elderly patients should be performed only after careful consideration of potential benefits, risks, and patient preferences.
- Diagnostic and therapeutic colonoscopy are more likely to benefit even very elderly patients, and in most cases should be performed if indicated.

Conflicts of Interest and Disclaimers None.

References

1. Zauber AG, Winawer SJ, O'Brien MJ, et al. Colonoscopic polypectomy and long-term prevention of colorectal-cancer deaths. N Engl J Med. 2012;366:687–96.
2. Harewood GC, Lieberman DA. Colonoscopy practice patterns since introduction of medicare coverage for average-risk screening. Clin Gastroenterol Hepatol. 2004;2:72–7.
3. Loffeld RJ, Liberov B, Dekkers PE. Yearly diagnostic yield of colonoscopy in patients age 80 years or older, with a special interest in colorectal cancer. Geriatr Gerontol Int. 2012;12:298–303.
4. Day LW, Walter LC, Velayos F. Colorectal cancer screening and surveillance in the elderly patient. Am J Gastroenterol 2011;106:1197–206;quiz 207.
5. Harewood GC, Lawlor GO, Larson MV. Incident rates of colonic neoplasia in older patients: when should we stop screening? J Gastroenterol Hepatol. 2006;21:1021–5.
6. Jemal A, Clegg LX, Ward E, et al. Annual report to the nation on the status of cancer, 1975–2001, with a special feature regarding survival. Cancer. 2004;101:3–27.
7. Smoot DT, Collins J, Dunlap S, et al. Outcome of colonoscopy in elderly African-American patients. Dig Dis Sci. 2009;54:2484–7.
8. Bat L, Pines A, Shemesh E, et al. Colonoscopy in patients aged 80 years or older and its contribution to the evaluation of rectal bleeding. Postgrad Med J. 1992;68:355–8.
9. Ure T, Dehghan K, Vernava 3rd AM, Longo WE, Andrus CA, Daniel GL. Colonoscopy in the elderly. Low risk, high yield. Surg Endosc. 1995;9:505–8.
10. Sardinha TC, Nogueras JJ, Ehrenpreis ED, et al. Colonoscopy in octogenarians: a review of 428 cases. Int J Colorectal Dis. 1999;14:172–6.
11. Clarke GA, Jacobson BC, Hammett RJ, Carr-Locke DL. The indications, utilization and safety of gastrointestinal endoscopy in an extremely elderly patient cohort. Endoscopy. 2001;33:580–4.
12. Lagares-Garcia JA, Kurek S, Collier B, et al. Colonoscopy in octogenarians and older patients. Surg Endosc. 2001;15:262–5. Epub 2000 Dec 12.
13. Arora A, Singh P. Colonoscopy in patients 80 years of age and older is safe, with high success rate and diagnostic yield. Gastrointest Endosc. 2004;60:408–13.
14. Syn WK, Tandon U, Ahmed MM. Colonoscopy in the very elderly is safe and worthwhile. Age Ageing. 2005;34:510–3.
15. Yoong KK, Heymann T. Colonoscopy in the very old: why bother? Postgrad Med J. 2005;81:196–7.
16. Karajeh MA, Sanders DS, Hurlstone DP. Colonoscopy in elderly people is a safe procedure with a high diagnostic yield: a prospective comparative study of 2000 patients. Endoscopy. 2006;38:226–30.
17. Duncan JE, Sweeney WB, Trudel JL, Madoff RD, Mellgren AF. Colonoscopy in the elderly: low risk, low yield in asymptomatic patients. Dis Colon Rectum. 2006;49:646–51.
18. Chatrenet P, Friocourt P, Ramain JP, Cherrier M, Maillard JB. Colonoscopy in the elderly: a study of 200 cases. Eur J Med. 1993;2:411–3.
19. Stevens T, Burke CA. Colonoscopy screening in the elderly: when to stop? Am J Gastroenterol. 2003;98:1881–5.
20. Akhtar AJ, Padda MS. Safety and efficacy of colonoscopy in the elderly: experience in an innercity community hospital serving African American and Hispanic patients. Ethn Dis. 2011;21:412–4.
21. DiPrima RE, Barkin JS, Blinder M, Goldberg RI, Phillips RS. Age as a risk factor in colonoscopy: fact versus fiction. Am J Gastroenterol. 1988;83:123–5.
22. Day LW, Kwon A, Inadomi JM, Walter LC, Somsouk M. Adverse events in older patients undergoing colonoscopy: a systematic review and meta-analysis. Gastrointest Endosc. 2011;74:885–96.
23. Ma WT, Mahadeva S, Kunanayagam S, Poi PJ, Goh KL. Colonoscopy in elderly Asians: a prospective evaluation in routine clinical practice. J Dig Dis. 2007;8:77–81.
24. Zerey M, Paton BL, Khan PD, et al. Colonoscopy in the very elderly: a review of 157 cases. Surg Endosc. 2007;21:1806–9.
25. Martinez JF, Aparicio JR, Company L, et al. Safety of continuous propofol sedation for endoscopic procedures in elderly patients. Rev Esp Enferm Dig. 2011;103:76–82.
26. Warren JL, Klabunde CN, Mariotto AB, et al. Adverse events after outpatient colonoscopy in the Medicare population. Ann Intern Med. 2009;150:849–57. W152.
27. Tsutsumi S, Fukushima H, Osaki K, Kuwano H. Feasibility of colonoscopy in patients 80 years of age and older. Hepatogastroenterology. 2007;54:1959–61.
28. Heuss LT, Schnieper P, Drewe J, Pflimlin E, Beglinger C. Conscious sedation with propofol in elderly patients: a prospective evaluation. Aliment Pharmacol Ther. 2003;17:1493–501.
29. Niehaus M, Tebbenjohanns J. Electromagnetic interference in patients with implanted pacemakers or cardioverter-defibrillators. Heart. 2001;86:246–8.
30. Nelson DB, McQuaid KR, Bond JH, Lieberman DA, Weiss DG, Johnston TK. Procedural success and complications of large-scale screening colonoscopy. Gastrointest Endosc. 2002;55:307–14.
31. Loffeld RJ, van der Putten AB. The completion rate of colonoscopy in normal daily practice: factors associated with failure. Digestion. 2009;80:267–70.
32. Cardin F, Andreotti A, Martella B, Terranova C, Militello C. Current practice in colonoscopy in the elderly. Aging Clin Exp Res. 2012;24:9–13.
33. Houissa F, Kchir H, Bouzaidi S, et al. Colonoscopy in elderly: feasibility, tolerance and indications: about 901 cases. Tunis Med. 2011;89:848–52.
34. George ML, Tutton MG, Jadhav VV, Abulafi AM, Swift RI. Colonoscopy in older patients: a safe and sound practice. Age Ageing. 2002;31:80–1.
35. Lukens FJ, Loeb DS, Machicao VI, Achem SR, Picco MF. Colonoscopy in octogenarians: a prospective outpatient study. Am J Gastroenterol. 2002;97:1722–5.
36. Jafri SM, Monkemuller K, Lukens FJ. Endoscopy in the elderly: a review of the efficacy and safety of colonoscopy, esophagogastroduodenoscopy, and endoscopic retrograde cholangiopancreatography. J Clin Gastroenterol. 2010;44:161–6.
37. Ko CW, Sonnenberg A. Comparing risks and benefits of colorectal cancer screening in elderly patients. Gastroenterology. 2005;129:1163–70.
38. Ladabaum U, Phillips KA. Colorectal cancer screening differential costs for younger versus older Americans. Am J Prev Med. 2006;30:378–84.
39. Levin B, Lieberman DA, McFarland B, et al. Screening and surveillance for the early detection of colorectal cancer and adenomatous polyps, 2008: a joint guideline from the American Cancer Society, the US Multi-Society Task Force on Colorectal Cancer, and the American College of Radiology. Gastroenterology. 2008;134:1570–95.

40. Rex DK, Johnson DA, Anderson JC, Schoenfeld PS, Burke CA, Inadomi JM. American College of Gastroenterology guidelines for colorectal cancer screening 2008. Am J Gastroenterol. 2009;104: 739–50.

41. Davila RE, Rajan E, Baron TH, et al. ASGE guideline: colorectal cancer screening and surveillance. Gastrointest Endosc. 2006;63:546–57.

42. Screening for colorectal cancer: U.S. Preventive Services Task Force recommendation statement. Ann Intern Med 2008;149:627–37.

43. Richards RJ, Crystal S. The frequency of early repeat tests after colonoscopy in elderly medicare recipients. Dig Dis Sci. 2010; 55:421–31.

44. Lin OS, Kozarek RA, Schembre DB, et al. Screening colonoscopy in very elderly patients: prevalence of neoplasia and estimated impact on life expectancy. JAMA. 2006;295:2357–65.

45. Kahi CJ, Azzouz F, Juliar BE, Imperiale TF. Survival of elderly persons undergoing colonoscopy: implications for colorectal cancer screening and surveillance. Gastrointest Endosc. 2007;66: 544–50.

46. Kahi CJ, van Ryn M, Juliar B, Stuart JS, Imperiale TF. Provider recommendations for colorectal cancer screening in elderly veterans. J Gen Intern Med. 2009;24:1263–8.

47. Koroukian SM, Xu F, Dor A, Cooper GS. Colorectal cancer screening in the elderly population: disparities by dual Medicare-Medicaid enrollment status. Health Serv Res. 2006;41: 2136–54.

48. DeCosse JJ, Tsioulias GJ, Jacobson JS. Colorectal cancer: detection, treatment, and rehabilitation. CA Cancer J Clin. 1994;44: 27–42.

Part III

Urologic/Urogynecoloic Aspects

Treatment Options for Stress Urinary Incontinence

Dudley Robinson and Linda Cardozo

Introduction

Urinary incontinence is a common and distressing condition which, although not life threatening, is known to have a significant effect on quality of life (QoL). The incidence of urinary incontinence increases with age and whilst SUI is more common in younger women many elderly women also complain of troublesome symptoms. With an increasingly elderly population urinary incontinence represents a significant burden on both primary and secondary healthcare and the incidence of SUI is likely to increase with increasing activity levels in this age group.

The term SUI may be used to describe the symptom or sign of urinary leakage on coughing or exertion but should not be regarded as a diagnosis. A diagnosis of (USI) may only be made after urodynamic investigation and this is defined as the involuntary leakage of urine during increased abdominal pressure in the absence of a detrusor contraction [1].

Epidemiology

A large epidemiological study of urinary incontinence has been reported in 27,936 women from Norway [2]. Overall 25 % of women reported urinary incontinence although only 7 % felt their symptoms to be significant. In addition the prevalence of incontinence was found to increase with age. When considering the type of incontinence 50 % of women complained of stress, 11 % urge and 36 % mixed incontinence.

D. Robinson • L. Cardozo (✉)
Department of Urogynaecology, Kings College Hospital,
Denmark Hill, London, UK
e-mail: Linda@lindacardozo.co.uk

A further analysis has also investigated the effect of age and parity on urinary incontinence. The prevalence among nulliparous women ranged from 8 to 32 % and increased with age. In general parity was associated with incontinence and the first delivery was found to be the most significant. The relative risk of SUI was 2.7 (95 %CI: 2.0–3.5) in the age group 20–34 years for primiparous women and 4.0 (95 %CI: 2.5–6.4) for multiparous women. There was a similar association for mixed incontinence although not for urge incontinence [3]. The authors concluded that parity was an important risk factor in younger women although this association was noted to disappear with age.

Pathophysiology

There are many different causes of SUI (Table 13.1) although when considering the pathophysiology the two commonest mechanisms are urethral hypermobility and intrinsic sphincter deficiency. Whilst the former is caused by a weakness in the pelvic floor musculature, pelvic fascia and pubourethral ligaments the latter is caused by pudendal nerve injury and subsequent damage to the intrinsic and extrinsic urethral sphincter.

The bladder neck and proximal urethra are normally situated in an intra-abdominal position above the pelvic floor and are supported by the pubourethral ligaments. Damage to either the pelvic floor musculature (levator ani) or pubourethral ligaments may result in descent of the proximal urethra such that it is no longer an intra-abdominal organ and this results in leakage of urine per urethram during physical stress.

More recently the 'integral theory' has been described by Petros and Ulmsten [4]. This hypothesis is based on previous studies which demonstrated that the distal and mid-urethra play an important role in the continence mechanism [5] and that the maximal urethral closure pressure is at the mid-urethral point [6]. This theory proposes that damage to the pubourethral ligaments supporting the urethra, impaired

© Springer Science+Business Media New York 2017
D.A. Gordon, M.R. Katlic (eds.), *Pelvic Floor Dysfunction and Pelvic Surgery in the Elderly*,
DOI 10.1007/978-1-4939-6554-0_13

Table 13.1 Causes of SUI

Urethral hypermobility
Urogenital prolapse
Pelvic floor damage or denervation
Parturition
Pelvic surgery
Menopause
Urethral scarring
Vaginal (urethral) surgery
Incontinence surgery
Urethral dilatation or urethrotomy
Recurrent urinary tract infections
Radiotherapy
Raised intra-abdominal pressure
Pregnancy
Chronic cough (bronchitis)
Abdominal/pelvic mass
Faecal impaction/constipation
Ascites
Obesity

support of the anterior vaginal wall to the mid-urethra, and weakened function of part of the pubococcygeal muscles, which insert adjacent to the urethra, are responsible for causing SUI.

Clinical Presentation

Women commonly complain of a multitude of lower urinary tract symptoms and these may be grouped into storage and voiding symptoms. Storage symptoms include frequency, urgency and nocturia in addition to stress and urgency incontinence. Voiding symptoms are less common in women and include hesitancy, poor stream and incomplete emptying, although may also be associated with symptoms of incontinence secondary to retention and overflow. Co-morbidities and polypharmacy are common in the elderly and some drugs are known to affect lower urinary tract function including diuretics, calcium antagonists, anti-depressants and α adrenergic antagonists. Consequently a thorough history and review of medication should be performed in all patients.

Clinical Signs

Whilst there are no specific clinical signs in women with urinary incontinence demonstrable urinary leakage may be noted as well as vulval excoriation and urogenital atrophy. A pelvic examination is also important to exclude the presence of urogenital prolapse, uterine fibroids or a pelvic mass, all of which may cause storage symptoms and incontinence.

In addition storage symptoms may also be associated with neurological conditions and therefore a basic neurological examination should be performed.

Investigations

Whilst many women with urinary incontinence may be managed initially with conservative measures all patients require a basic assessment in order to confirm the diagnosis as well as excluding any other underlying causes for lower urinary tract dysfunction (Fig. 13.1).

Urine Culture

A urinalysis should be performed and, if abnormal, a midstream specimen of urine (MSU) should be sent for microscopy, culture and sensitivity to exclude lower urinary tract infection.

Post Micturition Urinary Residual

Voiding difficulties may present with symptoms of frequency and urgency in addition to the symptoms of SUI. Clinical examination is only useful in excluding large urinary residuals and therefore a post micturition ultrasound of the bladder, or catheterisation, should be performed to exclude a chronic urinary residual.

Bladder Diary

All patients should complete a bladder diary in order to evaluate their fluid intake, voiding pattern and incontinence episodes. In addition to the number of voids and incontinence episodes, the mean volume voided over a 24-h period can also be calculated as well as the diurnal and nocturnal volumes. Analysis of bladder diaries is helpful both in making a diagnosis and also in monitoring progress with treatment.

Investigation in Secondary Care

Although many women complaining of urinary incontinence may be managed effectively in primary care on the basis of simple investigations alone, those women who complain of unusual or complex symptoms may benefit from further investigation (Fig. 13.2). In addition those women whose symptoms fail to improve with primary therapy may also benefit from further investigations to exclude other causes of lower urinary tract symptoms. Assessment in secondary care may involve urodynamic investigation and cystourethroscopy.

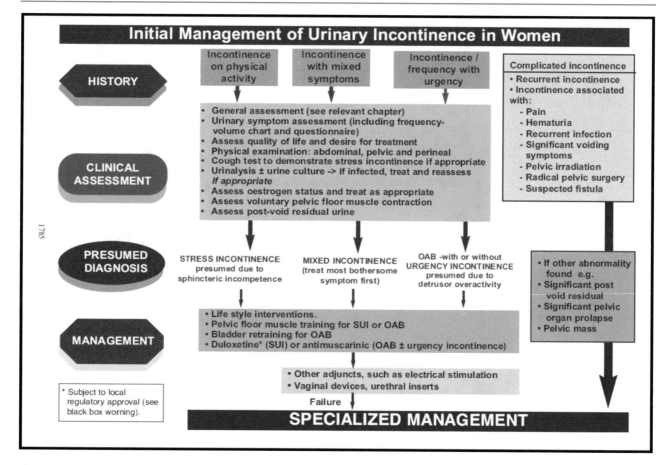

Fig. 13.1 Initial assessment of urinary incontinence (ICI Guidelines 2013) [7]

Whilst the diagnosis of urinary incontinence in primary care is subjective and based on symptoms alone further investigation in the secondary care setting allows a more objective urodynamic based diagnosis to be made.

Urodynamic Investigation

Urodynamics is the term used to describe lower urinary tract investigations that measure the ability of the bladder to store and expel urine. Urodynamic investigations include uroflowmetry, filling cystometry and pressure/flow voiding studies. Further investigation allows a urodynamic diagnosis to be made and, based on this, further management.

Cystourethroscopy

Although cystoscopy is not helpful in diagnosing USI, it may be used to exclude other causes for lower urinary tract symptoms such as a bladder tumour or calculus. In addition cystourethroscopy should be considered for all women complaining of the 'red flag' symptoms of haematuria, painful bladder syndrome and recurrent or continuous incontinence (Fig. 13.2).

Pad Test

A pad test may be used to document or confirm urinary incontinence although it is unable to distinguish between the types of incontinence. The test involves wearing a pre-weighed incontinence pad which is weighed before and after use. The difference in weight corresponds to the volume of urine lost. Both short- (1 h) and long-term pad tests (24–48 h) have been described although reliability has been shown to be greater for the longer term tests [7].

Quality of Life

Quality of Life (QoL) is assessed by the use of questionnaires completed by the patient alone or as part of the consultation and is useful to assess morbidity caused by urinary incontinence as well as evaluating treatment efficacy.

Generic questionnaires, such as the Short Form 36 [8], are general measures of QoL and are therefore applicable to a wide range of populations and clinical conditions whilst disease-specific questionnaires, such as the Kings Health Questionnaire (KHQ) [9] are designed to focus on lower urinary tract symptoms.

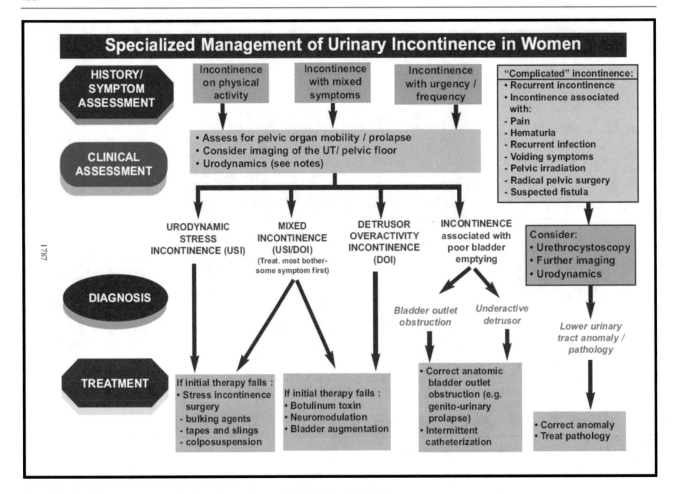

Fig. 13.2 Specialised assessment of urinary incontinence (ICI Guidelines 2013) [7]

Conservative Management

All women with urinary incontinence benefit from advice regarding simple lifestyle changes which they can use to help improve their symptoms. Often patients may drink too much and, if they complain of urinary symptoms, they should be told to reduce their fluid intake to between 1 and 1.5 l per day [10] and to avoid tea, coffee and alcohol. In addition there is also increasing evidence to suggest that weight loss may improve symptoms of urinary incontinence [11] in those who are overweight.

Pelvic Floor Muscle Training

Pelvic floor muscle training (PFMT) remains integral in the management of women with stress urinary incontinence with level 1, grade A evidence from five prospective randomized controlled trials with short-term cure rates between 35 and 80 % [12]. Supervised training is generally felt to be

more effective than unsupervised training [13] although benefits of biofeedback and electrical stimulation are less clear [14]. Consequently the International Consultation on Incontinence (ICI) [15] recommends that bladder retraining should be considered as first line treatment in all women with SUI.

Medical Management

Whilst historically several different drugs have been used anecdotally for the management of SUI duloxetine, a potent and balanced serotonin (5-hydroxytryptamine) and noradrenaline reuptake inhibitor (SNRI) is the only drug licensed for this indication and works by improving urethral striated sphincter activity via a centrally mediated pathway [16]. Duloxetine has been shown to be effective in the management of SUI and has demonstrated a reduction in incontinence episode frequency and a corresponding improvement in QoL [17] although nausea is a common side effect occurring in 25 % of women. Duloxetine has been shown to act synergistically with PFMT [18] and may also be useful in those women considering continence surgery [19].

Surgical Management

Many women who complain of symptomatic SUI and are found to have urodynamic stress incontinence (USI) following investigation, will require continence surgery. Whilst retropubic suspension procedures such as colposuspension and the Marshall–Marchetti–Krantz procedure have historically been shown to be associated with high cure rates and low complication rates more recently the description of the integral theory has led to the development of mid-urethral tape procedures which has revolutionised continence surgery.

Marshall–Marchetti–Krantz

The Marshall–Marchetti–Krantz [20] procedure is a suprapubic operation in which the paraurethral tissue at the level of the bladder neck is sutured to the periosteum and/or perichondrium of the posterior aspect of the pubic symphysis. This procedure elevates the bladder neck but will not correct any concomitant cystocele. It has been largely superseded by the Burch colposuspension because its complications include osteitis pubis in 2–7 % of cases.

Colposuspension

The Burch colposuspension has been modified by many authors, since its original description in 1961 [21] [Fig. 13.3]. Until relatively recently colposuspension has been the operation of choice in primary USI as it corrects both stress incontinence and a cystocele. However, it may not be suitable if the vagina is scarred or narrowed by previous surgery.

Whilst the colposuspension is now well recognised as an effective procedure for USI it is not without complications. Detrusor overactivity may occur de novo or may be unmasked by the procedure [22] and this may lead to long-term urinary symptoms. Voiding difficulties are common postoperatively and, although they usually resolve within a short time after the operation, long-term voiding dysfunction may result. In addition, a rectoenterocele may be exacerbated by repositioning the vagina [23]. However, the colposuspension is one of the few continence operations for which long-term data are available. Alcalay et al. [24] have reported a series of 109 women with an overall cure rate of 69 % at a mean of 13.8 years.

Bladder Neck Suspension Procedures

Endoscopically guided bladder neck suspensions [25–27] are simple to perform but are less effective than open suprapubic procedures and are now seldom used having been largely replaced by mid-urethral tape procedures. In all these operations a long needle is used to insert a loop of nylon on each side of the bladder neck; this is tied over the rectus sheath to elevate the urethrovesical junction. Cystoscopy is employed to ensure accurate placement of the sutures and to detect any damage to the bladder caused by the needle or the suture. In the Stamey procedure buffers are used to avoid the sutures cutting through the tissues, and in the Raz procedure a helical suture of Prolene is inserted deep into the endopelvic fascia lateral to the bladder neck to avoid cutting through. The main problem with all these operations is that they rely on two sutures and these may break or pull through the tissues. However, endoscopically guided bladder neck suspensions are quick and easy to perform. They

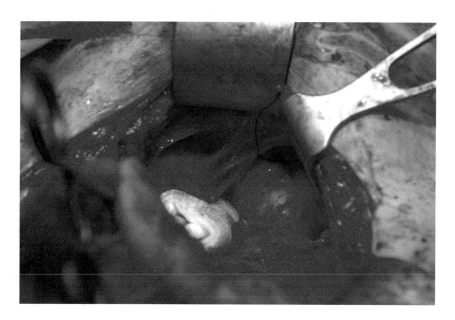

Fig. 13.3 Colposuspension: The bladder has been reflected medially and the first suture is placed in the paravaginal tissue

can be carried out under regional block and postoperative recovery is fast. Temporary voiding difficulties are common after long needle suspensions but these usually resolve and there are few other complications.

Laparoscopic Colposuspension

Minimally invasive surgery is attractive and this trend has extended to surgery for SUI. Although many authors have reported excellent short-term subjective results from laparoscopic colposuspension [28], early studies have shown inferior results to the open procedure [29].

More recently two large prospective randomised controlled trials have been reported from Australia and the United Kingdom comparing laparoscopic and open colposuspension. In the Australian study 200 women with USI were randomised to either laparoscopic or open colposuspension [30]. Overall there were no significant differences in objective and subjective measures of cure or in patient satisfaction at 6 months, 24 months or 3–5 years. Whilst the laparoscopic approach took longer (87 versus 42 min; $p<0.0001$) it was associated with less blood loss ($p=0.03$) and a quicker return to normal activities ($p=0.01$).

These findings are supported by the UK multicentre randomised controlled trial of 291 women with USI comparing laparoscopic to open colposuspension [31]. At 24 months intention to treat analysis showed no significant difference in cure rates between the procedures. Objective cure rates for open and laparoscopic colposuspension were 70.1 % and 79.7 %, respectively, whilst subjective cure rates were 54.6 % and 54.9 %, respectively.

These studies have confirmed that the clinical effectiveness of the two operations is comparable although the cost effectiveness of laparoscopic colposuspension remains unproven. A cost analysis comparing laparoscopic to open colposuspension was also performed alongside the UK study [32]. Healthcare resource use over the first six month follow-up period translated into costs of £1805 for the laparoscopic group versus £1433 for the open group.

Pubovaginal Sling

Sling procedures are often performed as secondary operations where there is scarring and narrowing of the vagina. The sling material can either be organic (rectus fascia, porcine dermis) or inorganic (Prolene, Mersilene, Marlex or Silastic). The sling may be inserted either abdominally, vaginally or by a combination of both. Normally the sling is used to elevate and support the bladder neck and proximal urethra, but not intentionally to obstruct it.

Sling procedures may be associated with a high incidence of side effects and complications. It is often difficult to decide how tight to make the sling. If it is too loose, incontinence will persist and if it is too tight, voiding difficulties may be permanent. Women who are going to undergo insertion of a sling must be prepared to perform clean intermittent self-catheterization postoperatively. In addition, there is a risk of infection, especially if inorganic material is used. The sling may erode into the urethra, bladder or vagina, in which case it must be removed and this can be exceedingly difficult.

Fig. 13.4 Tension free vaginal tape (TVT)

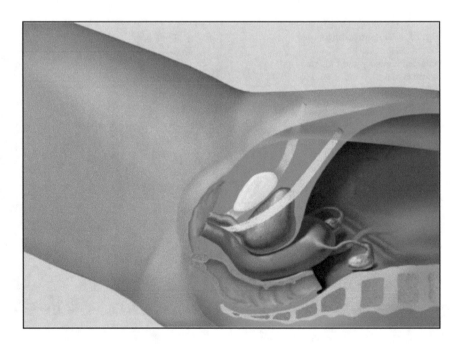

Retropubic Mid-Urethral Tape Procedures

The tension free vaginal tape (TVT) (Fig. 13.4) is a retropubic mid-urethral tape that was first described by Ulmsten et al. [33] and is now the most commonly performed continence procedure in the UK. A knitted 11 mm × 40 cm polypropylene mesh tape is inserted trans-vaginally at the level of the mid-urethra, using two 5 mm trocars. The procedure may be performed under local, spinal or general anaesthesia. Most women can go home the same day, although some do require catheterisation for short-term voiding difficulties.

Long-term efficacy data are supported by objective success rates of 90 % at 17-year follow-up [34] and the procedure has also been compared to open colposuspension in a multicentre prospective randomised trial of 344 women with USI [35]. Overall there was no significant difference in terms of objective cure; 66 % in the TVT group and 57 % in the colposuspension group. However, operation time, postoperative stay and return to normal activity were all longer in the colposuspension arm. Analysis of the long-term results at 24 months using a pad test, quality of life assessment and symptom questionnaires showed an objective cure rate of 63 % in the tension free vaginal tape arm and 51 % in the colposuspension arm. At 5 years there were no differences in subjective cure (63 % in the tension free vaginal tape group and 70 % in the colposuspension group), patient satisfaction and quality of life assessment. However, whilst there was a significant reduction in cystocele in both groups there was a higher incidence of enterocele, rectocele and apical prolapse in the colposuspension group [36].

The SPARC sling system is a minimally invasive sling procedure using a knitted 10 mm wide polypropylene mesh which is placed at the level of the mid-urethra by passing the needle via a suprapubic to vaginal approach [37]. The procedure may be performed under local, regional or general anaesthetic. A prospective multicentre study of 104 women with USI has been reported from France [38]. At a mean follow-up of 11.9 months the objective cure rate was 90.4 % and subjective cure 72 %. There was a 10.5 % incidence of bladder perforation and 11.5 % of women complained of de novo urgency following the procedure. More recently SPARC has been compared to TVT in a prospective randomised trial of 301 women [39]. At short-term follow-up there were no significant differences in cure rates, bladder perforation rates and de novo urgency. There was, however, a higher incidence of voiding difficulties and vaginal erosions in the SPARC group.

Transobturator Mid-Urethral Tape Procedures

The transobturator route for the placement of synthetic mid-urethral tapes was first described in 2001 [40]. As with the retropubic sling procedures transobturator tapes may be performed under local, regional or general anaesthetic and have the theoretical advantage of eliminating some of the complications associated with the retropubic route. However, the transobturator route may be associated with damage to the obturator nerve and vessels; in an anatomical dissection model, the tape passes 3.4–4.8 cm from the anterior and posterior branches of the obturator nerve, respectively, and 1.1 cm from the most medial branch of the obturator vessels [41]. Consequently nerve and vessel injury in addition to bladder injury and vaginal erosion remain a potential complication of the procedure.

The transobturator approach may be used as an 'inside-out' (TVT-O, Gynaecare) (Fig. 13.5) or alternatively an 'outside-in' (Monarc, American Medical Systems) technique and the evidence would suggest there is no difference in terms of efficacy between the two approaches [42]. In addition long-term follow-up studies suggest that the procedure is safe and durable [43]. A meta-analysis of the five randomised trials

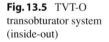

Fig. 13.5 TVT-O transobturator system (inside-out)

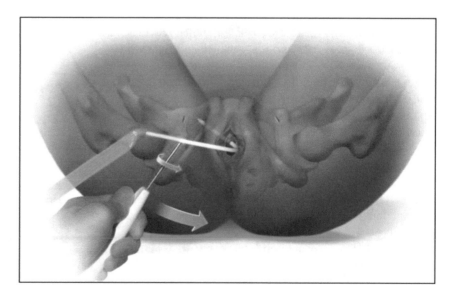

comparing TVTO with TVT and six randomised trials comparing TOT with TVT [44] suggests that overall cure rates were identical with the retropubic and transobturator routes. However, adverse events such as bladder injuries (OR 0.12; 95 % CI: 0.05–0.33) and voiding difficulties (OR 0.55; 95 % CI: 0.31–0.98) were less common, whereas groin pain (OR 8.28; 95 % CI: 2.7–25.4) and vaginal erosions (OR 1.96; 95 % CI: 0.87–4.39) were more common after the transobturator approach. These findings are also supported by a further meta-analysis comparing mid-urethral tapes with retropubic suspensions and pubovaginal sling procedures for SUI [45].

Single Incision Mid-Urethral Slings

More recently single incision mini slings have been developed as a more minimally invasive approach to managing SUI in the out-patient setting. Whilst there is an increasing evidence base to support their use at present there is a paucity of long-term efficacy data. A systematic review and meta-analysis has compared single incision tapes with mid-urethral tapes in nine randomised controlled trials in 758 women [46]. Overall the single incision tapes were associated with significantly lower patient reported and objective cure rates (RR 0.83; 95 %CI; 0.70–0.99 and RR 0.85; 95 %CI 0.74–0.97, respectively) although there was no difference in QoL improvement. Consequently, whilst the single incision mini tapes may offer a minimally invasive alternative to standard mid-urethral tapes current evidence would suggest that efficacy may be inferior and further long-term studies are required.

Urethral Bulking Agents

Urethral bulking agents are a minimally invasive surgical procedure for the treatment of USI inence and may be useful in the elderly and in those women with failed previous continence surgery and intrinsic sphincter deficiency. There are several different agents currently available (Macroplastique, Uroplasty; Bulkamid, Contura) and, whilst all tend to have lower efficacy than mid-urethral tape procedures [47], they may be performed under local anaesthesia in the clinic setting and are associated with lower morbidity. Macroplastique has previously been compared to collagen in a North American study of 248 women with USI ontinence. Outcome was assessed objectively using pad tests and subjectively at 12 months. Overall objective cure and improvement rates favoured Macroplastique over collagen (74 versus 65 %; $p = 0.13$). Whilst this difference was not significant subjective cure rates were higher in the Macroplastique group (41 versus 29 %; $p = 0.07$) [48].

Whilst success rates with urethral bulking agents are generally lower than those with conventional continence surgery they are minimally invasive and have lower complication rates meaning that they remain a useful alternative in selected women and also particularly in the elderly.

Conclusions

Urinary incontinence is a common condition which is known to have a significant impact on QoL. The incidence of incontinence tends to rise with increasing age and a significant number of elderly women complain of troublesome symptoms, many of which require further investigation and management.

With an increasingly aging population urinary incontinence will continue to have a major impact on the provision of healthcare both in the community and in secondary care. Whilst historically many women have regarded urinary symptoms to be common following childbirth, and part of the natural aging process, significant advances in the field of urogynaecology and urology have altered the perceptions of clinicians and patients. In addition, primary prevention of urinary incontinence, and patient education, will continue to be important and there is now good evidence to show that weight loss and lifestyle modifications play a significant role in the management of these women.

Whilst many women with SUI may be managed effectively based on symptoms alone in primary care those with refractory or complex symptoms benefit from further investigation in secondary care allowing a urodynamic diagnosis to be made.

All women who complain of SUI should be treated primarily with lifestyle changes and conservative measures including pelvic floor exercises. Those whose symptoms are not improved with conservative measures alone may find medical therapy with duloxetine useful in addition to pelvic floor muscle training although ultimately many women will benefit from continence surgery.

References

1. Haylen BT, de Ridder D, Freeman RM, Swift SE, Berghmans B, Lee J, Monga A, Petri P, Rizk DE, Sand PK, Schaer GN. An international urogynaecological association (IUGA)/international continence society (ICS) joint report on the terminology for female pelvic floor dysfunction. Int Urogynecol J. 2010;21:5–26.
2. Hannestad YS, Rortveit G, Sandvik H, Hunskar S. A community-based epidemiological survey of female urinary incontinence: the Norwegian EPINCONT study. Clin Epidemiol. 2000;53:1150–7.
3. Rortveit G, Hannnestad YS, Daltveit AK, Hunskaar S. Age and type dependent effects of parity on urinary incontinence: the Norwegian EPINCONT study. Obstet Gynaecol. 2001;98: 1004–10.

4. Petros P, Ulmsten U. An integral theory of female urinary incontinence. Experimental and clinical considerations. Acta Obstet Gynaecol Scand. 1990;153 Suppl:7–31.

5. Ingelman-Sundberg A. Urinary incontinence in women, excluding fistulas. Acta Obstet Gynaecol Scand. 1953;31:266–95.

6. Westbury M, Asmussen M, Ulmsten U. Location of maximal intraurethral pressure related to urogenital diaphragm in the female subject as studied by simultaneous urethra-cystometry and voiding urethrocystography. Am J Obstet Gynaecol. 1982;144:408–12.

7. Jorgensen L, Lose G, Thunedborg P. Diagnosis of mild stress incontinence in females: 24-hour pad weighing test versus the one-hour test. Neurourol Urodyn. 1987;6:165–6.

8. Lyons RA, Perry HM, Littlepage BNC. Evidence for the validity of the short form 36 questionnaire (SF-36) in an elderly population. Age Ageing. 1994;23:182–4.

9. Kelleher CJ, Cardozo LD, Khullar V, Salvatore S. A new questionnaire to assess the quality of life of urinary incontinent women. Br J Obstet Gynaecol. 1997;104:1374–9.

10. Swithinbank L, Hashim H, Abrams P. The effect of fluid intake on urinary symptoms in women. J Urol. 2005;174(1):187–9.

11. Subak LL, Wing R, West DS, Franklin F, Vittinghoff E, Creasman JM, Richter HE, Myers D, Burgio KL, Gorin AA, Macer J, Kusek JW, Grady D. PRIDE investigators weight loss to treat urinary incontinence in overweight and obese women. N Engl J Med. 2009;360(5):481–90.

12. Bo K. Pelvic Floor muscle training in treatment of female stress urinary incontinence, pelvic organ prolapse and sexual dysfunction. World J Urol. 2012;30(4):437–43.

13. Hay-Smith EJ, Herderschee R, Dumoulin C, Herbison GP. Comparisons of approaches to pelvic floor muscle training for urinary incontinence in women. Cochrane Database Syst Rev. 2011; 7:CD009508

14. Herderschee R, Hay-Smith EJ, Herbison GP, Roovers JP, Heineman MJ. Feedback or biofeedback to augment pelvic floor muscle training for urinary incontinence in women. Cochrane Database Syst Rev. 2011;7:CD009252

15. Moore K, Dumoulin C, Bradley C, Burgio K, Chambers T, Hagen S, Hunter K, Imamura M, Thakar R, Williams K, Vale L. Adult conservative management. In: Abrams P, Cardozo L, Khoury S, Wein A, editors. Incontinence. 5th ed. Health Publication, Editions 21, Paris, France; 2013. pp. 1101–228.

16. Thor KB, Katofiasc MA. Effects of Duloxetine, a combined serotonin and norepineephrine reuptake inhibitor, on central neural control of lower urinary tract function in the chloralose-anesthetised female cat. Pharmacol Exp Ther. 1995;74:1014–24.

17. Millard R, Moore K, Yalcin I, Bump R. Duloxetine vs. placebo in the treatment of stress urinary incontinence: a global phase III study. Neurourol Urodynam. 2003;22:482–3.

18. Ghoniem GM, Van Leeuwen JS, Elser DM, Freeman RM, Zhao YD, Yalcin I, Bump RC, Duloxetine/Pelvic Floor Muscle Training Clinical Trail Group. A randomised controlled trial of duloxetine alone, pelvic floor muscle training alone, combined treatment and no active treatment in women with stress urinary incontinence. J Urol. 2005;173:1647–53.

19. Cardozo L, Drutz HP, Baygani SK, Bump RC. Pharmacological treatment of women awaiting surgery for stress urinary incontinence. Obstet Gynaecol. 2004;104:511–9.

20. Marshall VF, Marchetti AA, Krantz KE. The correction of stress incontinence by simple vesicourethral suspension. Surg Gynaecol Obstet. 1949;88:509–18.

21. Burch J. Urethrovaginal fixation to Cooper's ligament for correction of stress incontinence, cystocele and prolapse. Am J Obstet Gynaecol. 1961;81:281.

22. Cardozo LD, Stanton SL, Williams JE. Detrusor instability following surgery for stress incontinence. Br J Urol. 1979;58:138–42.

23. Wiskind AK, Creighton SM, Stanton SL. The incidence of genital prolapse following the Burch colposuspension operation. Neurourol Urodyn. 1991;10:453–4.

24. Alcalay M, Monga A, Stanton SL. Burch colposuspension: 10–20 year follow-up. Br J Obstet Gynaecol. 1995;102:740–5.

25. Pereyra A. A simplified surgical procedure for the correction of stress incontinence in women. West J Surg. 1959;67:223.

26. Stamey T. Endoscopic suspension of the vesical neck for urinary incontinence. Surg Gynecol Obstet. 1973;136:547–54.

27. Raz S. Modified bladder neck suspension for female stress incontinence. Urology. 1981;17:82.

28. Liu CY. Laparoscopic retropubic colposuspension (Burch procedure): a review of 58 cases. J Reprod Med. 1993;38:526–30.

29. Burton G. A randomised comparison of laparoscopic and open colposuspension. Neurourol Urodyn. 1994;13:497–8.

30. Carey MP, Goh JT, Rosamilia A, Cornish A, Gordon I, Hawthorne G, Maher CF, Dwyer PL, Moran P, Gilmour DT. Laparoscopic versus open Burch colposuspension: a randomised controlled trial. BJOG. 2006;113:999–1006.

31. Kitchener HC, Dunn G, Lawton V, Reid F, Nelson L, Smith ARB on behalf of the COLPO study group. Laparoscopic versus open colposuspension- results of a prospective randomised controlled trial. BJOG 2006;113:1007–13.

32. Dumville JC, Manca A, Kitchener HC, Smith ARB, Nelson L, Torgerson DJ, on behalf of the COLPO study group. Cost effectiveness analysis of open colposuspension versus laparoscopic colposuspension in the treatment of urodynamic stress incontinence. BJOG. 2006;113:1014–22.

33. Ulmsten U, Henriksson L, Johnson P, Varhos G. An ambulatory surgical procedure under local anesthetic for treatment of female urinary incontinence. Int Urogynaecol J. 1996;7:81–6.

34. Nilsson CG, Palva K, Aarnio R, Morcos E, Falconer C. Seventeen year's follow up of the tension free vaginal tape procedure for female stress urinary incontinence. Int Urogynaecol J. 2013; 24:1265–9.

35. Ward K, Hilton P. United Kingdom and Ireland Tension Free Vaginal Tape Trial Group Prospective multicentre randomised trial of tension free vaginal tape and colposuspension as primary treatment for stress incontinence. BMJ. 2002;325:67.

36. Ward K, Hilton P, United Kingdom and Ireland Tension Free Vaginal Tape Trial Group. Tension free vaginal tape versus colposuspension for primary urodynamic stress incontinence: 5 year follow up. BJOG 2008;115:226–33.

37. Staskin DR, Tyagi R. The SPARC sling system. Atlas Urol Clin. 2004;12:185–95.

38. Deval B, Levardon M, Samain E, Rafii A, Cortesse A, Amarenco G, Ciofu C, Haab F. A French multicentre clinical trial of SPARC for stress urinary incontinence. Eur Urol. 2003;44:254–8.

39. Lord HE, Taylor JD, Finn JC, Tsokos N, Jeffery JT, Atherton MJ, Evans SF, Bremner AP, Elder GO, Holman CD. A randomised controlled equivalence trial of short term complications and efficacy of tension free vaginal tape and suprapubic urethral support sling for treating stress incontinence. BJU Int. 2006;98:367–76.

40. Delorme E. Transobturator urethral suspension: mini-invasive procedure in the treatment of stress urinary incontinence in women. Prog Urol. 2001;11:1306–13.

41. Whiteside JL, Walters MD. Anatomy of the obturator region: relations to a transobturator sling. Int Urogynaecol J Pelvic Floor Dysfunct. 2004;15:223–6.

42. Madhuvrata P, Riad M, Ammembal MK, Agur W, Abdel-Fattah M. Systemaic review and meta-analysis of 'inside-out versus 'outside-in' transobturator tapes in management of stress urinary

incontinence in women. Eur J Obstet Gynaecol Reprod Biol. 2012;162:1–10.

43. Abdel-Fattah M, Mostafa A, Familusi A, Ramsay I, N'dow J. Prospective randomised controlled trial of transobturator tapes in management of urodynamic stress incontinence in women: 3 year outcomes from the evaluation of Transobturator Tapes study. Eur Urol. 2012;62:843–51.

44. Latthe PM, Foon R, Toozs-Hobson P. Transobturator and retropubic tape procedures in stress urinary incontinence: a systematic review and meta-analysis of effectiveness and complications. BJOG. 2007;114:522–31.

45. Novara G, Artibani W, Barber MD, Chapple CR, Costantini E, Ficarra V, Hilton P, Nilsson CG, Waltregny. Updated systematic review and meta-analysis of the comparative data on colposuspensions, pubovaginal slings, and midurethral tapes in the surgical treatment of female stress urinary incontinence. Eur Urol. 2010;58:218–38.

*Recent Systematic Review of Continence Surgery

46. Abdel-Fattah M, Ford JA, Lim CP, Madhuvrata P. Single incision mini slings versus standard mid-urethral slings in surgical management of female stress urinary incontinence: a meta-analysis of effectiveness and complications. Eur Urol. 2011;60: 468–80.

47. Kirchin V, Page T, Keegan PE, Atiemo K, Cody JD, McClinton S. Urethral injection therapy for urinary incontinence in women. Cochrane Database Syst Rev. 2012;15:2:CD003881.

48. Ghoniem G, Bernhard P, Corcos J, Comiter C, Tomera K, Westney O, Herschorn S, Lucente V, Smith J, Wahle G, Mulcahy J. Multicentre randomised controlled trial to evaluate Macroplastique urethral bulking agent for the treatment of female stress urinary incontinence. Int Urogynaecol J. 2005;16(2):S129–30.

Overactive Bladder (OAB) in the Elderly with Contemporary Notions on Treatment Including Sacral Nerve Stimulation (SNS)

14

Rupinder Singh, Raymond Rackley, Sandip Vasavada, and David A. Gordon

Introduction

Overactive bladder (OAB) is a clinical syndrome that is defined by the trilogy of lower urinary tract symptoms. These include urinary urgency, with or without urge incontinence, urinary frequency (voiding eight or more times in a 24-h period), and nocturia (waking up during periods of deep sleep to void at night).

Overactive bladder as a symptom complex has the potential to inflict destructive effects on almost all aspects of ordinary life. The impingement on socialization is often intense. Patients suffering with overactive bladder tend to significantly restrict their daily activities which can lead to isolation with associated varying degrees of depression. Furthermore, when nocturia is the primary component, it can lead to serious sleep disturbance and diminished quality of life. Other deleterious effects of overactive bladder include impaired domestic and sexual function, as well as impaired work-related productivity.

At this point, one must acknowledge that all of these aspects of OAB have even more considerable consequences when we are dealing with an elderly population; especially, when significant medical comorbidities are associated. For

instance, an elderly woman with urinary urge incontinence (UUI) becomes a much higher risk for falls leading to debilitating fractures when compared to women without UUI.

All of the above, not withstanding, there are other significant concerns for the treatment of overactive bladder in elderly patients. A special challenge in this population are the issues associated with tolerability and safety of available oral medications. A clinician tasked with treating the elderly patient should try to choose a treatment that strikes the right balance between efficacy and safety. A proficient clinician also understands that making the correct diagnosis is immensely important before initiating any particular treatment. In order to do so, one must have at their disposal all available diagnostic modalities and an intimate knowledge of available treatment options [1–88].

Epidemiology

Prevalence

Not surprisingly, the prevalence of overactive bladder increases with age. It is expected that overactive bladder will become more common in the future as the average age of population living in the developed world is increasing. The rates of prevalence in the USA are all over the board. The American Urological Association (AUA) reports some studies that show rates as low as 7 % to others as high as 27–43 %. When we break out the gender gap, it looks like men range from 7 to 27 % while the rates in women go from about 9 % to a whopping 43 %. This would suggest that almost half of the female population in the USA may suffer with some type of significant lower urinary tract symptom. Urge incontinence was reported as being relatively higher in women when compared to men. Separately, an attempt at a large-

R. Singh
Department of Geriatric Pelvic Medicine and Neurourology, Department of Internal Medicine, Sinai Hospital of Baltimore, Baltimore, MD 21215, USA

R. Rackley
Department of Urology, Cleveland Clinic, Cleveland, OH, USA

S. Vasavada
Department of Urology, Center for Female Pelvic Medicine and Reconstructive Surgery, Cleveland Clinic, Cleveland, OH, USA

D.A. Gordon (✉)
Division of Pelvic Neuroscience, Department of Surgery, Sinai Hospital of Baltimore, Baltimore, MD 21215, USA
e-mail: dgordon@lifebridgehealth.org

© Springer Science+Business Media New York 2017
D.A. Gordon, M.R. Katlic (eds.), *Pelvic Floor Dysfunction and Pelvic Surgery in the Elderly*, DOI 10.1007/978-1-4939-6554-0_14

scale community based ongoing survey, constructed by a branch of the NIDDK was initiated with the acronym NOBLE (i.e., The National Overactive Bladder Evaluation). NOBLE looked at the prevalence and burden of overactive bladder in the USA and assessed variations in sex, age, and other demographic factors. According to the NOBLE study, the mean prevalence of overactive bladder is 16.9 % in women and 16.0 % in men. Likewise, this study notes that prevalence of overactive bladder increases with age. Their estimates suggest that the prevalence can be as high as 30 % after patients get beyond the 65 years of age marker.

Furthermore, similar results are reported for prevalence of urinary incontinence in the elderly. It is estimated that the elderly patients who are residents of long-term care facilities may have urinary incontinence prevalence of up to 50 %. In many cases, urinary incontinence was reported to be the primary cause of admission to the long-term care facility. Widespread misinformation in the general public unfortunately mandates that overactive bladder in the elderly is a normal aging process. Moreover, overactive bladder is a frequently underreported diagnosis, in part because patients believe that no effective treatment options are available for this disorder.

With respect to patients who meet the criteria for OAB, more than 40 % of those patients are "wet." that is clinical findings are consistent with UUI. Interestingly, it appears that OAB (wet) accounts for about 40–60 % of the total number of urinary incontinent patients in the USA. Risk factors for overactive bladder include but are not limited to obesity, excessive caffeine intake, and constipation. Poorly controlled diabetes along with poor functional mobility, and chronic pelvic pain may worsen the overactive bladder symptoms. Patients often have the symptoms for a considerable amount of time before seeking treatment. The condition is sometimes identified by the "at home" caregiver who pushes the patient to get formal diagnosis and treatment.

Quality of Life

New epidemiologic data now available supports the contention that overactive bladder can have a devastating impact on quality of life. Both OAB wet and dry cause significant reduction in quality of life. Within the realm of lower urinary tract symptoms, urinary urgency and UUI were reported to be as having more deleterious effects on patient's life when compared with more sensory based symptoms like frequency and nocturia. For instance, UUI is explicitly associated with depression and anxiety, work impairment, and social isolation. Community dwelling patients suffering with urinary incontinence of any kind (OAB or not) usually become progressively more reluctant to leave home, which puts them at increased risk for social isolation and depression. This certainly also limits their physical activity to a great degree, potentially increasing their risk of

physical disability. Finally, there have been many studies advocating that urinary incontinence can negatively impact quality of life in facility based patients as well.

Finally, severe nocturia, causing more than three awakenings per night may lead to bona fide sleep disturbances precluding the ability to resume a REM cycle. This in turn may lead to fatigue, impaired daytime function and even depression. Again, when nocturia becomes a central focus, the impact on quality of life will be great. However, it is important to remember that it is even more significant in the elderly.

Economic Impact

The economics of OAB often spark heated debate among experts but also as the cost of care increases, it helps drive the science of this symptom based syndrome. One large study completed in the year 2000 estimated the socioeconomic consequences of the overactive bladder syndrome to have a total cost of 12.6 billion US dollars.

Additionally, a 1995 study estimated that the total economic burden of all forms of urinary incontinence in the USA for the elderly (persons 65 years of age and older) approached 26.3 billion US dollar mark. The bulk of this cost was attributed to routine supportive care such as the use of the continence pads and reusable briefs, as well as costs associated with laundry and cleaning. It could be extremely burdensome for the elderly patients on a limited income to afford these amenities on long-term basis.

Workup/Evaluation of Overactive Bladder

Clinical Diagnosis

Initial diagnosis of the overactive bladder in the elderly in a primary care setting is based on detailed evaluation of the patient's signs and symptoms and by ruling out other possible causes.

What encompasses a complete evaluation for OAB? This should include a (1) comprehensive medical history, (2) pertinent physical examination, and a (3) urinalysis. Technically, it is only these three components that are absolutely necessary to make the diagnosis of OAB according to the NIDDK. In addition, it is most important to remember that it is the urinalysis that is the lynch pin of it all. It allows us to help differentiate *lower urinary tract symptoms* (LUTS) from infectious etiology. For example, if a patient presents with urinary urgency and urinary frequency to more than 10× in a 24-h period, the initial tendency of the professional healthcare provider would be to (not inappropriately) attach the OAB tag on this patient. This is especially true when the history and physical examination do not absolutely contradict the potential diagnosis of

OAB. At that point, one must move to the urinalysis to better elucidate the clinical scenario and formally make the diagnosis. So now let's assume that we move to NEEDING the urinalysis in the above-described patient. Let's say a patient presents with UUF and a PE consistent with OAB. The tendency is to place the diagnostic tag of OAB on this patient *if* we did not have a urinalysis that revealed significant pyuria and bacteriuria. In this case, the diagnosis of OAB cannot be made because UUF in this scenario is consistent with UTI not OAB! That is, in the final analysis, although OAB is a clinical diagnosis, the lynch pin of it all is the urinalysis. Lower urinary tract symptoms consistent with OAB in the face of a urinalysis suggesting UTI or diabetes or renal insufficiency will ALWAYS TRUMP the clinical symptoms and redirect the diagnosis.!

Other information that could be relevant in the initial assessment in the elderly patient should include a voiding diary and post-void residual urine volume (pVR) measurement. However, it is important to note that with respect to absolute criteria for OAB, it is the trilogy of (1) History, (2) PE, (3) U/A that is absolutely necessary! A pVR can lend significant information about potential neurogenic bladder BUT is *NOT* a requirement.

A comprehensive history taking is considered the most valuable part of clinical evaluation of the elderly patient with symptoms of overactive bladder. Focusing on these key symptoms can help differentiate between patients with overactive bladder and those suffering from stress incontinence (leakage of urine with coughing, sneezing, bending, and lifting, etc.). The clinician should also use history as a tool to differentiate between urinary incontinence associated with overactive bladder and other disorders including overflow incontinence and severe urethral insufficiency that may present in a similar fashion where incontinence is defined as urine leakage that is typically sensed by the patient as wetness.

When evaluating a male patient with potential overactive bladder, some special attention should be given to obstructive voiding symptoms that include hesitancy, poor urinary stream, straining to urinate, post-void dribbling, and incomplete emptying. These symptoms are more typical of benign prostatic hyperplasia or BPH but may have an etiologic association with overactive bladder in some patients. The association of OAB with bladder outlet obstruction goes hand in hand with the detrusor dysfunction that occurs with obstruction. This important concept and the associations that are intimately involved are reviewed in detail subsequently in the chapter that deals with obstructive repairs after stress urinary incontinence.

Transient urinary incontinence (TUI) is involuntary urine loss associated with other medical conditions. TUI is really a group of disorders that cause urinary incontinence. These disorders are commonly seen in elderly patients during an acute medical illness. By definition, TUI should improve with resolution of the underlying medical condition that triggered it in the first place. Therefore, taking a careful history to evaluate for any acute medical disorder as cause of incontinence is important.

Elderly patients frequently have multiple comorbidities requiring them to take multiple medications simultaneously. Polypharmacy therefore is a significant cause of urinary symptoms. Many medications can cause primary urinary symptoms or may exacerbate a preexisting bladder disorder. Careful review of all the medications a patient is taking at the time of evaluation and information about their potential side effects on the lower urinary system should be an essential part of history taking as well.

Physical Examination

Pertinent physical examination in an elderly patient with lower urinary symptoms can be a very useful tool in differentiating between overactive bladder and other causes of incontinence, especially in women. For example, a pelvic exam is an essential part for the evaluation of overactive bladder in women because it can be used effectively to make a diagnosis of stress incontinence. In addition, pelvic exam may diagnose stress incontinence in many women who may not be aware or deny having stress incontinence otherwise. Pelvic exam can also be used in evaluating lower urinary symptoms due to bladder prolapse, uterine prolapse, or vaginal mucosal atrophy in postmenopausal women.

Other Diagnostic Modalities

A subset of female patients presenting with overactive bladder symptoms may have recurrent urinary tract infections. It is therefore crucial to rule out a concurrent urinary infection that may mimic the symptoms of overactive bladder in such patients. It is the urinalysis that is paramount in this regard. Urinalysis, either by dipstick or by microscopic examination is considered the cornerstone of laboratory testing to check for potential urinary infections in all patients presenting with overactive bladder symptoms. In addition, urinalysis is also useful to check for the presence of microscopic hematuria and glucosuria. Microscopic hematuria in the absence of urinary infection requires further investigation with radiographic evaluation of the upper urinary tract as well as the evaluation of the lower urinary tract with a cystoscopy to rule out genitourinary pathology and potential malignancy. A reflux urine culture is recommended for patients with positive urinalysis and symptomatic UTI.

Other pertinent diagnostic evaluation for a patient with overactive bladder symptoms commonly utilized in the office setting is measuring the post-void residual urine volume. It is a fairly simple test that may help identify patients suspected of having overflow incontinence because urinary frequency and urgency are also the two readily reported symptoms by patients suffering from overflow incontinence. Post-void residual volume can be measured by either urethral catheterization, a bladder scanner, or by an abdominal ultrasound.

Yet, another useful way to gain important data is a patient kept bladder diary. This is an economical, simple, and non-invasive method to evaluate patients with voiding dysfunction. With this method, patients are instructed to carefully record their daily fluid intake and then record the time and volume of each void for up to 3–5 days. They are also encouraged to record and describe their symptoms associated with voiding that may help the clinician differentiate between urgency and stress incontinence. Examination of the compiled data can also be helpful in diagnosing frequency, nocturia, as well as the important differentiation between neuromuscular nocturia and nocturnal polyuria due to excessive fluid intake. Bladder diary also aids the clinician in treating the patient by providing valuable feedback.

As a final note for this section, it is important to remember that no matter how good the voiding diary is, there will be a subgroup of patients nevertheless, that will require more sophisticated testing such as complex urodynamic studies to make the accurate diagnosis and should be referred to a specialist trained to conduct such studies.

Treatment

Although overactive bladder symptoms in the most elderly patients can be successfully managed with either pharmacologic or non-pharmacologic methods alone, yet patients are frequently treated with a combination of both modalities.

Non-pharmacologic treatment includes simple but useful recommendations. For instance, dehydration can often exacerbate the overactive bladder symptoms in the elderly, and therefore, adequate daily fluid intake is an important aspect of non-pharmacologic therapy. Furthermore, patients are instructed to minimize the intake of caffeine, alcohol, and carbonated beverages that can irritate the bladder and worsen the overactive bladder symptoms. However, it is important to note that the American Urologic Association has set forth guidelines for treatment in OAB.

First-Line Treatments

1. Clinicians should offer behavioral therapies (e.g., bladder training, bladder control strategies, pelvic floor muscle training, fluid management) as first-line therapy to all patients with OAB.
2. Behavioral therapies may be combined with pharmacologic management.

Second-Line Treatments

1. Clinicians should offer oral antimuscarinics or oral ß3-adrenoceptor agonists as second-line therapy.
2. If an immediate release (IR) and an extended release (ER) formulation are available, then ER formulations should preferentially be prescribed over IR formulations because of lower rates of dry mouth.
3. Transdermal (TDS) oxybutynin (patch [now available to women ages 18 years and older without a prescription] or gel) may be offered.
4. If a patient experiences inadequate symptom control and/or unacceptable adverse drug events with one antimuscarinic medication, then a dose modification or a different antimuscarinic medication or ß3-adrenoceptor agonist may be tried.
5. Clinicians should not use antimuscarinics in patients with narrow angle glaucoma unless approved by the treating ophthalmologist and should use antimuscarinics with extreme caution in patients with impaired gastric emptying or a history of urinary retention.
6. Clinicians should manage constipation and dry mouth before abandoning effective antimuscarinic therapy. Management may include bowel management, fluid management, dose modification, or alternative antimuscarinics.
7. Clinicians must use caution in prescribing antimuscarinics in patients who are using other medications with anticholinergic properties.
8. Clinicians should use caution in prescribing antimuscarinics or ß3-adrenoceptor agonists in the frail OAB patient.
9. Patients who are refractory to behavioral and pharmacologic therapy should be evaluated by an appropriate specialist if they desire additional therapy.

Third-Line Treatments (Available Through Specialists)

Clinicians should discuss the patient's expectations from treatment and their willingness to participate in therapies other than pharmacotherapy. If the patient would not consider invasive treatment options, a referral to a specialist may not be warranted.

1. Specialists may offer intradetrusor botulinum toxin-A (100U) as third-line treatment in the carefully selected and thoroughly counseled patient who has been refractory to first- and second-line OAB treatments. The patient must be able and willing to return for frequent post-void residual evaluation and able and willing to perform self-catheterization if necessary.
2. Specialists may offer peripheral tibial nerve stimulation (PTNS) as third-line treatment in a carefully selected patient population.

3. Specialists may offer sacral neuromodulation (SNS) as third-line treatment in a carefully selected patient population characterized by severe refractory OAB symptoms or patients who are not candidates for second-line therapy and are willing to undergo a surgical procedure.

4. Practitioners and patients should persist with new treatments for an adequate trial in order to determine whether the therapy is efficacious and tolerable. Combination therapeutic approaches should be assembled methodically, with the addition of new therapies occurring only when the relative efficacy of the preceding therapy is known. Therapies that do not demonstrate efficacy after an adequate trial should be ceased.

Sacral Nerve Stimulation (SNS)

Introduction

Overactive bladder is essentially divided into two major categories according to the International Continence Society (ICS), (1) those without an underlying neurologic lesion which is known as idiopathic detrusor overactivity (IDO) and (2) those with an associated underlying neurologic lesion which is known as neurogenic detrusor overactivity (NDO). Not surprisingly, refractory IDO represents one of the most challenging problems in urology as well as a clinical problem that significantly erodes patient quality of life. Symptoms include urinary frequency, urgency, urge incontinence, and nocturia. Urge incontinence is caused by an involuntary bladder contraction and has many etiologies, including neurologic disease, bladder outlet obstruction, and senile and idiopathic causes. Obviously, the embarrassment and social stigma of incontinence is the predominant symptom which these patients seek to correct. Initial treatment for patients with overactive bladder without any remediable anatomic cause is anticholinergic therapy. For patients who are not candidates for, refractory to, or who cannot tolerate anticholinergic pharmacotherapy, options are limited. Augmentation cystoplasty, in which a piece of small or large intestine is used to enlarge the bladder, has traditionally been offered as a last resort. However, this is a major operation with significant potential short-term and long-term complications. As Leng and Chancellor [54] point out, even without complications most patients are troubled by the need for lifelong intermittent bladder catheterization after such reconstructive procedures. Neuromodulation offers an alternative to patients who have failed more conservative treatments and may be considering irreversible surgical options.

History

In the 1860s Giannuzzi stimulated the spinal cord in dogs and concluded that the hypogastric and pelvic nerves are involved in bladder regulation. In 1878, Saxtorph attempted to treat patients with urinary retention by directly stimulating the bladder with intravesical electrodes. Built on this foundation, the neuromodulation which we practice today has its roots in the 1960s work of Boyce, Dees, Caldwell [26] and

Table 14.1 Potential applications of electrical stimulation in the treatment of voiding dysfunction

Facilitate filling/storage		
Inhibit detrusor contractility	Vaginal	Neuromodulation
Increase bladder capacity	Anal	
Decrease UUF	Suprapubic	
	Posterior tibial	
	Common peroneal	
	Sacral roots	
	Intravesical	
Decrease noiceception	Vaginal	Neuromodulation anal
	Suprapubic	
	Sacral roots	
Increase outlet resistance	Vaginal	Direct stimulation
	Anal	
	Sacral roots	
Facilitate emptying		
Stimulate detrusor contraction (spinal cord injured patients)	Anterior sacral roots	Direct stimulation
Restore micturition reflex (idiopathic urinary retention)	Sacral roots	Neuromodulation

Adapted from A. Wein, Neuromuscular dysfunction of the lower urinary tract and its management, in P.C. Walsh et al. (2002) Campbell's Urology, 8th ed. (Philadelphia: Saunders), p. 981

Nashold [62], who experimented with various modes of bladder stimulation including a transurethral approach, direct detrusor stimulation, pelvic nerve and pelvic floor stimulation, and finally spinal cord stimulation. In the last century the pioneering work of Tanagho [47], Brindley [24], and Schmidt [70] demonstrated that stimulation of sacral root S3 generally induces detrusor and sphincter action and led to clinical trials of implantable devices to treat genitourinary disorders including erectile dysfunction, urinary incontinence, and urinary retention. The US Food and Drug Administration approved sacral nerve stimulation (SNS) for intractable urge incontinence in 1997, and for urgency frequency and non-obstructive urinary retention in 1999. Later labeling was changed to include "overactive bladder" as an appropriate diagnostic category. Since its inception, more than 20,000 InterStim neurostimulators (Medtronic Inc., Minneapolis, MN) have been implanted for the three approved indications for SNS of the lower urinary tract.

Putative Mechanism of Action of Sacral Neuromodulation

Two main theories exist regarding the mechanism of action of sacral neuromodulation. First, direct activation of efferent fibers to the striated urethral sphincter reflexively causes detrusor relaxation. Second, selective activation of afferent fibers causes inhibition at spinal and supraspinal levels. Accumulating evidence suggests that activation of somatic sacral afferent inflow at the sacral root level that, in turn, affects the storage and emptying reflexes in the bladder and central nervous system accounts for the positive effects of neuromodulation on both storage and emptying functions of the bladder. By monitoring somatosensory evoked potentials (SEP) during sacral neuromodulation, Malaguti et al. [58] concluded that sacral neuromodulation therapy works by sacral afferent activity and concomitant activation of the somatosensory cortex. Since sacral neuromodulation has been proven clinically effective for both storage (urgency frequency and urgency incontinence) and emptying (non-obstructive urinary retention) dysfunctions of the bladder, isolating the mechanism of action has been challenging.

Putative MOA of Sacral Neuromodulation in Overactive Bladder

The ability to volitionally store and evacuate urine is modulated by several centers in the brain. It is thought that patients with overactive bladder may have suffered an insult that effectively unmasks involuntary bladder contractions. Sacral neuromodulation of these primitive reflexes may restore nor-

mal micturition. Sacral neuromodulation may affect detrusor overactivity by suppressing or inhibiting interneuronal transmission in the bladder reflex pathway. This inhibition may, in part, modulate the sensory outflow from the bladder through the ascending pathways to the pontine micturition center (PMC), thereby, preventing involuntary contractions by modulating the micturition reflex circuit. In clinical practice, sacral neuromodulation improves abnormal bladder sensations, involuntary voids, and detrusor contractions. Interestingly, voluntary voiding is preserved. This may be due to selective avoidance of normal sensory ascending outflow pathways of the bladder from Aδ-fibers to the PMC, as well as initiation of the descending pathways from the PMC to sacral efferent outflow pathways.

Putative MOA of Sacral Neuromodulation in Urinary Retention

To allow for complete bladder emptying, detrusor contractions must be coordinated with urethral sphincteric relaxation. When the suprasacral pathways that coordinate sphincteric activity are altered, the guarding and urethral reflexes that allow for urine storage without leakage still exist and cannot be turned off. This may result in urinary retention and is seen in certain patients with spinal cord injury and detrusor sphincter dyssynergia. These patients have functional detrusor contractions but are unable to coordinate this with a relaxed urethral sphincter resulting in urinary retention. Inhibition of the guarding reflexes may improve urinary retention. Sacral neuromodulation is postulated to turn off excitatory flow to the urethral outlet and facilitate bladder emptying.

Electrical Stimulation for Storage Disorders

Patient Selection

Since many lower urinary tract symptoms and dysfunctions are secondary to neuromuscular etiologies, a thorough history and physical examination will often reveal the nature (acute vs. chronic) and help to classify the causes (neurogenic, anatomic, post-surgical, functional, inflammatory, and/or idiopathic). Urinalysis is routinely performed. Urine cytology should be considered in patients who present with refractory symptoms of dysuria, urgency or frequency as both bladder cancer and bladder carcinoma in situ may present with irritative bladder symptoms without hematuria. Urodynamic studies (UDS) including cystometrogram, pressure-flow studies, and electromyography (EMG) of sphincters and pelvic floor muscles are performed on a selected basis. Many patients without known neurologic disorders can be thoroughly evaluated with the use of a voiding diary and a focused history and physical examination of the pelvis. EMG is recommended in suspected cases of neurogenic bladder dysfunction, detrusor sphincter dyssynergia, or Fowler's syndrome and may be considered for evaluation of inappropriate pelvic floor muscle behavior. The pathophysiology of neurogenic bladders, as seen in patients with multiple sclerosis and spinal cord injury, can change with time and disease progression. As such, these patients will require reevaluation with urodynamics at regular intervals, or when symptoms change despite active medical intervention. Cystourethroscopy may be helpful. Urethral strictures and bladder neck contractures or fibrosis can be diagnosed. Bladder wall trabeculation may help to confirm a clinical suspicion of bladder outlet obstruction or neurogenic pathology. Baseline upper tract imaging is performed in patients with neurologic disease, or if indicated by physical or baseline studies or a patient's history.

Predictors of Success

Currently, sacral neuromodulation is prescribed for those patients with urgency, frequency, and urge incontinence who have failed traditional conservative measures such as bladder retraining, pelvic floor biofeedback, and medications and for whom more invasive procedures such as enterocystoplasty or urinary diversion might be inadvisable or has been declined. Recently, several studies have tried to more accurately identify which patients will or will not respond to sacral neuromodulation, however, predictive factors remain elusive. Koldewijn's [50] study found that neither gender nor patient age, history, or diagnosis was a predictor of success in sacral neuromodulation of lower urinary tract dysfunction. Urodynamic predictors of success have been equally hard to identify. One recent study found that both patients with and patients without demonstrable detrusor overactivity, or involuntary detrusor contractions noted on urodynamics, may have a positive response to sacral neuromodulation. To date only one published study has prospectively evaluated preoperative factors associated with cure in patients with intractable urge incontinence. Amundsen et al. [21] evaluated 105 patients between 2000 and 2003. Fifty-five were implanted and the average age at implantation was 60 years. Cure was defined as no daily leakage episodes after permanent implantation. Three factors were associated with lower cure rates: age greater than 55 years, three or more chronic conditions, and neurologic conditions. Individuals younger than 55 years had a cure rate of 65 % vs. 37 % for older individuals. Age older than 55 years and more than three chronic conditions were found to be independent risk factors for failure. The most common medical comorbidities present in this population included arthritis, hypertension, diabetes, and depression. Neurologic conditions included a history of back surgery in the majority of patients, multiple sclerosis,

Parkinson's disease, and cerebrovascular accident. The authors suggest that the aged population may have profound changes in the central neural control systems of the bladder as well as the bladder itself. Studies of cerebral function in older incontinent individuals using single photon emission computed tomography have reported that under perfusion is present in the frontal lobe. This is not seen in younger incontinent women. SNS targets spinal circuits. If the central control mechanism is impaired, it seems reasonable that SNS will be less efficacious.

Special Populations

Indications for neuromodulation are expanding. Several populations of patients with voiding dysfunction have some component of the indicated symptom complex that includes urgency, frequency, urge incontinence, or urinary retention. The current expansion of indications for neuromodulation has developed into areas of neurogenic bladder (*Parkinson's disease*, *multiple sclerosis*), spinal cord injury, and pediatric voiding dysfunction. Painful bladder syndrome, pelvic pain, fecal incontinence, and bowel disorders will be discussed elsewhere.

Multiple Sclerosis (MS)

Multiple sclerosis can cause a variety of voiding dysfunction scenarios including neurogenic detrusor overactivity, detrusor sphincter dyssynergy (DSD), areflexia, or any combination of these. Bladder problems affect up to 90–100 % of patients during the course of their disease. MS patients were excluded from the original sacral neuromodulation trials because of the theoretical change in the disease state that may be potentiated by neuromodulation. No prospective randomized trials exist on the use of neuromodulation in management of MS-related bladder dysfunction, but small series have shown encouraging results. It appears that the best candidates are ones with mild, non-progressive MS, with little functional decompensation who also have detrusor overactivity or retention but not areflexia.

Spinal Cord Injury (SCI)

Patients with spinal cord injury present with a variety of clinical and urodynamic findings ranging from detrusor areflexia to neurogenic detrusor overactivity with or without concomitant sphincteric dyssynergy. The goal of treatment of these patients is to prevent the urologic sequelae of SCI, such as infections, stones, and obstruction, while ensuring a bladder that functions well, empties at a low pressure to protect the kidneys, and maintains a good capacity and continence. Basic science data suggest that at least some communication should exist between sacral outflow and the pontine micturition center to allow processing for the reflexes that may be inhibited by the brain. Thus, patients with complete spinal cord lesions may not have the same potential benefit from neuromodulation as does one with an incomplete lesion. *However, this fact has yet to be proven clinically.* Few studies exist in neurogenic patients alone for whom sacral neuromodulation was performed. Andrews reported on a T8 paraplegic with urinary urgency and urge incontinence who underwent percutaneous tibial nerve stimulation. This patient experienced almost a twofold increase in bladder capacity.

Contraindications

There are several important contraindications to sacral neuromodulation. In patients with anatomic changes such as bony abnormalities of the sacrum, transforaminal access may be difficult or impossible. Patients with cognitive impairment rendering them incapable of operating the device or giving appropriate feedback regarding the level and comfort of stimulation are poor candidates. Finally, patients with physical limitations that prevent them from achieving normal pelvic organ function, such as patients with functional urinary incontinence and patients who are non-compliant, should not be offered this therapy.

Sacral neuromodulation is relatively contraindicated for those patients who have an anticipated need for future magnetic resonance (MR) imaging and patients who plan to become pregnant. The main concern with MRI and implantable stimulator/pacemaker-type devices is that heating of the leads has been demonstrated in vivo and in vitro. While some question the clinical significance of the small temperature changes with the leads, the potential exists to elicit nerve damage. Additionally, there is some concern that the magnetic field from MR imaging may damage the pulse generator. Many radiologists are reluctant to provide MR imaging services for patients with implantable electrical stimulation devices despite the anecdotal evidence that no adverse events have ever occurred when MR imaging has inadvertently or purposefully been done for emergent reasons or in small trials. Due to the unknown teratogenic potential of electrical stimulation it has been considered contraindicated in pregnant women with various voiding dysfunctions. One study that evaluated the effect of electrical stimulation on pregnant rats and their fetuses was unable to find any adverse effects and thus concluded that termination of pregnancy is not advised for prospective mothers when electrical stimulation has been performed unknowingly in early pregnancy. Women with electrical stimulation devices for pelvic health conditions who become pregnant may simply turn off their devices when considering and during pregnancy.

Surgical Protocol and Technique

The procedure consists of two semi-permanent stages with an optional "pre-screening stage." The programmable testing stage or formal Stage I is performed utilizing a quadripolar "Interstim Lead" which is placed surgically utilizing intravenous anesthesia or sedation. If adequate control is achieved, then the focus moves on to the surgical implantation of a programmable pulse generator which is formally considered Stage II. The entire process of combining Stage I and Stage II will take anywhere from 1 week to 4 weeks. Since its introduction, several modifications have been made in the technology, with resultant changes in the surgical technique. Although, at this point, it is for more of a historical perspective, it does highlight just how fast minimally invasive technology can evolve when a procedure has been spotlighted for its clinical merit. The most significant of these changes centered around the development of the "quadripolar tined lead." This was a dramatic technical advantage because it allowed for placement of programmable lead in a fashion that did NOT require formal anchoring to any anatomic fascial sheath. Although the procedure does require the delivery of a systemic anesthetic, *whether it is intravenous or spinal*, the entire procedure can be done percutaneously. The tined lead was introduced in 2002 and again offers the advantage of simplified placement of the lead through a percutaneous approach without the need for lead anchoring to the fascia [78]. The lead is secured through the action of the tines. Essentially, the tines provide a dual security purpose. Firstly, they are designed such that they will physically grasp adjacent soft tissues to provide and immediate level of positional stability. Secondly, the tines induce the deposition of "type I and type III" collagen formation around the lead to allow it to stay in position in a more permanent fashion. Another surgical modification was the movement of the location of the implantable pulse generator (IPG) unit from the lower anterior abdominal wall to the posterior gluteal region. For Stage I, preoperative intravenous antibiotics are given and standard aseptic techniques for the implantation of foreign bodies are implemented. The patient is placed in the prone position on the operating table and the buttocks are held apart using wide tape retraction so that the anus is visible during test stimulation. The anus and tape are prepped in a sterile fashion and then covered with a separate plastic drape until visualization of the anus is needed during the procedure. The patient's feet will also need to be visible during the procedure.

The S3 foramen, the desired location of the tined lead, can be localized via surface landmarks or fluoroscopic methods. The S3 foramen is generally located 2–3 cm off the midline on either side approximately 9–12 cm cephalad to the tip of the coccyx. If the sciatic notch can be palpated, this provides a useful landmark as well. A line is drawn connecting the sciatic notches bilaterally and an intersecting line is drawn at the midline of the sacrum. The S3 foramen can be located approximately one fingerbreadth lateral to the midline of the sacrum along the line connecting the sciatic notches. Less reliably, one can look for the least curved portion of the sacrum. In 2001, Chai et al. [27] introduced the use of the "cross-hair" fluoroscopic technique for S3 localization. Fluoroscopy is intended to help the surgeon identify a specific region to start attempting percutaneous access; it does not allow the surgeon to visualize the S3 foramen directly. More importantly, the use of lateral imaging allows the surgeon to determine the depth required for implanting the lead once the S3 foramen is identified.

At the previously marked S3 foramen, the foramen needle is inserted. Because the pelvic plexus and pudendal nerve run alongside the pelvis, the needle should be placed just inside the ventral foramen. Fluoroscopy is used to confirm needle position. The nerve is tested for the appropriate motor response: dorsiflexion of the great toe and bellows contraction of the perineal area. The so-called bellows reflex represents contraction of the levator muscles. The foramen needle is exchanged for the introducer sheath and the lead is passed so that the electrodes, numbered 0 through 3, are positioned with electrode 2 and 3 straddling the ventral surface of the sacrum. Test stimulation is repeated on each electrode and the responses are observed. An S3 response should be noted at a minimum of two of the four electrodes. Once satisfied with the position, the sheath is removed, releasing the tines that anchor the lead. Confirmation of an S3 sensory response, a sensation of stimulation in the perineum, is not required to confirm proper placement if the correct S3 motor response is observed. However, if a motor response is absent despite what appears to be fluoroscopically appropriate placement, the patient's sedation can be lightened and sensory responses can be elicited. Patient verification of the correct sensory response can then confirm proper localization (Table 14.2).

A 2–4 cm incision into the subcutaneous tissues in the upper lateral buttock is made below the beltline or below the level of the ischial wings for connecting the permanent lead to the percutaneous extension lead wire. If the screening trial is successful, this connection site will be the site of implantation for the IPG. The permanent lead is transferred to the medial aspect of the lateral buttock incision using the tunneling device. The lead is then connected to the extension wire and the tunneling device is used again to transpose the extension wire from the medial aspect of the incision to an exit point on the contralateral side of the back. This transfer and long tunnel reduces the occurrence of infection from the percutaneous exit site of the wire. The extension wire is connected to the external pulse generator. Patients are able to resume their normal activities immediately, but are advised to limit their excessive movement-related activities such as high impact exercises for the duration of the trial period. The external generator can be flexibly programmed for the duration of

Table 14.2 Sacral nerve responses

Nerve root	Sensory and motor responses
S-2	
Motor	Plantar flexion of entire foot and anal sphincter clamp
Sensory	Leg and buttocks
S-3	
Motor	Dorsiflexion of the great toe and a bellows reflex (anal wink)
Sensory	"Pulling" in scrotum, vagina, or perineum
S-4	
Motor	Bellows reflex only
Sensory	Sensation of pulling in the rectum only

the intended trial while the patient records their symptoms and bladder function in a voiding diary. If there is greater than 50 % improvement in the symptoms or voiding function, a Stage II procedure is performed. At the Stage II procedure, the IPG is placed. No fluoroscopy is required during Stage II when a permanent neuroelectrode has been placed for the Stage I procedure; however, if a PNE was performed for Stage I, then fluoroscopic confirmation of the neuroelectrode placement is advised. The buttock incision overlying the lead connections is opened, the percutaneous extension wire is removed, and the extension lead is secured to the permanent lead and subsequently to the IPG. The newer generation IPG is connected directly to the permanent lead without the need for an extension lead. The IPG pocket should be large enough to accommodate the IPG without tension and deep enough to prevent erosion and provide cosmetic results.

Here it is important to discuss the Optional "Pre-Screening Stage," more commonly known as a percutaneous sacral nerve root evaluation (S3 PNE). This is commonly done as an office based procedure which is frequently performed utilizing only local anesthesia. However, when sedation is administered, fluoroscopy can be utilized to help with localization. Again, as stated above, even with the S3 PNE, the S3 foramina can be localized via surface landmarks or fluoroscopic methods. More traditionally, it is located 2–3 cm off the midline on either side approximately 10 cm cephalad to the tip of the coccyx. If the sciatic notch can be palpated, this provides a useful landmark as well. A line is drawn connecting the sciatic notches bilaterally and an intersecting line is drawn at the midline of the sacrum. The S3 foramen can be located approximately one fingerbreadth lateral to the midline of the sacrum along the line connecting the sciatic notches. Less reliably, one can look for the least curved portion of the sacrum. In 2001, Chai et al. [27] introduced the use of the "cross-hair" fluoroscopic technique for S3 localization. Fluoroscopy is intended to help the surgeon identify a specific region to start attempting percutaneous access; it does *Not* allow the surgeon to visualize the S3 foramen directly.

Now that we have discussed the more well-documented ways to access the S3 formina, let me highlight a very reliable but less common technique. It is the "SCJ Proximal Progressive Technique" and it is my favorite method for the PNE. This technique is very reliable if the operator can confidently identify the initial reference point, which in this case is the "Sacrococcygeal Junction" (SCJ). It is important to note that this structure (the SCJ) is, in contradistinction, to the "tip of the coccyx." The tip of the coccyx is difficult to use as a reliable marker because the coccyx will often be pulled anteriorly in older patients since it is used as an attachment site for many pelvic floor muscles. In some cases, there is enough muscular tension on the coccyx to push it anteriorly, to an almost "perpendicular" position with respect to the sacrum. Consequently, the SCJ is easily palpated as the anteriorly pulled coccyx rounds up into the sacrum. Once the SCJ is palpated and marked, then the S3 foramina can be found by following a series of fingerbreadths. The first fingerbreadth cephalad to the SCJ would be the notch at S5, the next fingerbreadth cephalad would be the S4 foramina, the next one would be the S3 foramina from an abstract perspective. However, the human body is rarely abstract, and tissue depth and distance must be accounted for. Therefore, add another fingerbreadth to your walk up the sacrum *if* the approximate BMI of the patient is less than 20. If the BMI is more than 20, add two fingerbreadths. This should allow the operator to precisely drop the test lead into the third sacral foramina with confidence. Up to this point, the S3 PNE or "Pre-Screening Stage" has been looked upon with some degree of speculation in an optional sense, especially with respect to neuromuscular lower urinary tract dysfunction. The Stage I/Stage II combination procedure had taken hold on the urinary side, primarily because a very good clinical response to the S3 PNE did NOT necessarily translate to the same response upon conversion to a permanent qudripolar lead. So, to be sure of the clinical response, with the understanding that fractions of a millimeter on the nerve root side can mean a world of difference with respect to responses on the clinical side. So, the combination of a Stage I (perm trial) followed by (if positive) a Stage II implantation of pulse generator. The bottom line is that "testing" and maintaining the same lead would be optimal which had allowed the "Staged Implant Technique" to become preferred on the urinary side. Now, in 2016, with FDA approval of the fecal incontinence (FI) indication for SNS, the playing field changed with respect to the use of a pre-screening PNE. This is due at least in part to two major factors.

Bilateral Sacral Nerve Root Testing

There is no consensus as to whether one or two implanted S3 leads should be performed at the first stage. Bilateral implan-tation allows for testing of both the left and right S3 nerve roots. At the time of the second stage, the lead which produced the most robust response can be attached to the IPG and the other lead removed. Bilateral stimulation has been suggested for potential salvage of patients who have failed unilateral lead placement. The theory behind the additive effects of bilateral stimulation is based on animal studies that demonstrated bilateral stimulation yielded a more profound effect on bladder inhibition than did unilateral stimulation. The only clinical study comparing unilateral to bilateral test stimulation was unable to find any significant difference with regard to urge incontinence, frequency, or severity of leakage in the OAB group. The retention group patients had better parameters of emptying (volume per void) in bilateral as compared with unilateral stimulation. However, the numbers were too small in the retention group to make adequate conclusions. Studies are ongoing regarding bilateral stimulation for this indication.

Outcomes

Outcomes of SNS for the indications of idiopathic urgency frequency and urge incontinence are derived from two studies that have randomized patients to active or delayed therapy, as well as reports from numerous prospective and retrospective reviews of case series and registry databases. In 1999, Schmidt et al. [70] reported on SNS therapy in 76 patients with refractory urge incontinence. During the 6-month study period, at 16 different centers, patients were randomized to active or delayed therapy (control group). Of the 34 patients receiving active SNS therapy, 16 (47%) were completely dry, and an additional 10 (29%) demonstrated a greater than 50% reduction in incontinence episodes. In a similar study design, Hassouna et al. [41] reported the outcomes of SNS for refractory urgency frequency conditions in 51 randomized patients. At 6 months patients in the active SNS group showed improvement in the number of daily voids (16.9 ± 9.7 to 9.3 ± 5.1), volume voided (118 ± 74 to 226 ± 124 ml), degree of urgency (rank score of 2.2 ± 0.6 to 1.6 ± 0.9), and quality of life measures. At 6 months post implant, stimulators in the active group were turned off and urinary symptoms returned to baseline values. After reactivation of SNS, sustained efficacy was documented at 12 and 24 months. Limited but confirmational results of the earlier randomized trials have been obtained from prospective series and registry studies evaluating efficacy, safety, and quality of life measures. The results for the US registration trial that led to FDA approval for SNS reveal that 37 of 62 patients (60%) with refractory urgency frequency or urge incontinence achieved a 50% or more improvement in their condition.

Complications

The sacral nerve stimulation study group has published several reports on the efficacy and safety of the procedure for individual indications. The complications were pooled from the different studies based on the fact that the protocols, devices, efficacy results, and safety profiles were identical. Of 581 patients recruited, 219 underwent implantation of the InterStim system. The complications were divided into both percutaneous test stimulation related and post implant related problems. Of the 914 test stimulation procedures done on the 581 patients, 181 adverse events occurred in 166 of these procedures (18.2 % of the 914 procedures). The vast majority of complications were related to lead migration (108 events, 11.8 % of procedures). Technical problems and pain represented 2.6 % and 2.1 %, respectively, of the adverse events. For the 219 patients who underwent implantation of the InterStim system (lead and generator), pain at the neurostimulator site was the most commonly observed adverse effect at 12 months (15.3 %). Surgical revisions of the implanted neurostimulator or lead system were performed in 33.3 % of cases (73 of 219 patients) to resolve an adverse event. These included relocation of the neurostimulator because of pain at the subcutaneous pocket site and revision of the lead for suspected migration. Explantation of the system was performed in 10.5 % for lack of efficacy. One should consider the fact that, at the time, the generator was implanted in the lower abdomen. Everaert reported the complications related to SNS itself. Among the 53 patients who had undergone implantation of the quadripolar electrode (Medtronic InterStim, Model 3886 or 3080) and subcutaneous pulse generator in the abdominal site (Medtronic InterStim: Itrel 2, IPG) between 1994 and 1998, device-related pain was the most frequent problem, occurring in 18 of the 53 patients (34 %) and occurring equally in all implantation sites (sacral, flank, or abdominal). Pain responded to physiotherapy in eight patients and no explantation was done for pain reasons. Current-related complications occurred in 11 %. Fifteen revisions were performed in 12 patients. Revisions for prosthesis-related pain ($n=3$) and for late failures ($n=6$) were not successful. Hijaz et al. [43] reported the complications in a review of 214 patients who underwent SNS. Of the 214 patients, 161 underwent IPG implantation during a mean follow-up of 16 months. The second-stage explant and revision rate was 10.5 % and 16.1 %, respectively. The indications for explant were infection in 8 of 17 and failure to maintain response in 9 of 17. Revisions were performed for decreases in response (17/26), IPG site discomfort (4/26), draining sinus at the IPG site (4/26), and lead migration (1/26). It should be pointed out that the need for revision does not indicate unsuccessful treatment. As noted in the previous studies, all of the complications were minor, further solidifying the safety of this procedure. Hijaz et al. [43] have

also presented algorithms for troubleshooting of the SNS problems back in 2006. Generator site infection is best treated with explant of the whole system. Despite attempts to salvage some of these patients, follow-up revealed that the infection persisted in all and eventual explant was inevitable. The troubleshooting algorithm includes the search for causes of (a) pocket (IPG site) discomfort; (b) recurrent symptoms; (c) stimulation occurring in the wrong area of pelvis; (d) no stimulation; and (e) intermittent stimulation.

Selective Nerve Stimulation/The Pudendal Nerve

Sacral neuromodulation is thought to improve bladder storage by inhibiting the micturition reflex via electrical stimulation of sensory afferent fibers, in particular by depolarization of Aα and Aγ somatomotor fibers that affect the pelvic floor and external sphincter and thus inhibit detrusor activity. Many of the sensory afferent nerve fibers contained in the sacral spinal nerves originate in the pudendal nerve, thereby making the pudendal nerve an ideal target for neuromodulating inhibition of the micturition reflex. Direct pudendal nerve neuromodulation stimulates more pudendal afferents than SNS and may do so without the side effects of off-target stimulation of leg and buttock muscles. Thus, techniques for direct pudendal nerve stimulation at alternative locations to the sacral foramen are being developed.

Dorsal Genital Nerve

The most superficial, terminal branch of the pudendal nerve is the dorsal genital nerve (dorsal nerve of the penis in males, clitoral nerve in females). In both genders the dorsal genital nerve is located at the level of the symphysis pubis and is a purely sensory afferent branch carrying sensory information from the glans of the penis or clitoris. As a pure sensory afferent nerve branch of the pudendal nerve, the dorsal genital nerve contributes to the pudendal-pelvic nerve reflex that has been proposed as a mechanism of bladder inhibition. In experimental and clinical studies, direct electrical stimulation of the dorsal genital nerve appears promising in producing an inhibition of the micturition reflex. Results in laboratory animals and in persons with spinal cord injury have demonstrated that electrical stimulation of the dorsal genital nerves inhibits bladder contractions. Stimulation of the dorsal penile nerve has been tested in patients with spinal cord injury and has been shown to increase bladder volume and reduce bladder overactivity. Dorsal penile nerve stimulation was painless and no side effects noted. Similar experiments have shown that stimulation of the dorsal nerve of the penis abolishes reflexive bladder contractions and increases bladder capacity in persons with spinal injury. Feasibility trials using MedStim (Medtronic, Minneapolis, MN), an implantable neuroelectrode and pulse generator originally conceived by NDI, are under way for otherwise healthy patients with idiopathic detrusor overactivity.

Posterior Tibial Nerve

The posterior tibial nerve is a mixed sensory and motor nerve containing fibers originating from spinal roots L4 through S3 which modulate the somatic and autonomic nerves to the pelvic floor muscles, bladder and urinary sphincter. Based on translational findings of traditional Chinese acupuncture practices, McGuire et al. used transcutaneous stimulation of the common peroneal or posterior tibial nerve to inhibit detrusor overactivity. Percutaneous tibial nerve stimulation (PTNS) (Urgent PC, CystoMedix, Anoka, MN) is approved by the FDA. A small gauge stimulating needle is inserted approximately 5 cm cephalad to the medial malleolus and just posterior to the tibia. Electrical stimulation is then applied at a level just below the somatic sensory threshold for a total of 30 min. Sessions are repeated weekly for 10–12 weeks. PTNS is minimally invasive and well tolerated. Clinical trials using PTNS have been performed for detrusor overactivity with and without pelvic pain and for urinary retention. Overall, results are comparable to those seen with anticholinergic pharmacologic therapy. Proponents argue that relative to SNS, other surgical modalities, and chronic medical therapy, PTNS offers a much more economical alternative.

Sacral Neuromodulation for Emptying Disorders

Sacral neuromodulation using the InterStim system has been successful in patients with idiopathic urinary retention, i.e. without any anatomic obstructive component, also urinary retention after hysterectomy secondary to idiopathic afferent neurolysis of the bladder, and finally in patients with Fowler's syndrome, a syndrome of urinary retention in young, premenopausal women without overt neurologic disease. The success rate, however, is not as robust as that seen for the treatment of urgency, frequency, and urge incontinence. Additionally, improvement in patients with retention may not be as rapid as in patients undergoing sacral root stimulation for other reasons. Therefore, an extended Stage I trial is recommended. Furthermore, as previously described, bilateral lead placement sacral neuromodulation using the InterStim system has been successful in patients with idiopathic urinary retention, i.e. without any anatomic obstructive component, also urinary retention after hysterectomy secondary to idio-

pathic afferent neurolysis of the bladder, and finally in patients with Fowler's syndrome, a syndrome of urinary retention in young, premenopausal women without overt neurologic disease. The success rate, however, is not as robust as that seen for the treatment of urgency, frequency, and urge incontinence. Additionally, improvement in patients with retention may not be as rapid as in patients undergoing sacral root stimulation for other reasons. Therefore, an extended Stage I trial is recommended. Furthermore, as previously described, bilateral lead placement may prove to be more effective. A recent retrospective study looking at 29 patients with urinary retention due to a wide variety of etiologies found that those patients able to volitionally void more than 50 ml at presentation were more likely to proceed to Stage II and permanent implantation. Finally, a novel approach involving the placement of bilateral tined leads into the caudal epidural space was recently described for those patients with refractory urinary retention. This remains an experimental approach. A large, prospective randomized multi-center trial to evaluate the efficacy of sacral nerve stimulation for urinary retention was performed by Jonas. Of those patients evaluated with chronic, non-obstructive urinary retention, 68, or 38 %, proceeded to permanent implantation after PNE. Patients were randomly assigned to the treatment or control group, in which treatment was delayed for 6 months. Improvement in volitional voiding was seen in 83 % of patients who received the implant, and 69 % were able to discontinue intermittent catheterization entirely. At 18 months, 71 % of the patients available for follow-up had continued improvement. Aboseif evaluated the efficacy and change in quality of life in patients with idiopathic, chronic, non-anatomic, functional urinary retention. Thirty-two patients with idiopathic retention requiring intermittent catheterization underwent PNE. Twenty patients proceeded to permanent implantation. Eighteen of these patients were able to void and no longer required intermittent catheterization. Average voided volumes increased from 48 to 198 ml and post-void residuals decreased from 315 to 60 ml.

Summary

Overactive bladder as a syndrome is a collection of chronic, debilitating symptoms affecting the lower urinary tract that includes urinary urgency (with or without urge incontinence), frequency, and nocturia. It is significantly more prevalent in the elderly and is commonly underreported. Cornerstones of office-based workup of overactive bladder include complete medical history, physical exam, and urinalysis. Treatment of overactive bladder consists of non-pharmacologic as well as pharmacologic options. Antimuscarinic agents are the mainstay of pharmacologic therapy for overactive bladder. The newer, more selective agents can help reduce side effects in the elderly patients when used resourcefully.

Sacral neuromodulation (SNS) has enjoyed wide success in the field of voiding dysfunction with applications to a broad range of problems including both storage and emptying disorders. Due to refinements in technique and technology, it is a truly minimally invasive therapy which has provided inestimable quality of life improvements.

References

1. Staskin DR, Wein AJ, editors. New perspectives on the overactive bladder. Urology. 2002;60 Suppl:1–104.
2. DuBeau CE, Kiely DK, Resnick NM. Quality of life impact of urge incontinence in older persons: a new measure and conceptual structure. J Am Geriatr Soc. 1999;47:989–94.
3. Abrams P, Kelleher CJ, Kerr LA, Rogers RG. Overactive bladder significantly affects quality of life. Am J Manag Care. 2000;6(11 suppl):S580–90.
4. Brown JS, Vittinghoff E, Wymann JE, et al. Urinary incontinence: does it increase risk for falls and fractures? Study of Osteoporotic Fractures Research Group. J Am Geriatr Soc. 2000;48:721–5.
5. Gibbs RS. Danforth's obstetrics and gynecology, 10th ed. Philadelphia: Lippincott Williams & Wilkins; 2008. p. 890–1. ISBN 9780781769372.
6. Ghosh AK. Mayo Clinic internal medicine concise textbook. Rochester: Mayo Clinic Scientific Press; 2008. p. 339. ISBN 9781420067514.
7. Stewart WF, Van Rooyen JB, Cundiff GW, Abrams P, Herzog AR, Corey R, Hunt TL, Wein AJ. Prevalence and burden of overactive bladder in the United States. World J Urol. 2003;20(6):327–36. doi:10.1007/s00345-002-0301-4.
8. Stewart WF, Van Rooyen JB, Cundiff GW, et al. Prevalence and burden of overactive bladder in the United States. World J Urol. 1999;44:56–66.
9. Ouslander JG, Kane RL, Abrass IB. Urinary incontinence in elderly nursing home patients. JAMA. 1982;248:1194–8.
10. Coyne KS, Wein AJ, Tubaro A, et al. The burden of lower urinary tract symptoms: evaluating the effect of LUTS on health-related quality of life, anxiety and depression: EpiLUTS. BJU Int. 2009;103 Suppl 3:4.
11. Dubeau CE, Simon SE, Morris JN. The effect of urinary incontinence on quality of life in older nursing home residents. J Am Geriatr Soc. 2006;54:1325.
12. MacDiarmid SA, Gwynn E. Physical disability, an emerging complication of urinary incontinence. In: Society for urodynamics and female urology annual meeting, Bahamas, 22–25 Feb 2006.
13. Brown JS, McGhan WF, Chokroverty S. Comorbidities associated with overactive bladder. Am J Manag Care. 2000;6:S574–9.
14. Wein AJ, Rovner ES. The overactive bladder: an overview of primary care health providers. Int J Fertil. 1999;44:56–66.
15. Abrams P. Overactive bladder syndrome and urinary incontinence. Oxford: Oxford University Press; 2011. p. 7–8. ISBN 9780199599394.
16. Wagner TH, Hu T-W. Economic costs of urinary incontinence in 1995. Urology. 1998;51:355–61.
17. Fantl J, Newman D, Colling J, et al. Clinical practice guideline number 2: urinary incontinence in adults: acute and chronic management. Rockville: US Department of Health and Human Services, Agency for Health Care Policy and Research; 1996 (AHCPR publication 96–0682). update.
18. Chapple RC, MacDairmid SA. Urodynamics made easy. New York: Churchill Livingstone; 2000.
19. Andersson K-E. Potential benefits of muscarinic M3 receptor selectivity. Eur Urol Suppl. 2002;1:23–8.
20. Aboseif S, Tamaddon K, Chalfin S, Freedman S, Mourad MS, Chang JH, Kaptein JS. Sacral neuromodulation in functional urinary retention: an effective way to restore voiding. BJU Int. 2002;90:662–5.
21. Amundsen CL, Romero AA, Jamison MG, Webster GD. Sacral neuromodulation for intractable urge incontinence: are there factors associated with cure? Urology. 2005;66:746–50.
22. Andrews BJ, Reynard JM. Transcutaneous posterior tibial nerve stimulation for treatment of detrusor hyperreflexia in spinal cord injury. J Urol. 2003;170:926.
23. Bosch JL, Groen J. Sacral nerve neuromodulation in the treatment of patients with refractory motor urge incontinence: long-term results of a prospective longitudinal study. J Urol. 2000;163:1219–22.
24. Brindley GS. Electrical stimulation in vesicourethral dysfunction: general principles; practical devices. In: Mundy AR, Stephenson TP, Wein AJ, editors. Urodynamics: principles, practices, application. London: Churchill Livingstone; 1994. p. 481–8.
25. Brindley GS. The first 500 patients with sacral anterior root stimulator implants: general description. Paraplegia. 1994;32:795–805.
26. Caldwell KP. The electrical control of sphincter incompetence. Lancet. 1963;2:174–5.
27. Chai TC, Mamo GJ. Modified techniques of S3 foramen localization and lead implantation in S3 neuromodulation. Urology. 2001;58:786–90.
28. Cohen BL, Tunuguntla HS, Gousse A. Predictors of success for first stage neuromodulation: motor versus sensory response. J Urol. 2006;175:2178–80. discussion 2180–1.
29. Congregado Ruiz B, Pena Outeirino XM, Campoy Martinez P, Leon Duenas E, Leal Lopez A. Peripheral afferent nerve stimulation for treatment of lower urinary tract irritative symptoms. Eur Urol. 2004;45:65–9.
30. Cooperberg MR, Stoller ML. Percutaneous neuromodulation. Urol Clin North Am. 2005;32:71–8. vii.
31. Craggs M, McFarlane J. Neuromodulation of the lower urinary tract. Exp Physiol. 1999;84:149–60.
32. Dahms SE, Hohenfellner M, Thuroff JW. Sacral neurostimulation and neuromodulation in urological practice. Curr Opin Urol. 2000;10:329–35.
33. De Groat WC, Saum WR. Synaptic transmission in parasympathetic ganglia in the urinary bladder of the cat. J Physiol. 1976;256:137–58.
34. De Groat WC, Nadelhaft I, Milne RJ, Booth AM, Morgan C, Thor K. Organization of the sacral parasympathetic reflex pathways to the urinary bladder and large intestine. J Auton Nerv Syst. 1981;3:135–60.
35. Dees JE. Contraction of the urinary bladder produced by electric stimulation. Preliminary report. Invest Urol. 1965;2:539–47.
36. Fischer J, Madersbacher H, Zechberger J, Russegger L, Huber A. Sacral anterior root stimulation to promote micturition in transverse spinal cord lesions. Zentralbl Neurochir. 1993;54:77–9.
37. Fowler CJ. Neurological disorders of micturition and their treatment. Brain. 1999;122(Pt 7):1213–31.
38. Goh M, Diokno AC. Sacral neuromodulation for nonobstructive urinary retention—is success predictable? J Urol. 2007;178:197–9. discussion 199.
39. Govier FE, Litwiller S, Nitti V, Kreder Jr KJ, Rosenblatt P. Percutaneous afferent neuromodulation for the refractory overactive bladder: results of a multicenter study. J Urol. 2001;165:1193–8.
40. Griffiths D. Clinical studies of cerebral and urinary tract function in elderly people with urinary incontinence. Behav Brain Res. 1998;92:151–5.
41. Hassouna MM, Siegel SW, Nyeholt AA, Elhilali MM, van Kerrebroeck PE, Das AK, et al. Sacral neuromodulation in the treatment of urgency-frequency symptoms: a multicenter study on efficacy and safety. J Urol. 2000;163:1849–54.

42. Hedlund H, Schultz A, Talseth T, Tonseth K, van der Hagen A. Sacral neuromodulation in Norway: clinical experience of the first three years. Scand J Urol Nephrol. 2002;36 Suppl 210:87–95.

43. Hijaz A, Vasavada SP, Daneshgari F, Frinjari H, Goldman H, Rackley R. Complications and troubleshooting of two-stage sacral neuromodulation therapy: a single-institution experience. Urology. 2006;68:533–7.

44. Hohenfellner M, Schultz-Lampel D, Dahms S, Matzel K, Thuroff JW. Bilateral chronic sacral neuromodulation for treatment of lower urinary tract dysfunction. J Urol. 1998;160:821–4.

45. Hohenfellner M, Thuroff JW, Schultz-Lampel D. Sacral root stimulation to treat micturition disorders [sakrale neuromodulation zur therapie von Miktionsstorungen]. Aktuelle Urol. 1992;23:1–10.

46. Janknegt RA, Hassouna MM, Siegel SW, Schmidt RA, Gajewski JB, Rivas DA, et al. Long-term effectiveness of sacral nerve stimulation for refractory urge incontinence. Eur Urol. 2001;39:101–6.

47. Jonas U, Tanagho EA. Studies on the feasibility of urinary bladder evacuation by direct spinal cord stimulation. II. Poststimulus voiding: a way to overcome outflow resistance. Invest Urol. 1975;13:151–3.

48. Jonas U, Fowler CJ, Chancellor MB, Elhilali MM, Fall M, Gajewski JB, et al. Efficacy of sacral nerve stimulation for urinary retention: results 18 months after implantation. J Urol. 2001;165:15–9.

49. Klingler HC, Pycha A, Schmidbauer J, Marberger M. Use of peripheral neuromodulation of the S3 region for treatment of detrusor overactivity: a urodynamic-based study. Urology. 2000;56:766–71.

50. Koldewijn EL, Rijkhoff NJ, van Kerrebroeck EV, Debruyne FM, Wijkstra H. Selective sacral root stimulation for bladder control: acute experiments in an animal model. J Urol. 1994;151:1674–9.

51. Koldewijn EL, Rosier PF, Meuleman EJ, Koster AM, Debruyne FM, van Kerrebroeck PE. Predictors of success with neuromodulation in lower urinary tract dysfunction: results of trial stimulation in 100 patients. J Urol. 1994;152:2071–5.

52. Kruse MN, de Groat WC. Spinal pathways mediate coordinated bladder/urethral sphincter activity during reflex micturition in decerebrate and spinalized neonatal rats. Neurosci Lett. 1993;152:141–4.

53. Lee YH, Creasey GH. Self-controlled dorsal penile nerve stimulation to inhibit bladder hyperreflexia in incomplete spinal cord injury: a case report. Arch Phys Med Rehabil. 2002;83:273–7.

54. Leng WW, Chancellor MB. How sacral nerve stimulation neuromodulation works. Urol Clin North Am. 2005;32:11–8.

55. Madersbacher H. Conservative therapy of neurogenic disorders of micturition. Urologe A. 1999;38:24–9.

56. Madersbacher H, Fischer J. Sacral anterior root stimulation: prerequisites and indications. Neurourol Urodyn. 1993;12:489–94.

57. Maher MG, Mourtzinos A, Zabihi N, Laiwalla UZ, Raz S, Rodriguez LV. Bilateral caudal epidural neuromodulation for refractory urinary retention: a salvage procedure. J Urol. 2007;177:2237–40. discussion 2241.

58. Malaguti S, Spinelli M, Giardiello G, Lazzeri M, van den Hombergh U. Neurophysiological evidence may predict the outcome of sacral neuromodulation. J Urol. 2003;170:2323–6.

59. Martin ET. Can cardiac pacemakers and magnetic resonance imaging systems co-exist? Eur Heart J. 2005;26(2005):325–7.

60. McGuire EJ, Zhang SC, Horwinski ER, Lytton B. Treatment of motor and sensory detrusor instability by electrical stimulation. J Urol. 1983;129:78–9.

61. Minardi D, Muzzonigro G. Lower urinary tract and bowel disorders and multiple sclerosis: role of sacral neuromodulation: a preliminary report. Neuromodulation. 2005;8:176–81.

62. Nashold Jr BS, Friedman H, Boyarsky S. Electrical activation of micturition by spinal cord stimulation. J Surg Res. 1971;11:144–7.

63. Nashold Jr BS, Friedman H, Glenn JF, Grimes JH, Barry WF, Avery R. Electromicturition in paraplegia. Implantation of a spinal neuroprosthesis. Arch Surg. 1972;104:195–202.

64. Pettit PD, Thompson JR, Chen AH. Sacral neuromodulation: new applications in the treatment of female pelvic floor dysfunction. Curr Opin Obstet Gynecol. 2002;14:521–5.

65. Rijkhoff NJ, Wijkstra H, van Kerrebroeck PE, Debruyne FM. Selective detrusor activation by electrical sacral nerve root stimulation in spinal cord injury. J Urol. 1997;157:1504–8.

66. Roguin A, Zviman MM, Meininger GR, Rodrigues ER, Dickfeld TM, Bluemke DA, et al. Modern pacemaker and implantable cardioverter/defibrillator systems can be magnetic resonance imaging safe: in vitro and in vivo assessment of safety and function at 1.5 T. Circulation. 2004;110:475–82.

67. Ruud Bosch JL, Groen J. Treatment of refractory urge urinary incontinence with sacral spinal nerve stimulation in multiple sclerosis patients. Lancet. 1996;348:717–9.

68. Scheepens WA, de Bie RA, Weil EH, van Kerrebroeck PE. Unilateral versus bilateral sacral neuromodulation in patients with chronic voiding dysfunction. J Urol. 2002;168:2046–50.

69. Scheepens WA, van Koeveringe GA, de Bie RA, Weil EH, van Kerrebroeck PE. Urodynamic results of sacral neuromodulation correlate with subjective improvement in patients with an overactive bladder. Eur Urol. 2003;43:282–7.

70. Schmidt RA, Jonas U, Oleson KA, Janknegt RA, Hassouna MM, Siegel SW, van Kerrebroeck PE. Sacral nerve stimulation for treatment of refractory urinary urge incontinence. Sacral Nerve Stimulation Study Group. J Urol. 1999;162:352–7.

71. Schultz-Lampel D, Jiang C, Lindstrom S, Thuroff JW. Experimental results on mechanisms of action of electrical neuromodulation in chronic urinary retention. World J Urol. 1998;16:301–4.

72. Schultz-Lampel D, Jiang C, Lindstrom S, Thuroff JW. Summation effect of bilateral sacral root stimulation. Eur Urol. 1998;33:61.

73. Shaker HS, Hassouna M. Sacral nerve root neuromodulation: an effective treatment for refractory urge incontinence. J Urol. 1998;159:1516–9.

74. Siegel SW. Selecting patients for sacral nerve stimulation. Urol Clin North Am. 2005;32:19–26.

75. Siegel SW, Catanzaro F, Dijkema HE, Elhilali MM, Fowler CJ, Gajewski JB, et al. Long-term results of a multicenter study on sacral nerve stimulation for treatment of urinary urge incontinence, urgency-frequency, and retention. Urology. 2000;56:87–91.

76. South MM, Romero AA, Jamison MG, Webster GD, Amundsen CL. Detrusor overactivity does not predict outcome of sacral neuromodulation test stimulation. Int Urogynecol J. 2007;18(12):1395–8.

77. Spinelli M, Bertapelle P, Cappellano F, Zanollo A, Carone R, Catanzaro F, et al. Chronic sacral neuromodulation in patients with lower urinary tract symptoms: results from a national register. J Urol. 2001;166:541–5.

78. Spinelli M, Giardiello G, Gerber M, Arduini A, van den Hombergh U, Malaguti S. New sacral neuromodulation lead for percutaneous implantation using local anesthesia: description and first experience. J Urol. 2003;170:1905–7.

79. Swinn MJ, Kitchen ND, Goodwin RJ, Fowler CJ. Sacral neuromodulation for women with Fowler's syndrome. Eur Urol. 2000;38:439–43.

80. Van Balken MR, Vandoninck V, Gisolf KW, Vergunst H, Kiemeney LA, Debruyne FM, Bemelmans BL. Posterior tibial nerve stimulation as neuromodulative treatment of lower urinary tract dysfunction. J Urol. 2001;166:914–8.

81. Van Balken MR, Vandoninck V, Messelink BJ, Vergunst H, Heesakkers JP, Debruyne FM, et al. Percutaneous tibial nerve stimulation as neuromodulative treatment of chronic pelvic pain. Eur Urol. 2003;43:158–63. discussion 163.

82. Van Kerrebroeck EV, Scheepens WA, de Bie RA, Weil EH. European experience with bilateral sacral neuromodulation in patients with chronic lower urinary tract dysfunction. Urol Clin North Am. 2005;32:51–7.

83. Van Kerrebroeck EV, van der Aa HE, Bosch JL, Koldewijn EL, Vorsteveld JH, Debruyne FM. Sacral rhizotomies and electrical

bladder stimulation in spinal cord injury. Part I: clinical and uro-dynamic analysis. Dutch Study Group on Sacral Anterior Root Stimulation. Eur Urol. 1997;31:263–71.

84. Vandoninck V, van Balken MR, Finazzi Agro E, Petta F, Micali F, Heesakkers JP, Debruyne FM, Kiemeney LA, Bemelmans BL. Percutaneous tibial nerve stimulation in the treatment of overactive bladder: urodynamic data. Neurourol Urodyn. 2003;22:227–32.

85. Wang Y, Hassouna MM. Electrical stimulation has no adverse effect on pregnant rats and fetuses. J Urol. 1999;162:1785–7.

86. Wein A, Barrett D. Voiding function and dysfunction—a logical and practical approach. Year Book Medical. Chicago; 1988.

87. Wheeler Jr JS, Walter JS, Sibley P. Management of incontinent SCI patients with penile stimulation: preliminary results. J Am Paraplegia Soc. 1994;17:55–9.

88. Wheeler Jr JS, Walter JS, Zaszczurynski PJ. Bladder inhibition by penile nerve stimulation in spinal cord injury patients. J Urol. 1992;147:100–3.

Interstitial Cystitis: The Painful Bladder Syndrome

David A. Gordon and Haritha Pendli

Introduction

Cystitis is the inflammatory swelling of the bladder wall and is one of the dreaded eventualities of life as a female. However, in an effort to not be construed as sexist, it should be noted that, of course males are susceptible to cystitis but their attendant gross anatomy makes the initiation of this process much more challenging and much less likely. In any event, from a symptomatic perspective, cystitis translates as an unpleasant sensation deep in the anterior pelvis. The associated sensory phenomena of pain, pressure, and discomfort are quickly related to the urinary bladder with an even quicker desire by the patient for rapid eradication. This situation is most often implicated to some type of infectious agent, which incites a physiologic response that kicks off a cascade of events bringing inflammatory cells and inflammatory mediators to the bladder wall to face off with the infecting microorganisms. Hence begins the microscopic **"Battle Royale"**! Fortunately for most females, the prescription for relief is simple and essentially, beginning antibiotic therapy, which is targeted at the destruction of the microorganism. These agents work hand in hand with the host's natural inflammatory defense mechanisms to remove the infecting microorganism. Once successful eradication has been achieved, the host's natural physiologic response should "shut down" those inflammatory cascades and segue into the relief of her lower urinary tract symptoms. It is very important to note here that it is the "transmural inflammatory

reaction" at the level of the bladder wall that is primarily implicated in the genesis and perpetuation of these painful lower urinary tract symptoms, NOT the infecting microorganism! So, what happens if the antibiotic or the antiviral agent successfully achieves eradication of the offending microorganism BUT the host's natural inflammatory response does NOT subside? What is the patient left with? If this situation exists, then the patient is left with an active inflammatory reaction within the substance of a swollen, tender, erythematous bladder wall and hence "persistence of painful urinary urgency" WITHOUT an active offending microorganism! For a long time, this was considered an "oxymoron," i.e. cystitis without infection. *Nevertheless, essentially, what the patient is left with is a noninfectious inflammatory cystitis*. Perhaps, the most dreaded complication of all within this arena [1–52].

Although there may be several different types of *noninfectious inflammatory cystitis*, certainly, it would be the "interstitial subtype" that is by far the most studied and hence, the most well known. By definition, *"interstitial cystitis" (IC)* is a clinical syndrome characterized by daytime and nighttime urinary frequency and urgency with a pelvic pain component. A specific etiology has not been identified per se, but IC may be associated with several different subtypes, each with their own etiologic pathways. Moreover, the diagnostic criteria for the syndrome remain undefined. Furthermore, despite considerable research, universally effective treatments do not exist; therapy usually consists of various supportive, dietary, behavioral, pharmacologic, and interventional measures. Reconstructive bladder surgery is rarely indicated. As the syndrome of IC in the USA became more prevalent, it took on a greater proportion of the bulk practice of urology.

Consequently, in 2011 the American Urologic Association (AUA) created a subcommittee which composed and published its original guidelines statement by doing a systematic review of literature up to 2011. This original guidelines statement connects this subtype of noninfectious inflammatory cystitis with a "site specific" generalized pain syndrome. In

D.A. Gordon, M.D., FACS (✉)
Division of Pelvic Neuroscience, Department of Surgery,
The Sinai Hospital of Baltimore, 2401 W. Belvedere Ave,
Baltimore, MD 21215, USA
e-mail: dgordon@lifebridgehealth.org

H. Pendli, M.D.
The Maryland Institute for Pelvic Neuroscience, 1447 York Road,
Suite #406, Lutherville, MD 21093, USA
e-mail: harithapendli@yahoo.com

© Springer Science+Business Media New York 2017
D.A. Gordon, M.R. Katlic (eds.), *Pelvic Floor Dysfunction and Pelvic Surgery in the Elderly*,
DOI 10.1007/978-1-4939-6554-0_15

addition, the original statement stressed the use of objective measures for quantification of both lower urinary tract symptoms and bladder pain. Then, one of the counterparts to the AUA, the International Continence Society (ICS) coined the term "painful bladder syndrome" (PBS). By definition, PBS is *suprapubic pain that occurs with bladder filling and associated with increased daytime and nighttime frequency for at least 6 weeks, in the absence of proven urinary infection or other obvious pathology.* All of the above not withstanding, the definition of PBS by the ICS reserves the diagnosis of interstitial cystitis for patients with characteristic cystoscopic and histologic features of the condition. Subsequently, in 2014, the AUA amended their statement in favor of an evidence-based approach in an effort to provide a clinical framework for the diagnosis and management of IC. The AUA amendment in 2014 was ALSO used to help differentiate between three increasingly more common conditions which were now being seen more commonly by the general urologist in the USA. These included overactive bladder (OAB), urinary tract infection (UTI), and IC (Fig. 15.1).

Finally, one of the most important elements, for the provider, in dealing with patients with interstitial cystitis (IC) is education and emotional support. This syndrome is characterized by "flare and remission" and periodic exacerbations are managed individually because no long-term therapy has been shown to permanently prevent recurrent episodes. Finally, the mainstay of treatment options in this process is to palliate and alleviate uncomfortable LUT symptoms. Therapeutic interventions in this process are NOT necessarily "curative."

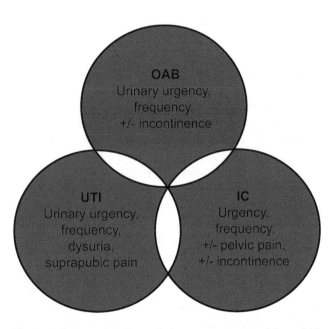

Fig. 15.1 Between three increasingly more common conditions which were now being seen more commonly by the general urologist in the USA: overactive bladder (OAB), urinary tract infection (UTI), interstitial cystitis (IC)

Evolution of Interstitial Cystitis (IC) Theory

IC has an older and more extensive history than one may expect. Its beginnings can be traced back to the nineteenth century. Interestingly, a *Philadelphia surgeon by the name of Joseph Parrish* may have stumbled on to an inadvertent description of the disease as he was attempting to treat bladder stones in a series of three women back in 1837. To his surprise, there were no stones ever recovered, but he went on to write a symptom trilogy of (1) severe urinary urgency, (2) urinary frequency, and (3) bladder pain. Interestingly, it was about 50 years later, in 1887 when *Dr. A.J. Skene* made a more valiant and descriptive attempt to describe this condition. Pathologically, it is characterized by a *nonspecific cellular and subcellular inflammatory response which destroys the mucous membrane of the urinary bladder in the absence of any infectious agent.* This destruction may be in part or in whole and may extend outward to the muscular coats of the bladder. Furthermore, he published these findings in his classic text, **"Diseases of the Bladder and Urethra in Women."** Idiomatically, it was via this piece of literature that practitioners started to use a more common phrase that still persists today in some circles, i.e. "urethral syndrome." Subsequently, in 1907, Dr. F. Nitze, a German surgeon describes a type of transmural bladder inflammation which was focused more acutely at the level of the mucosa and submucosa. These findings seemed to be consistent with the process described by Dr. Skene 25 years earlier. Nevertheless, Nitze coined this dysfunction "cystitis parenchymatosa." All of the above notwithstanding, it was 8 years later in **1915** when **Guy Hunner** took interest in this disease process with his description of characteristic *bladder wall ulcers in association with a symptom complex of urinary urgency and bladder pain.* He published his findings in the then *Boston Journal of Surgery* where he also describes an associated but rare type of inflammatory bladder ulcer. He goes on in the article and actually names the process ulcerative cystitis. His association with the entire issue does not stop here however. Hunner subsequently goes on to publish a follow-up article in the *American Journal of OB-GYN* 3 years later in 1918. The article was entitled the elusive ulcer and within its pages Hunner attempts to describe, in as much technical detail as he could muster, considering the state of the biological sciences in 1918, the concurrent inflammatory findings. *This included a strange but interstitial type of inflammation within the substance of the ulcer.* **Needless to say, within the next few years the term "interstitial cystitis" was born** and thrust into the urologic vernacular. Although this nomenclature is most often completely credited to Guy Hunner, he may or may not have been the first to coin the phrase. Hunner's description remained the state of the art for almost 30 years, until 1949 when Dr. J. Hand wrote the first comprehensive epidemiologic description of interstitial cystitis (IC). Here he breaks down the process to an initial inflammatory component followed by a delayed effect on the bladder wall elasticity. This initial inflammatory component is described as widespread, small, submucosal bladder hemorrhages known as petichiae. The late component is biomechanical compromise of bladder wall elasticity with translates clinically to a potentially significant decrease in bladder capacity which is now often characteristic of the condition.

It is my belief that the historical demographics of this syndrome are inextricably tied to its pathogenic and epidemiologic history. As one might imagine, considering both the evolution of American Medicine in the latter part of the twentieth century and the state of affairs of the optical science in medical endoscopy, trying to connect the symptom complex of urinary frequency, urinary urgency and bladder pain to the endoscopic finding of ulcerative cystitis was *rare* at best. Not surprisingly, the published demographics of the day reflect this. All things considered, it is probably fortunate because it is difficult for patients with this condition to lead productive and functional lives. O.K., the point is taken, *so enter Alan Wein, the chair of Urology at the University of Pennsylvania in 1978*. At that time, Dr. Wein began to generate lofty discussions and publications which centered around the concept of "Non Ulcerative Variants of Interstitial Cystitis" that seemed to go hand in hand with the changing demographics. Soon after this, Vicki Ratner, an orthopedic surgeon from California and Debra Slade, an east coast lawyer came together, and in 1984, the "Interstitial Cystitis Association" or ICA was born. This organization was also somewhat novel in that it brought together high level clinicians, clinical researchers, basic science researchers with patients who actually suffer with the disease, and gave them a forum for open discussion with the experts. The premise was to lay groundwork to try to piece together clinical concepts with "real time" clinical symptoms.

Epidemiology of IC with Historical Timeline

Attempting to develop an understanding of the burden that interstitial cystitis (IC) places on the US population is difficult at best. Trying to elucidate those risk factors which contribute to the disease as well as its sequelae is disjointed. In addition, pinpointing the specifics of IC as a disease entity is often erroneous because common entities such as UTI and overactive bladder (OAB) have overlapping clinical symptoms. To that end, it seems that our best information in the topic comes from several population based studies that have been published over the past quarter century. Moreover, it is extremely interesting to look at the evolving spectrum of population demographics in this country when it comes to IC. Let's take a look.

In *1971 Oravisto* used a mathematical formula to calculate the number of patients suffering with interstitial cystitis. The study was based out of Helsinki Finland. All of that notwithstanding, if this formula would have been used at that time to extrapolate against US population data at that time, the expected number of expected diagnosed cases of IC would have only come to about 21,000 cases. Obviously, knowing what we know today, this estimation is absolute folly. About a decade later, Vilheld in 1983, studying at the Urban Institute in Washington D.C. put together a population based study which ended up confirming many of the observations put forth by Oravisto. Moreover, he developed his own formula to predict the prevalence of IC in the USA. The population grids which he created estimated the entire potential IC population to be only 47,000 lives.

Interestingly, only 4 years later, in 1987, as we put forth Vilheld's formula to US diagnostics with respect to IC, there seemed to be a disconnect. An estimated 47,000–48,000 cases to be diagnosed was met with an actual 90,000 newly diagnosed cases of IC that year. This seemed to uphold the contention that the prevalence of interstitial cystitis seemed to be approximately 1.8–2.0 times the European prevalence. Moreover, the percentage of "real time" endoscopic diagnosis of IC as compared to those patients who present with bladder pain and sterile urine is about twenty percent (20 %). Thus by 1994, the NIH/NIDDK published a cross sectional population based survey which estimated the potential IC patient population at 500,000 women and about 50,000 men. During this period of time the medical community in this country was still evolving with respect to its acceptance and understanding of this disease. Consequently, the epidemiology and demographics were truly fluid, so by 1998, the Nurse Health Study (NHS) II had estimated the prevalence of IC in the USA to be approximately 267 per 100,000 population which would bring IC totals in the USA at about 850,000. Ultimately, these demographics were published in the Journal of Urology back in 1999. All of that not withstanding, by 2003, things were formally upregulated **again** with the unveiling of NHS III. Here the prevalence of IC in the USA was estimated to be approximately 371 per 100,000 population, which would bring population totals in the USA at between 1.0 and 1.5 million. Finally, there came **RAND**. The RAND IC Epidemiology Study (**RICE**) is *the largest IC epidemiology study ever undertaken* and completely changed our understanding of the prevalence of IC. This survey studied more than 100,000 familial groups of US women and revealed that 2.7–6.5 % of them may have IC! This translates to a whopping 3–8 million women.

From an epidemiologic perspective, Phil Hanno has identified other important factors to consider in this disease process, especially for clinical practitioners when it comes to creating a patient profile. Important factors include a median age of about 40 years. Almost 50 % of patient report a history

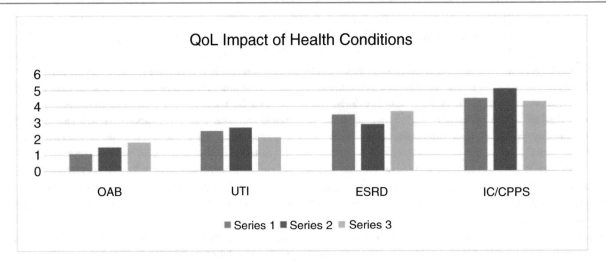

Fig. 15.2 Quality of life impact on health conditions. Series #1=IMPACT on general vitality; series #2=impact on mental health; series #3=impact on physical functioning. *OAB* overactive bladder, *UTI* urinary tract infection, *ESRD* end stage renal disease, *IC/CPPS* interstial cystitis/chronic pelvic pain syndrome

of childhood bladder problems and recurrent UTI. Their entire disease process is characterized by flare and remission with an average remission period of 8–12 months. Late deterioration of the disease process is unusual and quality of life (QoL) indicators suggest that patients with IC were lower than those with end stage renal disease who are currently on dialysis. Persons of Jewish origin made up 14 % of the IC population but only 3 % of the control population, a finding later substantiated by Koziol.

Finally, examination of the IC population yields some fairly consistent findings. These are that about 94 % of patients are white and approximately 90 % are female. Household size, marital status, number of male sexual partners, educational status, and parity were previously not statistically different between patients with interstitial cystitis and healthy controls. However, new data from the RAND interstitial cystitis cohort have shown that according to a standardized definition, women in that study were considerably more likely to be uninsured, less likely to be married, and had more children than others with the reported diagnosis of IC/BPS.

The condition is also dramatically under-reported in men. There is significant overlap of symptoms of IC/BPS to symptoms of patients with chronic prostatitis/chronic pelvic pain syndrome. In fact, 17 % of men were reported to have symptoms of both complexes. This supports the hypothesis that IC/BPS and chronic prostatitis/chronic pelvic pain syndrome share a common pathophysiology in men. However, many of these studies rely on the patient's self-reported symptoms, so estimates of incidence in men are likely higher than previously reported (Fig. 15.2).

Etiology and Pathogenesis

Although often times it seems that there is much confusion and not much to agree about in the world of IC, probably most experts would agree that the pathogenesis and etiology of interstitial cystitis remain unclear at best. However, maybe it is not so surprising considering that the most basic building block for any process has to the definition. If that is unclear or even in question, then everything that follows may come under its own level of scrutiny.

If one asks two different practitioners to describe the clinical parameters that make up interstitial cystitis, it often generates enigmatic responses. For example, even clinical experts may say, well, "I can't define it but I know it when I see it." The whole thing is grounded in lower urinary tract symptoms of urinary urgency and frequency on the backdrop of nongynecologic pelvic pain in the absence of any other clinical pathology. The National Institute of Diabetes & Digestive & Kidney Diseases (NIDDK) developed initial consensus criteria which were established for the diagnosis of IC back in the late 1980s. These criteria were not meant to define the disease, but to ensure that groups of patients to be studied academically would be done so in a comparable fashion. According to Phil Hanno, these criteria seemed to become almost a de-facto definition of the disease. The biggest negative associated with these early NIDDK criteria is that all of this is that what had initially been intended as a tool for research studies may have forced many patients to be left undiagnosed and potentially untreated if they did not meet the strict standards laid out. Fortunately, the NIDDK had developed a multi-institutional database study that later served to resolve this issue. The Interstitial Cystitis Data Base Study (*ICDB*) was a large, observational study designed to determine the treated history of IC patients and identify common patient characteristics. Entry requirements for the ICDB were considerably *less stringent* than the NIDDK criteria with the intention of being able to follow the progression of the disease, as well as to include all groups that might help identify the nature and the extent of the syndrome. The 24-point criteria are as follows:

1. Providing informed consent to participate in the study
2. Willing to undergo a cystoscopy under general or regional anesthesia, when indicated, during the course of the study
3. At least 18 years of age
4. Having symptoms of urinary urgency, frequency, or pain for more than 6 months
5. Urinating at least 7 times per day, or having some urgency or pain (measured on linear analog scales)
6. No history of or current genito-urinary tuberculosis
7. No history of urethral cancer
8. No history of or current bladder malignancy, high-grade dysplasia, or carcinoma in situ
9. Males: no history of or current prostate cancer
10. Females: no occurrence of ovarian, vaginal, or cervical cancer in the previous 3 years
11. Females: no current vaginitis, clue cell, trichomonas, or yeast infections
12. No bacterial cystitis in previous 3 months
13. No active herpes in previous 3 months
14. No antimicrobials for urinary tract infections in previous 3 months
15. Never having been treated with cyclophosphamide (Cytoxan)
16. No radiation cystitis
17. No neurogenic bladder dysfunction (e.g., due to a spinal cord injury, a stroke, Parkinson's disease, multiple sclerosis, spina bifida, or diabetic cystopathy)
18. No bladder outlet obstruction (determined by urodynamic investigation)
19. Males: no bacterial prostatitis for previous 6 months
20. Absence of bladder, ureteral, or urethral calculi for previous 3 months
21. No urethritis for previous 3 months
22. Not having had a urethral dilation, cystometrogram, bladder cystoscopy under full anesthesia, or a bladder biopsy in previous 3 months
23. Never having had an augmentation cystoplasty, cystectomy, cystolysis, or neurectomy
24. No significant urethral stenosis less than 12 French

Although not a true definition in the classic sense, these criteria allow the clinical practitioner to build a structural definition that facilitates being able to make the diagnosis. More importantly, this opens the door to allow for a substantive discussion with respect to the etiology of this disease process.

The pathogenesis and etiology of interstitial cystitis remain incompletely defined. It seems well accepted at this point that IC is NOT a single discreet entity. Moreover, there is *no* single pathological process that is universally present in IC. Consequently, it is logical that this *"syndrome of interstitial cystitis"* may well have multiple etiologies that result in the constellation of symptoms that include urinary urgency, general irritative voiding, and anterior pelvic pain. Essentially, one is left with an extremely complex pathological interaction of (**1**) changing epithelial permeability, (**2**) sensory nerve branch upregulation, (**3**) mast cell activation with intermittent degranulation, (**4**) the superimposition of multiple positive and negative feedback loops occurring simultaneously. All of this creating a vicious cycle which contributes to the chronicity of IC and explains the often times disappointing response to single-drug treatment. In the final analysis, after years of ICA facilitated expert roundtables, countless NIH funded consensus conferences and millions of dollars of basic and clinical research work there seems to be an increasingly accepted emerging theme that the process may be initiated from divergent pathophysiologic perspectives that lead to a Final Common Pathway of Uro-Epithelial Dysfunction. Furthermore, the role of the spinal cord, the central nervous system, and the pelvic floor in the pathogenesis and clinical manifestations of IC is now recognized. IC should NOT be considered to be an exclusively urologic condition. Depending on its pathophysiologic starting point, it may have neurogenic, pelvic floor, gynecologic and gastrointestinal manifestations. Essentially, there seem to be four (4) frequently quoted etiologic starting points that lead to final Uro-Epithelial Dysfunction. Although this may be considered a gross oversimplification by some experts, it is worthwhile to help bring things into perspective. It also helps explain why one may see two specific patients with the diagnosis of IC that present and behave so differently. So ICDB data suggest four pathways that break down in the trends as follows:

1. Neurogenic ~ (25 %)
2. Infectious ~ (30 %)
3. Allergic ~ (35 %)
4. AutoImmune ~ (10 %)

The "neurogenic patient" seems to generate an inflammatory response that leads to a preponderance of neurogenic inflammation and upregulation of unmyelinated "C" fibers. Once the "C" mediated sensory nerves leading to the bladder are upregulated, neurons in the dorsal root ganglia and spinal cord also release tachykinins (including substance P), leading to a state of neurologic "wind-up" manifested by visceral allodynia and hyperalgesia in the bladder and adjacent pelvic organs. Theoretically, the patient goes into "sympathetic overdrive" and explains why many IC patients have general smooth muscle hypertonicity leading to pelvic floor muscle spasm and dyspareunia and vulvodynia. Also, you will often see Raynauds phenomenon in this subgroup as well as gastrointestinal symptoms.

In the "allergic patient" one sees multiple hypersensitivities to both environmental allergens and medications. Essentially, these patients become "vasoactive" and very sensitive to inflammatory mediators. Mast cells contain vasoactive and inflammatory mediators (e.g., histamine, leukotrienes, prostaglandins, and tryptases), and they play a central role in the pathogenesis of neuroinflammatory conditions, including IC. Release of the granules into the interstitium (degranulation) occurs as part of an immunoglobulin E-mediated hypersensitivity reaction or in response to substance P, cytokines, bacterial toxins, allergens, toxins, and stress.

Mastocytosis occurs in 30–35 % of IC patients which is consistent with the allergic subtype defined by the ICDB. Increased levels of histamine, histamine metabolites, and tryptase occur in IC patients.

The "infectious patient" cultures in IC patients are routinely negative. However, the polymerase chain reaction (PCR) studies have frequently identified bacterial genetic material in IC. So, in essence, ONE episode of cystitis can cause bladder dysfunction that results in alterations in bladder permeability, neurogenic upregulation (purinergic, afferent, etc.), and mast cell recruitment and activation.

In the "autoimmune patient", IC has many features of an autoimmune disease—chronicity, exacerbations, and remissions, clinical response to steroids/immunosuppressives. This autoimmune relationship was first pointed out by Fister et al. with his observation that certain patients with IC had an association to lupus (SLE). In addition, there is a high prevalence of antinuclear antibodies, and association with other autoimmune syndromes such as thyroiditis. Current evidence suggests that autoimmune phenomena (bladder antibodies, etc.) are epi-phenomena that occur as a result of local bladder cellular damage.

Regardless of the component of origin, ultimately the final common pathway in patients with IC/BPS leads to damaged urothelium. When the surface glycosaminoglycan (GAG) layer is damaged (via a urinary tract infection (UTI), autoimmune phenomena, etc.), inflammatory mediators can "leak" into surrounding tissues, causing pain and lower urinary tract symptoms. Now the literature strongly support that IC's symptoms are associated with a defect in the bladder epithelium lining, allowing irritating substances in the urine to penetrate into the bladder—essentially, alter the electrophysiologic functioning of the GAG layer that overlays the bladder lining. Deficiency in this glycosaminoglycan (GAG) layer on the surface of the bladder results in increased permeability of the underlying submucosal tissues.

Numerous studies have noted the link between IC and anxiety, stress, hyper-responsiveness, and panic. This proposed association with interstitial cystitis is that the body's immune response may actually attack the bladder wall in affected patients. Biopsies on the bladder wall with its attendant vasculature often contain immune deposits and mast cells. Mast cells containing histamine packets gather when IC patients are faced with anxiety reactions or stressful situations. The body identifies the bladder wall as a foreign agent, and is attacked by the immune complexes. Essentially, the body attacks itself, which is the basis of autoimmune disorders. Additionally, IC may be triggered by an unknown toxin or stimulus which causes nerves in the bladder wall to fire uncontrollably. When they fire, they release substances called neuropeptides that induce a cascade of reactions that cause the release of substance P inducing bladder pain.

It should be noted here before we move on to the next phase that there is at least some historical precedent for subcategorizing IC based on the presence or absence of "ulceration." Obviously, the eponym that goes along with the ulcer bears the moniker of the author that ended up publishing perhaps the most noted article with respect to interstitial cystitis, i.e. Guy Hunner. Some experts call the ulcerative subtype of IC, the "classic" variety. The question as to whether the non-ulcerative variety of IC can progress to the ulcerative variety is frequently raised. Fortunately or unfortunately, any evidence in this regard is lacking. Although not absolute, the clinical presentation is also variable. Non-ulcerative patients present with a more diffuse pain syndrome and multiple systemic complaints. On the other hand, ulcerative patients tend to have more bladder muscle irritability and lower bladder capacity. The ulcerative type is rare, accounting for probably less than 10 % of cases in the USA Bladder biopsy findings show that the ulcerative lesion can be transmural, associated with marked inflammatory changes, granulation tissue, mast cell infiltration, and, in some cases, fibrosis. This classic ulcerative variety of interstitial cystitis can be associated with progressively smaller bladder capacity over time.

The Final Common Pathway

So, again, no matter where you are coming from, or what your starting point is, if the end result is cystitis, i.e. *bladder wall inflammation*, then there must be a discussion *regarding uro-epithelial dysfunction*. At this juncture, it doesn't really matter what type of cystitis it is, whether it be radiation cystitis, chemical cystitis or most importantly here, interstitial cystitis. Also, it should be noted that we have referenced several other publications as well as alluding ourselves to the concept of uro-epithelial dysfunction as the "final common pathway" in this disease state. Understanding that, it is really NOT enough to simply say "uro-epithelial dysfunction (UED)". What does that really mean? It sounds great! It's technical, literal, and descriptive, everything you could want out of medical terminology. Unfortunately, it is also complex, that is, a lot of moving biochemical parts. However, if we are using the term, there should at least be some general understanding. Now, most of the people who are reading this book are clinicians, not basic researchers. Even more significant is that they are clinicians who have to deal with some of these very difficult and complicated patients, so a general review of the key components of this "final common pathway" are in order.

The urinary bladder's epithelium or urothelium has been the subject of considerable interest and much research in recent years. However, what has changed dramatically in the last decade is the concept of the microscopic anatomy of this epithelial lining and how it does what it does. It is currently no longer considered just a simple barrier, or a nonspecific defense against microorganisms. It has been recognized, in and of itself, as a specialized tissue regulating complex bladder functions and playing a fundamental role in the pathogenesis of inflammatory cystitis. Suffice it to say, that you cannot really claim to understand interstitial cystitis without understanding some of the intricate inner workings of the urothelium.

For the past 15–20 years, researchers have been focusing on the urothelium as a physiologic organ. Essentially, the urothelium is divided up into two major components, the epithelium and subepithelium. Receptors and mediators that are active in the sub-epithelial layer have been studied, especially with respect to the purinergic or vanilloid neurotransmitters that they may utilize. Dysfunction at this level would be considered secondary uro-epithelial dysfunction.

Understanding the role of these subepithelial neurotransmitters will offer the opportunity for new therapeutic strategies. The urothelium from a histologic perspective is considered "transitional cell type." Transitional cell epithelium is graduated, with the most mature and well-differentiated cells ending up at the surface. In this case, those most superficial urothelial cells are known as umbrella-cells. Above the umbrella cell layer there is a thick layer of glycoproteins and proteoglycans, which together are called glycosaminoglycans (GAGs). They constitute a hydrophilic mucosal coating and act as a barrier against solutes found in urine. In recent years they have received special attention because injury to the GAG due to different noxious stimuli has been identified as the first step in the genesis of chronic inflammatory bladder diseases, such as recurrent urinary tract infections, chemical or radiation cystitis, interstitial cystitis, and/or bladder pain syndrome. It is important here to define the significance of the urothelium from a physiologic perspective and underline the role of glycosaminoglycans, in maintaining a layer of protection and insulation to the bladder wall. Finally, if one considers the GAG as the most superficial layer of the transitional cell epithelium in the

bladder and then examines it from a pathophysiologic perspective with respect to IC, it falls at the center of the disease process. Consequently, more descriptive semantics emerge and the term "uro-epithelial dysfunction" comes to the forefront.

So what if a patient develops an inflammatory cascade that eventually leads to UED, what are the pathophysiologic sequelae? The sequelae are increased permeability of the most superficial layers of the bladder wall. These would include the umbrella cell layer and its overlying GAG coating. Some common glycosaminoglycans (GAGs) are shown below. Obviously, heparin is synthetic GAG but very similar from a molecular perspective to their natural couterparts which are predominantly chondroitin and keratin sulfate as well as hyaluronic acid. It is important to remember that *functional GAG* allows for *impermeability*, which in turn gives protection to the underlying submucosal sensory nerves. When the inflammatory cycle, infectious or not leads to UED, the GAG becomes much more permeable and is often referred to as "leaky". This leaky GAG can then lead to the migration of microorganisms, urea and charged species (H+/K+) into the submucosa as noted in an ICDB subset analysis. By in turn, this yields to increased and inappropriate transmission of electrophysiologic impulses, often times upregulating the activity of sensory phenomena via both A-Delta fibers and unmyelinated "C" fibers. In addition to the above, physiologic GAG allows for the binding of a mono or bi-molecular layer of water that allows for insulation, protection, and a frictionless plane making it very difficult for micro-organism adherence (Fig. 15.3) permeability leads to the migration of micro-organisms, urea and charged species (H+/K+) into the submucosa as noted in an ICDB subset analysis. By in turn, this yields to increased and inappropriate transmission of electrophysiologic impulses, often times upregulating the activity of sensory phenomena via both A-Delta fibers and unmyelinated "C" fibers. In addition to the above, physiologic GAG allows for the binding of a mono or bi-molecular layer of water that allows for insulation, protection, and a frictionless plane making it very difficult for micro-organism adherence.

Light microscopic analysis of the most superficial layers of the bladder wall reveal a "haze" overlying the umbrella cell layer which appeared to be consistent with the GAG (Fig. 15.4). Consequently, it is very interesting to observe bladder biopsy specimens in patients with IC which suggest possible obvious histologic defects. Unfortunately, most likely, these observed defects are "artifact" and not real time. In fact, many authors including Dixon et al. in 1989, Wein and Levin in 1991 and Nickel et al. in 1993 all write about the inability to substantiate many of these biopsy findings. After more extensive study by many authors, Nickel et al. lead the charge that the GAG itself is physiologic. Moreover, any defect in GAG permeability is not histologic and cannot

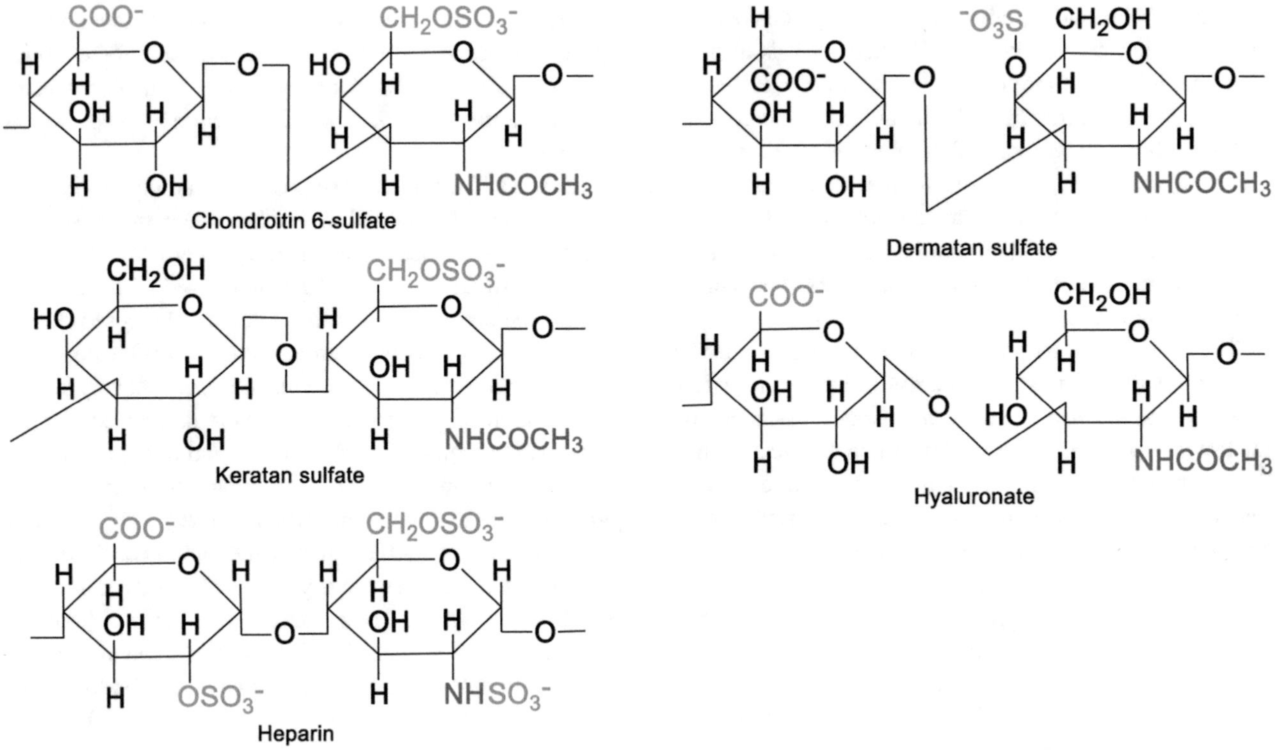

Fig. 15.3 Molecular Structure of GAG

Fig. 15.4 Light microscopic analysis of the most superficial layers of the bladder wall reveals a "haze" overlying the umbrella cell layer which appeared to be consistent with the GAG

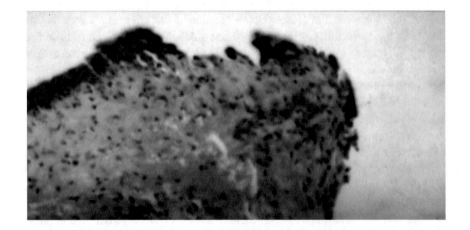

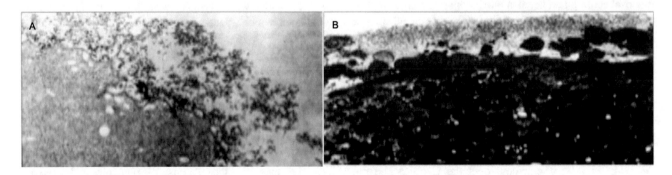

Fig. 15.5 (a) Physiologically inactive, compressed GAG; (b) physiologically active, hydrated GAG

be studied at a light microscopic level. In essence, to begin to understand GAG physiology, it must be examined at an electron microscopic level because a physiologically functional GAG must be appropriately charged on an electrophysiologic level to be able to attract and maintain 1–2 layers of water. This will allow "insulation" of the bladder wall submucosa from microorganisms and charged species and also allow for a "frictionless plane" which limits the ability of bacteria to adhere (Fig. 15.5a, b).

Genetics

Genetic studies are becoming an increasingly more important but are also an expense way to study disease processes. Initially, the push to move toward genetic evaluation first comes from observational protocols on a given population. In this case, if one compares the prevalence of interstitial cystitis (IC) among first-degree relatives of patients with IC with the prevalence of IC in the general population, there seems to be a skew. Often times the first evidence that a disease may have a genetic susceptibility is the demonstration of family aggregation of the process. Subsequently, Warren et al. at the University of Maryland looked at more than 2500 patients who had a formal diagnosis of IC. Here 3.9 % reported that they had 107 relatives (first-degree relatives) who were also diagnosed with the disease. These measurements, plus data-based assumptions of proportions of patients who actually met endoscopic requirements for the diagnosis of IC, suggest that women between the ages of 31–73 years old who were first-degree relatives of patients with IC themselves had a prevalence of IC of 995/100,000. A comparison of this with the number approximating the prevalence in the general population of American women of this age (60/100,000) indicates a risk ratio for IC in adult female first-degree relatives of 17. In essence, first-degree relatives of patients with IC have a prevalence of the disease which is 17 times that found in the general population. Previously reported genetic data based on observational population data suggest significant association of IC in monozygotic and dizygotic twins as well as a 9:1 preponderance of IC in females over males in the general population and a 3:1 to 4:1 in Jewish females versus females in the general population.

PAND or the panD locus is a gene map locus occurring at a site identified as 13q22–q32. It is important to note that panD is required for cell synthesis of panothenic acid, without which it is difficult for a cell to make recombinant DNA. Also, this locus is associated with a constellation of clinical disorders which include but is not limited to IC/PBS. In classical genetics many genes are known to have manifold effects, i.e., the gene seems to affect unrelated characteristics. An example of such a gene may be the locus 13q22 — 13q32 in humans which code for IC/PBS. Other component disorders associated with this gene locus are *migraine headaches, generalized panic dis-*

order, and mitral valve prolapse. All of these are commonly seen in association with IC. Thus, IC should be considered a pleiotropic disorder.

Diagnosis

The diagnosis of IC/PBS is often met with difficulty and confusion by both physician and patient. Part of the problem is that the clinical symptoms of this process can vary from patient to patient and sometimes even vary, based on the type of flare, within the same patient. Compounding the problem even further is that there really is no absolute with respect to a universally accepted or prescribed protocol to formally make this diagnosis. Consequently, in an attempt to promote some degree of interdisciplinary inclusivity, the NIH/NIDDK began to sponsor a series of consensus conferences to at least start to create a more widely accepted definition for diagnosis. Ultimately, between 1986 and 1987 the NIH/NIDDK released their "Research Criteria" for IC in an effort to be able to study the disease in an academic fashion. Surprisingly or not, it became almost a de-facto definition for the diagnosis of the disease by the mid to late 1980s.

NIH/NIDDK Research Criteria (Circa 1987)

1. Bladder pain on filling with relief on emptying
2. Urinary FREQUENCY at least 8× per day
3. Urinary urgency
4. Nocturia (at least one time per night)
5. Glomerulations and/or Hunner's ulcer visualizable @ cystoscopy under anesthesia @ pressures of 80 cm/H_2O for 3 min (NOT along the path of the scope) +/− B.Biopsy

Well, suffice it to say, the mystique of this whole disease process continues to manifest itself even after having introduced criteria that experts felt secure would clear up *all* confusion in diagnosis. Unfortunately, the 1987 criteria still seemed to engender a significant amount of research confusion *in patient recruitment* for the ICDB. So, then again, the following year in 1988. The NIH/NIDDK decided to hold a follow-up conference focused on making that selection process easier. To do that, they felt that perhaps "exclusion criteria" may be better suited for interstitial cystitis. This is what they came up with. You don't have IC if………

- Frequency less than 8 times per 24 h.
- Absence of nocturia
- Duration of symptoms less than 9 months
- Awake bladder capacity of greater than 350 cc
- In the presence of LUT stone disease
- TCC bladder
- Carcinoma in situ

- Previous pelvic XRT
- History of cyclophosphamide use
- Diagnosis of chronic prostatitis
- Any GYN malignancy
- Urethral diverticulum
- Active herpes
- Age under 18 years of age

Having noted all of the above, let's step back and look at this whole thing from above at 10,000 ft. If we assess the compendium of diagnostic possibilities here, there are essentially four components that should be considered as a physician when making the diagnosis. Firstly, clinically based on symptomology. Secondly, the endoscopic component. Thirdly, biochemically via tests and/or potential markers and finally, if all of the above fail, as would be echoed by the NIH/NIDDK consensus, the diagnosis should be made by exclusion.

So, first let's examine suggestive symptoms which would clue the diagnosis of IC. Classically, interstitial cystitis has a "triad" of lower urinary tract symptoms. These include: (1) urinary frequency, (2) urinary urgency, and (3) bladder/pelvic pain. If the symptomatic diagnosis is examined critically, the prevalence of symptoms within the triad can be broken down. The two most common lower urinary tract symptoms seen in IC are not surprisingly urinary frequency and urinary urgency. According to ICDB calculations, urinary urgency is the most common symptom seen in patients with IC, occurring at a penetration level of 91 %. Interestingly, urinary frequency is the second most common occurring 83 % of the time which may contribute to the conundrum since another very common syndrome known as overactive bladder (OAB) expresses itself with the same two presenting symptoms.

Again, not surprisingly, with the overlap of IC and OAB, *the symptomatic diagnosis of IC is confusing at best.* Furthermore the average patient has symptoms for 5 years and sees five separate clinicians before a diagnosis of IC is made. This in and of itself implies that clinicians have difficulty in making the diagnosis. Consequently, moving on to the endoscopic level for diagnostic consideration is an important superimposition. With the understanding that there is no "sine qua non" for IC at the symptomatic level, moving on to the "endoscopy component" adds another level of security. Unfortunately, lower urinary tract (LUT) endoscopy under local anesthesia adds nothing and may actually further inflame the situation. Essentially, if LUT endoscopy is to be done, it would be cystoscopy under anesthesia. This type of procedure is called a hydraulic bladder distension and is done as a protocol. The protocol would be to perform cysto-urethroscopy at rest and with pressure. The first part of the protocol is an endoscopic examination of the bladder and urethra at rest without pressure. Although there are no spe-

cific findings often times, there are focal areas of inflammation and submucosal hypervascularity. The second portion of the test is carried out under pressure. The bladder is filled under anesthesia at a pressure of 80 cm/H_2O pressure for 3 min. Then, the area is examined for a specific type of inflammatory response known as "glomerulation." Although, it is important to emphasize that even at this level, there is nothing pathomneumonic for IC. The glomerular response after hydraulic bladder distension is very characteristic and may help the clinician with difficult diagnostic dilemmas. This procedure stretches the muscular wall of the bladder and is often therapeutic as well as diagnostic. After hydraulic bladder distention procedures, a significant percentage of patients note increase in bladder capacity and decrease in their pelvic pain pattern. Although the reason for this effect is often hotly debated, there is physiologic rationale. These include (1) detrusor distention may de-functionalize certain key submucosal receptors such as vanilloid and purinergic subtypes which may mediate noxious sensory phenomena, (2) breakdown collagen crosslinking will enhance elasticity and increase capacity, and (3) distention may create a generalized neuropraxia, decreasing the pelvic pain pattern. The proportion of IC/BPS patients who experience relief from hydrodistention is currently unknown and evidence for this modality is limited by a lack of properly controlled studies. Nevertheless, it is important to remember that even though they are rare, complications do exist and include bladder rupture and sepsis which may be associated with prolonged, high-pressure hydrodistention. Finally, tissue has no role in the diagnosis of IC. Bladder biopsy may only confirm LUT inflammation in a nonspecific sense. However, tissue biopsy may be important to exclude carcinoma in situ as a potentially fatal entity presenting with primarily with irritative LUT symptoms like IC. By the late 1990s there was an emphasis towards newer and less invasive diagnostic modalities for IC. TO get away from some of the cumbersome NIH/NIDDK research recommendations. In 1998 Phil Hanno suggested that those NIH/NIDDK criteria were too restrictive and physicians in the community who were trying to stay on point with them, may be missing patients who actually suffer with IC. Consequently, biochemical aids for the diagnosis of IC came to the forefront. These would be (1) the potassium sensitivity test and (2) the collection of urinary biomarkers, especially the antiproliferative factor.

With a better understanding of the biochemical nature and physiologic function of the GAG as well as its implication into the role of the pathogenesis of IC, the "potassium sensitivity test (PST)" was presented. Based on uncovering the pathophysiology of "urothelial dysfunction," as the cornerstone of interstitial cystitis, the PST was devised as a minimally invasive alternative for the diagnosis of this disease. In essence, it is a simple test which consists of instilling a solution of potassium chloride into the bladder via a urinary catheter. The test should identify those patients with increased urothelial permeability by eliciting a "mild" degree of lower abdominal or pelvic discomfort. Unfortunately, the PST is no longer widely used in the USA, in part because multivariate data collection suggesting low sensitivity and specificity. In addition, it has turned out to be much more painful and much less accurate than suggested in its early clinical trials. The PST is usually touted as a predictive test in that it would be able to gauge the permeability of the most superficial of the urothelial layers, the GAG layer, which may be defective in IC patients. An important confounding factor in this regard is that other disease processes may also end up with a "final common pathway" that leads to uro-epithelial dysfunction. These would include processes such as "MS," "radiation cystitis," "chemotherapy (cytoxan) cystitis," "recent UTI", "obstructive BPH," etc. Consequently, in the final analysis, the PST is much more uncomfortable than previously expected and has fallen out of favor in most cases and at the very least should not be considered mainstream.

At about the same time that the PST was fading, much work was being done to try to identify stable functional urinary biomarkers that can be used as a diagnostic tool. Three urinary biomarkers were uncovered by Susan Keay at the University of Maryland in Baltimore. All of the biomarkers were able to be collected from the urine of affected patients. Two of the three were positively correlated with the disease, i.e. patients with IC had increasing concentrations of these factors in their urine. These were respectively: epidermal growth factor (EGF) and antiproliferative factor (APF). On the other hand, HB-EGF exhibited an inverse correlation in urine of interstitial cystitis patients, compared to controls. Now, it is important to note that EGF and HB-EGF are potent urothelial and smooth muscle cell mitogens, and enhance proliferation. In addition, they are produced by many different types of epithelial cells. HB-EGF is initially expressed as a transmembrane precursor (proHB-EGF), with the soluble form generated by the regulated metalloproteinase-dependent ectodomain shedding. All of the above not withstanding, the bottom line for EGF and HB-EGF is that they are products of complex biochemical reactions, they are often times difficult to assay and probably less accurate. Hence, APF seemed to be the marker that took "center stage" and was able to engender the greatest amount of research dollars. APF (*antiproliferative factor*) is a small glycosolated peptide with a chain length of 8 amino acids. APF is originally purified from the urine specimens of IC patients using high performance liquid chromatography [*xyz*]. The function of APF is to decrease cellular activity and turnover in the urothelium. It is easily collected and the activity of APF is detected in the urine of over 95 % of interstitial cystitis patients as compared to only 9 % of controls. The accumulation of APF in urine is capable of altering the physiology and behavior of uro-thelial cells. The physiologic effects of APF decrease the ability of uro-epithelial cells to turnover and reproduce. In addition, the most superficial cells of the urothelium are charged with the synthesis of GAG which is significantly inhibited. Moreover, the GAG that is made by the uro-epithelium which is chronically exposed to APF is dysfunctional, i.e. it is electrophysiologically impaired. Electrophysiologically impaired GAG has difficulty maintaining the physiologic charges necessary to attract H_2O molecules to sustain a hydrated GAG which is necessary for insulation and protection of the submucosa and substance of the bladder.

These physiologic effects are consistent with clinical observations of epithelial thinning and denudation observed in the bladder tissue of IC patients. Additional bladder dysfunction includes increased inflammatory infiltrates (e.g., mast cell and/or lymphocytic), which are correlated to the increased pain and cytokine production in IC/PBS bladder (*xyz*). It is important to note that APF is secreted from bladder epithelial cells derived from IC patients, but *NOT* from asymptomatic controls (xy). Even more importantly, the APF is ONLY secreted by bladder urothelial cells in affected patients. It is *NOT* secreted by urothelial cells collected from the renal pelvis. Consequently, because of all of these above factors, APF is still actively being sought after as a non-invasive, reliable diagnostic marker for interstitial cystitis.

The AUA Consensus-Based Guideline Statement for the Treatment of IC

Introductory Statement About the AUA Guidelines

The purpose of these guidelines is to provide direction to clinicians and patients regarding how to approach IC as a clinical entity. How to conduct a valid diagnostic process and, approach treatment with the goals of maximizing symptom control and patient quality of life (QoL) while minimizing AEs and patient burden. The strategies and approaches recommended by the AUA Guidelines were derived from evidence-based and consensus-based processes. The nomenclature utilized in IC can be a controversial issue at times in and of itself. Nevertheless, for the purpose of clarity the panel has decided to refer to the syndrome as IC/BPS (*bladder pain syndrome*) and to consider these terms synonymous. One must remember that the most effective approach for a particular patient is best determined by the individual clinician and patient. As the science relevant to IC/BPS evolves and improves, the strategies presented here will require amendment to remain consistent with the highest standards of clinical care.

Treatments Range from More Conservative to More Invasive

1. First-line therapies—patient education, behavioral therapy, dietary modification
2. Second line therapies—*pelvic floor physical therapy*, *oral medications, bladder instillations*
3. *Third line therapies—interventional treatment of Hunner's ulcers (laser, fulguration or Triamcinolone injection), hydraulic bladder distention*
4. Fourth line therapies—*neuromodulation (sacral root or pudendal branch)*
5. Fifth line therapies—*BTX-A, Cyclosporine A*
6. Sixth line therapies—*major surgical reconstruction (urinary diversion, augmentation), (+/cystectomy)*

It is beyond our scope to discuss all potential therapies in each category. In addition, some of these specific therapies are discussed by other authors in other sections of this text and it would be superfluous to duplicate them here. However, if a more in-depth discussion of a therapy takes place in another section, we will point that out and refer you there.

First-Line Therapies
Patient Education

This is often the least discussed and least emphasized of the first-line therapies, and perhaps any and all therapeutic options for IC. However, it may be the most important. Following each intervention, the patient is reassessed for response. Unfortunately, patients often get confused because the entire disease process is characterized by "flare and remission." In addition, therapies are often applied in a haphazard and placed in a "hit-or-miss" fashion. At times, the patient's anxiety level is so high that caregivers are pushed to combine numerous different therapies before the response to each therapy is truly assessed. This approach is sometimes partly driven by unrealistic patient demands and expectations regarding the success of various therapeutic interventions. All of this is directly related to misinformation secondary to inadequate patient education and support. Again, patients must receive plenty of reading material with visuals, graphics, and learning aids. These things combined with extensive counseling regarding the nature and prognosis of their condition and its response to therapy are critically important. Such counseling must be initiated prior to embarking on invasive interventions for which no proven overwhelming benefit may be achieved.

The Interstitial Cystitis Association (ICA) is the only nonprofit charitable organization dedicated solely to improving the quality of healthcare and lives of people living with interstitial cystitis (IC). Not surprisingly, "Education" is one of the ICA's cornerstones and the IC website bears it out. Patient's who suffer with IC are often referred to the sections on "virtual education" as well as its section on "support." There are many regularly meeting interstitial cystitis (IC) support groups located throughout the USA and around the world. These groups are open to all who wish to attend. To find out about a support group near you—see more at http://www.ichelp.org.

Diet

Research has found that there is a lot of variability among IC patients. Some people with IC report that certain foods appear to irritate their bladders and cause painful IC flares. And they find that making a few strategic changes to what they eat and drink can help to control IC symptoms including pain, frequency, and urgency. Other IC patients find that diet does affect their flares. Dietary modifications have been studied extensively as therapy for interstitial cystitis. These dietary measures focusing on the "low acid/low oxalate" variety can be effective when used alone, but they can also be complementary to virtually all other interventions for interstitial cystitis. When one combines "low acid/low oxalate diet" along with the educational measures previously described above the clinical results can be impressive. Some studies have reported that up to 90 % of patients expressed symptom exacerbations to food, beverage, and dietary supplements. Moreover, the flip side to this statement is also true, i.e. very high percentages of IC patients respond effectively to dietary therapy for IC.

There is a lot of information on the web promoting various diets for interstitial cystitis (IC). Both the IC clinical guideline of the American Urological Association (AUA) and the chronic pelvic pain practice bulletin of the American College of Obstetrical Gynecology (ACOG) recommend dietary modification as a useful approach for helping to manage IC and chronic pelvic pain—*see more at http://www.ichelp.org/living-with-ic/icdiet/#sthash.P01xBBxl.dpuf.*

Dietary Supplements, Calcium Glycerol Phosphate (Prelief)

Many patients report that certain foods and beverages exacerbate inflammatory lower urinary tract symptoms particularly in interstitial cystitis. Not surprisingly, and as would follow from what was outlined above, the foods that seem to cause the most problems are those that are the most acidic. Major culprits include tomato-based foods, cabbage, coffee, tea, citrus fruit, fruit juices and wine, especially red wine, probably secondary to the bitter tannins which are present. At first glance, removing these foods seems like such a simple solution to such a troublesome problem.

Dietary Supplements, Calcium Glycerol Phosphate (Prelief)

But when you think about the reality of eliminating many of your favorite foods from your life forever, any patient would wish there was an easier way.

The active ingredient in Prelief is calcium glycerophosphate, a dietary mineral that combines calcium and phosphorus in a 1:1 ratio. When it is added to acidic foods, the mineral acts as a base agent, actually bringing the pH of the food toward a neutral level. The mechanism of action would be considered "exogenous," not endogenous. That is, the biochemical reaction that takes place is outside of the body and actually occurs on the foodstuff itself, not the patient. This is an important distinction, because interfering with the body's natural acid–base metabolism can be disastrous. Furthermore, antacids which neutralize acid in the stomach often cause more problems than they solve. Even more importantly, there are minimal reported side effects following the use of Prelief. According to studies conducted by the manufacturer, calcium glycerophosphate was able to significantly reduce the acid level of common foods and beverages some by as much as 90 %. With just one tablet, the acid in an 8-ounce glass of iced tea was reduced by more than 90 %; a 6-ounce cup of coffee was reduced by 95 %; as well as an 8-ounce citrus drink. Three tablets reduced the acid in a 4-ounce glass of chardonnay by 80 % and the acid in 125 ml of bottled pasta sauce by 60 %.

Finally, urologic researchers, Tu, Gordon, Whitmore et al. at the Graduate Hospital in Philadelphia in the late 1990s studied the effects of Prelief on more than two hundred (200) patients with interstitial cystitis. When using it, 61 % of the participants reported a reduction in urinary urgency, and 70 % experienced less pain and discomfort when eating acidic foods.

Second Line Therapies
Pelvic Floor Physical Therapy

Pelvic floor physical therapy is an important component of therapy at this level. An in-depth discussion on this topic is extensively explored in the chapter dedicated to this concept and so, will not be included here.

Oral Medications: Elmiron, Amitriptyline, Hydroxyzine
Oral Medication: Elmiron

Elmiron is a negatively charged, synthetic sulfated polysaccharide. Essentially, it falls into a group of biochemicals known as glycosaminoglycans or GAGs. Chemically, Elmiron is pentosan polysulfate or PPS, (1->4)-β-Xylan 2,3-bis(hydrogen sulfate) with a 4 O-methyl-α-D-glucuronate (Fig. 15.6). Essentially, it is a two-chain molecule divided up into "alpha" and "beta" subunits. The alpha component is composed primarily of D-Xylose while the beta component is composed primarily of glucuronic acid. The molecule weighs between 4000 and 6000 daltons with a pH between 6 and 7 in aqueous solution. It is FDA approved in the USA for the relief of various medical conditions including thrombi and interstitial cystitis in humans. Various brand names for

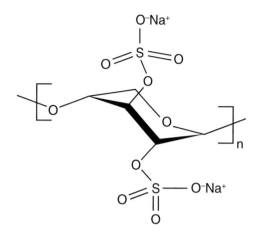

Fig. 15.6 Oral medication: elmiron: molecular makeup

the human drug include Elmiron, Anarthron, Fibrase, Thrombocid, and SP54. PPS is also sold under the brand name Comfora in India.

These GAGs have an affinity for mucosal membranes and physiologically "coat them" in an effort to make them electrophysiologically active. In this way, they can attract and attach a mono- or bi-molecular layer of H_2O to its surface which insulates and protects the urothelium and the submucosa below it. It is this GAG layer that gives mucus membranes their glistening appearance. But, it is also important to remember, as noted above in the section on pathophysiology that the natural lining of our bladder is GAG. More specifically, natural GAG is probably keratin or chondroitin sulfate whose biochemical structure is almost identical to "heparin sulfate." Not surprisingly then, by the late 1980s, as clinical research started to catch up with basic research, along with the understanding that the pathophysiologic crux in IC may be defective GAG, all lead to the belief that possible replacement of electrophysiologically intact GAG could help alleviate the lower urinary tract symptoms (LUTS) of urinary urgency and bladder pain. This was shown to be true with the instillation of heparin directly into the bladder. Now, having said all of that, as is the case with many drugs, there are pros and cons. With respect to GAGs in general, there is usually an attendant anticoagulant effect. In fact, many GAGs are used clinically as anticoagulants. Obviously, with IC, increasing bleeding tendency is not a characteristic that is usually sought after here. In fact, it should be guarded against. So, by the early 1990s, clinical researchers who focused on interstitial cystitis began to clamor for an agent that could be taken orally and attack the biochemical pathophysiology that make up the "final common pathway" that leads to clinical expression of the disease process. Consequently, in that regard, one must ask what are those pharmacologic characteristics that would be most coveted.

After examining this issue, it would seem the "ideal oral agent for IC" would have four key characteristics:

1. Renal excreted
2. Orally administered
3. GAG (to "*fill in or reactivate*" defects in the patient's existing GAG layer)
4. Without excessive anticoagulation effects

Well, if the old saying, "ask, and you shall receive" has any credence left, it was answered in October of 1996 when IVAX took pentosan polysulfate (Elmiron) to the FDA and was able to jump through all their hoops. Elmiron came into being and immediately was the answer to everyone's prayer, or at least that's what they thought. Certainly, it met all the criteria that the "experts" were clamoring for. However, as we amassed a more significant clinical experience, there seemed to be some issues that arose from a practical perspective.

Oral Medications: Amitriptyline

Amitriptyline HCl is an antidepressant with sedative effects. Its mechanism of action in man is not known. It is not a monoamine oxidase inhibitor and it does not act primarily by stimulation of the central nervous system (Fig. 15.7).

Amitriptyline inhibits the membrane pump mechanism responsible for uptake of norepinephrine and serotonin in adrenergic and serotonergic neurons. Pharmacologically this action may potentiate or prolong neuronal activity since reuptake of these biogenic amines is important physiologically in terminating transmitting activity. This interference with the reuptake of norepinephrine and/or serotonin may underlie its antidepressant activity.

Our review of the studies of clinical efficacy of the tricyclic compounds in the treatment of interstitial cystitis supports the general view that amitriptyline (and even imipramine) is more effective than placebo, and that amitriptyline may even be a little more effective than imipramine. Moreover, multiple review articles confirm the impression that we the authors have gained from other studies that clinical ratings of general improvement in the LUTS associated with interstitial cystitis are statistically significant and that the drug in slightly higher doses is a good deal more useful than placebo.

To this end, the "Interstitial Cystitis Collaborative Research Network," led by Lee Nyberg put together a well-received study specifically to look at amitriptyline in interstitial cystitis. Their results were published in the Journal of Urology back in 2010. Without "naming names," suffice it to say that all authors have a long and well-known history with respect to their expertise in dealing with patients suffering with IC. This is the first multicenter, randomized, relatively large-scale trial looking at the effectiveness of amitriptyline in interstitial cystitis/painful bladder syndrome (IC/PBS) patients. In spite of considering amitriptyline as one of the standard treatments for IC patients with grade "A" recommendation, surprisingly, the results did not show uniform improvement across all doses between placebo and the amitriptyline group. This trial included 271 patients who were randomized to two arms. All participants in both the placebo and amitriptyline arms underwent educational and behavioral modification programs, including symptom, fluid and diet management plus bladder training. The dose of the drug was increased from 10 to 25 mg, 50 mg, and then to a maximum dose of 75 mg over 4 weeks.

Outcome assessment was performed 12 weeks after randomization and was done by filling in a seven-point scale (from markedly worse to markedly improved). In addition to other forms of diaries and questionnaires to assess symptoms, in this study, improvement in LUTS was considered positive when the "seven-point scale" showed moderate or marked improvement. A total of 231 participants completed the study. Interestingly, and surprisingly, only those who managed to achieve a daily dose of at least 50 mg had a response rate of 77 % in the amitriptyline group compared to placebo (53 %), with p value <0.001, which is statistically significant. In conclusion, this study shows that considering amitriptyline at doses less than 50 mg as a standard treatment option with "grade A" recommendation in clinical practice should be challenged, and treatment guidelines should change in light of the results from this trial, with other options explored.

Another potentially fruitful area for further research with amitriptyline is that of augmentation of baseline therapy for IC. Anecdotally, and even with the addition of some wispy clinical evidence, TCAs may increase the durability of initial baseline protocol (multimodal medical therapy for IC) as an "add on agent" for those who receive even a short protocol period.

More importantly, these agents are safe when used with care. However, sometimes, side effects can be an issue. Some of the more commonly cited undesirable phenomena described by patients taking the drug are excessive somnolence, worsening depression, paradoxical anxiety, and rapid weight gain. All of these unwanted symptoms may be related

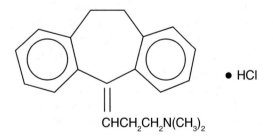

Fig. 15.7 Oral medication: amitriptyline: molecular makeup

to imipramine's effects on central adrenergic mechanisms, probably in hypothalamic and other diencephalic regions. However, if amitriptyline is properly used, that is, if the dosage is watched, then the side effects can be controlled by either reduction in dosage or corrective medication.

Oral Medications: Hydroxazine

Hydroxyzine (sold as Vistaril, Atarax) is an old drug by millennial standards. It is actually a first-generation antihistamine which was initially synthesized way back in 1956. At that time, Pfizer was able to navigate it through all of the regulatory processes and take it to market in the USA later that very same year. Interestingly, and probably secondary to its stability and tolerability, keep it in widespread use, still today. As an antihistamine, hydroxyzine is actually a derivative of piperazine. Hydroxyzine's antihistamine effect is due to its metabolite, cetirizine which is a potent H1 receptor antagonist and selective inhibitor of peripheral H1 receptors. This agent competes with histamine for binding at H1-receptor sites on the effector cell surface. The sedative properties of hydroxyzine occur as a result of suppression of certain subcortical regions of the brain. Additionally, but not surprisingly for an agent to be used in bladder disorders, there is an anticholinergic burden that it carries. Consequently, it is secondary to its central anticholinergic effects that make hydroxyzine effective in any type of agonistic bladder muscle disorder.

Interstitial cystitis is a painful subtype of inflammatory bladder disease that in and of itself has its own spectrum of patient profiles. As described above, the spectrum in IC can be roughly broken down into four subgroups. These include patients who have the allergic subtype. It is this subtype that seems to have a preponderance of patients who come back with histologically confirmed "detrusor mastocytosis."

The patients with mastocytosis differed from those without mastocytosis in that they were older, and had a higher frequency of hematuria, a higher frequency of a red, scarred and richly vascularized bladder at cystoscopy before distension, and a smaller cystoscopic bladder capacity. We conclude that by dividing patients with painful bladder into two groups according to the mast cell counts in the detrusor, certain differences in the clinical findings in the groups can be ruled out. However, in individual patients one cannot note with certainty to which pathological anatomical group the patient belongs, since great overlapping between the groups exists. Whether only patients with detrusor mastocytosis have interstitial cystitis depends on definitions and still remains an open question.

Intravesical Medications

Interstitial cystitis is a noninfectious inflammatory disease process that is characterized by flare and remission. As discussed above, treatment strategies usually start with hydrau-

lic bladder distention followed by oral medications, which in a majority of patients can maintain a stable socially acceptable lifestyle with a minimal pelvic pain component. However, periodically, there will be "breakthrough" inflammatory flares. For these cases, subjecting the patient back to systemic anesthetics for repeat "hydraulic bladder distention" or changing an oral medical protocol that has been effective in these challenging patients can be traumatic. Consequently, intravesical instillation of medications can be an extremely useful tool in suppressing these difficult flare responses. More importantly, there are several theoretical advantages to using intraveiscal treatment.

Some of the advantages for utilizing intravesical therapy in the treatment of refractory IC flares include: (1) the ability to deliver high concentrations of a drug directly to the bladder lining, (2) very low incidence intravesical agents being exposed to the systemic circulation and thus revealing an extremely low level of systemic side effects, (3) minimal incidence of drug interactions with the intravesical agents, and (4) direct interaction with defective inflamed urothelium with the potential for histological repair.

Intravesical Therapy: Heparin (GAG Enhancement)

As discussed above, the pathologic culmination of the final common pathway in IC is the genesis of a defective superficial portion of the urothelial layer. The biochemical nature of this part of the lining is made up primarily of glycosaminoglycan (GAG). Heparin is a systemic GAG that closely mimics that natural bladder lining and when instilled can be very effective in controlling clinical symptoms associated with IC flares. Parsons et al. suggest 1000 units of heparin be used intravesically three times per week in these situations. However, other authors utilize different doses. Some suggest increasing the heparin dose up to 2500 units. Whatever the case, or whatever the prescription, heparin can be a very useful tool. Finally, it is noteworthy to mention the use of chondroitin sulfate as an intravesical agent. This is a natural GAG and most closely mimics human bladder GAG which reveals high concentrations of both chondroitin sulfate and keratin sulfate.

Intravesical Therapy: Dimethyl Sulfoxide

Dimethyl sulfoxide (DMSO) was first synthesized in 1867 and is now used chiefly as an industrial solvent. However, it was not until 1964 that the remarkable medicinal properties of DMSO were identified. When applied to mammalian mucosa, the agent penetrates quickly and yields significant physiologic and pharmacologic actions, including suppression of inflammation, analgesia and bacteriostasis. As a result the drug has been used widely as treatment of troublesome urogenital disorders, and various postoperative pain syndromes. To date little, if any, local or systemic toxicity has been noted in the human after the administration of DMSO.

Intravesical dimethyl sulfoxide (DMSO) has been used in the treatment of interstitial cystitis, radiation cystitis, and even chronic prostatitis in males. Significant symptomatic relief has been achieved in the majority of patients treated with DMSO with no systemic or local toxicity has been noted. However, because of its simplicity and ease of administration, intravesical DMSO is often used effectively in IC clinical flares or those patients with severe LUTS after radiation or even those patients who have failed to respond to conventional therapy.

Intravesical Therapy: Combination Agents

Some healthcare providers recommend intravesical therapy with a combination of medications for difficult refractory IC flares. These agents are instilled into the bladder with a catheter, to reduce symptoms of pain and can be done in a clinician's office, or you can learn to self-administer the treatment at home. The treatment may be used as a single "rescue" treatment when symptoms are severe, or as a regularly scheduled treatment (e.g., three times per week for a period of weeks). The medications are in a liquid form and are a small amount (about 15 mL or 0.5 ounces). You hold the liquid in the bladder for as long as possible, and then urinate normally.

This type of combination of medications to be used for intravesical instillation are often called "COCKTAILS." Almost every provider who has an interest or specialization in treating these patients has their own version of what is the most effective combination of medications utilized in an intravesical fashion. Essentially, everyone has a "best cocktail" to be used in difficult IC flares. Almost every specialist will swear by their specific combination of concentrations of agents which usually include substances such as lidocaine, heparin, and sodium bicarbonate +/− antibiotic (often times gentamycin). It is believed that combining these agents helps to repair the bladder lining and decrease nerve sensitivity in the bladder. In some studies, approximately 80 % of patients had decreased pain for days after one treatment with heparin, sodium bicarbonate, and lidocaine. In addition, some patients experience reduced pain for days or weeks after bladder installations.

Third Line Therapies

According to the AUA Guidelines Committee, cystoscopy under anesthesia with short-duration, low-pressure (<80 cm/H$_2$O) hydrodistention may be undertaken. This third line course should be considered, if first- AND second-line treatments have *Not* provided acceptable symptom control and quality of life or if the patient's presenting symptoms suggest a more invasive approach is appropriate. Option (*Evidence Strength-Grade C*).

Also, if Hunner's lesions are present, then fulguration (with laser or electrocautery) and/or injection of triamcino-

lone should be performed. *Recommendation* (*Evidence Strength Grade C*).

Fourth Line Therapies

According to the AUA Guidelines Committee, intradetrusor botulinum toxin A (BTX-A) may be administered. As an aside, this can be done in an intramuscular fashion or a subcutaneous fashion, *if* other treatments have not provided adequate symptom control and quality of life or if the clinician and patient agree that symptoms require this approach. Patients must be willing to accept the possibility that post-treatment intermittent self-catheterization may be necessary. Option (*Evidence Strength-C*).

The AUA Guidelines Committee also suggest that a trial of sacral nerve root stimulation is not inappropriate at this level and may be performed when second and third line therapies have failed. If the trial is successful, then implantation of permanent implantable pulse generator may be undertaken. Again, this is only when other approved lines of therapy have not provided adequate symptom relief and quality of life or if the clinician and patient agree that symptoms require this approach. *Option* (*Evidence Strength-C*).

Fifth Line Therapies

At this point, the AUA Guidelines Committee suggest that Cyclosporine A may be administered as an oral medication if other treatments have not provided adequate symptom control and quality of life or if the clinician and patient agree that symptoms require this approach. *Option* (*Evidence Strength-C*).

Sixth Line Therapies

Major surgery (e.g., substitution cystoplasty, urinary diversion with or without cystectomy) may be undertaken in carefully selected patients for whom all other therapies have failed to provide adequate symptom control and quality of life (see caveat above in guideline statement #4). *Option* (*Evidence Strength-C*).

Conclusion

One must remember that IC/BPS can have a profound impact on the quality of life in patients who suffer with it. Furthermore, several epidemiologic studies have suggested that up to two-thirds of women with moderate to severe interstitial cystitis will see a major impairment in their quality of life and even more distressing is that over one third of those patients reported a significant impact in their sexual life. Furthermore, in 2012 a population based survey showed that among a group of adult women with moderate to severe symptoms of interstitial cystitis that 11 % reported suicidal thoughts or actions in the previous 2 weeks before interview. Other research has shown that the impact of IC/BPS on quality of life is severe and may be comparable to the quality of life experienced in end stage renal disease (ESRD) or rheumatoid arthritis.

Recognition of interstitial cystitis has grown dramatically over the past decade. The whole neuroinflammatory soft tissue component in the pelvis has lent tremendous credibility to the study and funding of this process. In fact, entire sections at both national and international urology and gynecology conferences have been dedicated to the entity in and of itself as well as addressing the heterogeneity that is inherent in the vast array of both diagnostic and therapeutic options available. Finally, to support the significant impingement that this disease process can put upon those men and women who suffer with it, the federal government as well as the center for Medicare and Medicaid (CMS) has now recognized this disease process with an Official Disability Code in the United States of America. Now, those patients who cannot hold down their job because of pelvic pressure, pelvic pain or even wetting their pants have an option. For more details, a list of physicians who dedicate all or part their practice to the diagnosis and treatment of IC are listed on the Interstitial Cystitis Association (ICA) website.

References

1. Dancel R, Mounsey A, Handler L. Medications used in IC. Am Fam Physician. 2015;91(2):116–7.
2. Hanno PM, Erickson D, Moldwin R, Faraday MM, American Urological Association. Diagnosis and management of interstitial cystitis, BPS, AUA guidelines amendment. J Urol. 2015; 193(5):1545–53.
3. Barr S. Diagnosis and management of IC. Obstet Gynecol Clin North Am. 2014;41(3):397–407.
4. Rourke W, Khan SA, Ahmed K, Masood S, Dasgupta P, Khan MS. Painful bladder syndrome/interstitial cystitis: aetiology, evaluation and management. Arch Ital Urol Androl. 2014;86(2):126–31. doi:10.4081/aiua.2014.2.126.
5. Jhang JF, Jiang YH, Kuo HC. Potential therapeutic effect of intravesical botulinum toxin type A on bladder pain syndrome/interstitial cystitis. Int J Urol. 2014;21 Suppl 1:49–55.
6. Kuo HC. Potential urine and serum biomarkers for patients with bladder pain syndrome/interstitial cystitis. Int J Urol. 2014;21 Suppl 1:34–41.
7. Meijlink JM. Interstitial cystitis and the painful bladder: a brief history of nomenclature, definitions and criteria. Int J Urol. 2014;21 Suppl 1:4–12.
8. Laviana A, Jellison F, Kim JH. Sacral neuromodulation for refractory overactive bladder, interstitial cystitis, and painful bladder syndrome. Neurosurg Clin North Am. 2014;25(1):33–46.
9. Offiah I, McMahon SB, O'Reilly BA. Interstitial cystitis/bladder pain syndrome: diagnosis and management. Int Urogynecol J. 2013;24(8):1243–56.
10. Neuhaus J, Schwalenberg T. Intravesical treatments of bladder pain syndrome/interstitial cystitis. Nat Rev Urol. 2012;9(12):707–20.
11. Elliott CS, Payne CK. Interstitial cystitis and the overlap with overactive bladder. Curr Urol Rep. 2012;13(5):319–26.
12. Quillin RB, Erickson DR. Management of interstitial cystitis/bladder pain syndrome: a urology perspective. Urol Clin North Am. 2012;39(3):389–96.
13. Quillin RB, Erickson DR. Practical use of the new American Urological Association interstitial cystitis guidelines. Curr Urol Rep. 2012;13(5):394–401.
14. Vesela R, Aronsson P, Andersson M, Wsol V, Tobin G. The potential of non-adrenergic, non-cholinergic targets in the treatment of interstitial cystitis/painful bladder syndrome. J Physiol Pharmacol. 2012;63(3):209–16.
15. FitzGerald MP, Payne CK, Lukacz ES, Yang CC, Peters KM, Chai TC, Nickel JC, Hanno PM, Kreder KJ, Burks DA, Mayer R, Kotarinos R, Fortman C, Allen TM, Fraser L, Mason-Cover M, Furey C, Odabachian L, Sanfield A, Chu J, Huestis K, Tata GE, Dugan N, Sheth H, Bewyer K, Anaeme A, Newton K, Featherstone W, Halle-Podell R, Cen L, Landis JR, Propert KJ, Foster HE Jr, Kusek JW, Nyberg LM; Interstitial Cystitis Collaborative Research Network. Randomized multicenter clinical trial of myofascial physical therapy in women with interstitial cystitis/painful bladder syndrome and pelvic floor tenderness. J Urol. 2012;187(6):2113–8.
16. Vij M, Srikrishna S, Cardozo L. Interstitial cystitis: diagnosis and management. Eur J Obstet Gynecol Reprod Biol. 2012; 161(1):1–7.
17. Friedlander JI, Shorter B, Moldwin RM. Diet and its role in interstitial cystitis/bladder pain syndrome (IC/BPS) and comorbid conditions. BJU Int. 2012;109(11):1584–91.
18. Whitmore KE, Theoharides TC. When to suspect interstitial cystitis. J Fam Pract. 2011;60(6):340–8.
19. Hanno PM, Burks DA, Clemens JQ, Dmochowski RR, Erickson D, Fitzgerald MP, Forrest JB, Gordon B, Gray M, Mayer RD, Newman D, Nyberg Jr L, Payne CK, Wesselmann U, Faraday MM, Interstitial Cystitis Guidelines Panel of the American Urological Association Education and Research, Inc. AUA guideline for the diagnosis and treatment of interstitial cystitis/bladder pain syndrome. J Urol. 2011;185(6):2162–70. Epub 2011 Apr 16.
20. Parsons CL. The role of a leaky epithelium and potassium in the generation of bladder symptoms in interstitial cystitis/overactive bladder, urethral syndrome, prostatitis and gynaecological chronic pelvic pain. BJU Int. 2011;107(3):370–5.
21. Foster Jr HE, Hanno PM, Nickel JC, Payne CK, Mayer RD, Burks DA, Yang CC, Chai TC, Kreder KJ, Peters KM, Lukacz ES, FitzGerald MP, Cen L, Landis JR, Propert KJ, Yang W, Kusek JW, Nyberg LM, Interstitial Cystitis Collaborative Research Network. Effect of amitriptyline on symptoms in treatment naïve patients with interstitial cystitis/painful bladder syndrome. J Urol. 2010;183(5):1853–8.
22. Shao Y, Shen ZJ, Rui WB, Zhou WL. Intravesical instillation of hyaluronic acid prolonged the effect of bladder hydrodistention in patients with severe interstitial cystitis. Urology. 2010;75(3): 547–50.
23. Chung MK, Jarnagin B. Early identification of interstitial cystitis may avoid unnecessary hysterectomy. JSLS. 2009;13(3):350–7.
24. Hanno PM, Chapple CR, Cardozo LD. Bladder pain syndrome/ interstitial cystitis: a sense of urgency. World J Urol. 2009;27(6): 717–21.
25. Forrest JB, Moldwin R. Diagnostic options for early identification and management of interstitial cystitis/painful bladder syndrome. Int J Clin Pract. 2008;62(12):1926–34.
26. Keay S. Cell signaling in interstitial cystitis/painful bladder syndrome. Cell Signal. 2008;20(12):2174–9.
27. Sairanen J, Hotakainen K, Tammela TL, Stenman UH, Ruutu M. Urinary epidermal growth factor and interleukin-6 levels in patients with painful bladder syndrome/interstitial cystitis treated with cyclosporine or pentosan polysulfate sodium. Urology. 2008;71(4):630–3.

28. Warren JW, Brown J, Tracy JK, Langenberg P, Wesselmann U, Greenberg P. Evidence-based criteria for pain of interstitial cystitis/painful bladder syndrome in women. Urology. 2008;71(3):444–8.

29. Dimitrakov J, Kroenke K, Steers WD, Berde C, Zurakowski D, Freeman MR, Jackson JL. Pharmacologic management of painful bladder syndrome/interstitial cystitis: a systematic review. Arch Intern Med. 2007;167(18):1922–9.

30. van de Merwe JP. Interstitial cystitis and systemic autoimmune diseases. Nat Clin Pract Urol. 2007;4(9):484–91.

31. Teichman JM, Moldwin R. The role of the bladder surface in interstitial cystitis/painful bladder syndrome. Can J Urol. 2007;14(4):3599–607.

32. Evans RJ, Sant GR. Current diagnosis of interstitial cystitis: an evolving paradigm. Urology. 2007;69(4 Suppl):64–72.

33. Forrest JB, Nickel JC, Moldwin RM. Chronic prostatitis/chronic pelvic pain syndrome and male interstitial cystitis: enigmas and opportunities. Urology. 2007;69(4 Suppl):60–3.

34. Sant GR, Kempuraj D, Marchand JE, Theoharides TC. The mast cell in interstitial cystitis: role in pathophysiology and pathogenesis. Urology. 2007;69(4 Suppl):34–40.

35. Nazif O, Teichman JM, Gebhart GF. Neural upregulation in interstitial cystitis. Urology. 2007;69(4 Suppl):24–33.

36. van Ophoven A, Hertle L. The dual serotonin and noradrenaline reuptake inhibitor duloxetine for the treatment of interstitial cystitis: results of an observational study. J Urol. 2007;177(2):552–5.

37. Bogart LM, Berry SH, Clemens JQ. Symptoms of interstitial cystitis, painful bladder syndrome and similar diseases in women: a systematic review. J Urol. 2007;177(2):450–6.

38. Berry SH, Bogart LM, Pham C, Liu K, Nyberg L, Stoto M, Suttorp M, Clemens JQ. Development, validation and testing of an epidemiological case definition of interstitial cystitis/painful bladder syndrome. J Urol. 2010;183(5):1848–52. Epub 2010 Mar 29.

39. Theoharides TC, Sant GR. Immunomodulators for treatment of interstitial cystitis. Urology. 2005;65(4):633–8.

40. Parsons CL. Successful downregulation of bladder sensory nerves with combination of heparin and alkalinized lidocaine in patients with interstitial cystitis. Urology. 2005;65(1):45–8.

41. Oyama IA, Rejba A, Lukban JC, Fletcher E, Kellogg-Spadt S, Holzberg AS, Whitmore KE. Modified Thiele massage as therapeutic intervention for female patients with interstitial cystitis and high-tone pelvic floor dysfunction. Urology. 2004;64(5):862–5.

42. Ratner V. Interstitial cystitis: a chronic inflammatory bladder condition. World J Urol. 2001;19(3):157–9.

43. Liebert M. Basic science research on the urinary bladder and interstitial cystitis: new genetic approaches. Urology. 2001;57(6 Suppl 1):7–8.

44. Van De Merwe JP, Arendsen HJ. Interstitial cystitis: a review of immunological aspects, etiology and pathogenesis, with a hypothesis. BJU Int. 2000;85(8):995–9.

45. Hunner GL. A rare type of bladder ulcer in women: report of cases. J Boston Med Surg. 1915;172:660–5.

46. Kim J, Freeman MR. Antiproliferative factor signaling and interstitial cystitis/painful bladder syndrome. Int Neurourol J. 2011;15(4):184–91.

47. Kim J, Keay SK, Freeman MR. Heparin-binding epidermal growth factor-like growth factor functionally antagonizes interstitial cystitis antiproliferative factor via mitogen-activated protein kinase pathway activation. BJU Int. 2009;103(4):541–6.

48. Chai TC, Zhang CO, Shoenfelt JL, Johnson Jr HW, Warren JW, Keay S. Bladder stretch alters urinary heparin-binding epidermal growth factor and antiproliferative factor in patients with interstitial cystitis. J Urol. 2000;163(5):1440–4.

49. Chai TC, Zhang C, Warren JW, Keay S. Percutaneous sacral third nerve root neurostimulation improves symptoms and normalizes urinary HB-EGF levels and antiproliferative activity in patients with interstitial cystitis. Urology. 2000;55(5):643–6.

50. Keay S, Zhang CO, Hise MK, Hebel JR, Jacobs SC, Gordon DA, Whitmore KE, Bodison S, Warren JW. A diagnostic in vitro urine assay for interstitial cystitis. Urology. 1998;52(6):974–8.

51. Keay S, Warren JW, Zhang CO, Tu LM, Gordon DA, Whitmore KE. Antiproliferative activity is present in bladder but not renal pelvic urine from interstitial cystitis patients. J Urol. 1999;162(4):1487–9.

52. Keay S, Kleinberg M, Zhang CO, Hise MK, Warren JW. Bladder epithelial cells from patients with interstitial cystitis produce an inhibitor of heparin-binding epidermal growth factor-like growth factor production. J Urol. 2000;164(6):2112–8.

Sacral Neuromodulation in Interstitial Cystitis

16

Chirag Dave, Kenneth M. Peters, and Michael Ehlert

Introduction

Collectively, pelvic pain syndromes represent one of the most prevalent and challenging disease entities encountered in medicine today. It is estimated that up to 15 % of women age 18–50 in the USA suffer from chronic pelvic pain. In the UK, the annual prevalence of women aged 15–73 presenting to primary care clinics for pelvic pain is comparable to both asthma and back pain, making it amongst the most common reasons for patient visits to their primary care physicians [1, 2]. The quality of life of patients with pelvic pain is reported to be worse than in patients with renal failure on hemodialysis [3]. Further, the diagnostic ambiguity inherent in broadly defined pelvic pain syndromes, coupled with a growing elderly population in the USA, has resulted in increased financial burden of the disease. Between 1992 and 2001 there was a twofold increase in the rate of hospital outpatient visits and a threefold increase in the rate of physician office visits related to interstitial cystitis (IC). Between 1994 and 2000, annual national expenditures for bladder pain syndrome (BPS) increased from $481 million to $751 million [4]. Given the limited efficacy of each individual treatment and the often complex co-morbid conditions that accompany the disease state, multi-modality treatment is required. This has led to the development of new technology and new research attempting to measure meaningful patient outcomes.

In 1997, the United States Food and Drug Administration (FDA) approved sacral neuromodulation (SNM) for urge incontinence, urgency frequency, and for non-obstructive urinary retention in 1999 and fecal incontinence in 2011 [5]. Although SNM has not been FDA approved for the treatment of IC/BPS, it is used regularly for urgency/frequency component of the syndrome and studies suggest that pain symptoms improve as well. This chapter will discuss the history, methodology, and outcomes associated with peripheral neurologic control of the bladder as well as the application of sacral, pudendal, and posterior tibial nerve stimulation for the treatment of IC/BPS.

History

In 1863 Gianuzzi stimulated the spinal cord in dogs and concluded that the hypogastric and pelvic nerves are involved in the regulation of the bladder. In 1878 Saxtorph was the first to attempt bladder stimulation when he treated patients with urinary retention by way of intravesical stimulation [6]. For nearly a century, the mainstay of treatment for overactive and painful bladder syndromes has consisted of non-invasive therapies such as behavioral modification, pelvic floor rehabilitation, and pharmacological therapy with at least 10 % of patients showing a poor response [3, 7]. Once these non-invasive therapies were exhausted, surgical procedures such as augmentation, enterocystoplasty, detrusor myomectomy, bladder denervation, and urinary diversion were employed, resulting in significant perioperative and long-term morbidity [7, 8]. As the understanding of bladder neurophysiology developed, alternative approaches were hypothesized and tested, until Tanagho and his group pioneered the initial investigations into electrical stimulation for neuromodulation in 1989 [9]. Neuromodulation is the electrical or chemical modulation of a nerve to influence the physiologic behavior of an organ and offers a minimally invasive, non-ablative, and reversible means to treat voiding dysfunction [7]. Since InterStim (Medtronic, Minneapolis,

C. Dave • M. Ehlert
Department of Urology, Beaumont Hospital, Royal Oak, MI, USA

K.M. Peters (✉)
Department of Urology, Beaumont Hospital, Oakland University William Beaumont School of Medicine,
3601 W. Thirteen Mile Road, Royal Oak, MI 48073, USA
e-mail: kmpeters@beaumont.edu

© Springer Science+Business Media New York 2017
D.A. Gordon, M.R. Katlic (eds.), *Pelvic Floor Dysfunction and Pelvic Surgery in the Elderly*,
DOI 10.1007/978-1-4939-6554-0_16

MN, USA) came to market in 1997, over 150,000 devices have been implanted for the treatment of urinary urgency, frequency, urge incontinence, urinary retention, and fecal incontinence. Continued research to improve technique and patient outcomes has been ongoing. The use of Interstim for other disorders has been well documented, including in the IC/BPS population.

Interstitial Cystitis/Bladder Pain Syndrome

Pain can be categorized into somatic, visceral, and neuropathic in origin. Somatic pain is well localized and most frequently described as sharp, burning, or aching. It originates from skin, muscles, soft tissue, bones, and joints and is transmitted along sensory afferents. Visceral pain is transmitted via sympathetic fibers of the autonomic nervous system and originates from internal viscous structures. It is poorly localized and perceived as dull or aching and may be associated with autonomic dysfunction [5]. Neuropathic pain is the result of an insult or injury to the peripheral or central nervous tissue leading to a pain syndrome characterized by dysesthesias, allodynia, and hyperesthesia [10]. In chronic pelvic pain, it has been postulated that a disease state damages a particular organ leading to somatic or visceral pain that eventually develops into neuropathic pain [5]. Chronic pelvic pain is a broad diagnosis of exclusion that likely encompasses many other pathologic states including interstitial cystitis/bladder pain syndrome (IC/BPS), chronic prostatitis (CP)/prostadynia (PD), coccygodynia, vulvodynia, and anorectal pain [11]. IC/BPS has received a great deal of attention due to the prevalence, cost, and associated morbidity. The Society for Urodynamics and Female Urology and the American Urological Association (AUA) define IC/BPS as

> An unpleasant sensation (pain, pressure, discomfort) perceived to be related to the urinary bladder, associated with lower urinary tract symptoms of more than six weeks duration, in the absence of other identifiable causes [12, 13].

The exact etiology of IC/BPS is poorly understood and many possible mechanisms have been proposed including autoimmune disorders, infection, pelvic floor dysfunction, toxins, and bladder wall defects [5]. One theory involves a defect in the urothelium or glygosaminoglycan layer and resulting exposure to a noxious stimulus, and subsequent mast cell activation [5, 11]. Upregulation of mast cell activity and increased sensory nerve fiber activity in the bladder leads to chronic inflammation and ultimately a neuropathic pain state [5]. Bladder afferent pathways normally send signals to the central nervous system indicating bladder fullness or discomfort and prompting a micturition reflex. The bladder afferent pathways are composed of small myelinated A-delta fibers and unmyelinated C-fibers. The A-delta fibers transmit signals indicating bladder fullness or wall tension

while C-fibers detect noxious stimuli and painful sensations. Normally, C-fibers are unresponsive to bladder distention. Neurologic or inflammatory diseases cause these "silent C-fibers" to become inappropriately sensitized to bladder distention and trigger micturition reflexes resulting in the urgency and frequency symptoms that accompany many dysfunctional voiding disorders [3, 5]. Interrupting this bladder hyperactivity by blocking C-fiber afferent activity in the spinal cord is a proposed mechanism of action for neuromodulation.

A majority of IC/BPS patients also suffer from pelvic floor dysfunction further contributing to pelvic pain, dyspareunia, voiding, and bowel dysfunction. The support for the pelvic organs comes primarily from the levator ani muscles which are situated beneath the vagina and urethra and consist of the pubococcygeus muscle anteriorly and the iliococcygeus muscle posteriorly. These muscles are palpable during pelvic examination and trigger points and taut musculature is frequently identified in IC/BPS patients. In a study of 70 patients with IC/BPS, 87 % had levator pain on pelvic examination [14]. The same study showed that half of these patients suffered from irritable bowel syndrome (IBS) and more than one third suffered from urge incontinence. Another study showed that myofascial pain and hypertonic bladder are present in up to 85 % of patients with IC/BPS [15]. The pelvic floor should be assessed in all IC/BPS patients, and if dysfunction is identified it should be included as target for multi-modality therapy.

Neuroanatomy

Normal voiding relies on intact neural pathways in the central nervous system. The bladder is naturally in a state of relaxation controlled by lumbar sympathetic relaxation of the bladder and excitation of the bladder base and urethra [3, 16]. The lumbar, pelvic, and pudendal nerves contain afferent and efferent axons. The sensation of bladder fullness is sent via afferent axons through the sacral spinal cord to the pontine micturition center. Once the signal is received, the efferent signal is sent via the parasympathetic nervous system at sacral spinal cord level S2–S4 prompting the bladder to contract while the urethra relaxes. Also important in normal voiding function is relaxation of the external urethral sphincter via the somatic nervous system (pudendal nerve). As mentioned earlier, interrupting afferent signals to the pontine micturition center is a proposed mechanism for neuromodulation [3, 17]. However, a number of reflex pathways, which bypass the pontine micturition center, have been described and are also potential targets for neuromodulation. In the vesicosympathetic reflex, bladder filling stimulates lumbar sympathetics and allows greater accommodation of filling. The guarding reflex is another feedback loop affecting continence whereby sphincter tone increases with bladder filling mediated by sympathetic and pudendal efferents to the bladder neck and external urethral sphincter, respectively [18]. Sacral afferents also synapse in the sacral spinal cord and communicate directly with bladder efferents and effectively bypass higher centers forming a bladder–bladder reflex [3, 18]. Disruption of any of these pathways can lead to classic symptoms of many voiding and bladder pain disorders including problems with storage and emptying. Problems with storage include urge incontinence (detrusor overactivity) and stress urinary incontinence (sphincter underactivity). Problems with emptying lead to retention and involve sphincter overactivity or detrusor underactivity [18]. Although the precise mechanism of neuromodulation is not understood, it appears to affect both spinal and cortical centers for voiding control.

Diagnosis and Treatment Algorithm of IC/ BPS

According to the AUA [12], the basic assessment of IC/BPS should include a history, physical, and laboratory exam to exclude other disorders such as bladder cancer, endometriosis, pelvic mass, or fistula and also to fulfill inclusion criteria for diagnosis. If the diagnosis is in doubt, cystoscopy and/or urodynamics should be considered. Treatment strategies should proceed using more conservative therapies first, with progressively less conservative therapies as needed to improve the patient's quality of life [16]. Multiple, simultaneous treatments may be considered; however, ineffective treatments should be stopped once a clinically meaningful interval has passed.

First line treatment should always include patient education about IC/BPS and special clarification that no single-treatment option has been effective for the majority of patients, thereby suggesting multiple therapeutic options. Patients should also be encouraged to use self-care practices, behavioral modifications, and stress management practices. Second line treatments include appropriate manual physical therapy techniques and multi-modal pain management approaches. Amitryptiline, cimetidine, hydroxyzine, or pentosan polysulfate may be administered with no preference for one treatment over the other. Dimethyl sulfoxide, heparin, or lidocaine may be used as an intravesical therapy. Third line treatments include cystoscopy and low-pressure hydrodistention which also allows for accurate assessment of maximum bladder capacity under anesthesia, which may be a predictor of poor treatment response. If Hunner's lesions are present, they should be fulgrated or triamcinolone may be injected. Fourth line treatment calls for a trial of neurostimulation while fifth line treatments include cyclosporine and intradetrusor botulinum toxin A, both of which have not been approved by the FDA. Finally, sixth line treatments include major surgery such as cystoplasty, or urinary diversion with or without cystectomy [12, 13]. As mentioned earlier, as many as 10 % of IC/BPS patients will not respond to more conservative first and second line treatments.

Patient Education

Patients with IC/BPS who choose to undergo neuromodulation should understand that treatment is primarily for the urgency/frequency component of their syndrome, but there is a possibility that nerve stimulation may also improve their pain. The procedure is performed in two stages so that improvement in symptoms can be observed prior to implanting a permanent device. Patients should be aware that symptom relief is not guaranteed and success is considered a 50 % improvement in overall symptoms, rather than complete resolution. The patients are informed that this is not a cure for their disease, rather a technique to manage their symptoms and once the unit is turned off, their symptoms will return [19]. Sacral abnormalities and obesity can make the location of the nerve technically challenging. However, a recent retrospective study showed no difference in treatment success between obese and non-obese patients [20]. Patients with cognitive deficits may have trouble managing the device and this should be considered when choosing to trial SNM. Voiding dysfunction is more prevalent in the elderly and although some studies have shown that older patients might have less efficacy with neuromodulation [16, 21], others have shown age to have no impact on outcomes [22]. Since SNM is performed in two stages to determine the efficacy prior to permanent implantation, it is reasonable to trial SNM in the elderly with refractory voiding dysfunction. Neuromodulation is contraindicated in pregnancy due to the risk of fetal loss or preterm labor, and patients with an implanted device who become pregnant should have the device turned off for the duration of the pregnancy [16]. Patients should also be counseled that MRI of the abdomen or pelvis or diathermy is contraindicated due to concerns of heating the electrodes, dislocation of the device or disruption of programming [23]. Patients should be screened separately at airports and be issued identification cards to inform others that the implant is in place.

Patients should know that neuromodulation is a two-stage procedure involving mild anesthesia and outpatient surgery. They should be screened for and counseled on anesthetic risk and usual complications of surgery. Patients should also be informed that there is a 100 % re-operation rate due to depletion of the IPG in 4–6 years post-implant. Also, a 15–20 % re-operation rate is expected due to technical difficulties based on the implantable nature of the device [19]. Patients should be required to keep voiding diaries prior to lead implantation as well as during the test period. After first stage lead placement, the patient will wear an external generator to adjust stimulation of the lead while they record the results. Second stage permanent implantation should only take place if there is a 50 % improvement in symptoms as documented in the voiding diaries. The lead should be removed from patients who do not respond to the test.

Sacral Neuromodulation

The S3 nerve root is the main target for sacral neuromodulation and is targeted via the S3 foramen resulting in changes to bladder storage function with low-amplitude electrical stimulation. Schmidt, Tanagho, and colleagues [9] originally developed the technique using a percutaneous placement of a single electrode that was then taped to the skin. The lack of fixation allowed movement of the lead and limitation of the length of trial. Patients who had a positive response would then have a large incision carried to the periosteum of the sacrum where it was anchored in place. Several other incisions were made to tunnel the cables and pocket the device, resulting in moderate morbidity [18]. Currently, sacral neuromodulation is a minimally invasive procedure. In 2003, Spinelli and colleagues described the placement of a lead with plastic tines that fixed the electrode in place without additional anchoring, thus allowing the same electrode to be used for testing and permanent implantation [24]. As a result, the re-operation rate dropped significantly. In an effort to mitigate cost and the need for IV sedation, alternative techniques were developed to allow outpatient testing. Two techniques have emerged to test the efficacy of SNM prior to implantation of a pulse generator. These include first stage lead placement (FSLP), which is performed under anesthesia in the operating room, and percutaneous nerve evaluation (PNE), which is performed in an office.

Percutaneous Nerve Evaluation (PNE)

PNE is an office-based technique that uses a temporary monopolar lead which is designed to be minimally traumatic and easy to retrieve. The procedure is performed as follows [16]:

1. The patient is placed in the prone position.
2. The S3 foramen is located without fluoroscopy by measuring 10 cm from the coccyx along the midline of the spine and then measuring 2 cm lateral and 3 cm superior to this point.
3. Local anesthetic is administered and the needle is introduced at a 30–60° angle.
4. Lead placement is confirmed by patient-reported sensation of stimulation in the vaginal, scrotal, or rectal area and flexion of the big toe.
5. The single electrode temporary lead is placed and then taped to the skin, connected to an external temporary pulse generator and worn by the patient for a test period of 3–7 days.

*A >50 % improvement in symptoms is considered a success, and a permanent lead and IPG can be placed.

The success rate of PNE has previously been reported to lie between 48 and 60 % [25, 26]. The benefits of PNE as an outpatient procedure include time efficiency, a shorter testing period, no anesthesia, and significant overall cost benefit. These benefits are weighed against several major limitations. The lead is a single electrode and is temporary; therefore, the tested effect is not necessarily reproducible during permanent lead placement. The lead can also easily migrate during the test period. Eight out of ten patients who failed PNE after an initial positive response went on to have successful SNM therapy when the permanent quadripolar lead was placed, suggesting that lead migration should not preclude permanent placement [25]. Borawski et al. reported that 46 % of patients receiving PNE responded to test stimulation and underwent implantation versus 88 % of patients receiving FSLP [27]. Numerous other studies have reached the same conclusion; however, there is no consensus on the optimal method to screen SNM candidates and is therefore deferred to the surgeon's clinical judgment.

First State Lead Placement (FSLP) [16]

1. The patient is brought to the operating room and placed in the prone position with pressure points padded.
2. The patient is placed under intravenous sedation and local anesthesia.
3. Using fluoroscopic guidance a directional guidewire is used to locate the intersection of the spinous process and the sacroiliac joint which, using a marking pen, is identified with a transverse line.
4. The entrance point to the S3 foramen is approximately 2 cm lateral and 3 cm superior to the point where the two lines cross. A needle is passed into the entrance point at a 30–60° angle to access the foramen.
5. S3 stimulation is confirmed by observation of bellows contraction of the pelvic floor and flexion of the great toe (bellows contraction alone suggests S4 stimulation; plantar flexion of the entire foot with heel rotation suggests stimulation of the S2 nerve root and the lead should be repositioned) [19].
6. Fluoroscopy is used to confirm placement of the needle.
7. A directional guide wire is placed and the tract is dilated using an introducer sheath.
8. The tined lead consisting of four cylindrical electrodes numbered 0–3 is deployed under fluoroscopy. Each electrode is stimulated individually and reflex responses are assessed with a goal of response on all four electrodes.
9. Lead position should be confirmed with fluoroscopy in the lateral and anterior–posterior positions.
10. A 1 cm incision is made and a subcutaneous pocket is made in the ipsilateral buttock for the potential site of the IPG if the test stage is successful.

11. The lead is then connected to a percutaneous extension lead, which is tunneled out of the contralateral buttock and connected to the temporary generator.
12. The pocket is closed and the external cords are secured with sterile 4 × 4 dressings and a bandage.

*A >50 % improvement in symptoms is considered a success, and a permanent lead and IPG can be placed (stage II).

Stage II/Permanent Implantation Involves the Following [16]

1. The pocket site is reopened, enlarged, and the lead is connected to a permanent IPG.
2. The connections of the device are confirmed in the operating room and the incision is closed with absorbable sutures.
3. Specific programs for stimulation of the leads are determined and set up postoperatively to determine the most optimal device settings.

Whether undergoing PNE or FSLP, patients may have a similar long-term therapeutic benefit suggesting similar specificity among techniques [28]. However, test to implant rate is considered a better way to measure screening efficacy. When comparing PNE to FSLP specifically in an IC/BPS population, Peters et al. [29] reported that the test to implant rate of patients receiving PNE was 52 % versus 94 % in the FSLP group. They also showed that assessing the sensory response during surgery reduced the re-operation rate from 43 to 0 %. Additionally, 96 % (25/26) of IC/BPS patients stated they would undergo an implant again and would also recommend the procedure to a friend.

Sacral Neuromodulation for IC/BPS

SNM is not currently FDA approved for IC/BPS, however it is used in this population with regularity for the urgency/frequency component of the syndrome and there is significant literature suggesting it may improve pelvic pain. In a prospective study of patients with refractory IC/PBS, at a mean of 14 months of follow-up, statistically significant improvements in daytime frequency, nocturia, and mean voided volume (111–264 ml) were observed and average pain decreased from 5.8 to 1.6 (scale of 0–10) on the Interstitial Cystitis Symptom and Problem Index score [30]. Peters and Konstandt reported that 20 of 21 patients with refractory IC followed for 15 months experienced moderate or marked improvement in pain after SNM with a statistically significant decrease in narcotic requirements [31]. In a long-term efficacy study, at a median 86-month follow-up on 30 patients with IC/PBS undergoing SNM, Marinkovic et al. reported a test to implant rate of 88 %

and a 64 % reduction in pain (visual analog scale) scores and improvement in voiding dysfunction [32]. In 2010 Gajewski et al. reported on 78 patients with IC/BPS after SNM followed for 62 months with a success rate of 72 % [33]. Powell and Kreder followed 22 IC/BPS patients after SNM for 59 months and more than 75 % reported sustained improvement in symptoms and a reduction in IC/BPS medications was observed [34]. Another randomized clinical trial showed decrease in visual analog pain scores of 49 %, a decrease in number of voids by 33 %, an increase in mean voided volume by 95 %, and a decrease in incontinence by 92 % among IC/BPS patients receiving SNM. In the same study, 100 % of the patients who received SNM said that they would undergo implantation again [35]. Srivastava et al. reviewed the efficacy of SNM in treating chronic pain in this patient population. In their literature review, most studies (8/10) showed a decrease in pain scores at long-term follow-up after permanent SNM [36]. In terms of safety, the most frequently reported adverse events include explantation, lead revision, and infection [36]. In summary, SNM is frequently used for patients with severe IC/BPS refractory to conservative therapy. It is a safe and reasonable option when conservative treatments have failed.

Pudendal Neuromodulation

Patients who are refractory to conservative therapies with inadequate (<50 %) response to SNM may benefit from pudendal neuromodulation (PNM). In 1989, Ohlsson used pudendal stimulation as an alternative for patients not responding to surface stimulation [37, 38]. In 2005, Spinelli et al. introduced the technically advanced procedure of accessing the primarily afferent sensory nerve which has since been refined and has become a popular off label treatment option for patients with refractory symptoms [16, 26]. Pudendal neruomodulation is not FDA approved for the treatment of lower urinary tract symptoms, however its safety and efficacy have been demonstrated in a number of different studies. The pudendal nerve is composed of fibers from S1–3, with most of the fibers contributed by S2 and S3 and thus an important contributor to bladder function as well as an ideal target for neuromodulation [7]. The pudendal nerve innervates the pelvic floor muscles, the external urethral and anal sphincters and pelvic organs. The optimal point of stimulation is at the level of the ischial spine [16]. The procedure is performed as follows [16]:

1. The patient is placed in the prone position, prepped and draped sterilely with pressure points padded.
2. Needle electrodes are placed into the anal sphincter at the 3 o'clock and 9 o'clock positions for intraoperative electromyography (EMG) monitoring.
3. The pudendal nerve can be accessed percutaneously through the ischiorectal space, by passing a foramen needle

just medial to the ischial tuberosity in a medial-to-lateral direction toward the ischial spine, and stimulated. Confirmation is by a compound muscle action potential (CMAP) on EMG and an anal wink.

4. Stimulation of the pudendal nerve is confirmed and visualized under fluoroscopy and the tined lead is placed using the directional guide wire and lead introducer, similarly to the sacral neuromodulation procedure.

5. Once the lead is positioned, tested, and deployed, it is tunneled to the standard IPG site in the upper buttock. A longer lead (41 cm) is needed to access the pudendal nerve and tunnel to the IPG site. The percutaneous extension lead is connected and tunneled out of the contralateral buttock.

6. Pudendal nerve stimulation is performed as a staged procedure and the criteria for success (≥50 % improvement in symptoms based on voiding diaries) must be met before permanent IPG implantation. Patients should be instructed to sit gently to avoid displacing the lead before tissue ingrowth has occurred.

In 2005, a randomized, prospective, single blinded crossover trial comparing SNM to PNM for voiding dysfunction showed that there was a statistically significant overall reduction in symptoms with PNM (63 %) versus SNM (46 %) and 79 % of the patients chose PNM as "superior." In a subset analysis of only patients with IC/BPS, 77 % of the patients chose PNM as "superior" [39]. Another study examining refractory patients who had PNM placed reported significant reductions in incontinent episodes, maximum cystometric capacity, bladder pressure on urodynamic studies, constipation, and fecal incontinence [7]. Finally, in a study of OAB and IC/BPS patients who had previously failed SNM, 41 out of 44 (93 %) of patients responded to PNM. Although less than 50 % of the patients reported marked improvement at 1 year, 88 % had the device in place, 83 % were using it, and 74 % would undergo the procedure again; 84 % of the patients stated that they would recommend PNM to a friend [40]. The limitations and safety profile of PNM are similar to that of SNM. PNM is a more technically challenging procedure than SNM and generally should be performed by an experienced, high volume surgeon [16]. In spite of such limitations, it has proven to be an extremely effective treatment option for refractory cases and the application continues to expand for the treatment of various dysfunctional voiding and pain disorders including IC/PBS [39].

Posterior Tibial Nerve Stimulation (PTNS)

Tibial nerve stimulation, initially described in 1983 by McGuire and colleagues, showed that electrical stimulation of the tibial nerve could efficaciously treat a variety of voiding dysfunctions [41]. Stoller and colleagues pioneered posterior tibial nerve stimulation when they designed a stimulator targeting the nerve just above the medial malleolus [7]. It was approved by the FDA in 2000 for the treatment of OAB and has the advantage of being performed in an office without anesthesia and lacking a permanent implant. PTNS has not been approved for the treatment of IC/BPS or chronic pelvic pain, however, several studies have demonstrated efficacy. The posterior tibial nerve originates from spinal roots L4 to S3 and serves as a peripheral mixed sensory motor nerve contributing directly to bladder and pelvic floor function [7, 16]. The procedure is performed as follows [16]:

1. The patient is positioned in the seated position.
2. A 34-gauge needle is inserted 3 cm into the skin (three fingerbreadths above the medial malleolus).
3. A grounding pad is placed on the arch of the ipsilateral foot.
4. The system is attached to the grounding pad and needle and the amplitude of the stimulation is increased until the large toe curls or the toes fan.
5. The stimulation session typically lasts for 30 min.

Studies have shown that 12 weekly sessions provide the best outcomes [16]. In a study of PTNS versus Sham for 12 weeks of therapy using a 7-point global response assessment to measure changes in patient symptoms showed that 54.5 % of patients reported improved responses from baseline versus 20.9 % in the Sham group [42]. In a prospective study of patients with chronic pelvic pain (CPP), after 12 weeks of PTNS, 60 % of patients had improvement of greater than 50 and 30 % of patients had improvement of 25–50 % in visual analog score (VAS) for pain, representing statistically significant improvements from baseline [43]. Van Balken et al. evaluated 33 patients with CPP undergoing 12 weeks of PTNS and reported that 100 % of the patients had significant improvement in quality of life and total pain rate intensity; 21 % of patients had mean VAS improvement of >50 % [44]. In a study of 13 patients with diagnosed IC/BPS enrolled for 10 weekly sessions of PTNS, there were no statistically significant changes in pain scores, voiding frequency and volumes, or in pain scores although several patients reported improvement, with one having complete resolution of symptoms [45].

As mentioned, the tibial nerve is an attractive target because it is easily accessible without the requirement of an operating room or anesthesia and therefore it has been widely adapted as a novel treatment for patients with a variety of dysfunctional voiding and pelvic pain syndromes including IC/BPS [16]. Larger randomized placebo controlled trials are necessary to assess long-term efficacy, particularly in the IC/PBS population [7]. Complications of PTNS are mild and include pain, bruising, bleeding, and tingling at the needle site. Further limitations include the time commitment involved in attending treatments, and difficulty obtaining insurance coverage [16].

Conclusion

Pelvic pain syndromes including IC/BPS are an extremely prevalent and expensive constellation of diseases that are amongst the most common reasons why patients visit their doctor. Treatment should always progress from the most conservative to least conservative therapies. SNM has emerged as a safe and efficacious treatment option for refractory IC/BPS and other dysfunctional voiding and pelvic pain disorders as evidenced by numerous well-designed studies. All physicians who treat this growing patient population should be well versed in the history, methodology, procedure, and outcomes associated with SNM as detailed in this chapter. Alternate methods of peripheral neurologic control of the bladder such as PNM and PTNS should be considered as the next step or as an adjunct to patients who have failed SNM. Neuromodulation has revolutionized the treatment of dysfunctional voiding and pelvic pain disorders and will likely continue to be a mainstay within the difficult treatment algorithm.

References

1. Coyne KS, Sexton CC, Irwin DE, Kopp ZS, Kelleher CJ, Milsom I. The impact of overactive bladder, incontinence and other lower urinary tract symptoms on quality of life, work productivity, sexuality and emotional well-being in men and women: results from the EPIC study. BJU Int. 2008;101(11):1388–95.
2. Coyne KS, Sexton CC, Vats V, Thompson C, Kopp ZS, Milsom I. National community prevalence of overactive bladder in the United States stratified by sex and age. Urology. 2011;77(5):1081–7.
3. Leng WW, Chancellor MB. How sacral nerve stimulation neuromodulation works. Urol Clin North Am. 2005;32(1):11–8.
4. Irwin DE, Milsom I, Hunskaar S, Reilly K, Kopp Z, Herschorn S, et al. Population-based survey of urinary incontinence, overactive bladder, and other lower urinary tract symptoms in five countries: results of the EPIC study. Eur Urol. 2006;50(6):1306–14. discussion 1314–5.
5. Hunter C, Dave N, Diwan S, Deer T. Neuromodulation of pelvic visceral pain: review of the literature and case series of potential novel targets for treatment. Pain Pract. 2013;13(1):3–17.
6. Daneshgari F, Abrams P. Future directions in pelvic neuromodulation. Urol Clin North Am. 2005;32(1):113–5. viii.
7. Peters KM. Alternative approaches to sacral nerve stimulation. Int Urogynecol J. 2010;21(12):1559–63.
8. Sherman ND, Jamison MG, Webster GD, Amundsen CL. Sacral neuromodulation for the treatment of refractory urinary urge incontinence after stress incontinence surgery. Am J Obstet Gynecol. 2005;193(6):2083–7.
9. Tanagho EA, Schmidt RA, Orvis BR. Neural stimulation for control of voiding dysfunction: a preliminary report in 22 patients with serious neuropathic voiding disorders. J Urol. 1989;142(2 Pt 1):340–5.
10. Kothari S. Neuromodulatory approaches to chronic pelvic pain and coccygodynia. Acta Neurochir Suppl. 2007;97(Pt 1):365–71.
11. Fariello JY, Whitmore K. Sacral neuromodulation stimulation for IC/PBS, chronic pelvic pain, and sexual dysfunction. Int Urogynecol J. 2010;21(12):1553–8.
12. Hanno PM, Burks DA, Clemens JQ, Dmochowski RR, Erickson D, Fitzgerald MP, et al. AUA guideline for the diagnosis and treatment of interstitial cystitis/bladder pain syndrome. J Urol. 2011; 185(6):2162–70.
13. Hanno P, Dmochowski R. Status of international consensus on interstitial cystitis/bladder pain syndrome/painful bladder syndrome: 2008 snapshot. Neurourol Urodyn. 2009;28(4):274–86.
14. Peters KM, Carrico DJ, Kalinowski SE, Ibrahim IA, Diokno AC. Prevalence of pelvic floor dysfunction in patients with interstitial cystitis. Urology. 2007;70(1):16–8.
15. Butrick CW. Interstitial cystitis and chronic pelvic pain: new insights in neuropathology, diagnosis, and treatment. Clin Obstet Gynecol. 2003;46(4):811–23.
16. Bartley J, Gilleran J, Peters K. Neuromodulation for overactive bladder. Nat Rev Urol. 2013;10(9):513–21.
17. Langley JN, Anderson HK. The innervation of the pelvic and adjoining viscera: Part II. The bladder. Part III. The external generative organs. Part IV. The internal generative organs. Part V. Position of the nerve cells on the course of the efferent nerve fibres. J Physiol. 1895;19(1–2):71–139.
18. Mayer RD, Howard FM. Sacral nerve stimulation: neuromodulation for voiding dysfunction and pain. Neurotherapeutics. 2008;5(1):107–13.
19. Peters KM. Neuromodulation, staged intervention, and new instruments. Atlas Urol Clin North Am. 2004;12:275–91.
20. Levin PJ, Wu JM, Siddiqui NY, Amundsen CL. Does obesity impact the success of an InterStim test phase for the treatment of refractory urge urinary incontinence in female patients? Female Pelvic Med Reconstr Surg. 2012;18(4):243–6.
21. Amundsen CL, Romero AA, Jamison MG, Webster GD. Sacral neuromodulation for intractable urge incontinence: are there factors associated with cure? Urology. 2005;66(4):746–50.
22. Peters KM, Killinger KA, Gilleran J, Boura JA. Does patient age impact outcomes of neuromodulation? Neurourol Urodyn. 2013; 32(1):30–6.
23. Chermansky CJ, Krlin RM, Holley TD, Woo HH, Winters JC. Magnetic resonance imaging following InterStim(R): an institutional experience with imaging safety and patient satisfaction. Neurourol Urodyn. 2011;30(8):1486–8.
24. Spinelli M, Giardiello G, Gerber M, Arduini A, van den Hombergh U, Malaguti S. New sacral neuromodulation lead for percutaneous implantation using local anesthesia: description and first experience. J Urol. 2003;170(5):1905–7.
25. Leong RK, De Wachter SG, Nieman FH, de Bie RA, van Kerrebroeck PE. PNE versus 1st stage tined lead procedure: a direct comparison to select the most sensitive test method to identify patients suitable for sacral neuromodulation therapy. Neurourol Urodyn. 2011;30(7):1249–52.
26. Spinelli M, Malaguti S, Giardiello G, Lazzeri M, Tarantola J, Van Den Hombergh U. A new minimally invasive procedure for pudendal nerve stimulation to treat neurogenic bladder: description of the method and preliminary data. Neurourol Urodyn. 2005;24(4):305–9.
27. Borawski KM, Foster RT, Webster GD, Amundsen CL. Predicting implantation with a neuromodulator using two different test stimulation techniques: a prospective randomized study in urge incontinent women. Neurourol Urodyn. 2007;26(1):14–8.
28. Peters KM, Killinger KA, Boura JA. Is sensory testing during lead placement crucial for achieving positive outcomes after sacral neuromodulation? Neurourol Urodyn. 2011;30(8):1489–92.
29. Peters KM, Carey JM, Konstandt DB. Sacral neuromodulation for the treatment of refractory interstitial cystitis: outcomes based on technique. Int Urogynecol J Pelvic Floor Dysfunct. 2003;14(4):223–8. discussion 228.
30. Comiter CV. Sacral neuromodulation for the symptomatic treatment of refractory interstitial cystitis: a prospective study. J Urol. 2003;169(4):1369–73.
31. Peters KM, Konstandt D. Sacral neuromodulation decreases narcotic requirements in refractory interstitial cystitis. BJU Int. 2004; 93(6):777–9.

32. Marinkovic SP, Gillen LM, Marinkovic CM. Minimum 6-year outcomes for interstitial cystitis treated with sacral neuromodulation. Int Urogynecol J. 2011;22(4):407–12.

33. Gajewski JB, Al-Zahrani AA. The long-term efficacy of sacral neuromodulation in the management of intractable cases of bladder pain syndrome: 14 years of experience in one centre. BJU Int. 2011;107(8):1258–64.

34. Powell CR, Kreder KJ. Long-term outcomes of urgency-frequency syndrome due to painful bladder syndrome treated with sacral neuromodulation and analysis of failures. J Urol. 2010;183(1):173–6.

35. Peters KM, Feber KM, Bennett RC. A prospective, single-blind, randomized crossover trial of sacral vs pudendal nerve stimulation for interstitial cystitis. BJU Int. 2007;100(4):835–9.

36. Srivastava D. Efficacy of sacral neuromodulation in treating chronic pain related to painful bladder syndrome/interstitial cystitis in adults. J Anaesthesiol Clin Pharmacol. 2012;28(4):428–35.

37. Wang S, Zhang S, Zhao L. Long-term efficacy of electrical pudendal nerve stimulation for urgency-frequency syndrome in women. Int Urogynecol J. 2013;25(3):397–402.

38. Carmel M, Lebel M, le Tu M. Pudendal nerve neuromodulation with neurophysiology guidance: a potential treatment option for refractory chronic pelvi-perineal pain. Int Urogynecol J. 2010;21(5):613–6.

39. Peters KM, Feber KM, Bennett RC. Sacral versus pudendal nerve stimulation for voiding dysfunction: a prospective, single-blinded, randomized, crossover trial. Neurourol Urodyn. 2005;24(7):643–7.

40. Peters KM, Killinger KA, Boguslawski BM, Boura JA. Chronic pudendal neuromodulation: expanding available treatment options for refractory urologic symptoms. Neurourol Urodyn. 2010;29(7):1267–71.

41. McGuire EJ, Zhang SC, Horwinski ER, Lytton B. Treatment of motor and sensory detrusor instability by electrical stimulation. J Urol. 1983;129(1):78–9.

42. Peters KM, Carrico DJ, Perez-Marrero RA, Khan AU, Wooldridge LS, Davis GL, et al. Randomized trial of percutaneous tibial nerve stimulation versus sham efficacy in the treatment of overactive bladder syndrome: results from the SUmiT trial. J Urol. 2010;183(4):1438–43.

43. Kim SW, Paick JS, Ku JH. Percutaneous posterior tibial nerve stimulation in patients with chronic pelvic pain: a preliminary study. Urol Int. 2007;78(1):58–62.

44. van Balken MR, Vandoninck V, Messelink BJ, Vergunst H, Heesakkers JP, Debruyne FM, et al. Percutaneous tibial nerve stimulation as neuromodulative treatment of chronic pelvic pain. Eur Urol. 2003;43(2):158–63. discussion 163.

45. Zhao J, Nordling J. Posterior tibial nerve stimulation in patients with intractable interstitial cystitis. BJU Int. 2004;94(1):101–4.

The Neurogenic Bladder and Hypertonic Pelvic Floor Muscle Dysfunction

17

David A. Gordon, Rohit Gossein, and Navpreet Rana

Introduction, Anatomy, and Physiology

Before we can begin any discussion dealing with the anatomy, physiology, or pathophysiology of the bladder, we must first be able to understand the bladder within the parameters of basic anatomic relationships, and to answer some simple questions, in practical terminology, regarding how and why the bladder is what it is.

The urinary bladder (Fig. 17.1) is an extra-peritoneal, visceral organ whose fundamental function in the human animal is storage. The urinary bladder has three points where its intrinsic integrity is breached. These are the two (2) ureteral orifices which let fluid into the bladder and the single (1) urethral opening at the level of the bladder neck, which lets fluid out of the bladder.

The location of the bladder varies by age. Usually up to the age of three, it is located mainly within the abdomen and later in adulthood within the pelvis proper. Its position in the adult pelvis varies mainly due to the differences of the surrounding accessory structures between genders. Table 17.1 details the surrounding structures of the bladder and are important for surgical instrumentation.

The vascular supply to the bladder is extensive. It is supplied by the internal iliac artery, via the superior and inferior branches. These later drain through the vesical veins and then into the internal iliac vein. It is important to note that vascular thrombosis of the anterior spinal artery, especially at the lumbosacral level, can affect bladder function primarily causing urinary retention. The lymphatic system at the base of the bladder surrounds into vesical plexus and drains immediately into the iliac and then ultimately para-aortic nodes (Fig. 17.2a, b).

From a microscopic perspective, the bladder is made up of layers of smooth muscle that stretch during the filling phase to accommodate increasing volumes of urine at low pressures. In addition, this muscle is protected by a lining of transitional cell epithelium which is further guarded by a layer of glycosaminoglycan (GAG). The normal capacity of the bladder is 400–500 cc. During urination, the bladder muscle (*the detrusor*) contracts, and two small circular muscles located in the area of the proximal urethra and bladder neck (the sphincter complex} relax at the same time that the bladder muscle contracts to allow urine to flow out. This coordinated muscular contraction/relaxation of the lower urinary tract, which may sound simple on the surface, is an extremely complex neuromuscular process that must work with microscopic precision. When this coordinated response does not work well, in a coordinated fashion, there can be significant risk to the intrinsic state of health of the renal units. We go into great detail describing the intricate neuromuscular process of micturition later in this chapter. Urine exits the bladder through the urethra, which carries it out of the body. Finally, the urethra is longer in men (16–18 cm) than in women (3.5–4.5 cm).

Uro-Philosophy 101, Structure and Function

The urinary bladder is a muscular sac (essentially a hollow muscle) in the pelvis (Fig. 17.3). That is, it is like a balloon made up of muscle cells. When empty, the bladder is about the size and shape of an upside down pear. It is located just above the inferior margin of the pubic bone and directly behind the body of that same bone. It is important to remember,

D.A. Gordon (✉)
Division of Pelvic NeuroScience, Department of Surgery, The Sinai Hospital of Baltimore, 2401 W. Belvedere Ave, Baltimore, MD 21215, USA
e-mail: dgordon@lifebridgehealth.org

R. Gossein
Department of Internal Medicine, Sinai Hospital of Baltimore/John's Hopkins University, Baltimore, MD, USA

N. Rana
University of New England, Biddeford, ME, USA

© Springer Science+Business Media New York 2017
D.A. Gordon, M.R. Katlic (eds.), *Pelvic Floor Dysfunction and Pelvic Surgery in the Elderly*,
DOI 10.1007/978-1-4939-6554-0_17

Fig. 17.1 Urinary bladder, (**a**) female and (**b**) Male

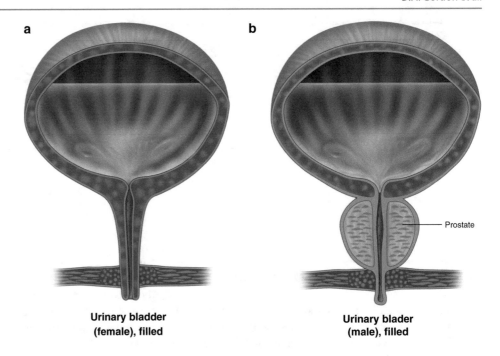

Urinary bladder (female), filled

Urinary blader (male), filled

Table 17.1 Structures around the bladder important for surgical instrumentation

Anterior	Symphysis pubis
Posterior	Rectum
Superior	Peritoneum
Inferior	Prostate and seminal vesicles (males)
	Pelvic floor musculature (females)

from a philosophical perspective, that as a muscle, *its natural function is to contract*. To be clear again, the bladder is a hollow muscle. Yet, when considering the bladder as an organ, which is the sum of all its parts, its philosophical nature would be considered primarily as a *storage vesicle*. Interestingly then, the nature of the structural building blocks, (smooth muscle cells), that make up the bladder are almost diametrically opposed to the philosophical nature of the bladder as a functional organ. Unusual but true. For the bladder to be most effective, this muscular organ must behave like a rubber balloon.

For a biologic naturalist, this natural conflict would be fascinating. However, before we totally wade into the uro-philosophy with respect to the structure and function of the bladder, let's take a trip back in time and remember some of the work of Charles Darwin during his travels on the HMS Beagle. Darwin proposed the scientific theory of a branching pattern of Evolution that resulted from a process that he called **Natural Selection**. This *"Natural Selection"* is essentially a series of adaptive changes to an organism in response to the stresses of nature, or even within an organism itself which continue over a long period of time and give rise to the diversity of form, as well as the alignment organic structure

and function. For example, as the needs of an organ (e.g., the bladder) within an organism change over time, the cellular composition and potentially, the neurologic innervation of that organ may modify its physiology so that structure and function remain in line from a physiologic perspective. Darwin could be considered a "Philosopher" as well as a "Naturalist" and the writings of Rene Descartes were very interesting to him. So, as Darwin tries to make sense of some of the findings that he encounters while on the Beagle, he superimposes Descartes' existentialist philosophy as he asks how it all translates to the human condition.

A hollow muscle (the bladder) whose nature is diametrically opposed to the nature of its component cellular makeup. So how does this happen? To allow this muscular organ to act like a storage balloon. In this case structure and function are not aligned. Although a hollow muscular conduit in the pelvis may be aligned in a fish, it is Not in a human. So if one accepts the Recapitulation Theory of Haeckel, i.e. "Ontogeny Recapitulates Phylogeny" then a hollow muscular conduit in a fish pelvis must become a storage organ in the human. How does this happen? The answer is "intense neuro-control" and in the case of the human bladder, it is "inhibitory neuro-control." It is this intense type of inhibitory neuro-control that allows divergent groups of muscles in the pelvis to act in a coordinated fashion and maintain urinary continence. Essentially, it is the concept of *Cortical Inhibition* that is what translates to "dryness" in the human condition.

To be able to be dry (not wet with urine) is to be able to maintain social acceptability as well as general health and well being. As Darwin has alluded to many times, in humans, as we come out of an aquatic environment and replace our scales or our mucus with skin (which cannot be chronically

a

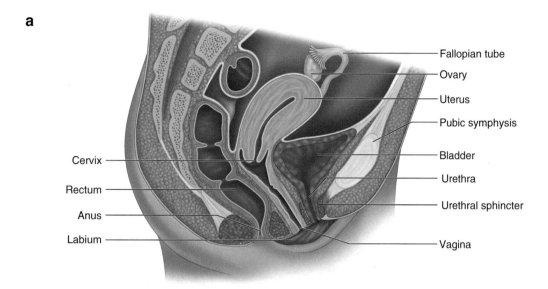

Fallopian tube
Ovary
Uterus
Pubic symphysis
Bladder
Urethra
Urethral sphincter
Vagina

Cervix
Rectum
Anus
Labium

b

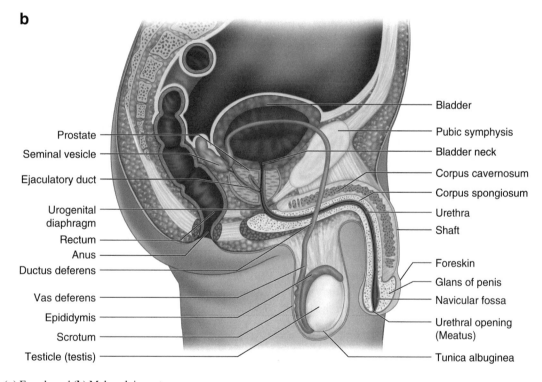

Bladder
Pubic symphysis
Bladder neck
Corpus cavernosum
Corpus spongiosum
Urethra
Shaft
Foreskin
Glans of penis
Navicular fossa
Urethral opening (Meatus)
Tunica albuginea

Prostate
Seminal vesicle
Ejaculatory duct
Urogenital diaphragm
Rectum
Anus
Ductus deferens
Vas deferens
Epididymis
Scrotum
Testicle (testis)

Fig. 17.2 (**a**) Female and (**b**) Male pelvic anatomy

wet), the ability to maintain dryness becomes even more important as a protection against excoriation and even worse, ulceration. This is especially true in those areas that are most affected by both the dampness of urine and the caustic effects of urea. Obviously, these high risk zones would be the perineum and the sacrum. I am sure we have all had the unwelcome opportunity to have to treat a large diameter, deep, infected sacral decubitus ulcer! Not a pleasant experience. Moreover, it can be a fatal one for the patient. Again, all highlighting the critical importance for an in-depth

understanding (from a neurophysiologic perspective) of cortical inhibition!

So, if this is so great and it all makes sense from a theoretical position, how do we know this is really the case? The answer is that we do not know for sure, and cannot know for sure, unless we have some way to measure and gauge these events from a physiologic and neuromuscular perspective. It sounds like a tall order, and a very complicated one at that. However, today we have developed incredibly intricate magnetic imaging studies combined with advanced physiologic

Fig. 17.3 Structure of the urinary bladder smooth muscle cells

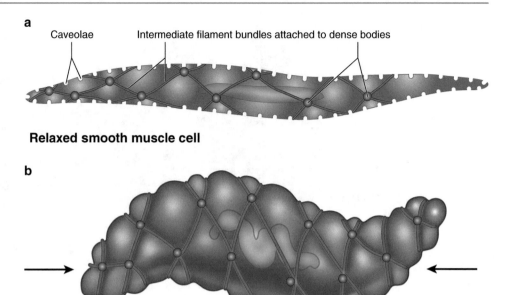

Relaxed smooth muscle cell

Contracted smooth muscle cell

staining techniques which have helped to clearly identify neuroanatomic parts of the brain and spinal cord. In addition, sophisticated electrophysiologic functional tests to reveal the neuromuscular responses of the bladder muscle in coordination with the pelvic floor musculature have become an integral part of how the neurogenic bladder is evaluated today in the form of urodynamic studies and pelvic floor muscle electromyography. The details of this type of testing are deferred from an in-depth breakdown here because they are discussed at length in another chapter Nevertheless, as advanced and sophisticated as all these tests are, they had to begin somewhere. The intricate functional neuromuscular detail is extracted from studies like *pelvic floor muscle electromyography. To have to guess,* it would seem likely that the use of this type of testing would have been initiated sometime after electricity became commonplace. So, maybe in the 1920s or 1930s?? Interestingly, the first attempts at assessing the neuromuscular function of the bladder were several decades before that. Essentially, Mooso and Pellicani performed the first documented simple cystometrogram in 1882.

> MOSSO and PELLACANI, in 1882, when the method of making continuous smoke-drum records had just been introduced by Marey, described a series of experiments upon the normal female human bladder. Their method was highly ingenious, and consisted of running records of the movements of a vessel of which the fluid contents communicated by tube and catheter with the interior of the bladder. The level of the fluid was kept constantly slightly above the level of the bladder and the record was therefore of variations of vesical volume and flow rates at constant pressure. From the OxfordJournals.org article published in July 1933.

Neuroanatomy and Neurophysiology of the Lower Urinary Tract

The lower urinary tract (LUT) physiology from a functional perspective is a concept that is commonly used to connote "the micturition cycle." Micturition comes from Latin roots, with the verb *micturire* which means to desire to void and should be used to express the entire process which includes both filling and emptying. The verb *to void* should be reserved for the actual act of emptying the bladder. The micturition cycle, as a term, is inclusive and comprehensive. Moreover, it implies two phases which include both filling and storage components. However, like so many other things in "real world" biology, they are not weighted evenly from a neuromuscular perspective. Nevertheless, more often than not, they are grouped together for the purposes of academic discussion. Actually, there is some logic to this because it ties together the circular spectrum of the way that our bodies handle liquid waste. Certainly, from a physiologic perspective highlighting the ties between filling and emptying is important because the musculature involved in this process (*the detrusor and the proximal urethral sphincteric complex*) must work in a coordinated fashion. So, it is very difficult to discuss intelligently how the group of muscles involved in voiding are behaving without understanding exactly what their muscular and soft tissue counterparts are doing in a simultaneous fashion, i.e. the complex interactions between the bladder, urethra, urethral sphincter, and nervous system. The micturition cycle is often discussed from a physiologic perspective. However, it may also **not** be unreasonable to break them up in a more philosophical discussion based on the human condition.

Acknowledging that the human condition requires social interaction for normal development, then being able to maintain some type of social structure is a requirement for man to prosper. To that end, for a human being to thrive in normal social situations, he or she **must be dry**! Essentially, for a human to be human, he or she must be able to maintain continence. So, here, we will break from tradition to look at the physiology of micturition from a philosophical perspective, one might split it into:

1. *The Physiology of Continence*
2. *The Physiology of Voiding*

Most importantly, the physiology of continence should take the preeminent position in that it accounts for over 95 % of the micturition cycle and is a core component for interactive human socialization, (maintaining dryness). To that end, let's open the discussion with the physiology of continence.

The Physiology of Continence

Storage of urine involves complex neural interactions between the bladder, urethra, urethral sphincter, and the brain and nervous system. The neural circuitry that controls this process is complex and highly distributed: it involves pathways at many levels of the CNS. The urinary bladder and urinary sphincter are the principal components of the lower urinary tract (LUT) responsible for continence.

In the most basic terms, the bladder is a hollow muscle whose function is to fill with fluid. Normally, that translates to a capacity of about 400–500 cc. At the same time, there is a continence zone (CZ) or sphinchteric complex which is located at the convergence of the bladder neck and proximal urethra. This sphincteric complex consists of an internal portion, which is a continuation of detrusor smooth muscle that thickens and converges to form the bladder neck area which is under tonic autonomic control from the sympathetic side. Proceeding in a more distal fashion, one runs into another constellation of high tone circular muscle surrounding the proximal urethra. This is the external component of the sphinchteric complex also known as the external sphinchter and rhabdoshpinchter which is composed of both striated and smooth muscle and must maintain contraction at rest. So, the achievement of urinary continence as a component of social acceptability is near the pinnacle of basic requirements for successful human interaction in modern society. As a general overview, it is a coordinated relationship that occurs with simultaneous bladder muscle (detrusor) relaxation along with chronic muscular contraction of both the

bladder neck *(internal urinary sphincter and the external urinary sphincter) and proximal urethra.* Here it is important to remember that, although extremely simplified, it is this descriptive overview that allows for urinary continence and the attendant maintenance of such, allows for social acceptability in the human condition. More importantly, it is this muscular state of affairs (allowing for continence) that is in place and active more than 90 % of the life time total. Consequently, it is considered by many experts to be the "tonic" situation. Now, taking into account all of the above, eventually, the bladder will reach its awake capacity which should lead to the desire to void. Voiding occurs when the external urinary sphincter relaxes as the initial **voluntary** trigger which is immediately followed by relaxation of the bladder neck, which is then almost immediately coordinated with a bladder muscle *(detrusor)* contraction, allowing for the unobstructed expulsion of urine.

This section is dedicated to the "All Important" Physiology of Continence (Fig. 17.4a, b), but before we get deep into its inner workings and tonic control we should set the back drop of continence as a whole. Remember, the micturition cycle is overseen and coordinated through both the autonomic and somatic nervous systems. Since the autonomic nervous system breaks down to the sympathetic and parasympathetic systems, the micturition cycle really falls under an integrated trilogy of neurologic pathways, i.e. somatic, sympathetic and parasympathetic.

To review, the sympathetic nervous system in the pelvis allows for bladder muscle relaxation with simultaneous tonic contraction of the sphincters. This is mediated through the hypogastric nerve, and these signals originate from the spinal cord at levels T10–L2. The parasympathetic system allows for bladder contraction and internal sphincter relaxation. This is mediated through the pelvic nerve, and these signals originate from the spinal cord levels at S2–S4. The somatic (voluntary) system allows for the control of the striated sphincter which is mediated through the pudendal nerve (S2–S4). All three of these systems are part of reflex pathways and are under the influence of higher centers (cerebrum and brainstem, pons micturition center). So, understanding the active presence of these three neurologic pathways underscores the preeminent position of **detrusor stability** in the maintenance of dryness and in turn socially acceptability.

The physiology of continence is under tonic sympathetic control but from a comprehensive perspective, it includes both sympathetic and somatic functions. The discussion of sympathetic control is in itself complex because it takes into account two (2) separate anatomic levels. These are: *(1) the bladder muscle* and *(2) the bladder neck musculature.* Sympathetic input to the bladder and the bladder neck musculature *(including the internal sphinchter)* is mediated by adrenergic receptors. The majority of receptors here belong to

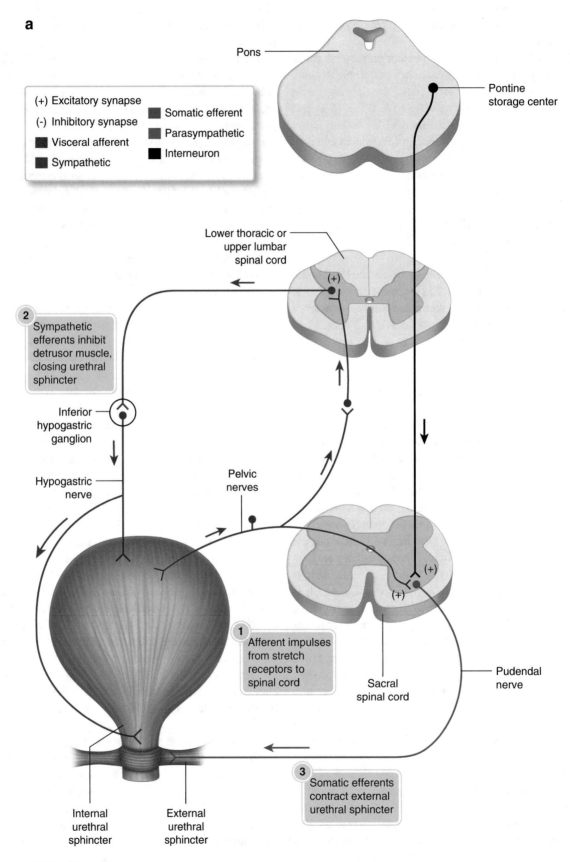

a

Pons

Pontine
storage center

(+) Excitatory synapse
(-) Inhibitory synapse
■ Visceral afferent
■ Sympathetic
■ Somatic efferent
■ Parasympathetic
■ Interneuron

Lower thoracic or
upper lumbar
spinal cord

(+)

2
Sympathetic
efferents inhibit
detrusor muscle,
closing urethral
sphincter

Inferior
hypogastric
ganglion

Hypogastric
nerve

Pelvic
nerves

1
Afferent impulses
from stretch
receptors to
spinal cord

(+)

(+)

Pudendal
nerve

Sacral
spinal cord

3
Somatic efferents
contract external
urethral sphincter

Internal
urethral
sphincter

External
urethral
sphincter

Fig. 17.4 (**a, b**) Physiology of continence

b

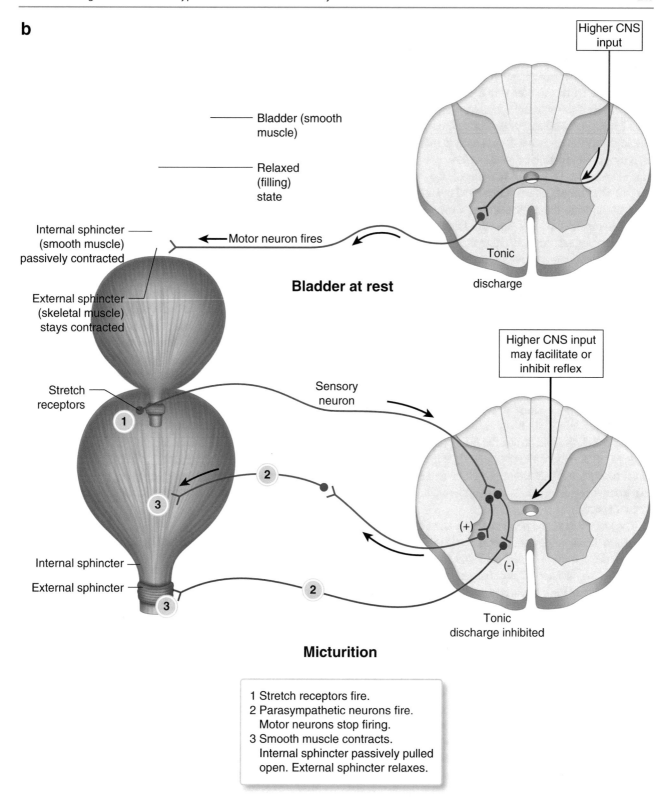

Higher CNS input

Bladder (smooth muscle)

Relaxed (filling) state

Internal sphincter (smooth muscle) passively contracted

← Motor neuron fires

Bladder at rest

Tonic discharge

External sphincter (skeletal muscle) stays contracted

Higher CNS input may facilitate or inhibit reflex

Stretch receptors

Sensory neuron

1

2

3

(+)

Internal sphincter

External sphincter

(-)

2

3

Tonic discharge inhibited

Micturition

1 Stretch receptors fire.
2 Parasympathetic neurons fire.
   Motor neurons stop firing.
3 Smooth muscle contracts.
   Internal sphincter passively pulled
   open. External sphincter relaxes.

Fig. 17.4   (continued)

the family of alpha receptors. However, this includes a super selective receptor subtype known as the alpha-1-a receptor. These alpha-1 adrenergic receptors at the bladder neck communicate via postganglionic fibers and utilize *norepinephrine* as its transmitter which results in tonic muscular contraction of the internal sphinchter, allowing for bladder neck apposition with a mucosal seal and subsequent dryness. In addition, the sympathetic nervous system inhibits detrusor activity via stimulation of *beta-3-adrenergic receptors* with *norepinephrine*. The use of norepinephrine here versus epinephrine has been confirmed in animal models. Finally, sympathetic input to the LUT also has a role in the inhibition of parasympathetic input into the bladder, thus inhibiting stimulatory signals from reaching the detrusor which further stabilizes the detrusor muscle. *So, to sum it all up,* as the sympathetic system via the thoracolumbar cord fires, it sends stimuli out through the hypogastric nerve to their nerve endings where norepinephrine will be released and stimulate three (3) separate receptor subtypes. These are, the beta 3 receptor at the level of the bladder muscle to enhance stability and elasticity, the alpha-1-a receptor at the level of the bladder neck in an effort to maintain apposition and a mucosal seal, thirdly, norepinephrine will stimulate presynaptic parasympathetic nerve endings to prevent acetylcholine release which would stimulate bladder muscle contraction, which would be undesireable during the filling phase. It is the combination of all these events that allow for the bladder muscle to act like the walls of a rubber balloon and enhance its role as a storage vesicle which is an integral role in the physiology of continence.

The last piece of the neuromuscular puzzle to review with respect to the physiology of continence is the somatic nervous system. Here, motor neurons originate from Onuf's nucleus, located on the anterior horns of the sacral spinal cord at levels S2–S4, and send their axons into the pudendal nerve that stimulate the striated muscle of the external sphincter to contract via the release of acetylcholine. This acetylcholine then binds to post-junctional nicotinic receptors, resulting in contraction of the external sphincter. Both alpha-receptors and serotonin 5-HT2 receptors are located in Onuf's nucleus and facilitate the storage reflex. So, in summation:

"The Physiology of Continence" that is the ability to store urine in a competent fashion is regulated by *two separate storage reflexes*—the (1) sympathetic (autonomic) reflex and the (2) somatic (guarding) reflex which is mediated by small myelinated A-delta fibers which are coordinated by the spinobulbospinal pathway. *Let's look at the sympathetic pathway first.* This neurologic route begins with an impulse to store urine emanating from the periphery (bladder). Sensation from the bladder wall initiates afferent activity. This afferent activity travels in the pelvic nerves to the spinal cord via the S3 level at which time it is gated and sent up to the L1–L3 level via either the tract of Lesseur or the lateral spinotha-

lamic tract. At that point, sympathetic activity is initiated and transmitted out from the "thoracolumbar cord" via the hypogastric nerve, which leads to a blockage of excitatory parasympathetic stimulation of the bladder. After this sympathetic barrage is sent out, that afferent impulse continues up the spinal cord to the brainstem, specifically the micturition center located in the pons and then to higher centers in the cerebrum for assessment. During this time, more sympathetic activity is generated which leads postganglionic neurons to release noradrenaline, which binds to beta-3-adrenoreceptors in the detrusor, leading to detrusor stability and elasticity and most importantly prevention of parasympathetic agonism.

The second storage reflex, the somatic storage (guarding) reflex occurs in response to certain variable stimuli including sudden increases in intra-abdominal pressure. In this reflex, afferent activity travels along the myelinated A-delta fibers in the pelvic nerve to the sacral spinal cord, where efferent somatic urethral motor neurons in Onuf's nucleus are located. Afferent activity which has continued up the cord via the aforementioned ascending tracts is also relayed to the periaqueductal gray (PAG) via the pontine micturition center (PMC). The PMC sends impulses to motor neurons in Onuf's nucleus, and axons from these neurons travel in the pudendal nerve and stimulate the rhabdosphincter to contract which would enhance the mucosal seal, increase outlet resistance, and maintain continence. Finally, what all of this means is that when these pathways operate appropriately, the patient remains socially acceptable and most importantly, DRY!!

The Physiology of Continence (Peripheral NeuroControl)

The peripheral control of continence is a rapidly growing area within the arena of NeuroScience as a whole. There is so much work being done in this arena that you could almost dedicate an entire book just to this topic. Unfortunately, we do not have that luxury here, so I will ask the reader's indulgence in my attempt to condense this very important piece of neuro-control in the pelvis as I do my best to highlight and adequately cover those most important aspects.

Peripheral Control of Continence (The Urothelium)

It is very important for the clinician treating those patients with neuromuscular dysfunction in the lower urinary tract to understand the role of the dense neural network within the soft tissue which lies just below the bladder mucosa. Now this special area has been coined the "suburothelium." This network is comprised of mostly afferent fibers which serve as mechanoreceptors from the bladder wall and transmit primarily sensory stimuli dealing with bladder fullness and bladder pain to the sacral spinal cord. All this is accomplished via the utilization of two (2) major types of neurons. These are the A-Delta fibers and unmyelinated "C" fibers. The "C" fibers are charged primarily with the conduction of noxious feelings of pain and pressure. Therefore, the *A*-Delta fibers are the "primary" in the area and are predominant within "conditions of health." So, in essence, it is these A-Delta fibers that carry sensations of bladder pressure and fullness that are *not* noxious.

Peripheral Control of Continence (The Functional Syncytium)

It is important to remember here that the bladder wall functions as a major sense organ within the anatomic pelvis. The moniker given to this sense organ is "The Functional Syncytium" and from a microscopic anatomic perspective, it consists of both the urothelium and the soft tissue lying just beneath, known as the "suburothelium." This functional syncytium works together through intercellular communications achieved with "neurotransmitters" to convey the feelings of pressure and temperature. Both acetylcholine (ACh) and ATP are utilized in abundance by the bladder wall urothelium as it distends during urine storage in an effort to facilitate continence. From a neurologic perspective, it is proposed that the Ach released from the urothelium during periods of bladder storage acts on muscarinic receptors in the suburothelium and the detrusor to stimulate and maintain bladder wall tone and a consistent level of compliance.

In addition, it speaks to a possible autocrine role for Ach released by the urothelium and accepted by suburothelial receptors. Once these suburothelial muscarinic receptors are activated by Ach from the urothelium, they release UDIF (urothelial derived inhibitory factor) which in turn decreases detrusor tone to provide that degree of muscular antagonism to allow for fine-tuning the degree of bladder wall tone to create a fluctuating level of detrusor compliance as the bladder volume constantly changes during filling. Furthermore, Ach released by the urothelium activates two (2) nicotinic signaling pathways which work via a negative feedback mechanism. These pathways are mediated by Alpha-7 (α7, inhibitory) and Alpha-3 (α3, excitatory) nicotinic receptors, which facilitate urine storage and bladder emptying, respectively.

This "Functional Syncytium", as an entity to help the bladder wall maintain its sensory role is as stated above not only dependent on Ach and its attendant muscarinic receptors for functionality but also ATP. With respect to ATP as a sensory neurotransmitter, there are two (2) receptor lines that are important. One receptor is primary and the other is works in a facilitatory fashion. The primary purinergic receptor with a functional role in mechanosensation from the bladder wall is the P2X3 receptor which is an ATP gated purinergic receptor. Essentially, the cascade is as follows, ATP released

from the urothelium will find and activate the P2X3 receptor in the suburothelium which in turn will send signals of stretch and fullness through the sacral spinal cord and then up to the brainstem. The second receptor works to facilitate the action of the P2X3 receptor. It also is purinergic in nature and its class was formerly known as a vanilloid receptor, specifically the VR1 receptor. Today it is known as Transient Receptor Potential Vanilloid 1 (TRPV-1). This receptor, when activated, mediates the activity of unmyelinated nerves (C-fibers) in the suburothelium and facilitates the activity of myelinated nerves in the same area below the urothelium. So, in sum, the activity of these TPRV-1 receptors facilitates the transmission of bladder filling via the P2X3 receptors relationship with myelinated A-Delta fibers. However, the activity of the TPRV-1 receptors via unmyelinated "C" fibers is enhanced dramatically as fullness takes on an uncomfortable nature. The final part of this "Functional Syncytium" is that there is a cell mediator in the suburothelium known as the "interstitial cell." This cell aids with the sensations of bladder wall distention and fullness. Now, it is understood that this cell is actually a specialized type of myofibroblast and although not completely understood, it is integral in this entire cascade of purinergic neuromuscular sensory function from the pelvis.

The Physiology of Voiding

The total amount of time that a human being spends voiding, that is, actually passing urine from the body, is a small fraction of the total time that our bodies activate those neurologic pathways which allow for continence. So, it should not be surprising that the length of the section on "Voiding Physiology" reflects that natural tendency.

The voiding reflex involves the pontine micturition center (PMC) as well as other regions in the brain, including the hypothalamus and the cerebral cortex. So, if the reader can indulge another bit of oversimplification as we follow an impulse down the spinal cord through the sacral cord and to the bladder muscle, this is it. The efferent side begins with a bladder that is full or near full. At that time, the idea of voluntary control is initiated at higher centers in the cerebral cortex and hypothalamus. This neurologic data is transmitted back to the micturition center in the pons. The PMC organizes and distributes these neurologic impulses since the PMC controls the delegation of descending pathways. Once the neuro-stimulation from higher centers is organized in the pons, it is shipped out to the corticospinal tract which sends impulses downward via the corticospinal tract through the thoracolumbar cord to end up at the sacral cord. As the impulse travels down from the brainstem toward the sacrum, it passes through the thoracolumbar cord, which is one of the bastions for sympathetic outflow. As this descending signal passes through this part of the cord, it suppresses sympathetic outflow which destabilizes the detrusor muscle by withdrawing Beta-3 stimulation and prepares it for contraction while simultaneously relaxing the internal urinary sphinchter via withdraw of Alpha tone at the bladder neck which begins decreasing outlet resistance. Upon arrival of this impulse in the sacral cord, there are two (2) distributive pathways it may take, (1) somatic or (2) parasympathetic.

Firstly, with respect to the somatic component, as the impulse descends into the sacral cord, it is directed to the anterior horn of level (S2–S4) in the area of Onuf's nucleus. The sacral roots of S2–S4 coalesce to form the pudendal nerve, which carries the impulse outward toward the external (voluntary striated) urethral sphincter (EUS). An initial somatic spike is immediately followed by withdrawal of somatic stimulation to the EUS which triggers the initiation of voiding via the second distributive pathway which is parasympathetic.

Secondly, the parasympathetic component of the impulse descends and utilizes the intermediolateral column of the sacral cord to send out the parasympathetic signal to the "pelvic ganglion." This nerve cluster is parasympathetic in nature and collects and collates these impulses before they allow them to fire out via the pelvic nerve to the neuromuscular junction at the level of the detrusor muscle, thus releasing Ach and allowing for detrusor contraction and bladder emptying.

Site Specific Neurogenecity

Spinal Cord Injury (SCI)

The ability to voluntarily initiate voiding involves a trigger type relaxation of the proximal urethral continence zone which is essentially the sphincter complex series of heterogeneous circular musculature which extends from the proximal urethra up through the bladder neck. This is followed almost simultaneously by an escalating detrusor contraction. This series of neuromuscular phenomena occurring in almost simultaneous sequence, as we have reviewed above, is known as the micturition reflex. Experimental studies in animals have shown that this voiding reflex is coordinated by spinobulbospinal pathway which passes through pontine micturition center (PMC) positioned in rostral brainstem. Spinal pathways connecting the PMC to the sacral cord have to be intact for this reciprocal response. Transection of the spinal cord disrupts this spinobulbospinal pathway communication with PMC, which eliminates voluntary control of voiding and the reciprocal bladder and sphincter response, resulting in an areflexic or hyporeflexic bladder during the period of "spinal shock" causing urinary retention. However, this process is followed by slow re-initiation of the infantile sacral reflex pathways over a period of time, without any inhibitory control from higher centers, causing neurogenic detrusor overactivity or (NDO). It is important to remember that only sacral reflex activity is preserved and will return after the period of spinal shock.

Theory regarding neurogenic lower urinary tract dysfunction (NLUTD) in spinal cord injury classifies the disorder into four major types (and a special fifth classification):

1. detrusor hyperreflexia in combination with hyperreflexive (spastic) sphincter, this condition is also known as detrusor sphincter dyssynergia (DSD)
2. detrusor hyporeflexia in combination with a hyperreflexive (spastic) sphincter
3. detrusor hyporeflexia (areflexia) in combination with a hyporeflexive (flaccid) sphincter
4. detrusor hyperreflexia in combination with sphincter hypo-normoreflexia
5. The non-neurogenic neurogenic bladder (variants of Hinman's syndrome)
   hypertonic pelvic floor muscle dysfunction

Type 1 dysfunction is most frequently seen in supraconal lesions. *Type 2* is usually observed in conal lesions. *Type 3* is seen in cauda equina lesions, while *Type 4* is typically observed in suprapontine lesions. In incomplete suprasacral lesion, synergistic relaxation of the external sphincter may be preserved. Balanced voiding may occur but urgency and urge incontinence usually persist.

Micturition reflex is initiated by small myelinated afferents (Aδ) and unmyelinated afferents (C-fibers). SCI at lower thoracic level (T8–T12) or suprasacral micturition center eliminates both reflexes, however, in weeks to months long latency C-fiber reflex reappears, and Aδ-fiber never recovers. It is the re-development of these C-fibers which causes automatic micturition in paraplegic animals. This is the underlying pathophysiology of NDO, and reflex bladder contractions in the experimental models.

The insufficient emptying of the bladder induces recurrent UTI, nephrolithiasis, hydronephrosis, and finally renal failure. Lower motor neuron lesions or injury to the sacral micturition center (S1–S4) results in the loss of parasympathetic control of the bladder detrusor and a somatic denervation of the external urethral sphincter, with associated loss of afferent pathways. In a complete lesion, conscious awareness of bladder fullness will be lost and the micturition reflex is absent. As a result one would experience stress incontinence and urinary retention. Stress incontinence is a result of incompetent urinary sphincter with significant reduction of maximal urethral pressure. However, in some patients paradoxic obstruction of the external urethral sphincter has been observed, secondary to a fibrotic degeneration of the muscle, and this is mainly because of a systemic disease. Also, in the lower motor neuron SCI, due to some unknown reason it has been observed that the bladder neck remains open even during the filling phase, and further contributing to overflow and stress incontinence. Repeated studies have revealed that suprasacral lesions are associated with detrusor hyperreflexia and/or detrusor sphincter dyssynergia (DSD) in 94.9 %, and sacral lesions with detrusor areflexia in 85.7 % of cases.

Brain Lesions

Voiding dysfunction is very prevalent in patients with history of stroke or other neurological disorders. Spinal cord lesions at certain levels may lead to impaired coordination of the bladder and with the outlet (i.e., the CZ and paraurethral musculature), while suprapontine lesions rather lead to urinary urge incontinence due to detrusor hyperactivity (NDO).

Normal micturition reflex is coordinated by the PMC or the M-region, which are both located in the dorsal pontine tegmentum. The inhibitory input from the medial frontal lobe controls the excitability of the PMC. Therefore, a lesion above the PMC produces uninhibited bladder, resulting in detrusor overactivity. On the other hand, lesion between the PMC and the sacral cord produces spastic bladder. In an analysis 49 % of 39 patients with brainstem stroke suffered from lower urinary tract dysfunction, majority being nocturnal urinary frequency, voiding difficulty and urinary retention. These cases suggested lower urinary tract control is located in the dorsolateral pons area, including the pontine reticular nucleus and reticular formation, adjacent to the medial parabrachial nucleus and the locus coeruleus. In the most recent study 30 cases of brainstem infarctions were analyzed. In this subpopulation, 70 % of these patients had lower urinary tract symptoms, comprising of 46.7 % storage disorders and 23.3 % emptying disorder. Patients with emptying disorders were more prevalent with medullary lesions (55.6 %) and storage disorder was common in patients with pontine lesions (61.9 %). To evaluate how the central nervous system site impacts the lower urinary tract function, prospective study was conducted. This study included 60 patients with cerebrovascular accidents, where 47 % presented with retention and overflow incontinence 40 % complained of detrusor hyperreflexia, and 13 % had frequency and urgency despite normal urodynamic study. The cause of retention was due to detrusor hypoflexia in majority of the patients, and mainly it was due to *cerebellar lesion*. Detrusor hyperreflexia was seen in patients with lesions in basal ganglia, internal capsule, and cerebral cortex. Out of these 60 patients, 40 had ischemic and 20 had hemorrhagic infarcts. The majority of patients with hemorrhagic infarcts presented with areflexic detrusor, on the other hand ischemic infarcts majority presented with detrusor hyperreflexia. It is important to address that the urodynamic study in these individuals was done acutely after their CVA, as a result detrusor areflexia which was reported would be expected as a consequence of neurogenic shock. This would be expected during this period. However, it is very important to note that detrusor hyporeflexia or areflexia would *not* be expected in mature lesions above the brainstem.

Of these 60 patients, 8 had frontoparietal lesions, out of which 6 presented with detrusor hyperreflexia. Inhibitory control of the motor area designated to the detrusor is on the superomedial area of the frontal lobe and the genu of the corpus callosum. Therefore, frontal and frontoparietal lesions would lead to loss of the normal cortical inhibitory influence resulting in detrusor hyperreflexia. The patients with lesions in internal capsule also showed detrusor hyperreflexia, and this is because various ascending and descending tracts pass from here, and thus lesion mimics frontoparietal lesion. Infarcts in cerebellar area show detrusor areflexia with no effect on the external urethral sphincter. The cerebellum derives sensory input from the detrusor and pelvic floor musculature through spinocerebellar tracts, but it does not initiate contraction, but rather modulates the effect of cerebral cortex and the brain stem detrusor nuclei. The net effect of this modulation normally leads to suppression of reflex detrusor contraction, as a result one would expect to have hyperreflexic detrusor in response to cerebellar dysfunction, but rather opposite happens, and that relationship is not well understood.

Systemic Diseases

Parkinson's Disease

Parkinson's disease is a progressive degenerative neurological movement disorder. Parkinson's involves the malfunction and even death of vital nerve cells in the brain. The neurons which are primarily affected are neurons in an area of the brain called the substantia nigra. Many of these dying neurons produce dopamine, a chemical that sends messages to the part of the brain that controls movement and coordination. As the disease progresses, the amount of dopamine produced in the brain decreases, leaving a person unable to control movement normally. The symptoms that patients typically express are motor features such as resting tremor, bradykinesia, cogwheel rigidity, and postural instability. Other non-motor symptoms include dysphagia, constipation, orthostatic hypotension, depression, sexual dysfunction, and lower urinary tract symptoms. In Parkinson's disease bladder symptoms usually occur at advanced stages of the disease, however being an elderly patient, other conditions tend to influence continence and emptying, especially obstruction in older men being a common cause. In the PRIAMO study, which was conducted to assess the non-motor symptoms and their impact on quality of the patients, it was determined that majority patients had symptoms in the psychiatric domain, but lower urinary tract symptoms were also very common in about 57.3 %, which included urgency (35 %) and nocturia (35 %). Interestingly, urinary urge incontinence was less common but may be secondary to the tendency for this demographic to be older males which often have a component of outlet obstruction from BPH.

Under normal conditions, the net output from the basal ganglia inhibits the thalamus, and dopaminergic striatal activity induces selective disinhibition. It is believed that in Parkinson's disease this disinhibition cannot be performed due to degeneration of nigrostriatal dopaminergic neurons resulting in non-selective motion such as "tremor." In addition to that, Parkinson's disease is associated with decreased input of sensory information to the cortex, as a result patients have reduced ability to integrate and separate sensory input as the disease progresses.

Some studies have shown that patients who received deep-brain stimulation (DBS) of the subthalamic nucleus, suggested that lower urinary tract symptoms are associated with cortical dysfunction in Parkinson's disease. This implies that frontal cortical areas are unable to stimulate the pontine micturition center which disrupts the integration of sensory input from the bladder. Also, basal ganglia have an inhibitory effect on micturition reflex, and detrusor overactivity develops after cell loss in the substantia nigra. some studies have shown that treatment with 1-methyl-4-phenyl-1,2,3,6-tetrahydropyridine (MPTP), can generate a neuromuscular situation that is consistent with overactive bladder or detrusor overactivity. However, selective dopamine D1 receptor agonists have been successfully used to suppress detrusor overactivity.

Multiple Sclerosis (MS)

Multiple sclerosis (MS) is a potentially disabling disease of the brain and spinal cord (central nervous system). In MS, the immune system attacks the protective sheath (myelin) that covers nerve fibers and causes communication problems between your brain and the rest of your body. Eventually, the disease can cause the nerves themselves to deteriorate or become permanently damaged. Multiple sclerosis (MS) is the most common progressive neurological disorder often affecting younger patients. MS is an autoimmune disease, where communication between the central nervous system and other parts of the body is affected. This communication defect is because of loss of myelin, causing disruption in the ability of the nerves to conduct electrical impulses and communicate. Just based on the shear numbers and volume of fibers involved, it is the inhibitor fibers that are most significantly affected. This will create a disinhibited state, allowing for involuntary bladder muscle activity. Bladder dysfunction has been well recognized as an important physical disability in MS patients. Studies in past have shown that approxi-

mately 75 % of all patients with MS will develop urinary dysfunction during the course of their disease. The urinary dysfunction symptoms include frequency, urgency, and urge incontinence. These symptoms are a result of neurogenic detrusor overactivity (NDO), neurogenic detrusor underactivity, and/or detrusor sphincter dyssynergia (DSD) which tends to develop as a result of neurological change, most often from spinal cord involvement. Obstructive symptoms have been observed as well, resulting in urinary retention in 25 % of these cases. Lesions in particular region of the central nervous system cause associated symptoms observed in these patients. If the lesion is confined to subcortical white-matter, detrusor overactivity will be much prevalent in those patients, on the other hand if the lesion involves spinal cord, one would see detrusor overactivity and detrusor sphincter dyssnergia (DSD).

Multiple System Atrophy (MSA) and Detrusor Dysfunction

Multiple system atrophy (MSA), formerly known as *The Shy Drager Syndrome* is a neurodegenerative disorder and manifests in the age group of 50–60 years. The clinical symptoms resemble very much like that of Parkinson's disease. Patients often have autonomic failure (orthostatic hypotension, bowel and bladder disturbances, sexual dysfunction), parkinsonism, cerebellar ataxia, pyramidal tract signs. MSA is classified into two subtypes, based on their patient's motor features, either MSA-P (parkinsonism) or MSA-C (cerebellar). The majority of the MSA patients have lower urinary tract symptoms, although actual study percentages range from 45 % to 95 %. The nature of pelvic symptomatology centers around urgency, frequency, urge incontinence to large residual volume post micturition.

Urodynamic evaluation showed that patients with MSA often have detrusor over activity as the underlying cause of overactive bladder symptoms. This is mainly because of neuronal loss in nigrostriatal dopaminergic system, cerebellum, pontomedullary raphe, and frontal cortex. Incomplete bladder emptying is also seen, but that usually happens with progression of the illness. One of the studies demonstrated increase in mean post void residual between the first and fifth years of the disease. Open bladder neck and weakness of urethral sphincter muscles also contribute to incontinence. Denervation of the striated sphincter results from a loss anterior horn cells in the Onuf's nucleus of the sacral spinal cord.

Detrusor Dysfunction in Diabetes

Normal bladder function is attained by proper communication between sensory and motor pathways present both in peripheral and central nervous system. Bladder dysfunction seen in diabetic patients caused by peripheral neuropathy is often urinary retention. This is because there is destruction of primarily sensory nerves going to the bladder, which results in bladder distension often without sensation. This distension is because of lack of detrusor contraction, and patients develop overflow incontinence. Bladder dysfunction in diabetes can occur in varied ways, that is, diabetic cystopathy, detrusor overactivity, and urge urinary incontinence. Onset of bladder dysfunction in diabetics usually occurs in advanced stages of the disease. Patients usually remain asymptomatic during early stages. The initial lower urinary tract pathology to represent usually is impaired bladder sensation. Micturition reflexes are delayed due to decrease in bladder sensation, which results in increasing bladder capacity and urinary retention. Patients usually are asymptomatic at this stage, but one starts noticing frequent urinary tract infections due to urine retention, and slowly symptoms of straining, hesitation, and weak stream start to develop.

The prevalence rate of bladder dysfunction increases with the chronicity of the diabetes mellitus. Rate of bladder dysfunction is about 25 % after 10 years of diabetes, and >50 % after 45 years of diabetes.

Spina Bifida Affect on Bladder Dysfunction

Spina bifida is a major congenital defect which occurs because of incomplete closure of the backbone and membranes during embryonic development. It affects multiple organ systems, including the urinary bladder. More than 90 % of affected individuals have neurogenic bladder. This is because the nerves in the spinal cord that control the bladder detrusor muscles do not form properly. Consistent urinary incontinence is seen in children because of external sphincter function alteration from denervation. Detrusor sphincter dyssynergia leads to detrusor hypertrophy which causes obstruction, and affects the storage capability of the bladder. This may facilitate a situation that can lead to recurrent urinary tract infections, which in turn may lead to kidney dysfunction. A study showed newborns with myelomeningocele, 55 % had detrusor sphincter dyssynergia, 18 % had synergy, and 27 % had absent activity.

Treatment Options in Neurogenic Bladder

To discuss treatment options for patients with neurogenic bladder is a challenging task. In and of itself, this topic could account for an entire chapter or even more. Nevertheless, we will try to treat this topic in a concise fashion, yet as comprehensively as possible. The correct therapy or combination of therapies should be determined by assessing multiple factors. These would include clinical lower urinary tract symptoms (primarily incontinent vs primarily retentive), consideration must also be given to the type and extent of nerve damage associated with the underlying neurologic condition. Therapies for neurogenic bladder fall into six cat-

egories: (1) physical-psychological, (2) electrical-stimulatory, (3) drug therapy, (4) CIC, (5) surgery, and (6) biologic neuromodulation using Botox.

Physical-Psychological Therapy/Timed Voiding

Physical-psychological therapy is more commonly known as timed voiding. It combines "will power" and exercise. The patient is asked to keep a voiding diary, which is a daily record of the amount and time of fluid intake, times of urination, and episodes of leakage. The record creates a pattern that may initially allow patients to determine the times of the day they should be in close proximity to a bathroom. These are also the times when a patient should attempt to urinate. The intervals between voiding times are gradually extended as the patient gains control over voiding. This conditioning is often coupled with physical exercises, principally Kegel exercises, which strengthen the pelvic musculature. The Valsalva maneuver, an exertion used to pass stool, may also be sufficient to empty a bladder.

Sacral Nerve Root Stimulation

As discussed in previous chapters, the lumbosacral plexus is the controlling factor with respect to bladder and pelvic floor musculature. Therefore, it is not surprising that trying to electro-physiologically manipulate the way that these roots process neurologic stimuli can have a profound effect on the neuromuscular functioning of the bladder and the pelvic floor. Again, this is discussed in detail in Chapter xyz. Nevertheless, it is easy to describe that small electrode ridden leads are placed under the skin over the lower back in close proximity to the S2–S4 nerve roots. Then, a test phase proceeds during the course of a 2- to 3-week period where neuromuscular responses are recorded. If those responses are favorable, then a small stimulator disc loaded with the appropriate software is implanted in a minor surgical procedure just beneath the skin at the convergence of the "lumbo-sacral and gluteal regions." The stimulator delivers electrical impulses that mimic those that would normally be delivered by nerves if they were behaving normally. The device has been approved by the US Food and Drug Administration to treat urge incontinence, urgency-frequency syndromes, and urinary retention in patients in whom other therapies have failed.

Drug Therapy

There are as yet no drugs that target specific muscles such as the detrusor or sphincteric complex and pelvic floor musculature. However, there are classes of drugs that reduce involuntary bladder muscle spasm and other drugs that control pelvic floor muscle contractions. These agents are discussed at length in previous chapters so they will not be expounded upon here. It is important to note here that these drugs can sometimes be effective in appropriately selected neurogenic bladder conditions. Essentially, there are three (4) major classes of drugs used to treat neuromuscular bladder disorders. These are: (1) anticholinergic agents, (2) antimuscarinic agents, (3) tricyclic agents, and (4) sympathomimetic agents.

Anticholinergic Agents

Anticholinergic drugs are agents that act at the level of the cholinergic ganglion, thus the name "anticholinergic." They are widely considered to be first line medical therapy in women with urge incontinence. They work to inhibit involuntary bladder contractions and may be useful in treating lower urinary tract symptoms associated with sensory dysfunction. All anticholinergic drugs have similar performance profiles and toxicity. Potential adverse effects of all anticholinergic agents include blurred vision, dry mouth, heart palpitations, drowsiness, and facial flushing. When anticholinergic drugs are used in excess, acute urinary retention in the bladder may occur.

- Propantheline bromide (Pro Banthine)
  Adult dosing is 15 mg PO tid/qid. Pediatric dosing, not established.
  Propantheline bromide is a pregnancy category C drug.
- Dicyclomine hydrochloride (Bentyl)
  Adult dosing is 10–20 mg PO tid. Pediatric dosing, not established.
  Dicyclomine hydrochloride is a pregnancy category B drug.
- Hyoscyamine sulfate (Levsin/SL, Levsin, Levsinex)
  Adult dosing is 0.125 mg PO q4h. Pediatric dosing, not established.
  Hyoscyamine sulfate is a pregnancy category C drug.

Antimuscarinic Agents

These agents are most commonly grouped together with the anticholinergic agents and technically they are. That is, these agents modulate receptors that are primarily parasympathetic and utilize acetylcholine as their neurotransmitter. However, and most importantly, it is the preferential site of action that separates these two (2) groups of molecules. True anticholinergic agents primarily act at the level of the cholinergic ganglion while antimuscarinic agents have a preferential affinity for the neuromuscular junction. Essentially, these are "musculotropic" agents that relax the smooth muscles of the end organ, in this case the urinary bladder by exerting a

direct spasmolytic action on the smooth muscle of the bladder, these antispasmodic type drugs have been reported to increase bladder capacity and effectively decrease or eliminate urge incontinence. All of these agents are tertiary amines except for Trospium which is a quaternary amine. The quaternary structure makes this molecule very polar and hence does not cross membranes like the BBB very well. The adverse-effect profile of these drugs is similar to that of anticholinergic agents.

- Oxybutynin chloride (Ditropan IR, Ditropan XL)
  Ditropan XL achieves steady-state levels over a 24-h period and avoids first-pass metabolism. Medical studies have shown that oxybutynin chloride reduces incontinence episodes by 83–90 %. The total continence rate has been reported to be 41–50 %. In clinical trials, only 1 % stopped taking Ditropan XL because of dry mouth, and less than 1 % stopped taking Ditropan XL due to CNS adverse effects.
  Dosing of Ditropan XL is 5–15 mg PO qd. Pediatric dosing has not been established.
- Tolterodine L-tartrate (Detrol LA)
  Dosing of Detrol LA is 4 mg po qd. Pediatric dosing has not been established.
- Trospium (Sanctura)
  Adult dosing is 20 mg PO bid; In patients with a CrCl <30 mL/min, dosing is 20 mg po @ hs. Pediatric dosing has not been established.
- Fesoterodine (Toviaz)
  Adult dosing is 4 mg PO qd; it may be increased to 8 mg/qd. Pediatric dosing has not been established.
- Solifenicen (Vesicare)
  Adult dosing is 5 mg po qd; it may be increased to 10 mg/qd. Pediatric dosing has not been established.

Centrally Acting Agents, Tricyclic Antidepressant Drugs

Historically, these drugs were used to treat major depression; however, they have an additional use that is not FDA approved treatment of bladder dysfunction. They function to increase norepinephrine and serotonin levels. In addition, they exhibit anticholinergic and direct muscle relaxant effects on the urinary bladder.

- Imipramine hydrochloride (Tofranil)
  Adult dosing is 10–50 mg PO qd/tid; the range is 25–100 mg qd.
  Pediatric dosing has not been established
- Amitriptyline hydrochloride (Elavil)
  It increases circulating levels of norepinephrine and serotonin by blocking their reuptake at nerve endings and is ineffective for use in urge incontinence.

However, it is extremely effective in decreasing symptoms of urinary frequency in women with pelvic floor muscle dysfunction.

Adult dosing is 10 mg po @hs. Pediatric dosing has not been established.

Sympathomimetic Agents (Beta III Agonists)

There is only a limited amount of historical data with these drugs because of its fairly recent FDA approval in July of 2012. Currently, there is only one agent that is FDA approved. The drug goes to the chemical name of mirabegron and is traded as Myrbetriq and is approved by the FDA for the treatment of bladder dysfunction. The mechanism of action is to functionally increase norepinephrine levels at the detrusor muscle. In addition, they do *not* exhibit any of the anticholinergic side effects seen with agents in other classes.

- Mirabegron, (Myrbetriq)
- Adult dosing is 10–50 mg PO qd/tid; the range is 25–100 mg qd.
- Pediatric dosing has not been established.

CIC

Catheterization is not infrequently employed to ensure complete bladder drainage. It involves the insertion of a thin tube through the urethra and into the bladder. A number of patients can learn to insert the catheter themselves. The therapy is called clean intermittent catheterization (CIC). Exceptional sanitary procedures must be followed as the risk of urinary tract infection is significant with any type of catheterization. Another therapy, indwelling catheterization, places a catheter in the bladder for extended periods. These prevent bladder distension by continually draining urine into a bedside collector. Again, infection is a concern.

Surgery

There are two broad categories of surgical procedures used in neurogenic bladder (NGB) today. These are the (1) the artificial urinary sphincter and (2) ilea urinary diversion.

The artificial urinary sphincter (AUS) (Fig. 17.5) is a mechanical prosthetic device. Essentially, they function to make the bladder neck and bladder outlet competent. The device consists of a cuff that fits around the bladder neck, a pressure regulating balloon, and a pump that inflates the cuff. The balloon is placed beneath the abdominal muscles. The pump is placed in the labia in women and in the scrotum for men. Other locations include placement beneath the skin of the abdominal wall or thigh. Activation of the pump diverts fluid from the cuff to the balloon allowing the sphincter muscle to relax and urine to pass. The cuff automatically reinflates automatically in 3–5 min. It is very important to note here that patient selection is paramount in the neurogenic bladder arena. This is because the precise type of neurogenic bladder has to be elucidated. For example, if the patient has a

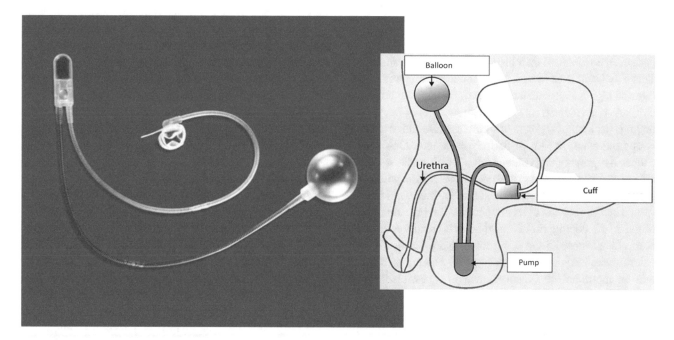

Fig. 17.5 Artificial urinary sphincter. With permission from Pariser J, Cohen AJ, Rosen AM, Bales GT. Artificial Urinary Sphincter: Patient Selection and Surgical Technique. In: Sandhu JS, ed. Urinary Dysfunction in Prostate Cancer Springer, New York 2015; pp: 71–92; and Bauer RM, Hubner KW. Moderne operative Therapiemöglichkeiten der männlichen Belastungsinkontinenz. Der Urologe 2014;53(3):339–345

Type IV NGB after CVA, the patient should be hyperreflexic and generate much higher bladder filling pressures, usually with significant involuntary detrusor muscle activity. Consequently, any attempt to increase outlet resistance or close the bladder neck against significant involuntary bladder muscle activity should be avoided. To that end, an AUS would not be a good choice. Moreover, it would not only not be a good choice, it should be considered "contraindicated" because an active AUS in this scenario would put the upper tracts (renal units) at risk. However, if the patient with the general diagnosis of NGB with urinary incontinence underwent the appropriate diagnostic workup including electrophysiologic testing such as urodynamic studies and pelvic floor muscle electromyography and revealed what would be considered a Type III NGB, that might be a good candidate for the AUS and would *not* put the kidneys at risk. In this case, the patient could have a normoreflexic or hyporeflexic detrusor with an incompetent bladder neck.

Some type of reconstructive urinary diversion has to be considered when all else fails with respect to therapy for NGB when one is left with a patient that is not only socially unacceptable but also may potentially have compromised upper tracts (renal units) as well as an excoriated and/or ulcerated perineum. There are many options in this regard (too many to discuss individually here), but ileal urinary diversion is the choice that is most often selected. Ileal urinary diversion is a surgical technique that was developed near the end of the Second World War, in the mid-1940s. The physician who created this surgical technique is a man named Eugene M. Bricker. Consequently, the procedure was formerly referred to as the Bricker Pouch, after its inventor. Basically, it is a form of incontinent urostomy and even after all this time is still the most utilized technique for the diversion of urine in patients with neurogenic bladder, or in patients who have had their bladder removed for malignancy. This may be, at least in part, due to its very low complication rate and high patient satisfaction level. To create an ileal conduit, one must identify an appropriate segment of ileum. The ileum is the longest segment of small intestine and as a whole is approximately 3.5 m or 350 cm in length. One should choose a segment that positioned at a location that would be able to easily be brought to the marked stomal site with minimal effort and without tension. Usually, this would come from a healthy section of its midportion. Having said that, its initial 25 cm coming off of the jejunum is usually avoided as is the distal most 25 cm of terminal ileum because this is where excess bile salts are reabsorbed. Having said all of this, an approximately 30 cm segment of accessible ileum is selected for the pouch.

More than 30 cm of intestine is avoided because excessive amounts of urea and nitrogen are absorbed back into the systemic circulation which can ultimately compromise renal function. This is even more significant when renal function begins at a compromised level. To that end, the most distal portion of the resected segment of ileum is then brought out through a marked opening (a stoma) in the marked position on the abdominal wall. The residual small bowel is reanastamosed with the residual terminal ileum, usually seated inferior relative to the anastomosis. Finally, in the creation of an ileal conduit, the ureters are resected as close to the ureterovesical junction as possible. Then the ureters are brought up into the wound and connected to the ileal pouch surgically in the most accessible and tension free fashion as possible. This portion of the procedure is known as the creation of the *ureteroenteric anastomosis*. Although many of these procedures may initially appear to create a burden, they have the purpose of preventing kidney damage. If left untreated, *neurogenic bladder* could lead to renal disease (kidney failure) which requires either a kidney transplant or dialysis to maintain life.

Biologic Neuromodulation Using BoTox

As discussed in the previous sections, developing neurogenecity at the bladder muscle level can be a debilitating circumstance for any patient. The symptoms of neurogenic bladder (NGB) can range from detrusor underactivity to overactivity, depending on the site of neurologic insult. Certainly, the overactive detrusor would be more common, more cumbersome, and more complicated because its clinical sequelae cuts to the quick of a "human being's essence" with respect to their level of social acceptability, potentially even throwing them back to an infancy like situation requiring the use of pads and diapers to try to contain urine leakage, one of our most intimate and basic functions. The appropriate therapy is predicated upon accurate diagnosis through a careful medical and voiding history together with a variety of clinical examinations. The bottom line is that these patients will often "run the table" as far as the treatment ladder goes. Nevertheless, suffice to say that if these patients fail to reach clinical success with medication and behavioral therapy, the minimally invasive option of biologic neuromodulation using Botox is a good next step, before moving onto more major surgery.

Botulinum toxin (abbreviated either as BTX or BoTNA) is produced by *Clostridium botulinum,* a gram-positive anaerobic bacterium. The clinical syndrome of botulism leads to a painful paralysis leading to diaphragmatic dysfunction and eventual respiratory failure. Interestingly, medical science has been fascinated with this very deadly disease as well as the micro-organism which is responsible. Interestingly, the history of the use of botulinum toxin in medicine is circuitous, insightful as well as creative. So not surprisingly, someone who could combine the scientific discipline of medicine with the creativity associated with poetry. To that end, Justines

Fig. 17.6 Ileal urinary diversion

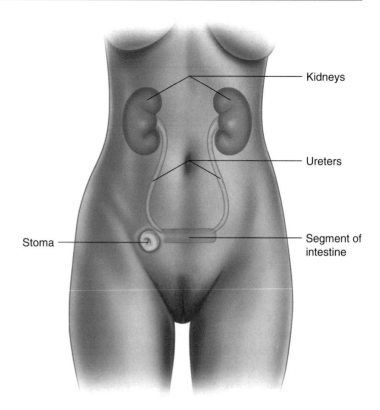

Kerner (1786–1862) fit the bill, a physician and a poet who first floated the idea of using small aliquots of the toxin as a medical therapy. The historical timeline for the use of BTX in medicine is outlined below (Fig. 17.6).

Historical Timeline for BoTox

- Approximately about 1860, Justines Kerner, proposed the idea of using the toxin for medical purposes.
- In 1870, Muller (another German physician) coined the name botulism. The Latin form is *botulus*, which means sausage.
- In 1895, Professor Emile Van Ermengem, of Belgium, first isolated the bacterium *Clostridium botulinum.*
- In 1946, Dr. Edward J Schantz succeeded in purifying BoNT-A in crystalline form—cultured *Clostridium botulinum* and isolated the toxin.
- In 1949, Dr. Burgen's group discovered that botulinum toxin blocks neuromuscular transmission.
- About 1955, Dr. Vernon Brooks discovered that when BoNT-A is injected into a hyperactive muscle, it blocks the release of acetylcholine from motor nerve endings
- In 1973, Dr. Alan B. Scott, of Smith-Kettlewell Eye Research Institute, used BoNT-A in monkey experiments; in 1980, he used BoNT-A for the first time in humans to treat strabismus.

- In December 1989, BoNT-A (BOTOX®) was approved by the US Food and Drug Administration (FDA) for the treatment of strabismus, blepharospasm, and hemifacial spasm in patients aged younger than 12 years.
- On December 21, 2000, BoNT-A received FDA approval for treatment of cervical dystonia.
- On July 21, 2011, the FDA approved incobotulinumtoxinA (Xeomin) for temporary improvement in the appearance of moderate-to-severe glabellar lines, or frown lines between the eyebrows, in adult patients.
- On August 24, 2011, the FDA approved onabotulinumtoxinA (BOTOX®) injection for the treatment of urinary incontinence due to detrusor overactivity associated with a neurologic condition.

Preparations

Botulism can occur following ingestion of contaminated food, *if* the bacteria has been present long enough, with colony counts high enough, to make the toxin. There are seven different serological subtypes of botulinium toxin, (BTX). These are types A, B, C D, E, F, and G, which are antigenically and serologically distinct but structurally similar. Human botulism is caused mainly by types A, B, E. Types C and D cause toxicity only in animals. The different toxins all possess specific potencies, so, if multiple preparations are being used, then care is required to avoid technical errors. The approved preparations with indications are as follows:

- *Onabotulinum Toxin-A (BoTox)*—Approved for cervical dystonia, blethorospasm, hyperhidrosis, *neurogenic detrusor overactivity* (NDO), cosmetic therapy
- *Abobotulinum Toxin-A (Dysport)*—Cervical dystonia, moderate to severe glabellar lines.
- *Incobotulinum Toxin-A (Xeomin)*—Cervical dystonia, blepharospasm, moderate to severe glabellar lines.
- *Rimabotulinum Toxin-B (Myobloc)*—Cervical dystonia

Mechanism of Action (Fig. 17.7)

The BoTox is a dual chained (150 kD) molecule connected with a disulfide bridge *(image above)*. The heavy chain (~100 kD—amino acids 449–1280) provides cholinergic specificity at its "C" terminus and is responsible for binding the toxin to receptors at the presynaptic nerve ending. More importantly, it promotes the mechanism by which the light chain gets across the endosomal membrane and into the cytosol of the cholinergic nerve ending. The light chain (~50 kD-amino acids 1–448) acts as a zinc (Zn^{2+}) endopeptidase similar to tetanus toxin with proteolytic activity located at the N-terminal end. The light chain is the functional portion of the BoTox molecule that acts as a chemical sword to facilitate cleavage. Before, we dive into the biochemical specifics, we should review the normal situation. Remember that the presynaptic nerve terminal functions to release ACh into the cleft of the neuro-muscular junction. The neurotransmitter Ach is stored in vesicles which must attach to the inner membrane of the nerve ending to facilitate expulsion into the neuromuscular junction. Neuronal stimulation is the event that kicks off a cascade which will activate a series of proteins to aid in the attachment of the Ach vesicle to the presynaptic membrane. These proteins are known as the SNARE complex. Once the Ach is released into the synapse at the neuromuscular junction, it initiates a postsynaptic muscular contraction.

When Botox is injected into the neuromuscular junction, the dual chain molecule targets the presynaptic nerve ending. The "C" terminus of the heavy chain targets receptors on the outer membrane of the nerve terminal. After binding is complete, the Botox molecule enters the cytosol of the nerve ending via a process known as "receptor mediated endocytosis." When this process is complete, the toxin is then floating within a receptor bubble, inside the cell. Soon after entry, the light chain of the Botox molecule is released into the cytosol of the nerve terminal where it seeks out and finds the SNARE complex of proteins *(the SNARE complex functions in facilitating the release of Ach from the nerve terminal into the synapse)*. Specifically, this *"sword like"* light chain will cleave the SNARE protein known as *SNAP 25*. This will help prevent the release of Ach into the neuromuscular junction, thus inhibiting muscle contraction.

Botox as Therapy for Neurogenic Detrusor Overactivity

Neurogenic detrusor overactivity (NDO) is a simple phrase for a complex issue. The site specific reasons have been outlined above and need not be reiterated here. However, it is worthwhile to note that the final common pathway to the source of neurogenicity at the level of the detrusor is the "loss of cortical inhibition" which allows for involuntary detrusor activity. It is this "cortical dysinhibition" that allows for the clinical sequelae of NDO, the most distressing of which is "urinary urge incontinence" (UUI). Essentially, UUI is unexpected urine loss which is associated with involuntary detrusor muscle contraction.

Botox has been used to treat urinary incontinence for many years. It acts to decrease involuntary muscular contractions of the bladder. This type of bladder muscle activity can arise from routine pelvic muscle overactivity, which commonly occurs in women with aging and estrogen deficiency. In addition, Botox can be used to treat more refractory

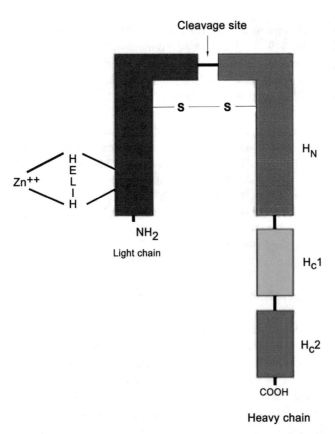

Fig. 17.7 Molecular confirmation

neurogenic detrusor overactivity in patients with underlying neurologic disease or injury.

Botox needs to be injected into the muscle of the bladder. This is done in the clinic or operating room. First the bladder is flushed with a local anesthesia, via a catheter, which is allowed to thoroughly numb the bladder. Then a scope is passed up the urethra (urine channel) into the bladder. A small needle is placed through the scope and several injections are made into the bladder designed to spread Botox throughout the muscle of the bladder. Most patients tolerate this procedure well.

Botox acts to decrease the strength of the bladder's natural contraction. So, not surprisingly, one potential side effect of this is incomplete bladder emptying or if the BoTox effect is more significant, even complete urinary retention. In other words, if the Botox works to well and patients cannot void on their own. If this residual urine is high enough, or if the patient cannot void at all, then a catheter has to be placed permanently or periodically (CIC) in order to drain their bladder. This complication is rare in patients with overactive bladder, because we limit the amount of Botox we inject. There have been very few instances of Botox ever causing systemic weakness. This is a theoretical risk associated with Botox therapy, but extremely uncommon.

Botox is a well-tolerated treatment and the application of this therapy ranges from simple conditions like overactive bladder to treatment of severely spastic bladders from neurologic disease. In many instances, Botox can be injected in a short procedure in our clinic. The therapy lasts for 6–8 months and then is re-injected. There is no limitation to the duration of using this type of therapy.

Suggested Reading

1. Adamson AS, Gelister J, Hayward R, Snell ME. Tethered cord syndrome: an unusual cause of adult bladder dysfunction. Br J Urol. 1993;71:417–21.
2. Ahlberg J, Norlen L, Blomstrand C, Wikkelso C. Outcome of shunt operation on urinary incontinence in normal pressure hydrocephalus predicted by lumbar puncture. J Neurol Neurosurg Psychiatry. 1988;51:105–8.
3. Allen TD. Psychogenic urinary retention. South Med J. 1972;65:302–4.
4. Andrew J, Nathan PW. Lesions of the anterior frontal lobes and disturbances of micturition and defaecation. Brain. 1964;87:233–62.
5. Betts CD, D'Mellow MT, Fowler CJ. Urinary symptoms and the neurological features of bladder dysfunction in multiple sclerosis. J Neurol Neurosurg Psychiatry. 1993;56:245–50.
6. Brindley GS. The first 500 patients with sacral anterior root stimulator implants: general description. Paraplegia. 1994;32:795–805.
7. Chancellor MB, Blaivas JG. Multiple sclerosis. In: Chancellor MB, Blaivas JG, editors. Practical neuro-urology. Boston: Butterworth-Heinemann; 1995. p. 119–37.
8. de Groat WC. Nervous control of the urinary bladder of the cat. Brain Res. 1975;87:201–11.
9. de Groat WC. Central neural control of the lower urinary tract. In: Bock G, Whelan J, editors. Neurobiology of incontinence. Chichester: Wiley; 1990. p. 27–56.
10. Escaf S, Cavallotti C, Ricci A, Vega JA, Amenta F. Dopamine D1 and D2 receptors in the human ureter and urinary bladder: a radioligand binding and autoradiographic study. Br J Urol. 1994;73:473–9.
11. Fowler CJ, Christmas TJ, Chapple CR, Parkhouse HF, Kirby RS, Jacobs HS. Abnormal electromyographic activity of the urethral sphincter, voiding dysfunction, and polycystic ovaries: a new syndrome? Br Med J. 1988;297:1436–8.
12. Greenstein A, Matzkin H, Kaver I, Braf Z. Acute urinary retention in herpes genitalis infection: urodynamic evaluation. Urology. 1988;31:453–6.
13. Griffiths DJ, McCracken PN, Harrison GM, Gormley EA, Moore K, Hooper R, et al. Cerebral aetiology of urinary urge incontinence in elderly people. Age Ageing. 1994;23:246–50.
14. Hassouna MM, Elhilali MM. Role of the sacral root stimulator in voiding dysfunction. World J Urol. 1991;9:145–8.
15. Hattori T, Sakakibara R, Yasuda K, Murayama N, Hirayama K. Micturitional disturbance in cervical spondylotic myelopathy. J Spinal Disord. 1990;3:16–8.
16. Holstege G, Griffiths D, de Wall H, Dalm E. Anatomical and physiological observations on supraspinal control of bladder and urethral sphincter muscles in the cat. J Comp Neurol. 1986;250:449–61.
17. Khan Z, Hertanu J, Yang WC, Melman A, Leiter E. Predictive correlation of urodynamic dysfunction and brain injury after cerebrovascular accident. J Urol. 1981;126:86–8.
18. Lapides J, Diokno AC, Gould FR, Lowe BS. Further observations on self-catheterization. J Urol. 1976;116:169–71.
19. Margolis G. A review of literature on psychogenic urinary retention. [Review]. J Urol. 1965;94:257–8.
20. Mochizuki H, Saito H. Mesial frontal lobe syndromes: correlations between neurological deficits and radiological localizations. [Review]. Tohoku J Exp Med. 1990;161 Suppl: 231–9.
21. Neurogenic bladder dysfunction in lumbar intervertebral disc prolapse. Br J Urol. 1992;69:38–40.
22. Resnick NM, Yalla SV. Detrusor hyperactivity with impaired contractile function: an unrecognized but common cause of incontinence in elderly patients. JAMA. 1987;257:3076–81.
23. Sakakibara R, Hattori T, Yasuda K, Yamanishi T. Micturitional disturbance after acute hemispheric stroke: analysis of the lesion site by CT and MRI. J Neurol Sci. 1996;137:47–56.
24. Sirls LT, Zimmern PE, Leach GE. Role of limited evaluation and aggressive medical management in multiple sclerosis: a review of 113 patients. J Urol. 1994;151:946–50.
25. Staskin DS, Vardi Y, Siroky MB. Post-prostatectomy continence in the parkinsonian patient: the significance of poor voluntary sphincter control. J Urol. 1988;140:117–8.
26. Thor K, Kawatani M, de Groat WC. Plasticity in the reflex pathways to the lower urinary tract of the cat during postnatal development and following spinal cord injury. In: Goldberger ME, Gorio A, Murray M, editors. Development and plasticity of the mammalian spinal cord. Padova: Liviana Press; 1986. p. 65–110.
27. van Kerrebroeck PE, Koldewijn EL, Debruyne FM. Worldwide experience with the Finetech-Brindley sacral anterior root stimulator. Neurourol Urodyn. 1993;12:497–503.
28. Ventimiglia B, Patti F, Reggio E, Failla G, Morana C, Lopes M, et al. Disorders of micturition in neurological patients. J Neurol. 1998;245:173–7.
29. Schurch B, Tawadros C, Carda S. Dysfunction of lower urinary tract in patients with spinal cord injury. Handb Clin Neurol. 2015;130:247–67.
30. Bauer SB, Labib KB, Dieppa RA, et al. Urodynamic evaluation of boy with myelodysplasia and incontinence. Urology. 1977;10:354–62.

31. Weld KJ, Dmochowski RR. Association of level of injury and bladder behavior in patients with post-traumatic spinal cord injury. Urology. 2000;55:490–4.

32. Burney TL, Senapati M, Desai S, Choudhary ST, Badlani GH. Acute cerebrovascular accident and lower urinary tract dysfunction: a prospective correlation of the site of brain injury with urodynamic findings. J Urol. 1996;156:1748–50.

33. Hald T, Bradley WE. The nervous control of the urinary bladder. In: The urinary bladder: neurology and urodynamics. Baltimore: Williams & Wilkins; 1982. p. 48–57.

34. Borrie MJ, Campbell A, Caradoc-Davies TH, Spears GF. Urinary incontinence after stroke: a prospective study. Age Ageing 1986;15:177.

35. Bradley WE. Innervation of the male urinary bladder. Urol Clin North Am. 1978;5:279.

36. Barone P, Antonini A, Colosimo C, et al. The PRIAMO study: a multicenter assessment of nonmotor symptoms and their impact on quality of life in Parkinson's disease. Mov Disord. 2009; 24(11):1641–9.

37. de Groat WC, Yoshimura N. Plasticity in reflex pathways to the lower urinary tract following spinal cord injury. Exp Neurol. 2012;235:123–32.

38. Vizzard MA. Neurochemical plasticity and the role of neurotrophic factors in bladder reflex pathways after spinal cord injury. In: Weaver LC, Polosa C, editors. Progress in brain research. vol. 152. Elsevier; 2006. p. 97–115.

39. de Groat WC, Kawatani M, Hisamitsu T, Cheng CL, Ma CP, Thor K, Steers W, Roppolo JR. Mechanisms underlying the recovery of urinary-bladder function following spinal-cord injury. J. Auton. Nerv. Syst. 1990;30: S71–8.

40. de Groat WC, Nadelhaft I, Milne RJ, Booth AM, Morgan C, Thor K. Organization of the sacral parasympathetic reflex pathways to the urinary bladder and large intestine. J Auton Nerv Syst. 1981;3(2–4):135–60.

41. Loewy AD, Saper CB, Baker RP. Descending projections from the pontine micturition center. Brain Res. 1979;172:533–8.

42. Nour S, Svarer C, Kristensen J, Paulson OB, Law I. Cerebral activation during micturition in normal men. Brain. 2000;123:781–9. doi:10.1093/brain/123.4.781.

43. Sakakibara R. Lower urinary tract dysfunction in patients with brain lesions. Handb Clin Neurol. 2015;130:269–87.

44. Yum KS, Na SJ, Lee KY, Kim J, Oh SH, Kim YD, Yoon B, Heo JH, Lee KO. Pattern of voiding dysfunction after acute brainstem infarction. Eur Neurol. 2013;70(5–6):291–6.

45. Betts C. Bladder and sexual dysfunction in multiple sclerosis. In: Fowler CJ, editor. Neurology of bladder, bowel and sexual dysfunction. Boston: Butterwoth Heinemann; 1999. p. 289–308.

46. de Sèze M, Ruffion A, Denys P, Joseph PA, Perrouin-Verbe B, and the International Francophone Neuro-Urological expert study group (GENULF). The neurogenic bladder in multiple sclerosis: review of the literature and proposal of management guidelines. Mult Scler. 2007;13(7):915–28.

47. Coon EA, Sletten DM, Saurez MD, Mandrekar JN, Ahlskog JE, Bower JH, Matsumoto JY, Silber MH, Benarroch EE, Fealey RD, Sandroni P, Low PA, Singer W. Clinical features and autonomic testing predict survival in multiple system atrophy. Brain. 2015;138(Pt 12).

48. Benarroch EE. New findings on the neuropathology of multiple system atrophy. Auton Neurosci. 2002;96(1):59–62.

49. Panicker JN, Fowler CJ, Kessler TM. Lower urinary tract dysfunction in the neurological patient: clinical assessment and management. Lancet Neurol. 2015;14:720–32.

50. Benarroch EE, Schmeichel AM, Low PA, et al. Involvement of medullary serotonergic groups in multiple system atrophy. Ann Neurol. 2004;55(3):418–22.

51. Ito T, Sakakibara R, Yasuda K, et al. Incomplete emptying and urinary retention in multiple-system atrophy: when does it occur and how do we manage it? Mov Disord. 2006;21(6):816–23.

52. Sakakibara R, Hattori T, Uchiyama T, et al. Videourodynamic and sphincter motor unit potential analyses in Parkinson's disease and multiple system atrophy. J Neurol Neurosurg Psychiatry. 2001; 71(5):600–6.

53. Burn DJ, Jaros E. Multiple system atrophy: cellular and molecular pathology. Mol Pathol. 2001;54(6):419–26.

54. Mukerji G, Waters J, Chessell IP, Bountra C, Agarwal SK, Anand P. Pain during ice water test distinguishes clinical bladder hypersensitivity from overactivity disorders. BMC Urol. 2006;6:31.

55. Yamaguchi C, Sakakibara R, Uchiyama T, Liu Z, Yamamoto T, Ito T, et al. Bladder sensation in peripheral nerve lesions. Neurourol Urodyn. 2006;25:763–9.

56. Sakakibara R, Uchiyama T, Kuwabara S, Mori M, Ito T, Yamamoto T, et al. Prevalence and mechanism of bladder dysfunction in Guillain–Barre' syndrome. Neurourol Urodyn. 2009;28:432–7.

57. Sasaki K, Yoshimura N, Chancellor MB. Implications of diabetes mellitus in urology. Urol Clin North Am. 2003;30:1–12.

58. Niakan E, Harati Y, Comstock JP. Diabetic autonomic neuropathy. Metabolism. 1986;35:224–34.

59. Lloyd JC, Wiener JS, Gargollo PC, et al. Contemporary epidemiological trends in complex congenital genitourinary anomalies. J Urol. 2013;190:1590.

60. Bauer SB, Hallett M, Khoshbin S, et al. Predictive value of urodynamic evaluation in newborns with myelodysplasia. JAMA. 1984;252:650.

61. Carr MC. Neuropathic bladder in the neonate. Clin Perinatol. 2014;41(3):725–33. doi:10.1016/j.clp.2014.05.017. Epub 2014 Jul 18. Review.

62. OxfordJournals.org, July 1933.

Biology of Pain and Pathophysiology of Pelvic Pain Syndrome

Pooja Lakshmin and David A. Gordon

Why Study Pain? What Is the Impact and Need to Understand the Pathology?

Complaints of pain are the most common reason for patient presentation to ambulatory medical settings [1], and account for about 35 million office visits annually [2]. In a majority of cases, the pain will respond to a simple treatment modality or, better yet, will spontaneously remit; however, in one-fourth of cases, the symptoms become chronic [1]. Chronic pain is pervasive, and physicians from many different medical specialties will treat patients who suffer from chronic pain. Moreover, the fact that patients who suffer from chronic pain can present to a variety of different physicians makes the treatment of chronic pain particularly difficult.

Chronic pelvic pain is defined as pain of at least six months' duration that occurs below the umbilicus and is severe enough to cause functional disability or require treatment [3]. In the USA, this problem accounts for approximately 10 % of all ambulatory referrals to a gynecologist and is a common indication for diagnostic and therapeutic surgery [4]. The frequency of the different causes of chronic pelvic pain is greatly influenced by local patient population, referral patterns, and specialty focus of the practice. The literature on the causes of pelvic pain is conflicting: one study found that gastrointestinal and urological problems were more common than gynecological conditions in women with chronic pelvic pain syndromes [5, 6], while another study found that two-thirds of causes of pelvic pain are related to

endometriosis and adhesions [7]. Causing more difficulty in making a diagnosis of chronic pelvic pain, no correlation has been found between the intensity of pain and the amount of tissue damage observed. Research does consistently report that patients who suffer from chronic pain report physical functional loss, vegetative depression symptoms, and varying family dynamics [8]. Pelvic pain symptoms may be due to multiple factors and pain can be the result of several medical comorbid conditions. The specific cause of the chronic pain is often elusive, becoming a source of frustration for patients and health-care providers [9].

What Is Pelvic Pain? How Do We Separate the Objective and Experiential?

As discussed, often there is not a direct correlation between the intensity of the pain experience and the amount of tissue damage observed. According to the International Association for the Study of Pain, pain is defined as "an unpleasant sensory and emotional experience associated with actual or potential tissue damage, or described in terms of such damage" [10]. Thus, pain is a complex perception that incorporates emotional and psychological processes that do not detract from the fact that pain itself is also a sensory phenomenon at the neurological level [11]. Pain is something that is interpreted in the brain, while nociception is the sensory physiological response to noxious stimulation that can potentially generate pain perception. Thus, there is an important distinction between neural responses to noxious stimulation (which can occur in sensory nerves) and the perception of their activity (which can be interpreted by the brain as pain). We will discuss the complex neurophysiology of this process later in this chapter.

From a psychiatric perspective, in the past, there was a dualistic approach to diagnosing chronic pain—definable in its physical versus psychological origins. In the case of psychological pain, psychiatric labels were involved, i.e.,

P. Lakshmin
Department of Psychology, Rutgers, The State University of New Jersey, Room 304, Smith Hall, Newark, NJ 07102, USA
e-mail: plakshmin@psychology.rutgers.edu

D. A. Gordon (✉)
The Division of Pelvic Neuroscience, Department of Surgery, The Sinai Hospital of Baltimore, 2401 W. Belvedere Ave, Baltimore, MD 21215, USA
e-mail: dgordon@lifebridgehealth.org

© Springer Science+Business Media New York 2017
D.A. Gordon, M.R. Katlic (eds.), *Pelvic Floor Dysfunction and Pelvic Surgery in the Elderly*,
DOI 10.1007/978-1-4939-6554-0_18

Psychogenic Pain Disorder from the DSM-III [12] or Somatoform Pain Disorder from the DSM-III-R [13]. Emotional distress and cognitive issues typically accompany physical pain. Moreover, there typically will be significant social and interpersonal difficulties in patients who suffer from chronic pain. Because of these factors, it is difficult for providers to distinguish "psychogenic" from "organic" pain. Psychogenic pain is defined as physical pain that is caused, increased, or prolonged by mental, emotional, or behavioral factors [14].

Thus, there was a change in the requirement for the exclusion of a physical cause of the pain in the newer model of psychiatric diagnosing, which embraces the idea that there is a complex interplay between biological and psychological factors that contribute to the pain experience by precipitating, exacerbating, or maintaining pain. The DSM-IV-TR [15] acknowledges that pain can be associated with medical conditions, psychological factors, or both. One commonality that is widespread in understanding the phenomenology of pain disorders is that there are negative stereotypes associated with chronic pain, and there may be a suspicion by the physician that the patient is disingenuous, exaggerating, or faking.

When treating a patient who suffers from chronic pain, it is important to use a "bio-psycho-social" approach to evaluation. Rather than dichotomizing between physical and psychological origins, the *biopsychosocial approach* maintains the focus on the patient's experience. In chronic pain, patients are likely to experience fear and anxiety, as well as alarm about what the pain signifies, and concerns over being able to alleviate it. There is often a strong need for controlling the symptoms. Specifically in chronic pain patients, psychological and social factors play a role in the overall pain experience [16]. Patients may start to avoid or procrastinate certain activities because of fear that pain will be elicited. There may be a decline in the patient's interests, social life, and interpersonal relationships. Psychological vulnerabilities can be a significant issue in this scenario.

Pathophysiology of Pelvic Pain in Women

The pathophysiology of chronic pelvic pain syndromes is diverse, as there are many different etiologies. Common causes of chronic pelvic pain in women include gynecologic, urologic, gastrointestinal, musculoskeletal, neurological, immunological, and mental health pathology. The pathological processes can also be divided into different categories based on mechanism including: inflammatory (infective), inflammatory (non-infective), mechanical, functional, neuropathic, and musculoskeletal.

Gynecological etiology of pelvic pain syndromes is common. *Endometriosis* is the most common diagnosis made at the time of gynecological laparoscopy for the eval-

uation of chronic pelvic pain. Overall, about one-third of women who undergo laparoscopy because of these symptoms will ultimately be diagnosed with endometriosis [17]. Endometriosis is defined as the presence of endometrial glands and tissue in locations other than the uterine endometrium. It is thought to be caused by retrograde dissemination of endometrial tissue fragments through fallopian tubes during menstruation, with implantation on the ovary or other peritoneal structures, or blood borne or lymphatic-borne dissemination of endometrial fragments. It is characteristically responsive to hormonal variations of the menstrual cycle. It occurs most often in the pelvic region, with the ovary being the most common site, followed by uterine ligaments, recto-vaginal septum, and pelvic peritoneum. The clinical manifestation of endometriosis includes severe menstrual related pain [18].

Pelvic inflammatory disease (PID) is another common cause of pelvic pain in women. This is an acute infection of the upper genital tract structures, including any or all of the uterus, fallopian tubes, ovaries, and neighboring pelvic organs. This condition typically affects young, sexually active women. It is a community acquired infection, initiated by a sexually transmitted agent such as Neisseria gonorrhoeae and Chlamydia trachomatis [19]. The pathology of PID is related to disruption of the normal vaginal flora. Typically, the endo-cervical canal serves as a barrier protecting the normally sterile upper genital tract from the organisms of the vaginal ecosystem. Disturbance of this barrier allows the vaginal bacteria access to the upper genital organs, thus causing PID [20]. Some studies show that dense adhesions may limit organ motility and thereby cause visceral pain in the pelvis [21]. This has also been found in laparoscopic studies [22].

Leiomyoma, or more commonly called fibroids, are the most common uterine tumor. Fibroids are a benign neoplasm with a very low risk of malignant transformation. Histologically, they are estrogen sensitive, and because of this they will often increase in size during pregnancy, and decrease in size during menopause. Clinically, women that suffer from fibroids will complain of menorrhagia (increased menstrual bleeding), prolonged bleeding, pelvic pressure and pain. They are the single most common reason for hysterectomy and are clinically apparent in up to 25 % of women [23].

Dysmenorrhea is the medical condition of pain during menstruation that interferes with daily activities. Two different types characterize it: primary and secondary dysmenorrhea. Primary dysmenorrhea is diagnosed when the symptoms have been present since menarche, when the pain starts on the first day of the period and where identifiable pathology is absent. Secondary dysmenorrhea occurs later in menstrual life. In this case, pain can build up even before the onset of menstruation, and a specific pathology, such as endometriosis, is more common [18].

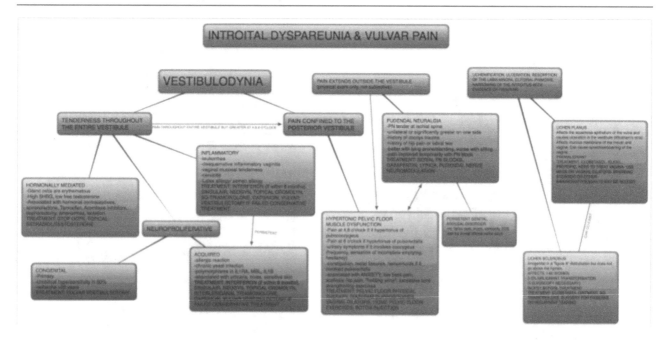

Fig. 18.1 Introital dyspareunia and vulvar pain. A schematic diagram of different etiologies for vulvar pain, including vestibulodynia (previously known as vulvar vestibulitis syndrome), which is thought to be vulvodynia localized to the vestibule region. Modified from Andrew Goldstein, MD

Vulvar pain syndromes include the diagnosis of localized, provoked vulvodynia (formally known as vulvar vestibulitis). It is characterized by severe pain provoked by focal touch or pressure of the vulva, and the vulvar vestibule is the most common site of pain (commonly termed vestibulodynia) [24]. The exact pathogenesis for *vulvodynia* has not yet been established, and it is thought that various factors may play a role, including genetic, inflammation, allergy, pelvic floor dysfunction, and neurologic sensitization [25]. Figure 18.1 shows a depiction of one conceptualization of the various pathophysiologic etiologies of vestibulodynia and dyspareunia.

Persistent genital arousal disorder (PGAD) is a clinical condition characterized by intense genital arousal occurring in the absence of subjective desire or interest. Typical sufferers of PGAD are women who experience intrusive, unsolicited, and spontaneous episodes of genital arousal that are not relieved by orgasms. These symptoms often prevent the women from functioning adequately in home or work-life, as the symptoms can last for hours or for days. The syndrome, first termed and characterized by Leiblum and Nathan [26] as Persistent Sexual Arousal Syndrome (PSAS), was then renamed to clarify that the disorder is a problem of genital, rather than sexual, arousal. Complaints by PGAD sufferers typically include clitoral tingling, irritation, vaginal congestion, vaginal contractions, throbbing, pressure, pain, and in some cases, spontaneous orgasms [27]. Many women who suffer from this condition often feel shame and embarrassment in discussing their symptoms with healthcare providers. Women that suffer from PGAD can be premenopausal, peri-menopausal, or post-menopausal. Furthermore, there is

some similarity between PGAD and vulvodynia. In both conditions, there is little certainty about etiology. Women who suffer from PGAD or vulvodynia often suffer for long periods of time before seeking medical care, and in many cases, these women are told that their condition is "in their head." Both conditions, like all pelvic pain disorders, are highly distressing and emotionally consuming [28]. It has recently been noticed that Tarlov cysts, which form on the genital sensory nerve roots, and are thought to contain aberrant genital sensory nerve fibers, may abrade the sacral bone and cause the symptoms of PGAD. This supports the theory of characterizing PGAD as a neurological condition. The most common symptoms caused by Tarlov cysts include pain in the perineum, vagina, penis, buttock, sacrum, and dyspareunia, proctalgia, bladder dysfunction, urinary dysfunction, and bowel dysfunction [29]. Figures 18.2 and 18.3 show a sagittal view of sacral Tarlov cysts taken from MRI [29]. Figures 18.2 and 18.3 show a sagittal view of a sacral Tarlov cysts taken from MRI.

Other notable causes of pelvic pain originating from a gynecologic etiology include: pelvic congestion syndrome [30], adenomyosis, ovarian cancer, ovarian remnant and residual ovary syndrome, leiomyoma [31], dysmenorrhea, dyspareunia (discussed later in this chapter), or postsurgical neuropathy.

The urinary tract is another common system that is a source of pain in women who have chronic pelvic pain. Interstitial cystitis and painful bladder syndrome are known to be a common cause of chronic pelvic pain. The pathology of interstitial cystitis is well studied and is thought to be a

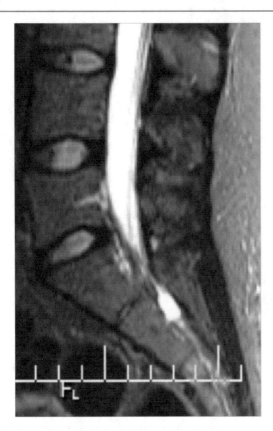

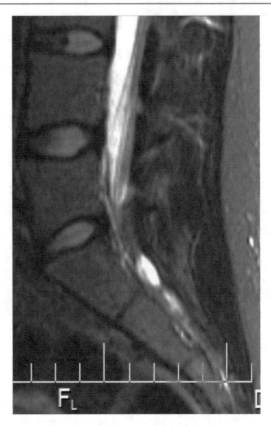

Fig. 18.2 Sagittal views of Tarlov cysts: MRI image of a sacral Tarlov cyst. Tarlov (peri-neural) cysts occur on general dorsal nerve roots and produce paresthesias. They have been associated with persistant genital arousal disorder, which can present with genital discomfort and pain. With permission from Komisaruk BR and Lee H-J. Prevalence of sacral spinal (Tarlov) cysts in persistent genital arousal disorder. J Sex Med 2012; 9:2047–2056 © Elsevier

Fig. 15.3 Sagittal views of Tarlov cysts: MRI image of a sacral Tarlov cyst. Tarlov (peri-neural) cysts occur on general dorsal nerve roots and produce paresthesias. They have been associated with persistant genital arousal disorder, which can present with genital discomfort and pain. With permission from Komisaruk BR and Lee H-J. Prevalence of sacral spinal (Tarlov) cysts in persistent genital arousal disorder. J Sex Med 2012; 9:2047–2056 © Elsevier

chronic inflammatory condition of the bladder that in turn causes pelvic pain, irritable bladder, urinary frequency, and exaggerated urge to void [32]. The literature seems to suggest that while the patient's symptoms may overlap with those of urinary tract infection (UTI), many patients are culture negative [33]. The condition is also thought to be associated with central nervous system up-regulation, and patients will often exhibit bladder hyperalgesia and allodynia. Some literature suggests that in patients with interstitial cystitis, those who have a history of abuse tend to have greater pain intensity than non-abused patients. One theory proposes that this is linked to the hypothalamic–pituitary–adrenal axis abnormality that is reported in traumatized individuals [34]. Other common urinary tract etiologies for chronic pelvic pain in women include recurrent urinary tract infection, urethral diverticulum, and bladder neoplasia.

Gastrointestinal causes of pelvic pain are also common. These include irritable bowel syndrome, inflammatory bowel disease, diverticular colitis, colon cancer, chronic intestinal pseudo-obstruction, chronic constipation, and celiac disease. Irritable bowel syndrome is a chronic or intermittent abdom-

inal pain syndrome associated with bowel functions, in the absence of any organic causes. Some studies report that irritable bowel syndrome is the most common diagnosis in primary care populations with chronic pelvic pain [9, 35]. Inflammatory bowel disease, i.e., Crohn's disease, is characterized by fatigue, diarrhea with cramping abdominal pain, with or without gross bleeding. Pathophysiology of this condition is marked by a transmural inflammatory process, leading to fibrotic strictures that then lead to obstructions. Ulcerative colitis, also an inflammatory bowel disease, has similar clinical manifestations; however, rectal bleeding is more common with ulcerative colitis than in Crohn's disease. The pathology of diverticular colitis is linked to the histologic and endoscopic findings, which may vary from mild inflammation to chronic, active inflammation resembling inflammatory bowel disease. The pathogenesis is not fully known.

Musculoskeletal pathology is linked to pelvic pain. Women with fibromyalgia often present to their primary care doctors or gynecologists with pelvic pain as the main complaint. Fibromyalgia is a common cause of chronic musculoskeletal pain and it is one of a group of soft issue pain disorders. It is not associated with tissue inflammation and the exact etiology is unknown. Often, there are no obvious abnormalities on exam, and laboratory and radiologic studies are normal. For this reason, fibromyalgia has often been considered to be "psychogenic" or "psychosomatic" [36, 37]. Recent literature suggests that fibromyalgia may be a disorder of pain regulation, or "central sensitization" (discussed later in this chapter). Fibromyalgia and irritable bowel syndrome share commonalities in central nervous system pain processing characteristics [38]. Initially thought to be a muscle disease in origin, some experts now believe that the muscle pathology is secondary to pain-induced inactivity. There is evidence that these alterations in central nervous system processing are responsible for many of the features of fibromyalgia, while genetic and environmental factors interact to promote a state of chronic central and peripheral nervous system hyperirritability [39].

Other musculoskeletal causes of chronic pelvic pain include pelvic floor muscle myalgia (including coccydynia, piriformis/levator ani syndrome). Research shows that women with chronic pelvic pain have decreased thresholds to pain in the pelvic floor muscles, which suggests that pelvic floor tension myalgia may be a direct sequela of chronic pelvic pain due to other disorders like endometriosis or interstitial cystitis [40]. Other causes include incorrect posture, chronic abdominal wall pain, or osteitis pubis. Chronic abdominal wall pain may be related to a muscular injury or strain or a nerve injury (iliohypogastric, ilioinguinal, genitofemoral, lateral femoral cutaneous, pudendal). Pathology of the nerves can also cause pain that is referred to visceral organs [41]. *Myofascial pelvic pain syndrome* originates from trigger points in skeletal muscle. Referred pain and sometimes autonomic phenomena can occur when the hyperirritable spots are compressed [42]. Clinically, this diagnosis is described as a disorder in which pelvic pain is caused by short, tight, and tender pelvic floor muscles, usually with hypersensitive trigger points. The pain associated with this may occur in the pelvis, vagina, vulva, rectum or bladder, or even more distal areas including the thighs, buttocks, or

Table 18.1 Sensory fields of the genital nerves in women

Genital structure	Sensory nerve
Clitoris	Pudendal nerve
Perigenital skin	Pudendal nerve, pelvic nerve
Vagina	Pelvic nerve
Cervix	Pelvic nerve, hypogastric nerve, vagus nerve
Uterus	Hypogastric nerve, vagus nerve

The female genital tract is innervated by a rich nerve supply. Genital sensation is thought to be distributed among the hypogastric, pelvic, pudendal, and vagus nerves. The sensory field itself is the part of the genital system that is supplied by the nerves that innervate it, and there is overlap among the genital organs. These nerves are important in conveying painful as well as pleasurable sensations from the female genitals: whether it is childbirth, or orgasm. Courtesy of B. R. Komisaruk

lower abdomen. Other common symptoms include a sense of achiness, heaviness, burning, as well as overactive bladder, constipation, or dyspareunia. Table 18.1 indicates the sensory distribution of the nerves innervating the female genitalia. These nerves are important in conveying painful as well as pleasurable sensations. Many experts believe that most, if not all, women with chronic pelvic pain have some degree of myofascial pelvic pain syndrome [43].

Sexual Pain Disorder

Sexual pain disorders refer to conditions of genital pain that interfere with intercourse. The diagnosis of *dyspareunia* refers to painful sexual intercourse, due to medical or psychological causes. This type of pelvic pain is much more common in women than in men. In most cases, there is an original physical origin for the disorder. In some cases, the patient's pelvic floor musculature can contract involuntarily, and this is termed vaginismus. Approximately 15 % of women have chronic dyspareunia that is poorly understood, infrequently cured, and rarely discussed in the healthcare setting [44, 45]. There is increasing evidence for the role of neuropathic pain mechanisms in the pathophysiology of sexual pain, and some experts argue for both vaginismus and dyspareunia to be classified as pain disorders. These problems can affect women of any age, and depending on the healthcare provider that is visited, the patient may receive a conflicting diagnosis, further complicating the treatment of chronic pelvic pain. A description of the treatment variabilities for vulvar pain has been published elsewhere [46]. The most recent reiteration of the Diagnostic and Statistical Manual of Mental Disorders (the DSM-5) [47] has notably combined dyspareunia and vaginismus into a new diagnosis: genitopelvic pain/penetration disorder. There has been debate about whether these pain conditions are better served as pain disorders or sex disorders and there is a strong case for the removal of dyspareunia from the DSM altogether, arguing that the chronicity and the partial response to tricyclic antidepressants support that conclusion that chronic dyspareunia is an example of chronic pain [48].

The Role of Mental Health and Pain: Depression, Trauma, and Anxiety

The psychological and mental health role that pain plays in patients who suffer from chronic pelvic pain is significant. Patients with chronic pain have a relatively high incidence of physical or sexual abuse. It has been reported that up to 47 % of women with chronic pelvic pain disclose a history of physical or sexual abuse [49–51]. One study assessed the history of *physical and sexual abuse* in childhood and adulthood in women with chronic pelvic pain, women with chronic pain in other locations, and a control group of women. The study found that 39% of women with chronic pelvic pain had been physically abused during childhood, and that this percentage was significantly higher than that observed in women with other chronic pain conditions (18.4% or controls: 9.4%). The prevalence of childhood sexual abuse (as distinct from physical abuse) did not differ among the groups studied. Thus, the literature suggests that pelvic pain itself is unlikely to be specifically and psychodynamically related to sexual abuse, but that the pernicious and unpredictable nature of abuse may promote the chronic nature of the pain symptoms [49]. We also know that *depression* seems to occur more frequently in women with chronic pelvic pain [52], and though it is not clear if depression and chronic pelvic pain are causally related, some researchers believe that some cases of chronic pelvic pain may be a variant type of depression [53]. Other leading experts hold that stressful life experiences, such as childhood sexual abuse, could cause the symptoms of chronic pelvic pain and depression [54]. In a study of 25 women with chronic pelvic pain and a control group, the patients with chronic pelvic pain showed a significantly higher prevalence of major depression, substance abuse, adult sexual dysfunction, somatization, and history of childhood and adult sexual abuse than the control group [54]. Another school of thought reports that depression may increase the risk that a trauma leads to chronic pelvic pain [55].

Pelvic Pain in Men: A Brief Overview

In men, the pathophysiological basis for chronic pelvic pain has been largely linked to the prostate (thus, the term chronic "prostatitis"), and as in women, in many instances the etiology is unknown. Bacterial infection is often suspected, particularly in the inflammatory subset of chronic prostatitis, yet a bacterial etiology has not been consistently identified. In men, many cases of chronic pelvic pain are thought to be related to an imbalance toward increased pro-inflammatory, and decreased anti-inflammatory, cytokines. Moreover, it seems that autoimmune process may be involved and experimental evidence indicates that this may be under hormonal influence. Also similar to this condition in women, psychological stress may produce measurable biochemical changes and influence the pain process as a whole [56].

What Is the Biology of Pain?

Now that we have addressed the most common clinical conditions that are characterized by chronic pelvic pain, let's discuss in more detail the biology and neuroscientific basis of pain perception. As discussed earlier in this chapter, pain describes the unwelcome sensory or emotional experience associated with actual or potential tissue damage. Pain is unlike many other somatic, sensory modalities in that it has an urgent and primitive quality, possessing both affective and emotional components. As we learned in this chapter, the way that the human body manifests chronic pain is diverse, and people who suffer from pain can present to their healthcare providers in a variety of ways. Chronic pain, in many respects, may be a disease of the nervous system, not merely a symptom of some other disease process.

The perception of pain is subjective and is influenced by many factors; two people can be faced with identical stimuli and have very different responses. We see this clinically in that one woman may have severe menstrual pain and bleeding secondary to uterine fibroids, and another may not have such a severe response. As we have mentioned, pain is not the direct expression of a sensory event but rather the product of elaborate processing in the central nervous system. This, the psychological or "psychogenic" aspect of pain, and how this is characterized in clinical medicine becomes significant. Pain, by its nature, is a subjective experience [57]. Persistent pain can be characterized as either nociceptive or neuropathic. *Nociceptive pain* results from the activation of nociceptors in response to tissue injury, and is usually accompanied by inflammation. *Neuropathic pain* results from direct injury to nerves in the peripheral or central nervous system.

There is a general pathway that is activated when a human being experienced something that could be painful. It begins with a noxious stimulus activating a nociceptor. *Nociceptors* are free nerve endings of primary sensory neurons, and they function in the periphery of the human body, including the skin, joints, and muscles. Signals from the nociceptors are then conveyed to neurons in the dorsal horn of the spinal cord. There are several types of nociceptors, including thermal (sensing extreme temperatures), mechanical (activated by intense pressure), and polymodal nociceptors. A fourth class, called silent nociceptors is found in the viscera, and is activated by inflammation, contributing to the pain conditions of hyperalgesia and central sensitization (discussed later in this chapter). After the nociceptor receives a stimulus, it sends a receptor potential, which then triggers an afferent (sensory) action potential. There are four neurotransmitters that are thought to be important for generating this action potential: glutamate, substance P, glycine, and aspartate. There are different types of fibers that terminate on the dorsal horn of the spinal cord, carrying pain sensations from the nociceptors. The A delta group fibers respond primarily to sharp pressure or heat. These are fast acting, myelinated fibers. The C fiber group is slower, and responds to pressure, heat or cold, or noxious chemicals. This is a more long lasting, burning pain, like the type one feels with a sunburn. The A delta fibers carry the sharp burst of initial pain (also more localizable:

"epicritic" pain), while the C fibers carry the longer more burning (less localizable, "protopathic") pain.

These C fibers have also been found to convey pain-blocking effects. Vaginal stimulation activates the pelvic nerve [58], which consists of predominantly C fibers, and produces analgesia in women [59]. It was found that permanent destruction of the C fibers in the neonatal rat (with capsaicin) abolishes the analgesic effect of vaginal stimulation when the rats mature [60].

As discussed above, the uncontrolled activation of these nociceptors is associated with some pathological conditions: allodynia and hyperalgesia. People with *allodynia* feel pain in response to stimuli that are normally innocuous, e.g., the movement of joints in a patient with fibromyalgia, or sunburned skin. Patients with allodynia do not feel pain constantly; in the absence of a stimulus, there is not pain. By contrast, patients with *hyperalgesia*, which can be defined as an exaggerated response to noxious stimuli, report persistent pain in the absence of stimuli. Allodynia and hyperalgesia may also be related to central sensitization, which is discussed below.

The Ascending Pain Pathway

The *ascending pain pathway* relays neural impulses from the spinal cord to several brain structures, including the thalamus and cerebral cortex. The main pain pathway through which pain is transmitted from the body to the brain is the *ventral spinothalamic tract*. There are also as many as four other accessory pathways that can carry information about pain from the spinal cord to the brain. Depending on the pathway, they produce different responses that one would typically associate with pain. Projections to the reticular formation of the midbrain produce arousal, projections to the amygdala are thought to produce the emotional responses associated with pain, and projections to the hypothalamus are thought to activate hormonal and cardiovascular responses. These pathways can be crossed and uncrossed while ascending up the spinal cord. Because there are multiple pathways by which the pain is generated and perceived and, it makes pain itself a difficult condition to treat [61].

As we discussed above, when the nerve fibers reach the dorsal horn of the spinal cord they synapse and the second order neurons cross over and ascend to the thalamus via the spinothalamic pathway, also known as the ventro-lateral pathway. There they synapse with the third order neurons that project to the sensory cortex. In the thalamus, the target nuclei are in the ventral posterior nuclear complex: the ventral posterior medial nuclei (VPM) and the ventral posterior lateral nuclei (VPL).

Information about noxious and thermal stimulation of the face goes through a different sensory pathway, i.e., the spinal trigeminal tract. The first order axons originate from the trigeminal ganglion cells, which carry information from nociceptor and thermoreceptors from the face into the brainstem. The fibers enter the pons and descend to the medulla. They then synapse onto the spinal nucleus of the trigeminal complex in the caudal medulla, and then ascend via the trigeminal lemniscus through the middle medulla, mid-pons, and midbrain until they synapse at the contralateral thalamus. Information from the face is sent to the VPM, while information from the rest of the body is sent to the VPL. Once this pain pathway synapses in the thalamus, they project to the primary and secondary somatosensory cortex. The *primary somatosensory cortex* is thought to be responsible for sensory discrimination of pain, while the secondary somatosensory cortex is thought to be important for the recognition of pain and the memory of past pain. The cerebral cortex is important for processing the perception of pain, and bringing this sensation into conscious experience.

Moreover, as we have discussed, the experience of pain is neither a function of the magnitude of tissue damage nor the strength of the neural impulse. The experiential setting during with the injury occurs and the emotional components play a large role in the experience of pain. For example, the pain that one might experience during a generally accepted "emotionally positive" experience such as childbirth is frequently considered much more tolerable than the pain experienced during a generally accepted "emotionally negative" experience, such as the traumatic pain associated with a car wreck. Thus, treating conditions that are associated with "**Chronic Pain**" requires an individualized approach, as no two patients will experience pain in the same fashion.

For more details on the mechanisms of action of neurotransmitters and a detailed description of the sensory pathways, see Basbaum and Jessell's Chap. 24 Pain in The Principles of Neural Science 5th edition by Kandel.

The Descending Pain Pathway

There are also *descending pain pathways* that project from the brain to the spinal cord and then inhibit nociceptive activity. These descending pathways suppress the transmission of pain signals from the dorsal horn of the spinal cord to higher brain centers. The periaqueductal gray (PAG) surrounds the cerebral aqueduct, and is a major component of this system. Stimulation of PAG has been shown to produce analgesia, but no change in the ability to detect temperature, pressure, or touch. The neurons in the PAG end on cells in the medulla, including serotonergic cell bodies of the raphe nucleus. These serotonergic neurons descend to the spinal cord where they inhibit nociceptive responses. Other cells in the PAG project to the locus coeruleus in the midbrain, which synthesizes norepinephrine; these cells project down the spinal cord where they also inhibit nociception [57].

As we discussed, the perception of pain is controlled by cortical mechanisms: the cingulate gyrus and the insular cortex both contain neurons that are activated strongly by nociceptive somatosensory stimuli [57–61]. Researchers have found that no single area of the brain generates the sensation of pain. Instead, emotional and sensory components create the mosaic of activity that leads to pain. These findings are especially important to the concept of a biopsychosocial modality for treating chronic pain. Research has shown that when people are hypnotized so that the painful stimulus is not experienced as unpleasant, activity in only some areas of the brain is suppressed, suggesting that the stimulus is still experienced at the physiologic level, but it does not hurt.

The *gate control theory of pain*, proposed in the 1960s by Ronald Melzack and Patrick Wall is based on evidence that psychological as well as physical factors control our response to, and interpretation of, pain. They suggest there is a gating system in the dorsal horn of the spinal cord through which pain information passes on its way to the brain. The opening and closing of the gate can be affected by many factors, one of which is via the descending pathway. Information from the descending pathway from higher brain centers closes the gate by releasing serotonin and noradrenaline, which stimulates inhibitory neurons in the dorsal horn, thus attenuating pain transmission. This is important in our understanding that the subjective experience of pain is dependent on an individual's beliefs, behavioral skills, and coping strategies. These different mechanisms can contribute to the maintenance, exacerbation, or attenuation of pain perception.

Central sensitization may play a role in increasing responsiveness of the CNS to input from receptors [62–64]. This view of chronic pelvic pain is thought to account for chronic pain in the absence of peripheral pathology [65] and the discrepancy between the amount of tissue damage seen and severity of pain and disability experienced by patients who suffer from chronic pelvic pain syndromes [66]. There may be a hypersensitive state that leads to amplification of perception of peripheral stimuli, painful perception of nonnoxious stimuli (allodynia) and increased sensitivity for painful stimuli (hyperalgesia) [67, 68].

Are There Sex-Related Differences in Perception of Pain?

In terms of gender and the experience of pain, we know that men and women tend to cope differently with stress. Pain can be classified as a stressor, and coping with pain can be defined as an attempt to manage a stressful situation [69].

The literature seems to consistently support that, in general, men are more inclined to use active, problem-focused coping skills, while in contrast, women are more inclined to use emotion focused coping: expressing feelings, seeking social support, and blaming themselves [70]. Literature has shown that female chronic pain patients tend to engage in more catastrophizing than male chronic pain patients [71]. This is an interesting phenomenon, especially given that we know women go through many "physiological" painful events in their life—including childbirth and menstruation.

Catastrophizing, which can be defined as a perceived lack of control, excessive worry about the future, and a tendency to view life as overwhelming, has been identified as an important variable in chronic pain. This behavioral tendency is a key factor in the relationship between chronic pain and negative affect [72]. The association between pain and mood, or affective response, is well documented in the literature. In the National Health and Nutrition Examination Survey, pain and depressive symptoms tended to be more evident in women reporting chronic pain than in men [73]. We know that catastrophizing is implicated in the severity of pain that is experienced by female endometriosis patients. For this reason, the way that healthcare providers approach patients who suffer from chronic pelvic pain is critical [74].

Pelvic Pain in Sociocultural Context

The female pelvic region, because of its key role as a sexual and reproductive organ, is powerfully invested with personal, psychosocial, and cultural symbolism. Thus, when we consider chronic pelvic pain in a clinical setting, we must consider the cultural and societal constructs in which this condition exists. It is impossible to experience pelvic pain without also experiencing the psychosocial and cultural implications. Over history, female reproductive organs have been perceived by the medical profession and society in general as troublesome and expendable [75]. In the context of chronic pelvic pain, this cultural ideal becomes quite important; the USA has had the highest rate of hysterectomy in the world. There is an avid discourse in the field of women's reproductive and sexual health discussing the role of "pathologizing" female reproductive and sexual organs [76]. Many women who suffer from chronic pelvic pain, whether it is endometriosis or Persistent Genital Arousal Disorder [77], face a double edged sword in that they are faced with a medical culture that is in many ways "pathologizing" areas of their body that have important roles (and what does that pathologizing imply for these womens' body and self image?) while these women also face the pressures of their complaints being viewed by healthcare providers as "all being in their heads" or "exaggerating." It is a difficult position, and in the field of chronic pelvic pain, these issues are significant [78]. The notion that one's sexuality or reproductive machinery is "broken" or "inadequate" is deeply entrenched in the psychological schema of chronic pelvic pain. In this context, pleasure becomes important and can be immensely healing.

What About Pleasure? Is It All About Avoiding Pain?

Jeremy Bentham stated: "Nature has placed mankind under the governance of two sovereign masters, pain and pleasure. It is for them alone to point out what we ought to do, as well as to determine what we shall do (1789). His statement seems to indicate that all good feelings are pleasures, and that "pain" could describe all that humankind sought to avoid, is poignant. In the medical field, pain (unlike pleasure) is the subject of a vast amount of neuroscientific and medical research. Pain research is primarily concerned with pain in relation to nociception. Functional brain imaging has been used in an attempt to objectively measure pain, and the most consistent brain regions to become activated are the insula, thalamus, and dorsal anterior cingulate cortex [79]. But what do we make of *pleasure*, especially in relation to women who suffer from pelvic pain? Research shows that vaginal stimulation can produce pleasure, pain, and analgesia [80]. Moreover, when women self-apply vaginal stimulation in a way that feels pleasurable, the magnitude of the analgesia increased [81]. We also know that vaginal stimulation can be painful, in the case of dyspareunia [82]. Stressors are not necessarily "unpleasurable": there is an intense physiological stress response characterized by a doubling of the heart rate and blood pressure, indicating activation of the sympathetic division of the autonomic nervous system, which typically occurs during orgasm [81], and is an example of a pleasurable stress response. Komisaruk and Whipple conclude that the pleasurable component of vaginal stimulation could be an adaptive mechanism [83]. They measured the effect of specifically pleasurable vaginal self-stimulation on the perception of pain. In these studies, pain thresholds were measured by gradually increasing compression applied to the fingertips; the pain detection threshold was defined by the force at which the women first stated that they felt pain. The women applied vaginal self-stimulation with a non-vibrating sterilized smooth plastic cylinder. The researchers found that when the women in the study applied steady pressure to the anterior vaginal wall, their pain thresholds increased significantly by a mean of over 40 %. When they were asked to apply the stimulus specifically in a way that felt pleasurable to them, their pain thresholds increased by over 80 %. Four out of the ten women in this study experienced orgasm at the time, at which point the pain threshold increased by over 100 %. There was no change in the tactile thresholds measured by

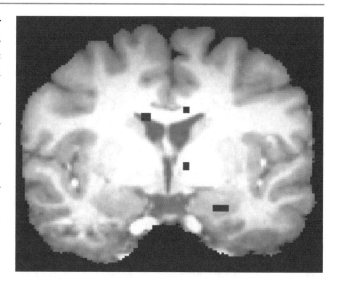

Fig. 18.4 Intense activation sites during orgasm. fMRI (functional magnetic resonance imaging) is a useful technology to capture brain activity during human orgasm. The fMRI method is based on the increased blood flow that supplies neurons when they become active. This image, taken at Rutgers University—Newark Orgasm Laboratory, indicates high-threshold activation in the thalamus and amygdala (*Red coloring*) during human orgasm. Courtesy Rutgers University—Newark Orgasm Laboratory, unpublished

von Frey fibers, indicating that the vaginal self-stimulation induced analgesia, rather than anesthesia. In more recent studies of women using fMRI, Komisaruk has found that the insular cortex and anterior cingulate cortex in the forebrain are activated during orgasm (see Fig. 18.4 for fMRI image of the high threshold activation during human orgasm) [84]. Other researchers have also reported that these cortical regions are activated during pain [85]. Thus, these findings suggest that there may be an active inhibitory component that occurs between orgasm and pain in the insula and anterior cingulate cortex, indicating that they are both important for pain and pleasure. Given the unique experience of women's pelvic or genital pain, and the findings that genital stimulation and orgasm can attenuate pain perception, evidently there is a unique and important aspect in the biology of pain that is also tied to the biology of pleasure.

Women with pelvic pain suffer from a disturbance in their sexual life. A 2013 study assessing 182 patients with deep infiltrating endometriosis collected data on satisfaction, orgasm, desire, and pelvic pain interference with sex. The results of the study demonstrated that women with this type of pelvic pain have sexual function impairment, which is correlated with a decrease in the overall well-being score. They found that the presence of dyspareunia and vaginal endometriotic lesions seemed to be involved with sexual dysfunction [86]. This information is important when we treat patients who suffer from chronic pelvic pain, because the ability to experience pleasure affects our health.

Many studies in recent years have shown that sexual activity has health benefits. These studies, while correlational, emphasize the important notion that women who experience pelvic pain have a need for sexual pleasure as well. One study suggests that women who reported past sexual enjoyment lived longer than those who did not report sexual enjoyment [87]. This is in contrast to men, for whom the frequency of intercourse is the only significant positive predictor of longevity. There is also evidence that the incidence of heart attack in women was correlated with the inability to be aroused sexually, to experience orgasm, and with sexual dissatisfaction [88], while in men, more frequent ejaculations were reported to have a protective effect on general health [89] and reduced incidence of prostate cancer [90].

In summary, chronic pelvic pain is diverse medical condition that requires a sophisticated treatment approach by the healthcare provider. As we have discussed in this chapter, the pathophysiologic basis of chronic pelvic pain in women is broad and can encompass urologic, gynecologic, neurologic, musculoskeletal, or psychological etiologies. Because of the complex nature of chronic pain, it may be that there are multiple pain modalities presenting in one patient at the same time. Thus, it is of utmost importance to employ a Bio-psycho-social modal to approaching diagnosis and therapy in these patients. Moreover, we have discussed the neurobiology of chronic pain, and the neurologic pathways, from nociceptor, to spinal cord, to the thalamus, finally leading to transmission of neural impulses to the somatosensory cortex, and the perception of pain. Finally, we discussed the importance of pleasure and quality of sexual function for women who suffer from chronic pelvic pain.

Key Points

- Pain is defined as "an unpleasant sensory and emotional experience associated with actual or potential tissue damage, or described in terms of such damage." Messages about tissue damage are perceived by receptors called nociceptors, and then transmitted to the spinal cord via small myelinated fibers and very small unmyelinated fibers. From the spinal cord, the neural messages are carried to the brainstem, thalamus, and cerebral cortex and ultimately perceived as pain.
- A Bio-psycho-social response is needed when treating chronic pelvic pain as chronic pain presents in a heterogeneous fashion. The experiential setting during which the injury occurs and the emotional components play a large role in the experience of pain. Thus, treating chronic pain conditions requires an individualized approach, as no two patients' experience of pain is quite the same.
- The conscious perception of pain happens in the brain, however, there is no one brain region that generates pain.

The experience of pain is neither a function of the magnitude of tissue damage (at the level of nociception) nor the strength of the neural impulse, and chronic pain may be a disease of the nervous system, not merely a symptom of a disease process.
- Etiologies of chronic pelvic pain syndromes are diverse, including gynecologic, urologic, gastrointestinal, musculoskeletal, and psychiatric.
- Chronic pain is a psychosocial stressor. Men and women tend to cope with it differently. Men typically take an active, problem-focused approach, while women utilize emotion focused coping, social support, and expressing feelings.
- People who suffer from chronic pain report physical functional loss, vegetative depression symptoms, and varying family dynamics. Women with chronic pelvic pain have a higher incidence of depression, and there is also an association with trauma.
- The notion that one's sexuality or reproductive machinery is "broken" or "inadequate" is deeply entrenched in the psychological schema of chronic pelvic pain. Women with chronic pelvic pain report difficulty experiencing sexual pleasure; yet, research indicates that sexual pleasure is associated with longevity in women. In this context, pleasure becomes important and can be immensely healing.

References

1. Schappert SM. National Ambulatory medical care survey: 1989 summary. Natl Vital Stat Rep. 1992;13:1–80.
2. Knapp DA, Koch H. The Management of new pain in office-based ambulatory care: national ambulatory medical care survey, 1980 and 1981. Adv Data. 1984;97:1–9.
3. Engeler D, Baranowski AP, Elneil S, Hughes J, Messelink EJ, Olivera P, et al. Guidelines on Chronic Pelvic Pain European Association of Urology. 2012. Available from: http://www.uroweb.org/gls/pdf/24_chronic_Pelvic_Pain_LRMarch 23th.pdf.
4. Reiter R. A profile of women with chronic pelvic pain. Clin Obstet Gynecol. 1990;33(1):130.
5. Zondervan KT, Yudkin PL, Vessey MP, Dawes MG, Barlow DH, Kennedy SH. Patterns of diagnosis and referral in women consulting for chronic pelvic pain in the UK primary care. Br J Obstet Gynaecol. 1999;106(11):1156.
6. Demir F, Ozcimen EE, Oral HB. The role of gynecological, urological, and psychiatric factors in chronic pelvic pain. Arch Gynecol Obstet. 2012;286(5):1215–20.
7. Neis K, Neis K. Chronic pelvic pain: cause, diagnosis, and therapy from a gynaecologist's and an endoscopist's point of view. Gynecol Endrocrinol. 2009;25(11):757–61.
8. Rock J, Jones H. Te Linde's operative gynecology. 10th ed. Lippincott Williams and Wilkins; 2008.
9. Zondervan KT, Yudkin PL, Vessey MP, Jenkinson CP, Dawes MG, Barlow DH, et al. Chronic pelvic pain in the community - symptoms, investigations, and diagnoses. Am J Obstet Gynceol. 2001;184(6):1149.
10. Merksey H, Bogduk N. Classification of chronic pain: descriptions of chronic pain syndromes and definitions of pain terms. 2nd ed. Seattle International Association for the study of Pain; 1994.

11. Pain and disability: clinical, behavioral, and public policy perspectives. Osterweis M, Kleinman A, Mechanic D, editors. Washington: National Academy Press; 1987.
12. American Psychiatric Association. Diagnostic and statistical manual of mental disorders. 3rd ed. Washington: American Psychiatric Association; 1980.
13. American Psychiatric Association: diagnostic and statistical manual of mental disorders. 3rd ed. Revised ed. Washington: American Psychiatric Association; 1987.
14. Merksey H, Spear FG. The concept of pain. J Psychosom Res. 1967;11(1):59–67.
15. American Psychiatric Association: diagnostic and statistical manual of mental disorders. 4th ed. Text Revision ed. Washington: American Psychiatric Association; 2000.
16. Dersh J, Polatin PB, Gatchel RJ. Chronic pain and psychopathology: research findings and theoretical considerations. Psychosom Med. 2002;64:773–86.
17. Howard F. The role of laparoscopy in the evaluation of chronic pelvic pain: pitfalls with a negative laparoscopy. J Am Assoc Gynecol Laparosc. 1996;4(1):85.
18. Stones RW. Female genital pain. In: Fillingim RB, editor. Sex, gender and pain. Seattle: IASP Press; 2000.
19. Gradison M. Pelvic inflammatory disease. Am Fam Physician. 2012;85(8):791–6.
20. Eschenbach DA. Acute pelvic inflammatory disease: etiology, risk factors and pathogenesis. Clin Obstet Gynecol. 1976;19(1):147.
21. Medicine Pcotasfr. Pathogenesis, consequences, and control of peritoneal adhesions in gynecological surgery. Fertil Steril. 2007;88(1):21.
22. Howard FM, El-Minawi AM, Sanchez RA. Conscious pain mapping by laparscopy in women with chronic pelvic pain. Obstet Gynecol. 2000;96(6):934.
23. Stewart EA. Uterine fibroids. Lancet. 2001;357:293.
24. Friedrich EGJ. Vulvar vestibulitis syndrome. J Reprod Med. 1987;32(2):110.
25. Baggish MS, Miklos JR. Vulvar pain syndrome: a review. Obstet Gynecol Surv. 1995;50(8):618.
26. Leiblum SR, Nathan SG. Persistent sexual arousal syndrome: a newly discovered pattern of female sexuality. J Sex Marital Ther. 2001;27:365–80.
27. Leiblum SR, Seehus M. FSFI Scores of women with persistent genital arousal disorder compared with published scores of women with female sexual arousal disorder and healthy controls. J Sex Med. 2009;6:469–73.
28. Leiblum SR. Persistant genital arousal disorder. In: Leiblum SR, editor. Perplexing, distressing, and under recognized. 4th ed. New York: The Guildford Press; 2007.
29. Komisaruk BR, Lee HJ. Prevalence of sacral spinal (Tarlov) cysts in persistant genital arousal disorder. J Sex Med. 2012;9:2047–56.
30. Beard RW, Reginald PW, Wadsworth J. Clinical features of women with chronic lower abdominal pain and pelvic congestion. Br J Obstet Gynaecol. 1988;95(2):153.
31. Lippman SA, Warner M, Samuels S, Olive D. Uterine fibroids and gynecologic pain symptoms in a population based study. Fertil Steril. 2003;80(6):1488.
32. Stanford EJ, Dell JR, Parsons CL. The emerging presence of interstitial cystitis in gynecologic patients with chronic pelvic pain. Urology. 2007;69(4 supplement):53.
33. Dell JR. Interstitial cystitis/painful bladder syndrome: appropriate diagnosis and management. J Women's Health. 2007;16(8):1181–7.
34. Mayson BE, Teichman JM. The relationship between sexual abuse and interstitial cystitis/painful bladder syndrome. Curr Urol Rep. 2009;10(6):441–7.
35. Williams RE, Hartmann KE, Sandler RS. Recognition and treatment of irritable bowel syndrome among women with chronic pelvic pain. Am J Obstet Gynceol. 2005;192(3):761.
36. Sarzi-Puttini P, Atzeni F, Mease PJ. Chronic widespread pain: from peripheral to central evolution. Best Pract Res Clin Rheumatol. 2011;25(2):133–9.
37. Schimdt-Wilcke T, Clauw DJ. Fibromyalgia: from pathophysiology to therapy. Nat Rev Rheumatol. 2011;7(9):518.
38. Staud R. Abnormal pain modulation in patients with spatially distributed chronic pain: fibromyalgia. Rheum Dis Clin North Am. 2009;35(2):263.
39. Dadabhoy D, Crofford LJ, Spaeth M, Russell IJ. Biology and therapy of fibromyalgia: evidence based biomarkers for fibromyalgia syndrome. Arthritis Res Ther. 2008;10(4):211.
40. Tu FF, Fitzgerald CM, Kuiken T, Farrell T, Harden RN, Norman HR. Comparative measurement of pelvic floor pain sensitivity in chronic pelvic pain. Obstet Gynecol. 2007;110(6):1244.
41. Loos MJ, Scheltinga MR, Mulders LG, Roumen RM. The Pfannenstiel incision as a source of chronic pain. Obstet Gynecol. 2008;111(4):839.
42. Sharp HT. Myofascial pain syndrome of the abdominal wall for the busy clinician. Clin Obstet Gynecol. 2003;46(4):783.
43. Srinivasan AK, Kaye JD, Moldwin R. Myofascial dysfunction associated with chronic pelvic floor pain: management strategies. Curr Pain Headache Rep. 2007;11(5):359.
44. Rosenbaum TY. Muscloskeletal Pain and sexual function in women. J Sex Med. 2010;7(2 Pt 1):645–53.
45. Schultz WW, Basson R, Binik Y, Eschenbach D, Wesselmann U, Lankveld JV. Women's sexual pain and its management. J Sex Med. 2005;2(3):301–16.
46. Binik YM, Bergeron S, Khalife S. Dysparuenia and vaginismus: so called sexual pain. In: Leiblum SR, editor. Principles and practice of sex therapy. 4th ed. New York: The Guildford Press; 2007.
47. American Psychiatric association. Diagnostic and statistical manual of mental disorders. 5th ed. Washington: American Psychiatric Association; 2013.
48. Binik YM. Should dyspareunia be retained as a sexual dysfunction in DSM-V? A painful classification decision. Arch Sex Behav. 2005;34(1):11–21.
49. Rapkin AJ, Kames LD, Darke LL, Stampler FM, Naliboff BD. History of physical and sexual abuse in women with chronic pelvic pain. Obstet Gynecol. 1990;76(1):92.
50. Walling MK, Reiter RC, O'Hara MW, Milburn AK. Abuse history and chronic pain in women: prevalences of sexual abuse and physical abuse. Obstet Gynecol. 1994;84(2):193.
51. Meltzer-Brody S, Leserman J, Zolnoun D, Steege J, Green E, Teich A. Trauma and posttraumatic stress disorder in women with chronic pelvic pain. Obstet Gynecol. 2007;109(4):902.
52. Lorencatto C, Petta CA, Navarro MJ, Bahamondes L, Matos A. Depression in women with endometriosis with and without chronic pelvic pain. Acta Obstet Gynecol Scand. 2006;85(1):88.
53. Blumer D, Heilbronn M. Chronic pain as a variant of depressive disease: the pain prone-disorder. J Nerv Ment Dis. 1982;170(7):381.
54. Walker E, Katon W, Harrop-Griffiths J, Holm L, Russo J, Hickok LR. Relationship of chronic pelvic pain to psychiatric diagnosis and childhood sexual abuse. Am J Psychiatry. 1988;145(1):75.
55. Randolph ME, Reddy DM. Sexual functioning in women with chronic pelvic pain: the impact of depression, support, and abuse. J Sex Res. 2006;43(1):38.
56. Pontari M, Ruggieri M. Mechanisms in prostatitis/chronic pelvic pain syndrome. J Urol. 2004;272:830–45.
57. Basbaum AI, Jessell TM. Pain. 5th ed. In: Kandel ER, editor. McGraw-Hill Professional; 2012.
58. Komisaruk BR, Adler NT, Hutchison J. Genital sensory field: enlargement by estrogen treatment in female rats. Science. 1972;178:1295–8.
59. Komisaruk BR, Whipple B. The role of vaginal stimulation-produced analgesia in reproductive processes. In: Genazzani AR,

Nappi G, Facchinetti F, Martignoni E, editors. Pain and reproduction. Casterton Hall, UK: The Parthenon Publishing Group; 1988.

60. Rodriguez-Sierra JF, Skofitsch G, Komisaruk BR, Jacobowitz DM. Abolition of vagino-cervical stimulation-induced analgesia by capsaicin administered to neonatal, but not adult rats. Physiol Behav. 1988;44:267–72.

61. Kolb B, Whishaw IQ. An introduction to brain and behavior. 4th ed. New York: Worth Publishers; 2014.

62. Janicki TI. Chronic pelvic pain as a form of complex regional pain syndrome. Clin Obstet Gynecol. 2003;46:797–803.

63. Nijs J, Houdenhove BV, Oostendorp RA. Recognition of central sensitization in patients with musculoskeletal pain: application of pain neurophysiology in manual therapy practice. Man Ther. 2010;15:135–41.

64. Meyer R, Campbell JN, Raja SN. Peripheral neural mechanisms of nociception. In: Wall P, Melzack R, editors. Textbook of pain. 3rd ed. Edinburgh: Churchill Livingstone; 2012 1995.

65. As-Sanie S, Harris RE, Napadow V, Kim J, Neshewat G, Kairys A, et al. Changes in regional gray matter volume in women with chronic pelvic pain: a voxel based morphometry study. Pain. 2012;153:1006–14.

66. Neziri AY, Haesler S, Peterson-Felix S, Muller M, Arendt-Nielsen L, Manresa JB, et al. Generalized expansion of nociceptive reflex receptive fields in chronic pain patients. Pain. 2010;151:798–805.

67. Baranowski AP. Chronic pelvic pain. Best Pract Res Clin Gastroenterol. 2009;23:593–610.

68. Serap K, Hermans L, Willems T, Roussel N, Meeus M. Central sensitization in urogynecological chronic pelvic pain: a systematic literature review. Pain Physician. 2013;16:291–308.

69. Lazarus RA, Folkman S. Stress, appraisal, and coping. New York: Springer; 1984.

70. Vingerhoets AJ, Heck GIV. Gender, coping and psychosomatic symptoms. Psychol Med. 1990;20(1):125–35.

71. Geisser ME, Robinson ME. Catastrophizing, depression, and the sensory, affective and evaluative aspects of chronic pain. Pain. 1994;58:79–83.

72. Jensen I. Coping with long-term musculoskeletal pain and its consequences: is gender a factor? Pain. 1994;57:167–72.

73. Magni G. Prospective study on the relationship between depressive symptoms and chronic musculoskeletal pain. Pain. 1990;56:289–97.

74. Deguara CS, Pepas L, Davis C. Does minimally invasive surgery for endometriosis improve pelvic symptoms and quality of life? Curr Opin Obstet Gynecol. 2012;24(4):241–4.

75. Scully D, Bart P. A funny thing happened on the way to the orifice: women in gynecology textbooks. In: Huber J, editor. Changing women in a changing society. Chicago IL: University of Chicago Press; 1973

76. Lostein LM. Female sexuality and feminine development: Freud and his legacy. Adv Psychsom Med. 1985;12:57–70.

77. Goldstein I, De EJB, Johnson J. Persistent sexual arousal syndrome and clitoral priapism. In: Goldstein I, Meston C, Davis S, Traish AM, editors. Women's sexual function and dysfunction: study, diagnosis and treatment. London: Taylor and Francis; 2006.

78. Grace VM. Problems of communication, diagnosis, and treatment experienced by women using the New Zealand health service for chronic pelvic pain: a qualitative analysis. Heath Care Women Int. 1995;16(6):521–35.

79. Tracey I. Nociceptive processing in the human brain. Curr Opin Neurobiol. 2005;15:478–87.

80. Komisaruk BR, Whipple B. The suppression of pain by genital stimulation in females. Ann Rev Sex Res. 1995;6:151–86.

81. Whipple B, Komisaruk BR. Analgesia produced in women by genital self-stimulation. J Sex Res. 1988;24:130–40.

82. Meana M, Binik YM. Painful coitus: a review of female dyspareunia. J Nerv Ment Dis. 1994;182:264–72.

83. Komisaruk BR, Whipple B. How does Vaginal stimulation produced pleasure, pain and analgesia. In: Fillingim RB, editor. Seattle; 2000.

84. Komisaruk BR, Whipple B, Crawford A, Grimes S, Liu WC, Kalnin A, et al. Brain activation during vaginocervical self-stimulation and orgasm in women with complete spinal cord injury: fMRI evidence of mediation by the vagus nerves. Brain Res. 2004;1024:77–88.

85. Casey KL, Morrow TJ, Lorenz J, Minoshima S. Temporal and spatial dynamics of human forebrain activity during heat pain: analysis by positron emission tomography. J Neurophysiol. 2001;85:951–9.

86. Montanari G, Donato ND, Benfenati A, Giovanardi G, Zannoni L, Vicenzi C, et al. Women with deep infiltrating endometriosis: sexual satisfaction, desire, orgasm and pelvic problem interference with sex. J Sex Med. 2013;10(6):1559–66.

87. Palmore EB. Predictor of longevity difference: a 25 year follow-up. Gerontologist. 1982;22:513–8.

88. Abramov LA. Sexual life and sexual frigidity among women developing acute myocardial infarction. Psychosom Med. 1976;38:418–25.

89. Davey-smith G, Frankel S, Yarnell J. Sex and death: are they related? Findings from Caerphilly Cohort Study. BMJ. 1997;315:1641–4.

90. Giles GG, Severi G, English DR, McCredie MR, Borland R, Boyle P, et al. Sexual factors and prostate cancer. Br J Urol. 2003;92:211–6.

Chronic Pelvic Pain: Pudendal Neuralgia and Therapeutic Neural Blockade

Rupinder Singh, Edward T. Soriano, and David A. Gordon

Introduction

When it comes to sources of chronic pelvic pain, the list is voluminous and comes from many angles. However, neuro-inflammatory causes of pelvic pain are among the rarest. Nevertheless, if one examines the emerging disciplines that encompass neuromuscular pelvic floor disorders, then the painful clinical syndrome that evolves from inflammation along the course of the pudendal nerve is becoming very significant and will be discussed at length below. Here, it is important to note that the precise etiology of pudendal neuralgia is coming under question. Currently, mainstream thought is that this type of inflammation around a segment of the pudendal nerve (*arguably the most important nerve coursing through the pelvis*) is proposed to be a type of *ischemic neuritis* that can occur when compressed by a spastic musculature that makes up the pelvic floor or along an anatomically tunneled segment. This tunneled segment is known as *"Alcock's canal."* Consequently, the pathology of this clinical scenario most often centers around compression or entrapment as it passes through this tunnel. Not surprisingly, the syndrome is known as "Alcock's syndrome" and "pudendal nerve entrapment" (PNE).

The word *pudendal* originates from Latin *pudenda*, which means the external genitals. It is essentially derived from *pudendum*, which literally means *"parts to be ashamed of."* The pudendal nerve is the principal nerve of the muscular pelvis and perineum. It is a mixed nerve which is responsible for carrying both motor and sensory fibers to and from the pelvic area in both sexes. It carries sensory signals from the external genitalia, skin around the anus, and perineum in both males and females. In addition, it supplies motor innervation to various pelvic muscles including the male or female external urethral sphincter as well as the external anal sphincter.

Neuroanatomy of the Pudendal Nerve

The pudendal nerve is a paired nerve, which means that there are two of these nerves in the human pelvis, one the left side of the pelvis and one on the right side. On either side of the body, pudendal nerve is derived from the *ventral rami* of the second, third, and fourth *sacral spinal nerves* (Fig. 19.1), with fourth sacral spinal nerve being the chief contributor. The pudendal nerve forms as the three roots converge immediately above the upper border of the *sacrotuberous ligament* and the *coccygeus muscle* (Fig. 19.1). The three roots transform into two cords once the middle and the lower roots join to form the lower cord, and these in turn merge to form the proper pudendal nerve just proximal to the *sacrospinous ligament* (Fig. 19.1).

The pudendal nerve courses between the *piriformis* and the *coccygeus* muscles before it leaves the pelvis through the lower part of the *greater sciatic foramen* (Fig. 19.2). Next, it passes over the lateral part of the *sacrospinous ligament* (Fig. 19.1). It then reenters the pelvis through the *lesser sciatic foramen* (Fig. 19.2). Once the pudendal never reenters the pelvis, it is accompanied by the *internal pudendal artery* and the sheath of the *obturator fascia*. The sheath of the obturator fascia containing the pudendal nerve and the internal pudendal vessels here is termed the *pudendal canal*. The pudendal canal is also recognized by its other well-known name "Alcock's canal," termed after the Irish anatomist *Benjamin Alcock* who first documented it in the year 1836.

R. Singh
Department of Geriatric Pelvic Medicine and Neurourology, Sinai Hospital of Baltimore, Baltimore, MD, USA

E.T. Soriano
Pain Management Services, Sinai Hospital, Baltimore, MD, USA

D.A. Gordon (✉)
Division of Pelvic NeuroScience, Department of Surgery, The Sinai Hospital of Baltimore, 2401 W. Belvedere Ave, Baltimore, MD 21215, USA
e-mail: dgordon@lifebridgehealth.org

© Springer Science+Business Media New York 2017
D.A. Gordon, M.R. Katlic (eds.), *Pelvic Floor Dysfunction and Pelvic Surgery in the Elderly*,
DOI 10.1007/978-1-4939-6554-0_19

Fig. 19.1 Pudendal nerve
anatomy. From: http://www.
pudendalhope.info/sites/
default/files/Health
OrganisationforPudend
ChronicPainBro1-2.jpg

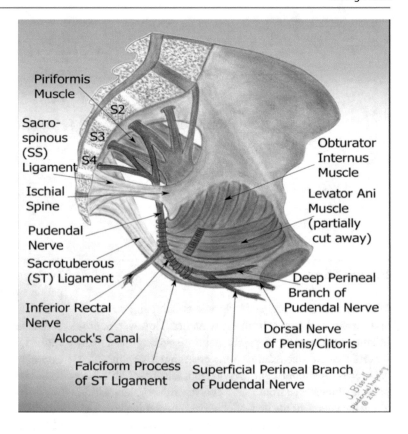

Fig. 19.2 Possible pudendal
nerve entrapment by the
sacrospinous ligament/
sacroiliac joint complex.
From: https://
jointpreservation.wordpress.
com/category/ligamenttendon/

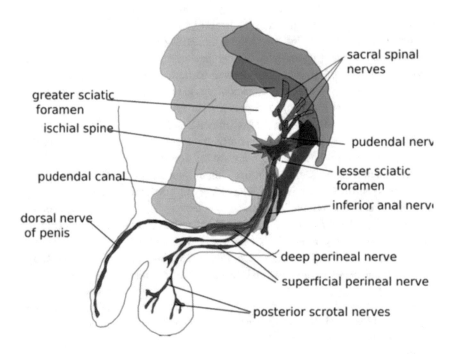

After entering the pudendal canal, the pudendal nerve divides into its terminal branches. It first gives off the *inferior anal nerve* (Fig. 19.1), then the *perineal nerve* (Fig. 19.1), before finally terminating as the *dorsal nerve of the penis* in males or the *dorsal nerve of the clitoris* in females (Fig. 19.1).

Neurophysiology of the Pudendal Nerve

The pudendal nerve functionally is a mixed nerve that contains both motor and sensory fibers. Furthermore, it contains *sympathetic* fibers but lacks *parasympathetic* fibers. The dorsal nerve of the penis/clitoris, which is a terminal branch of the pudendal nerve, carries the sensory information from the penis in males or the clitoris in females (Fig. 19.1). In addition, the *posterior scrotal branch* of the pudendal nerve in males or the *posterior labial branch* in females carries sensory information from the posterior scrotum or the posterior labia, respectively. A branch of the pudendal nerve also carries sensory information from the anal canal via its sensory terminal branches. Pudendal nerve is also responsible for the afferent component of penile erection in males as well as clitoral erection in females. The pudendal nerve additionally plays a role in facilitating ejaculation via its sympathetic fibers.

The motor fibers in the pudendal nerve are responsible for innervating the muscles of the pelvic floor and the perineum including the *bulbospongiosus, ischiocavernosus, levator ani* muscle group, either *pubourethralis* in males or *pubovaginalis* in females, the *external anal sphincter*, and the male or female *external urethral sphincter*. Since the pudendal nerve supplies motor fibers to the external urethral sphincter as well as the external anal sphincter in both males and females, it plays an integral part in the voluntary voiding as well as defecating mechanisms.

Pathophysiology of Pudendal Neuralgia

Here, it is important to note that the precise etiology of *pudendal neuralgia* is coming under question. Currently, mainstream thought is that this type of inflammation around a segment of the pudendal nerve (*arguably the most important nerve coursing through the pelvis*) is proposed to be a type of *ischemic neuritis* that can occur when compressed by either spastic pelvic floor muscles or along an anatomically tunneled segment. This tunneled segment is known as "*Alcock's canal.*" Consequently, the pathology of this clinical scenario most often centers around compression or entrapment as it passes through this tunnel. Not surprisingly, the syndrome is known as "Alcock's syndrome," "pudendal nerve entrapment" or PNE. The two most important narrow sites responsible for anatomic nerve entrapment are around the ischial spine between the *sacrospinous* and the *sacrotuberous* ligament (Fig. 19.1), and in the *Alcock's canal* (Fig. 19.1).

Today, the term *pudendal neuralgia (PN)* is often used *interchangeably* with "pudendal nerve entrapment." However, there is *no* evidence to support equating the presence of this syndrome with a diagnosis of pudendal nerve entrapment, meaning that it is possible to have all the symptoms of PNE *without* having any structural, static anatomic compression. This is supported by a 2009 literature review. Essentially, all of the symptoms of pudendal neuralgia are presumed to be absolutely secondary to an anatomic compression or entrapment. Now there are many parameters that bring this line of

pathophysiology into question. In addition, a 2015 study of 13 normal female cadavers found that the pudendal nerve was attached or fixed to the sacrospinous ligament in all cadavers studied, suggesting that the diagnosis of pudendal nerve entrapment may be overestimated.

The pudendal nerve is implicated in a multitude of pathological conditions. It is vulnerable to injury by being compressed, entrapped, and overstretched resulting in temporary or irreversible nerve injury. All of these circumstances lead to inflammation around the "pudendal nerve," essentially "pudendal neuritis." It is this type of neural inflammation about the pudendal nerve that leads to the classic symptom complex usually associated with pudendal nerve entrapment, especially pain associated with prolonged sitting causing chronic compression of the pudendal nerve. Common activities that increase the risk of nerve entrapment include professional bicycling, horseback riding, long drives, and pelvic mass, notably *sacrococcygeal teratoma.*

On the other hand, stretch injury to the pudendal nerve may be caused by any condition that causes the pelvic floor to be overstretched, such as difficult childbirth or strenuous squatting exercise, and chronic straining during defecation with chronic constipation. Furthermore, systemic diseases like chronic diabetes mellitus and multiple sclerosis can damage the pudendal nerve by causing demyelination leading to significant pudendal neuropathy. Clinical insults to pudendal nerve by any mechanism may also lead to significant urinary or fecal incontinence.

Pudendal neuralgia or "*Alcock's syndrome*" is a rare cause of chronic pelvic pain in the primary care setting. Again, pudendal neuralgia has a multifactorial etiology. It may be secondary to being squeezed by spastic pelvic floor musculature, or by compression within a small anatomic canal or by either inflammatory or mechanical insult to the nerve and finally by an inflammatory cycle created by biochemically caustic sacral cysts (*Tarlov's cysts*). *The resultant pain is commonly positional and is exacerbated by prolonged sitting.* Other frequently reported clinical signs and symptoms include *genital numbness, sexual dysfunction*, pain with intercourse, *fecal incontinence*, and urinary incontinence. Furthermore, patients may describe their symptoms as a vague pain, stabbing pain, burning sensation, pin pricking, twisting pain, cold sensation, and pulling sensation. Other specific anatomical areas involved may include the rectum, anus, urethra, and the perineum. Gender specific symptoms in women may include pain in the vagina and vulva, the *labia majora*, and *labia minora*, and the clitoris. Similarly, in men these symptoms include pain in the penis and the scrotum. Paresthesia and pain symptoms may encompass other anatomical landmarks including the groin, inner part of the leg, buttocks, and the lower abdomen. Patients may perceive pain and paresthesia in only one of these areas, several areas, or in all of the above-mentioned areas. Patients may also experience hyperesthesia and allodynia in the involved areas (hypersensitivity/extreme sensitivity to the slightest touch), which may prevent them from wearing certain clothing.

Furthermore, patients can present with voiding dysfunction, which may include hesitancy, extreme urgency, or frequency. Bowel dysfunction may also ensue and cause painful defecation, and chronic constipation. Sexual dysfunction in women specifically can include extreme pain with penetration and for men symptoms can include erectile dysfunction as well as pain with orgasm.

Pathophysiology of Pudendal Neuralgia in Tarlov's Cysts

Sacral cysts, first described by I.M. Tarlov in 1938 are occasionally found incidentally in the course of radiological examination of the lumbosacral spine for various disorders. Review of the literature on Tarlov cysts, which develop at the distal limits of the dural sheath, a thinned extension of the dura mater, which encapsulates not only the brain and spinal cord, but also the dorsal and ventral nerve roots. This thinned dural sheath includes the epineurium and terminates near the dorsal root ganglia. At that point, the perineurium (*contiguous with the pia/arachnoid*) balloons out under pressure of the cerebrospinal fluid (CSF), perhaps in part because of the absence of constraint by the proximally overlying dura mater. The perineurial wall contains spinal nerve root fibers and ganglion cells and the fibers may be present in the cyst cavity itself. It is described that the neck of this fluid-filled balloon structure is constricted, creating a one way "ball-valve" structure that allows CSF to enter, but not leave readily. As the volume of CSF changes in response to postural and positional changes, e.g., from supine to sitting, or in response to the Valsalva maneuver, sensory nerve root fibers in the cyst wall can stretch or compress against adjacent bone or the nerve roots, thereby producing abnormal sensations.

The S2 and S3 dorsal roots convey sensory phenomena along the course of the pelvic and pudendal nerves. These nerves innervate the external and internal genitalia which could generate the abnormal sensations. When these sensations are uncomfortable, they fall into the category classified as pain. When these sensations are stimulatory, they may initiate "persistent genital arousal disorder."

Symptoms of Tarlov cysts include pain in perineum, vagina, penis, buttock, leg, lower back, sacrum, or coccyx, dyspareunia, proctalgia, bladder dysfunction, urinary incontinence, micturition disorders, *bowel incontinence*, *radicular pain (neuralgia)*, loss of sensibility, muscle weakness or *paresis,* and *dysesthesias* which are essentially abnormal sensations noted in the absence of appropriate or associated stimulation. Also, paresthesias can occur in the thigh or foot, most often described as burning sensations. Tarlov cysts less than 1.0 cm in diameter are often reported as asymptomatic

and symptomatic cysts less than 2.0 cm are now frequently managed non-surgically with injections or sacral neuromodulation (see Figs. 19.2 and 19.3). It seems plausible that despite differences in terminology, there is a degree of congruence between these two sets of symptomatology.

Persistent Genital Arousal Disorder (PGAD)

It is important to remember that even involuntary genital arousal can be painful. PGAD is a complex pathology with multiple etiologies and with variably effective therapies. This syndrome is perplexing and characterized by high levels of genital arousal occurring in the absence of subjective interest or desire. PGAD sufferers are women who experience involuntary, intrusive, painful and seemingly spontaneous genital arousal that can be unrelenting. This arousal can persist for hours, days, or even longer, despite attempts to relieve it with sexual activity or orgasm, which at best provide only brief relief from the symptoms. Attempts to quell the genital arousal by engaging in masturbation or sexual activity may lead to brief relief, no relief, or even more arousal and activation.

Neurodiagnostic Evaluation in Pudendal Neuralgia

Pudendal neuralgia is a diagnosis of exclusion. All other potential causes of pelvic pain and other related symptoms have to be ruled out before the definitive diagnosis of pudendal neuralgia is made. A detailed medical history and pertinent physical exam are considered the two most important diagnostic tools in diagnosing pudendal neuralgia. Once the preliminary diagnosis of pudendal neuralgia is made via history and physical exam, it can be confirmed by utilizing a local nerve block. This technique can be used to simultaneously to confirm the diagnosis and initiate treatment, whereby the pudendal nerve is blocked by a local anesthetic to see if symptoms can be eliminated by numbing the nerve at specific sites.

Furthermore, pudendal nerve *motor latency* test can be utilized to measure the pudendal nerve conduction velocity. During the pudendal motor latency test, electrodes are fixed in the muscles of the perineum and the rectum. Next, the pudendal nerve is stimulated with an electric probe. The average speed of the stimulus transmission is measured and recorded. The average stimulus transmission is often significantly slower in patients suffering from pudendal neuralgia.

Treatment of Pudendal Neuralgia

When conservative measures such as avoidance of postures/activities that exacerbate symptoms, physical therapy, and medical management fail to provide relief, a combined anesthetic and steroid pudendal nerve block injection is used for both diagnosis and treatment. For instance, if the pain is relieved immediately following the injection, it suggests that the pudendal nerve is the likely source of symptoms. The hope is that if the inflammatory process is suppressed that that the threshold for neural depolarization will decrease and the sensory component of the nerve will begin to fire in a fashion which is more closely aligned to its normal equilibrium. This may take several injections so it is not surprising for symptoms to return when the anesthetic and steroids wear off initially, again highlighting the need for repeated nerve blocks. Patients may require two to three nerve blocks before sufficient symptomatic relief is achieved after reduction in inflammation.

General Concepts of Neural Blockade

Neural blockade dates back to the late 1800s when Dr. Carl Koller injected cocaine during ophthalmic surgery. Plexus blocks and peripheral nerve blocks were subsequently performed by Dr. William Halstead followed by subarachnoid and extradural cocaine injections by Drs. Leonard Corning and Heinrich Quincke. Eventually, safer anesthetic agents and techniques were developed. Intrathecal, epidural, plexus, sympathetic nerve and peripheral nerve blocks have now become routine in both anesthesia and in the treatment of acute and chronic pain syndromes.

Nerve blocks are performed for a variety of reasons. In the management of pelvic pain, nerve blocks can serve both diagnostic and therapeutic purposes. Diagnostic blocks can be performed for the purpose of localizing the pain generating neural pathways as well as determining if a patient may be a candidate for other neuroablative therapies. Therapeutic nerve blocks are performed in an attempt to disrupt the nociceptive input from the periphery to the dorsal horn of the spinal cord. This nociceptive input has the potential of creating changes at the spinal cord level which can contribute to the development of chronic pain states. The wind-up phenomena at the spinal cord level has been well described. Wind-up may underlie the continuation of pain sensation despite a reduction in the actual number of action potentials generated from the nociceptive C-fibers. These changes at the spinal cord can then lead to central sensitization. With central sensitization low frequency action potentials into the CNS by nociceptive neurons increase synaptic activity in the dorsal horn of the spinal cord. Changes in the central nervous system include synaptic plasticity, changes in microglia, astrocytes, involvement of N-methyl D-Aspartate (NMDA) activation, and gene transcription. Central sensitization in which the central nervous system alters and amplifies pain may act to uncouple the stimulus response relationship that defines nociceptive pain. Therefore, managing a chronic centralized pain syndrome by treating the peripheral tissues

that initiated the original nociceptive input generally fails. Aggressive, early treatment of acute pain is necessary to help reduce the risk of development of these central nervous system changes, which lead to wind-up and central sensitization. Local anesthetics, by blocking the action potentials from C-fibers, may help "reset" the pain generating nociceptive fibers and, hopefully, reduce the probability of developing a chronic neuropathic pain syndrome from an acute pain syndrome. Diagnostic and therapeutic blocks are directed based upon the clinical presentation of the patient's pain. Shows the anatomic structures and corresponding plexi or nerves which can be blocked to relieve pain.

Anesthetic Properties in Neural Blockade

Local anesthetics have been used for over 100 years for neural blockade. Anesthetics are divided into amides and esters, although today the amides are used almost exclusively in clinical practice. Lidocaine and bupivacaine are by far the most common anesthetics used in neural blockade. The clinical pharmacology of local anesthetics is beyond the scope of this chapter, but some basic concepts should be understood by the clinician performing nerve blocks. Briefly, the resting cell membrane has a selective permeability to potassium ions (K+) allowing for a net efflux of K+ outside the cell and with a positive charge relative to inside the axonal neuroplasm. This accounts for the negative resting potential of approximately −60 to −70 mV. During depolarization of an axon there is a selective permeability to Na+ ions allowing for an influx of Na+ ions into the cell, causing an alteration in the inner cell potential. This allows for transmission of an impulse along the axon. Repolarization occurs as the force of Na+ influx diminishes and voltage dependent K+ channels open allowing an efflux of K+ ions outside the cell membrane eventually restoring the cell to its resting state.

Local anesthetics prevent nerve conduction by blocking the influx of Na+ ions through the cell membrane, thereby blocking the change in the potential difference between the inside and outside of the cell membrane required to cause cell depolarization. Lidocaine tends to have a rapid onset of action and duration of between 1 and 2 h. Bupivacaine has a slower onset of action but a more prolonged duration between approximately 4–6 h. Bupivacaine also tends to have a greater differential between sensory and motor blockade. This can be beneficial in peripheral mixed somatic nerve blocks, particularly in an outpatient setting, by limiting motor block while obtaining adequate sensory nerve blockade. The therapeutic benefits of anesthetic agents, however, may not be limited to their ability to block neural impulse conduction. Local anesthetics may also have anti-inflammatory properties.

Systemic side effects need to be taken into consideration while performing nerve blocks. Inadvertent intravascular injections can cause potentially serious side effects. A toxic dose of lidocaine is approximately 4.5 mg/kg although there are risks of side effects at a dose of 1.5 mg/kg. Symptoms of lidocaine toxicity include lightheadedness, dizziness, perioral or tongue paresthesias, headaches and, at high concentrations, seizures. Cardiovascular effects, including dysrhythmias, are possible, but are less common than CNS effects. Bupivacaine has greater potential cardiovascular effects than does lidocaine. The toxic dose of bupivacaine is approximately 2.5 mg/kg. Inadvertent intravascular injection of bupivacaine has been known to cause significant cardiovascular side effects including hypotension and arrhythmias with cardiovascular collapse and death. The cardiovascular side effects of bupivacaine are due to its high affinity for the myocardial Na+ channel.

While local anesthetic toxicity is rare, these potentially serious side effects may be limited by using image guided, site specific, and low volume injections with fluoroscopic or ultrasound guidance. By injecting contrast under live fluoroscopic visualization prior to the injection of anesthetic one can reduce the risk of inadvertent direct vascular injection. Under ultrasound guidance the injection site can be directly visualized around the intended nerve or fascial plane. In addition, before injecting large doses of anesthetics or when performing multiple injections, the maximum dose of anesthetic based upon the patient's weight should be considered.

Somatic Nerve Blocks

Somatic nerve blocks are often utilized in chronic pelvic pain. Chronic pudendal neuralgia has been well documented. The pudendal nerve is a somatosensory nerve derived from the S2–S4 nerve roots. It provides sensory innervation to the anus, perineum, penis, or clitoris and provides motor supply to the pelvic floor musculature. The nerve can become irritated, and a painful neuropathy created, if the nerve becomes entrapped at the attachment of the sacrospinous ligament to the ischial spine or in the pudendal canal. Irritation of the pudendal nerve can cause perineal pain involving the penis, scrotum, labia, perineum, and anorectal regions. A diagnostic criteria has been offered for pudendal neuralgia which includes pain in the territory of the pudendal nerve from the anus to the penis or clitoris; pain predominantly experienced while sitting; pain with no objective sensory impairment and, finally, pain relieved with a diagnostic pudendal nerve block.

Various techniques to block the pudendal nerve have been described including blind techniques, CT and fluoroscopically guided techniques and, more recently, ultrasound guided techniques. In the last decade, ultrasound has gained more popularity as it allows for soft tissue and nerve visualization and limits patient and operator radiation exposure.

Ultrasound allows for the direct visualization of the critical landmarks: the ischial spine, pudendal artery, sacrospinous ligament, sacrotuberous ligament, and the pudendal nerve. The target for the injection is between the sacrotuberous and sacrospinous ligaments. The pudendal nerve runs in close proximity to the sciatic nerve. Use of a peripheral nerve stimulator is suggested to reduce the chance of a sciatic nerve block. 4 ml of 0.25 % bupivacaine with or without steroid can then be injected. A study by Bellingham et al. found no significant difference in outcomes between fluoroscopic and ultrasound guided injections. If patients with pudendal neuropathy benefit temporarily with diagnostic and/or therapeutic injections, pulsed radiofrequency neuroablation has been demonstrated to be of benefit. In addition, there has been a case report of successful treatment of urinary urgency and hesitancy accompanied by pain in the perineum in an elderly male after undergoing pulsed radiofrequency treatment of the pudendal nerve.

The ilioinguinal, iliohypogastric, and genitofemoral nerves may contribute to chronic pelvic pain, particularly with pain after surgical procedures or trauma. The ilioinguinal, iliohypogastric, and genitofemoral nerves can all be blocked using ultrasound guidance. Blind techniques have been known to have a high failure rate. Typically, the ilioinguinal and iliohypogastric nerves are blocked together. Above the iliac crest the nerves travel from deep to superficial and pierce the transversus abdominis muscle to lie between the transversus abdominis and the internal oblique in 90 % of cases. Using ultrasound, the abdominal wall is scanned approximately 5 cm cranial to the anterior superior iliac spine. Generally, at this level, the ilioinguinal and iliohypogastric nerves are reliably located between the transversus abdominis and internal oblique. The external oblique is also visualized at this level. Color Doppler can be utilized to visualize the deep circumflex artery, which may be in the same fascial plane as the nerves. Generally, 6–8 ml of 0.25 % bupivacaine is adequate to block both nerves.

The genitofemoral nerve block has been well described by Soneji et al. and is performed by performing ultrasound scanning along the inguinal canal generally with the probe two fingerbreadths lateral to the pubic tubercle and the probe held perpendicular to the inguinal canal. The femoral artery is located and traced cephalad where it travels deep and transitions to the external iliac artery at which point the contents of the inguinal canal can be visualized. The nerve may be either within or outside the spermatic cord in males and, therefore, injection of approximately 4 ml of 0.25 % bupivacaine with or without steroid in injected both inside and outside the spermatic cord. In females a total of 5 ml of injection fluid is deposited within the inguinal canal around the round ligament. Cryoablation of the genitofemoral nerve after successful diagnostic block has also been described in the literature for chronic inguinal pain.

Trigger Point Therapy

Myofascial trigger points were first termed by Dr. Janet Travell in 1942, though similar phenomena have been described dating back to the sixteenth century. When first described *myofascial trigger points* (*MTrPs*) were defined as "being a *focus of hyperirritability* in a muscle or its fascia referring pain in a specific pattern." Currently *MTrPs* are generally accepted to be discrete, focal, hyperirritable spots located in a taut band of skeletal muscle. In addition to local pain they may produce referred pain, motor dysfunction, or autonomic phenomena. MTrPs are grossly *classified as being one of two types.* An active MTrP is an actively symptomatic trigger point; while a latent trigger point does not trigger pain without being stimulated, though it may restrict movement or cause muscle weakness. Active MTrPs are always tender, prevent muscle lengthening, may refer pain or autonomic reactions on direct compression, and create a local twitch response. On exam an LTR is a visible or palpable contraction as the tense muscle fibers of the trigger point contract, these can be observed visually, recorded electromyographically, or visualized using diagnostic ultrasound.

Myofascial trigger points form the basis of myofascial pain syndrome, and can play a role in many other pain syndromes as well. Myofascial pain syndrome is a chronic pain syndrome that is caused by multiple trigger points or fascial constriction which can occur in many distinct areas of the body and causing a variety of different symptoms.

Whether active or latent, MTrPs are thought to form through a multifactorial process. These mechanisms include trauma, joint, muscle, and postural dysfunction, sleep disturbances, emotional and mental disturbances, and vitamin deficiency or insufficiencies. As with all tissues in the body, skeletal muscle contains nociceptors. These nociceptors are unique in that they require a large amount of stimulation before they fire which assures they will not relay painful signals during normal muscle contractions, stretches, or pressure. MTrPs typically cause painful signals secondary to their persistent noxious stimulation, leading to both spontaneous and referred pain. This pain may be related to noxious stimuli arising from local elevations in inflammatory mediators and neuropeptides. Recent studies have shown that active MTrPs have increased calcitonin gene related peptide (CGrP), substance P, TNF-a, and IL-B, IL-6, and IL-8.

In clinical practice MTrPs are largely diagnosed by identifying taut bands and the local twitch response. Their presence or that of referred pain or reproduction of symptoms has been shown to increase the specificity of the diagnosis, and clinical outcomes are significantly improved when a local twitch response, LTR, is observed prior to intervention. In some practices EMG may be used to aid in trigger point diagnosis and management. Diagnostically, LTR contractions can be recorded as high amplitude polyphasic discharges. Surface EMG can also be used to assist in assessing muscle behavior at rest and performing functional tasks, as well as aid in muscle awareness and postural training.

There are many *applications with respect to MTrPs in Pelvic Medicine.* Myofascial trigger points often effect postural muscles including the back and pelvic girdle and can be associated with visceral organ dysfunction either through a viscero-somatic or somato-visceral reflex mechanism. MTrPs of the pelvic floor may be identified in as many as *85% of patients with urological, colorectal, or gynecological pelvic pain syndromes* with symptoms including bowel, bladder, and sexual dysfunction in addition to pain. Many urologic and gynecologic disease processes including interstitial cystitis, bladder pain syndrome, vulvodynia, chronic prostatitis, and chronic pelvic pain syndrome include vague symptoms of pain which may be related to feedback cycles from MTrPs. Symptoms from these disease states may be related to MTrPs found in the abdominal wall or pelvic muscles. Some suspect that these urologic syndromes are a part of a spectrum which progresses through years of self-reinforcing chronically progressive myofascial and trigger point dysfunction.

The pain associated with these disease states may be *propagated through a convergence of afferent C and A-delta fibers although it is usually heavily "C" weighted.* This aberrant sensory phenomena emanate from the dysfunctional organ and pelvic floor musculature via second order neurons in the spinal cord. Ultimately, when enough of this unmyelinated painful aberrant sensory input barrages the sacral spinal cord, the normal electrophysiologic gating mechanism can be over run and disrupted. This then can lead to an antidromic impulse, in which a nerve fires in a retrograde fashion may be propagated to the affected organ (bladder, prostate, vagina, etc.) through dorsal root reflexes, axon reflexes, or some yet unknown mechanism. Research on interstitial cystitis suggests inflammation found in this disease process may be related to a neurogenic origin in which antidromic propagation causes an increased number of nociceptors, as well as the release of CGrP, substance P, and other inflammatory markers listed earlier leading to mast cell degranulation in the mucosa, which may be found in this disease. The urologic syndromes outlined may classically be difficult to treat as they are likely more multifactorial in cause, and although MTrPs may appear somewhat abstract they likely play an important role in the formation and propagation of these and other disease states.

Treatment of MTrPs

The *first line of management* for MTrPs should be to treat underlying perpetuating factors to prevent the potential for recurrence. These factors include emotional and sleep disturbances, physical and postural dysfunctions, and nutritional deficiency or insufficiencies. After correcting underlying factors nonpharmacologic treatments should then be explored, and can include behavior modification with transvaginal or transrectal biofeedback, bowel and bladder control, physical therapy, massage, heat and ice therapy, and transcutaneous electric nerve stimulator (TENS unit).

Trigger point injections and dry needling are reserved for physician treatment and are typically used as adjuvant therapy to more conservative treatments outlined earlier. MTrP injection and dry needling are both options to treat symptomatic active trigger points. Although dry needling has been proven to be as effective as trigger point injections, injections are generally more commonly used as post injection soreness has been shown to be less intense and of a shorter duration when injected with local anesthetic. This supports the idea that the therapeutic effect is the actual mechanical disruption of the MTrP; breaking the positive feedback loop, diluting, and removing metabolites and nociceptive substances through the vasodilation effect of local anesthetic, and the release of endorphins.

The approach to MTrP assessment begins with a physical exam performed via rectum or vagina with the patient in the lithotomy or semi-prone Sim's position. A manual exam using a sweeping motion from posterior to anterior should be performed to identify taut bands, LTRs, and radiation or reproduction of symptoms. Pelvic floor muscles commonly associated with MTrPs include the sphincter ani, levator ani, coccygeus, and on exam should be assessed in addition to the pubourethralis, vaginalis, rectalis, iliococcygeus, obturator internus, and piriformis muscles. Further examination can include adductor muscles of the medial thigh, lumbar paraspinal muscles, and gluteal muscles. Reproduction of all or part of the patient's pain, LTR, or palpation of a taut band can warrant treatment.

Prior to injecting a trigger point, the clinician should ensure they have all the necessary equipment to complete the procedure. Rubber gloves and alcohol will be needed to clean the skin at the entry site, as well as a 3–5 ml syringe and 21–26 gauge needle of varying length depending on the muscle to be injected. It is important to use a long enough needle, and avoid inserting to its hilt, which is the weakest part and may result in breaking off as a foreign body. For anesthetic agent, lidocaine or procaine can be used based on preference, though procaine has the distinction of being the least myotoxic of all local anesthetics.

In general, for MTrPs outside of the pelvic floor once a trigger point has been located it can be injected by isolating the point between the first and second digits and advancing the needle while warning the patient of potential reproduction of symptoms. After entering the point withdraw the plunger to confirm placement outside of a vessel, and inject a small amount of local anesthetic. Tension should be maintained on the skin and the clinician should move the needle in various directions to disrupt the MTrP, and remove the needle when the LTR or taut band is no longer palpable, or the symptoms resolve. Following the procedure the patient should be prompted to stretch the affected muscle to promote muscle elongation, and removal of inciting substances.

There are three basic approaches described to address pelvic floor MTrPs. These include vaginal, subgluteal, and perineal approaches outlined in Fig. 19.1. The first approach is the subgluteal approach and follows a path inferior and medial to the ischial tuberosities, similar to a perineal nerve block, but directed towards a finger palpating and stabilizing the MTrP rectally or vaginally. The second approach is a perineal approach in which the needle is directed through the perineum and towards the MTrP palpated and held in place either by a palpating finger in the vagina or rectum. The final approach is transvaginal, in which the needle is inserted through the vagina towards an MTrP palpated and held in place through a palpating finger in the rectum. This final transvaginal approach has the added benefit of being closer and allowing easier access to deeper musculature. As with all MTrPs, despite method of approach the same protocol should be followed including withdrawal of plunger to assure proper placement outside of a vessel, followed by injection of a small amount of local anesthetic after which the point should be mechanically disrupted. This process should be repeated until no further MTrPs are elicited, and may treat 5–10 points if needed, and making sure to stretch or manipulate the area following the procedure to promote muscle elongation, and removal of inciting substances.

Although myofascial trigger point injections are relatively benign, there are some contraindications that should be considered. Although there are only a few considerations that must be made before injecting a patient, again, one should be familiar with the relative contraindications. These relative contraindications include patients with a history of bleeding disorder or on anticoagulation, some practitioners may choose to hold aspirin prior to the procedure though these appear to be preference. True contraindications would include a patient with a current infection, or if their MTrP is secondary to acute trauma, in which case the patient should be monitored for recovery, and if the MTrP still exists should be treated at that point. A patient with an allergy to a particular injection agent should be assessed for possible alternative use, or treated alternatively with dry needling technique. Generally patients should be given at least 3–5 days for treatment to work and should not be retreated within this time frame. In addition to this if the patient has failed three successive treatments alternative pathologies and alternative treatments should be considered.

Post injection complications are relatively rare and shared with other similar injection type procedures. These include infection, needle breakage, and hematoma formation.

These can be avoided by maintaining proper aseptic technique, and to apply pressure briefly post injection to stop any local bleeding which may be present. More serious complications include intravascular injection of anesthetic agents leading to systemic toxicity, seizure, arrhythmia, or nerve damage if injected intraneurally. These complications highlight the importance of making sure of correct placement of needle before injecting agents.

Summary

MTrPs have been identified with nearly every musculoskeletal pain problem including pelvic pain and other urologic syndromes. Classically MTrPs are defined as taut bands of muscle referring pain, and producing a local twitch response on examination. Although originally described by Dr. Janet Travell in 1942 trigger points have been undergoing an increasing amount of research, including studies on urologic manifestations. Many urologic pathologies may be interrelated with myofascial trigger points, either being created, or compounded by MTrPs.

Treatment for MTrP should include identifying and treating the underlying pathologic lesions that are responsible for the MTrP formation and activation. The MTrP should be managed conservatively first through physical therapy modalities, failing that more aggressive therapy should be started including trigger point injections.

Suggested Reading

Harper D. "Pudendum". Online etymology dictionary. Retrieved 3 Mar 2016.

Agur AMR, Dalley AF, Grant JCB. Grant's atlas of anatomy. 13th ed. Philadelphia: Wolters Kluwer Health/Lippincott Williams & Wilkins; 2013. ISBN 978-1-60831-756-1.

Standring S (editor in chief). Gray's anatomy: the anatomical basis of clinical practice, 39th ed. Elsevier; 2004. ISBN 978-0-443-06676-4.

Shafik A, el-Sherif M, Youssef A, Olfat ES. Surgical anatomy of the pudendal nerve and its clinical implications. Clin Anat. 1995; 8(2):110–5.

Wolff BG, et al., editors. The ASCRS textbook of colon and rectal surgery. New York: Springer; 2007. ISBN 0-387-24846-3.

Oelhafen K, Shayota BJ, Muhleman M, Klaassen Z, Tubbs RS, Loukas M. Benjamin Alcock (1801-?) and his canal. Clin Anat. 2013;26(6):662–6. doi:10.1002/ca.22080.PMID22488487.

Neill, editor-in-chief, Jimmy D. Knobil and Neill's physiology of reproduction, 3rd ed. Amsterdam: Elsevier; 2006. ISBN 0-12-515400-3.

Babayan RK, Siroky MB, Oates RD. Handbook of urology diagnosis and therapy, 3rd ed. Philadelphia: Lippincott Williams & Wilkins; 2004. ISBN 978-0-7817-4221-4.

Penson DF. Male sexual function: a guide to clinical management. Ann Int Med. 2002;134:300.

Drake RL, Vogl W, Tibbitts, Adam W.M. Mitchell; illustrations by Richard; Richardson, Paul. Gray's anatomy for students. Philadelphia: Elsevier/Churchill Livingstone; 2005. ISBN 978-0-8089-2306-0.

Howard FM. The role of laparoscopy in chronic pelvic pain: promise and pitfalls. Obstet Gynecol Surv. 1993;48:357–87.

http://www.pudendalhope.info/sites/default/files/HealthOrganisationforPudendChronicPainBro1-2.jpg

Tarlov IM. Perineurial cysts of the spinal nerve roots. Arch Neurol Psychiatry. 1938;40:1067–74.

Langdown AJ, Grundy JR, Birch NC. The clinical relevance of Tarlov cysts. J Spinal Disord Tech. 2005;18:29–33.

Komisaruk BR, Whipple B, Beyer-Flores C. The science of orgasm. Baltimore: The Johns Hopkins University Press; 2006.

Leiblum SR, Nathan SG. Persistent sexual arousal syndrome: a newly discovered pattern of female sexuality. J Sex Marital Ther. 2001;27:365–80.

Leiblum S, Nathan S. Persistent sexual arousal syndrome in women: a not uncommon but little recognized complaint. J Sex Rel Ther. 2002;17:191–8.

Leiblum S. Persistent genital arousal disorder: what it is and what it isn't. Contemp Sex. 2006;40:8–13.

Leiblum S, Seehuus M, Goldmeier D, Brown C. Psychological, medical, and pharmacological correlates of persistent genital arousal disorder. J Sex Med. 2007;4(5):1358–66.

Leiblum S. Persistent genital arousal disorder. In: Leiblum S, editor. Principles and practices of sex therapy. New York: Guilford Press; 2007. p. 54–83.

Goldstein I, De EJB, Johnson J. Persistent sexual arousal syndrome and clitoral priapism. In: Goldstein I, Meston C, Davis S, Traish, editors. Women's sexual function and dysfunction: study, diagnosis and treatment. London: Taylor & Francis; 2006. p. 674–85.

Leiblum S, Seehuus M, Brown C. Persistent genital arousal: disordered or normative aspect of female sexual response? J Sex Med. 2007;4:680–9.

Goldmeier D, Leiblum S. Interaction of organic and psychological factors in persistent genital arousal disorder in women: a report of six cases. Int J STD AIDS. 2008;19:488–90.

Leiblum SR, Seehuus M. FSFI scores of women with persistent genital arousal disorder compared with published scores of women with female sexual arousal disorder and healthy controls. J Sex Med. 2009;6:469–73.

Part IV

Gynecologic/Urogynecologic Aspects

Sushma Srikrishna, Ganesh Thiagamoorthy, and Linda Cardozo

Pelvic Organ Prolapse in the Older Woman

Pelvic organ prolapse (POP) is a common condition with a significant deleterious impact on quality of life. This condition is more commonly seen in the elderly population, affecting 37 % of women over the age of 80 [1]. There are several factors involved in the aetiopathogenesis. Age related vascular changes impair circulation to tissue and combined with the decreased elasticity of collagen with age, the older woman is at increased risk of POP [2]. Loss of vaginal rugae becomes apparent 2–3 years after the menopause. This occurs secondary to increased collagen breakdown which is considered to be a factor in the aetiology of POP [3–6]. Respiratory function steadily declines from 25 years of age and the strength of pulmonary muscle decreases significantly impairing effective cough. Due to the reduced ability to clear ones' airway, coughs may become more frequent and stronger in order to achieve expectoration. This increases intra-abdominal pressure worsening prolapse and also raising concerns regarding prolonged surgery and anaesthetic morbidity [7]. Disability, social isolation and poor nutrition may lead to poorer mobility, increased constipation and delayed presentation before help is sought.

The lifetime risk of undergoing surgery to treat POP is 11 % [8]. Currently 33 % of neonates survive until the age of 80 years. It has been predicted this will rise to 50 % by 2050 [9]. As the life expectancy of women is greater than that of men, the proportion of women in the elderly population will increase even further. Surgery for POP accounts for approximately 20 % of elective major gynaecological surgery and this increases to 59 % in elderly women [10]. By 2030, there will be approximately 39.9 million women in this age group, with a rate of growth almost double that of the general population. Overall, individuals aged 65 years and older will represent 19 % of the population by 2030, compared with 12.4 % of the population in 2000. In addition, women more than 80 years of age are the fastest growing segment of society. As both the incidence and prevalence of prolapse surgery increase with age, pelvic organ prolapse (POP) becomes an increasingly bothersome disorder in this patient population.

The management of POP is symptom driven, therefore, if POP does not cause significant bother it rarely needs active intervention. Exceptions obviously exist, for example, if a prolapse has become ulcerated, management is required to prevent infections and severe sequelae. A procidentia can cause renal dysfunction secondary to kinking off the ureters. Review by a specialist with the aid of a validated quality of life questionnaire such as the International Consultation on Incontinence Questionnaire—Vaginal Symptoms (ICIQ-VS) is essential. These assessment tools will help assess bother, as well as the frequency and severity of urinary, bowel and sexual symptoms [11]. Common presentations of POP are outlined in Table 20.1. A detailed history should be taken to enquire about all of these symptoms.

After a relevant history, it is essential to perform a thorough examination. Pelvic examination should be carried out at maximum Valsalva with an empty bladder whilst the woman is both supine and standing to fully assess the extent of any prolapse and the compartments affected [12–14]. There are many grading systems to document urogenital prolapse. The most popular amongst general gynaecologists is the severity assessment of mild, moderate and severe [15]. The International Urogynecological Association and International Continence Society have recommended the pelvic organ prolapse quantification (POP-Q) system as it has been shown to be reproducible and reliable [16].

There are a number of investigations which may need to be carried out in a woman with POP. If co-existing lower urinary symptoms are highlighted during the initial history, a mid-stream urine (MSU) sample should be tested, and if

S. Srikrishna (✉) • G. Thiagamoorthy • L. Cardozo
Department of Urogynecology, King's College Hospital,
Denmark Hill, London SE5 9RS, UK
e-mail: sushmasrikrishna@hotmail.com

© Springer Science+Business Media New York 2017
D.A. Gordon, M.R. Katlic (eds.), *Pelvic Floor Dysfunction and Pelvic Surgery in the Elderly*,
DOI 10.1007/978-1-4939-6554-0_20

Table 20.1 Common presentations of pelvic organ prolapse

1. Bulge/pressure symptoms (worse at the end of the day, better on lying down)
a. Something coming down the vagina
b. Lump/bulge seen or felt in the vagina
c. Lower backache
d. Lower abdominal dragging sensation
2. Bladder symptoms
a. Recurrent UTI
b. Urinary incontinence
c. Voiding dysfunction
3. Bowel symptoms
a. Tenesmus
b. Need to digitate to defecate
4. Symptoms related to sexual function
a. Dyspareunia
5. Others
a. Vaginal discharge
b. Rarely vaginal bleeding

surgery is contemplated, urodynamics (UDS) should be performed. The MSU is useful to screen for infection, calculi or cancer. A simple bladder scan to assess post void residual is an important part of the investigations. A significant residual, usually over 100 ml, can predispose a woman to recurrent urinary tract infections. Most will improve with treatment of the prolapse but in some cases clean intermittent self-catheterisation (CISC) may be indicated [10]. Pre-operative UDS is useful to rule out concomitant voiding dysfunction, stress urinary incontinence, and detrusor overactivity. Imaging is beneficial to exclude a pelvic mass as a cause of prolapse and to assess the integrity of renal tract when conservative management is considered. Where symptoms of obstructed defaecation are noted, investigations of bowel function may also be warranted such as defecatory proctography and anorectal physiology studies.

The main aim of treatment is to improve the woman's quality of life. Not only should surgery relieve symptoms of prolapse such as the awareness of a vaginal bulge, but ideally restore or maintain bladder, bowel and sexual function [17]. Management is individualised depending upon presenting symptoms and lifestyle. Treatment options may be incorrectly limited in the elderly with the misconception that surgery should be avoided. A woman's age should not be a factor for avoidance of surgical treatment. Her current state of health and expectations are most important and realistic counselling which addresses these is essential.

The first line of management in POP is conservative lifestyle modifications. POP is exacerbated by increased intra-abdominal pressure with studies confirming that chronic cough, constipation, lifting weights and obesity all increase the risk [18–22]. Therefore, lifestyle modifications to reduce these such as weight loss strategies and smoking cessation

classes can improve the situation and reduce the chance of worsening prolapse. Anaemia, benign joint hypermobility syndrome, vitamin D deficiency and incidence of fractures have all been found to be associated with an increased risk of POP [23–25]. It has been proposed that the suboptimal collagen status associated with POP may similarly involve bone collagen thus increase the risk of fractures. Although it is difficult to prove a causal relationship between vitamin D deficiency and POP, it may be worth considering treating this deficiency as a primary care preventative measure which may also reduce the risk of worsening POP.

Other than lifestyle modifications, pelvic floor muscle training (PFMT) can play an important role in the management of POP. Women with moderate prolapse have been found to have significantly lower PFM contraction strength [26]. PFMT directed by a specialist physiotherapist has been shown objectively to improve POP by one stage on average [27] and subjectively significantly reduce symptom frequency and bother of POP. This is thought to be secondary to the statistically significant change in resting position of the bladder and rectum in those who have undertaken PFMT [28].

The use of oestrogen in the treatment of POP remains controversial. Studies have shown that POP in postmenopausal women has been associated with lower oestrogen levels and an increase in oestrogen receptors in the uterosacral and cardinal ligaments [29]. This may imply that the supportive structures of the uterus are affected by the lack of oestrogen and therefore upregulate production of receptors rendering the tissue more sensitive to oestrogen replacement. This theory is further reinforced by some limited evidence that systemic oestrogen replacement reduces risk of prolapse and may improve POPQ scores [30]. Low dose vaginal oestrogen has been found to be a very effective treatment of postmenopausal atrophic vaginitis [31, 32]. Vaginal oestrogen mainly has a local effect and results in minimal systemic absorption which reduces the incidence of systemic side effects including endometrial stimulation. As a result of this, adjuvant progestogen are not required. This reduces the risk of thrombosis.

Few studies have investigated the impact of local vaginal oestrogen supplementation with regard to breast cancer recurrence. It has been shown to increase serum E2/E3 and decrease LH and FSH [33, 34], but not associated with increased risk of recurrence of breast cancer [35]. Both the largest trials assessing the safety of hormone replacement therapy (HRT) in women after breast cancer, 'Stockholm' and 'HRT After Breast Cancer- Is It Safe?' (HABIT), regarded use of LDVO only as part of the non-treatment arms [36, 37]. Table 20.2 describes different LDVO preparations which are currently available.

The final conservative management tool is a pessary. A pessary mechanically supports the prolapsing organ and limits its descent into the vagina. By relieving the pressure on the

Table 20.2 Low dose vaginal oestrogen preparations

Type of oestrogen	Mode of administration	Trade name
Oestriol	Cream 0.01 %	Gynest
	Cream 0.1 %	Ovestin
	Pessary 0.5 mg	OrthoGynest
Oestradiol	Tablet 10 mcg	Vagifem
	Tablet 25 mcg	Vagifem
	Ring	Estring

Table 20.3 Factors affecting surgical management of prolapse

1. Patient preference
2. Sexual activity
3. Isolated vault prolapse
4. Multiple previous surgeries
5. Concomitant intra-abdominal pathology
6. Co-existing Lower urinary tract symptoms
7. Planned staged procedure

supporting structures and the pelvic organs, symptoms of POP are improved. Pessaries and surgery have been shown to be equally effective at relieving symptoms of POP. The demographics of the women choosing either option may be different however. Those choosing pessaries tend to be slightly older and suffer less bothersome symptoms related to bowel emptying, sexual function and quality of life [38]. Pessaries are more ideal for women who are awaiting, are unfit for, or do not wish to undergo surgery. There is limited evidence available to aid decision making with regard to which pessary is best. A randomised crossover trial comparing the gelhorn and ring pessary found both equally effective in improving symptoms and impact of prolapse [39]. Sexual function can be grossly affected by prolapse and the loss of sexuality is not an inevitable aspect of aging. The majority of healthy people remain sexually active on a regular basis until advanced old age [40]. Sexuality of the older women is more dependent on basic conditions like general well-being, physical and mental health, quality of relationship, or life situation [41]. Age increases the chances of the woman suffering poorer health secondary to age related diseases and thus may decrease desire but is not an independent factor for decreased sexuality. Menopause does decrease desire but may have an adverse impact because of discomfort. Women who are sexually active have been found on examination to have less evidence of vaginal atrophy [42]. If POP does not cause problems during intercourse, sexual function can be maintained whilst using a pessary if the patient uses a ring pessary or one which she can remove before intercourse. Sexuality has an important role in older women's lives and if POP does cause discomfort to either party during intercourse, surgical treatment may well be indicated.

Surgery remains the definitive treatment of POP. Age itself is not a contraindication to any type of anaesthesia. The sensitivity to drugs increases with age whilst metabolism and clearance of drugs decreases with age. The effect of aging on the cardiovascular, respiratory, immune and clotting systems increases the risks of intra- and post-operative morbidity. The mean overall complication rate for POP surgery is 3.8 % with cardiovascular events the most common [43]. Almost 6 % of women suffer short-term urinary retention requiring catheterisation [44]. Catheterisation may increase the likelihood of decreased mobility, venous throm-

boembolism and urinary tract infection (UTI). UTIs are a common cause of temporospatial disorientation which occurs in 4.6 % of older women post POP surgery. The objective success rate in women over 75 years of age was 87.6 %, however highlighting the viability of surgery for POP in the elderly [43]. There was no difference in POP treatment failure rates in women who were 65 years of age or more when compared to women under 65 [45]. Administration of low dose vaginal oestrogen after POP surgery via an estradiol-releasing ring is feasible and results in improved markers of tissue quality postoperatively compared to placebo and controls [46]. At Kings College Hospital NHS Foundation Trust, we routinely recommend either the topical cream or oestradiol vaginal tablets.

Surgical repair of POP depends on the compartment which is affected. The exact operation which is performed is determined by a number of factors (Table 20.3). The commonest route used to repair POP is transvaginal. Other routes include transanal/perineal, abdominal, laparoscopic and robotic. There are no high quality clinical trials to guide the operating surgeon regarding the best operation.

In patients with recurrent prolapse, one may consider repeat surgery with native tissue, repeat surgery with mesh augmentation or colpocleisis. Both the latter require a fully informed detailed consultation with the patient in view of the increased risks or cessation of sexual activity, respectively. POP repair with mesh augmentation compared to using native tissue only has been shown to reduce the recurrence of POP by up to 30 % but has a significantly higher serious complication rate. (Cochrane) Complications include prominence, exposure or extrusion of the mesh, alongside the formation of fistulous tracts. This can lead to vaginal bleeding, vaginal discomfort, dyspareunia, lower urinary tract or even bowel symptoms. Colpocleisis is the surgical closure of the vagina up to the introitus. This relieves symptoms of prolapse but precludes sexual intercourse.

Patients suffering from stress incontinence together with POP may consider the benefits of concomitant insertion of a mid-urethral sling such as the tension free vaginal tape (TVT) at the same time as the POP repair. There has been a large body of evidence supporting this practice [47–49]. For some women, reduction of the prolapse may expose underlying 'occult' stress incontinence. Pre-operative urodynamics may highlight this and as long as the patient is fully counselled, they may wish to be managed with either an interval or concomitant procedure.

Conclusion

POP in the elderly is becoming increasingly prevalent as the population ages. The modern older woman expects to remain active and maintain a good quality of life and as there have been few studies of prolapse management specifically in the elderly more are required. Neither surgery nor anaesthesia is contraindicated in the elderly and studies suggest that the results of surgery are the same in older women as they are in younger women. Regardless of age, each patient should be assessed individually with a holistic multi-compartment approach and the risk benefit ratios of every treatment considered.

Key Points

- Pelvic organ prolapse is more common in elderly patients.
- The commonest symptom is vaginal bulge (bulge sensation or the sensation of something coming down through the vaginal introitus).
- Diagnosis can be confirmed with vaginal examination to identify the presence, compartments affected, extent and potential complications of POP
- Different treatment options are available, including observation, lifestyle management, physiotherapy and use of pessaries, as well as surgical options
- Management should be tailored on an individual basis, based on symptoms, desire for treatment and comorbidity
- Pessaries and colpocleisis are the treatment options used more often in elderly patients than in the general population.

References

1. Morley GW. Treatment of uterine and vaginal prolapse. Clin Obstet Gynecol. 1996;39(4):959–69.
2. Gosain A, DiPietro LA. Aging and wound healing. World J Surg. 2004;28(3):321–6.
3. Sturdee DW, Panay N. Recommendations for the management of postmenopausal vaginal atrophy. Climacteric. 2010;13:509–22.
4. Phillips CH, Anthony F, Benyon C, et al. Collagen metabolism in the uterosacral ligaments and vaginal skin of women with uterine prolapse. BJOG. 2006;113:39–46.
5. Moalli PA, Talarico LC, Sung VW, et al. Impact of menopause on collagen subtypes in the arcus tendineous fasciae pelvis. Am J Obstet Gynecol. 2004;190:620–7.
6. Tinelli A, Malvasi A, Rahimi S, et al. Age-related pelvic floor modifications and prolapse risk factors in postmenopausal women. Menopause. 2010;17:204–12.
7. Sharma G, Goodwin J. Effect of aging on respiratory system physiology and immunology. Clin Interv Aging. 2006;1(3):253–60.
8. Olsen AL, Smith VJ, Bergstrom JO, et al. Epidemiology of surgically managed pelvic organ prolapse and urinary incontinence. Obstet Gynecol. 1997;89(4):501–6.
9. Mathers CD, Murray CJL, Lopez AD, et al. Global patterns of healthy life expectancy for older women. J Women Aging. 2002;14(1–2):99–117.
10. Luesley DM. Obstetrics and gynaecology: an evidence-based text for MRCOG, 2nd ed. Hodder Arnold, 09/2010. 97.2
11. Abrams P, Cardozo L, Khoury S, Wein A. International consultation on urological disease, 5th Edition, Paris, 2013.
12. Silva WA, Kleeman S, Segal J, et al. Effects of a full bladder and patient positioning on pelvic organ prolapse assessment. Obstet Gynecol. 2004;104(1):37–41.
13. Visco AG, Wei JT, McClure LA, et al. Effects of examination technique modifications on pelvic organ prolapse quantification (POP-Q) results. Int Urogynecol J Pelvic Floor Dysfunct. 2003;14(2):136–40.
14. Barber MD, Lambers A, Visco AG, et al. Effect of patient position on clinical evaluation of pelvic organ prolapse. Obstet Gynecol. 2000;96(1):18–22.
15. Porges RF. A practical system of diagnosis and classification of pelvic relaxations. Surg Gynecol Obstet. 1963;117:769–73.
16. Bump RC, Mattiasson A, Bø K, Brubaker LP, et al. The standardization of terminology of female pelvic organ prolapse and pelvic floor dysfunction. Am J Obstet Gynecol. 1996;175(1):10–7.
17. Srikrishna S, Robinson D, Cardozo L. A longitudinal study of patient and surgeon goal achievement 2 years after surgery following pelvic floor dysfunction surgery. BJOG. 2010;117(12):1504–11.
18. Saks EK, Harvie HS, Asfaw TS, et al. Clinical significance of obstructive defecatory symptoms in women with pelvic organ prolapse. Int J Gynaecol Obstet. 2010;111(3):237–40.
19. Braekken IH, Majida M, Ellström Engh M, et al. Pelvic floor function is independently associated with pelvic organ prolapse. BJOG. 2009;116(13):1706–14.
20. Miedel A, Tegerstedt G, Maehle-Schmidt M, et al. Nonobstetric risk factors for symptomatic pelvic organ prolapse. Obstet Gynecol. 2009;113(5):1089–97.
21. Whitcomb EL, Rortveit G, Brown JS, et al. Racial differences in pelvic organ prolapse. Obstet Gynecol. 2009;114(6):1271–7.
22. Washington BB, Erekson EA, Kassis NC, et al. The association between obesity and stage II or greater prolapse. Am J Obstet Gynecol. 2010;202(5):503.
23. Scherf C, Morison L, Fiander A, et al. Epidemiology of pelvic organ prolapse in rural Gambia, West Africa. BJOG. 2002;109(4):431–6.
24. Pal L, Hailpern SM, Santoro NF, et al. Association of pelvic organ prolapse and fractures in postmenopausal women: analysis of baseline data from the Women's Health Initiative, Estrogen Plus Progestin trial. Menopause. 2008;15(1):59–66.
25. Mastoroudes H, Giarenis I, Cardozo L, et al. Prolapse and sexual function in women with benign joint hypermobility syndrome. BJOG. 2013;120(2):187–92.
26. Moen MD, Noone MB, Vassallo BJ, et al. Pelvic floor muscle function in women presenting with pelvic floor disorders. Int Urogynecol J Pelvic Floor Dysfunct. 2009;20(7):843–6.
27. Stupp L, Resende AP, Oliveira E, et al. Pelvic floor muscle training for treatment of pelvic organ prolapse: an assessor-blinded randomized controlled trial. Int Urogynecol J. 2011;22(10):1233–9.
28. Braekken IH, Majida M, Engh ME, et al. Can pelvic floor muscle training reverse pelvic organ prolapse and reduce prolapse symptoms? An assessor-blinded, randomized, controlled trial. Am J Obstet Gynecol. 2010;203(2):170.
29. Lang JH, Zhu L, Sun ZJ, et al. Estrogen levels and estrogen receptors in patients with stress urinary incontinence and pelvic organ prolapse. Int J Gynaecol Obstet. 2003;80(1):35–9.

30. Vardy MD, Lindsay R, Scotti RJ, et al. Short-term urogenital effects of raloxifene, tamoxifen, and estrogen. Am J Obstet Gynecol. 2003;189(1):81–8.

31. Mainini G, Scaffa C, Rotondi M, et al. Local estrogen replacement therapy in postmenopausal atrophic vaginitis: efficacy and safety of low dose 17 beta-estradiol vaginal tablets. Clin Exp Obstet Gynecol. 2005;32(2):111–3.

32. Cardozo L, Bachmann G, McClish D, et al. Meta-analysis of estrogen therapy in the management of urogenital atrophy in postmenopausal women: second report of the Hormones and Urogenital Therapy Committee. Obstet Gynecol. 1998;92:722–7.

33. Keller PJ, Riedmann R, Fischer M, et al. Oestrogens, gonadotropins and prolactin after intra-vaginal administration of oestriol in postmenopausal women. Maturitas. 1981;3(1):47–53.

34. Kendall A, Dowsett M, Folkerd E, et al. Caution: vaginal estradiol appears to be contraindicated in postmenopausal women on adjuvant aromatase inhibitors. Ann Oncol. 2006;17(4):584–7.

35. Dew JE, Wren BG, Eden JA. A cohort study of topical vaginal estrogen therapy in women previously treated for breast cancer. Climacteric. 2003;6(1):45–52.

36. Holmberg L, Anderson H. HABITS (hormonal replacement therapy after breast cancer—is it safe?), a randomised comparison: trial stopped. Lancet. 2004;363:453–5.

37. Von Schoultz E, Lars E. Menopausal hormone therapy after breast cancer: the Stockholm randomized trial. J Natl Cancer Inst. 2005;97(7):533–5.

38. Kapoor DS, Thakar R, Sultan AH, et al. Conservative versus surgical management of prolapse: what dictates patient choice? Int Urogynecol J Pelvic Floor Dysfunct. 2009;20(10):1157–61.

39. Cundiff GW, Amundsen CL, Bent AE, et al. The PESSRI study: symptom relief outcomes of a randomized crossover trial of the ring and Gellhorn pessaries. Am J Obstet Gynecol. 2007;196(4):405.e1–8.

40. Kaplan HS. Sex, intimacy, and the aging process. J Am Acad Psychoanal. 1990;18(2):185–205.

41. Hartmann U, Philippsohn S, Heiser K, et al. Low sexual desire in midlife and older women: personality factors, psychosocial development, present sexuality. Menopause. 2004;1:726–40.

42. Leiblum S, Bachmann G, Kemmann E, et al. Vaginal atrophy in the postmenopausal woman. The importance of sexual activity and hormones. JAMA. 1983;249:2195–8.

43. Menard JP, Mulfinger C, Estrade JP, et al. Pelvic organ prolapse surgery in women aged more than 70 years: a literature review. Gynecol Obstet Fertil. 2008;36(1):67–73.

44. Ghezzi F, Uccella S, Cromi A, et al. Surgical treatment for pelvic floor disorders in women 75 years or older: a single-center experience. Menopause. 2011;18(3):314–8.

45. Sung VW, Joo K, Marques F, et al. Patient-reported outcomes after combined surgery for pelvic floor disorders in older compared to younger women. Am J Obstet Gynecol. 2009;201:534.e1–5.

46. Karp DR, Jean-Michel M, Johnston Y. A randomized clinical trial of the impact of local estrogen on postoperative tissue quality after vaginal reconstructive surgery. Female Pelvic Med Reconstr Surg. 2012;18(4):211–5.

47. Yip SK, Pang MW. Tension-free vaginal tape sling procedure for the treatment of stress urinary incontinence in Hong Kong women with and without pelvic organ prolapse: 1-year outcome study. Hong Kong Med J. 2006;12(1):15–20.

48. Partoll LM. Efficacy of tension-free vaginal tape with other pelvic reconstructive surgery. Am J Obstet Gynecol. 2002;186(6):1292–5; discussion 1295–8.

49. Lo TS. Combined pelvic reconstructive surgery and transobturator tape (monarc) in women with advanced prolapse and urodynamic stress incontinence: a case control series. J Minim Invasive Gynecol. 2009;16(2):163–8.

Robotic Pelvic Surgery: Historical Perspective, Single-Site Robotic Surgery and Robotic Sacral Colpopexy

Ray Bologna, Shane Svoboda, and Samantha Staley

Introduction

The rapid advancement of technology over the past 100 years, especially when we contemplate it in the context of man's historical footprint is staggering. It is even more awe inspiring, when we look at the past 30 years. This exponential growth of technology has transformed myth and sometimes even fantasy into the *realities of daily life*. Ancient civilizations could only dream of having automated devices at their disposal and now, we almost take them for granted. The rise of the computer has enabled spectacular progress in almost every aspect of modern society. To say nothing about the fact that computing power doubles every 18 months. Cellular phones and inexpensive computers bring the internet to even the most rural areas of under-developed countries with the implication of putting "real time data" at the fingertips of almost every human being on the planet. Still, what this means with respect to the spread of education around the world via the ability to learn at a distance is almost unfathomable. The microchip, the emergence of genetic engineering and biotechnology must also be considered revolutionary developments, occurring in the second half of this last century. However, in the wake of all of this comes a series of possibilities that link art and science like never before, and at the forefront of this convergence is the science of "robotics." Android robots can fluctuate from feats of great strength and endurance, to being able to mimic the finest and most subtle motions of human activity. Having said all of this, it is important to remember that no single civilization, culture, or era can be credited for modern robotics as many cultures, sciences, and artistic endeavors *inspired imaginations* that made the dreams of fiction into possibility.

Historical Evolution

Mechanical humanoid figurines, created for entertainment in ancient China go back to almost 1000 BC. Subsequently, hundreds of years later, the Greek inventor Archytas Armentum (circa 400 BC) designed a mechanical bird made of wood that could fly up to 200 m on its own, propelling itself with what would be considered a type of a steam engine. Although in and of itself, the wooden bird is an isolated event, it stirred the spirit of creativity in men who were so inclined and paved the way for an Arabic inventor, Ismail al Jazari. Al Jazari (1136–1206) is best known for writing the Arabic text The Book of Knowledge of Ingenious Mechanical Devices written in 1206. Here he was able to create designs for the construction of several automated machines and invented the first programmable robot for entertainment purposes by designing a band with automated humanoid sounds, put in the form of music.

Any serious discussion of robotics cannot begin without an examination of Leonardo da Vinci who has appropriately been attributed with inspiring modern robotics for so many reasons that they would be too numerous to address individually here. However, because of his artistic insight which went far beyond his years, superimposed on the jealousy that he engendered among his contemporaries, he almost never made it.

Leonardo was born on April 15, 1452, in a farmhouse nestled amid the rolling hills of Tuscany. Born out of wedlock to respected Florentine notary Ser Piero and a young peasant woman named Caterina. The bond was doomed to failure before it started. Consequently, to attain any chance

R. Bologna (✉)
Department of Urology, Cleveland Clinic Akron General, 320 W. Exchange Street, Akron, OH 44302, USA
e-mail: raybologna@gmail.com

S. Svoboda
Department of Surgery, Sinai Hospital, Baltimore, MD, USA

S. Staley
Department of Urology, Cleveland Clinic Akron General, Akron, OH, USA

© Springer Science+Business Media New York 2017
D.A. Gordon, M.R. Katlic (eds.), *Pelvic Floor Dysfunction and Pelvic Surgery in the Elderly*,
DOI 10.1007/978-1-4939-6554-0_21

of survival, let alone, success, he had to be raised by his father's family in nearby Vinci, the Tuscan town from which his surname is derived. Hence, he became known in perpetuity as Leonardo da Vinci.

The science of robotics actually begins with the motto that Leonardo wrote for himself as a guide. "A good artist must be a thinker and must have two sacred missions: firstly, *to study the intricacies of the human body* and secondly, *to attempt to understand the human soul.*" "The former is easy, the latter hard, for it must be expressed by gestures and the movement of the limbs." This latter could be construed as the earliest attempt to grasp the science of robotics. To accurately depict gestures and movements of the human being. Not an easy task, but to this end, da Vinci began to seriously study anatomy. Actually, his anatomic studies yielded some of the most accurate anatomic drawings, still useable today. Leonardo's obsession with human anatomy pushed him to critically dissect human bodies during the 1480s. His drawings of a fetus in utero, the heart and vascular system, sex organs, bony tissue, and other muscular structures are some of the first on human record. These dissections paved the way for him to design the first mechanical, (robotic) knight and his most famous treatise on Anatomy and Proportions with the "Vitruvian Man."

Leonardo passed in 1519 but his works, writings and ideas paved the way for others to follow his path. By the 1540s the works of da Vinci had become familiar to an Italian clockmaker of both Italian and Spanish descent named Gianello Torriano. The ideas of da Vinci inspired Torriano to create what was called at that time, automatons and were the first machines to mimic human movements. The most successful automaton was created in the late 1550s and named the Lute Player Lady. This device is 44 cm in height and can strum the lute while turning her head and walking forward. She has survived all these centuries and is now displayed in the Kunstkammer museum in Vienna.

Some consider Pierre Jaquet-Droz to be one of the forefathers of the personal computer. He was born to a family of wealthy Swiss watchmakers and was sent to the University of Basel to study philosophy and theology. His family had hopes that he would enter the priesthood but Pierre had a natural affinity for the physical sciences and soon switched his course direction to math and physics where he was able to study under the famous Daniel Bernoulli. Bernoulli felt Pierre to have an affinity for what would be considered "mechanical physics." Nevertheless, after graduation Pierre returned to the family business where he was asked to work on their line of "pendulum clocks." He did not really feel that this was where his expertise lied and so he moved to "automation mechanics" and developed a line of time pieces that was highly technical and very attractive to some of their "higher end" customers. Not surprisingly, in 1759 Pierre undertook a journey to Spain to present to the Court of King

Ferdinand VI of Spain where he first demonstrated his automata. Included in his presentation was a clock with a shepherd playing on a flute, and a dog guarding a basket of apples. When King Ferdinand tried to take one of the apples, the mechanical dog began barking so naturally, that one of the King's own dogs began to bark back in response. At that time, everyone in the room believed that the entire event was an act of witch craft and ran out of the room, all of them quickly making the "sign of the cross" as they left. The Minister of Marine was the only one that stayed, and asked the shepherd what time it was, but did not receive an answer. Jaquet-Droz remarked that he probably did not understand Spanish and suggested that he be addressed in French. The question was repeated and the shepherd replied immediately. At that point, the frightened Minister hurried away. Jaquet-Droz became concerned about getting arrested by the Inquisition as a sorcerer. Consequently, he immediately invited the Grand Inquisitor to come and reassess the situation and revealed the inner mechanism of his devices. He demonstrated that the mechanism was moved entirely by natural means. Jaquet-Droz's so-called Shepherd's Clock is still on display in one of the King of Spain's palace museums. Subsequently, he created an eerily capable robot in 1772 called "The Writer" that contained a robot capable of writing whatever the user desired by using interchangeable cams, one with each letter of the alphabet. The android, made of 6000 pieces, is sitting on a Louis-XV-style stool, holding a quill (goose feather) that dips into the inkwell, and then he shakes it slightly before beginning to draw letters on paper with the pen. Additional androids were developed by Jaquet-Droz and his son Henri-Louis capable of drawing and playing musical pieces.

The astonishing automated mechanisms of Jaquet-Droz fascinated the world's most important people: the royal families of Europe, China, India, and Japan. The automata were initially exposed in Chaux-de-Fonds, attracting an important crowd (writers of the day reported that people flocked from all over the country to see such extraordinary works of whimsy and technical skill), but the dedication will come with the road show: Geneva (1774), Paris (1775), then Brussels, London, Russia and Madrid, where the automats will be sold to a collector in 1787.

Up to this point, these devices were called by various names, including android or humanoid. The term robot was not really used routinely until the nineteenth century and comes from the Czech word robota meaning forced labor and is derived from the term rab, meaning slave. The use of the term robota first appears in "Rossum's Universal Robot," a play by Karel Capek that describes artificial people who are created to perform mundane tasks to allow real people more leisure time until people use them for malice. These characters warn of modernization and rapid growth of the world that will eventually lead to robots with increasing capabilities that will eventually revolt against their human makers. This fear is a common theme in television and movies today such as The Matrix and Terminator, in which machines become self-aware and realize that their human creators are the problem and should be eliminated to save the world. As we create more advanced technologies these fictional depictions ask an important question: will our own curiosity and hubris be the downfall of man? Is there such a thing as science fiction, or simply scientific eventuality?

In 1942, Isaac Asimov used the term robotics to denote this field of study and outlined the three (3) Rules of Robotics as a safeguard against robotic rebellion against their masters. (1) A robot may not injure a human being, or, through inaction, allow one to come to harm. (2) A robot must obey all orders given to it from humans, except where such orders would contradict the First Law. (3) A robot must protect its own existence, except when to do so would contradict the First Law or the Second Law. These laws continue to pertain to robots used in surgery and the concept of non-maleficence. The robot remained a concept of fiction outside the realm of entertainment until 1951 when Raymond Goertz designed the first tele-operational master–slave manipulator in order to handle hazardous radioactive materials. This initiated the development of other robots for tasks deemed too hazardous for human workers [1–3].

The concept of telepresence is important in the historical development of robotics. Telepresence is the sensation that a person is in one location while being in another. The use of robotics in manufacturing allowed hazardous or unwanted tasks to be performed in a more accurate method.

The scientific definition of a robot is a reprogrammable, computer-controlled mechanical device equipped with sensors and actuators. The first robot used to replace a human worker was the Unimate in 1961. This machine was able to store commands with six degrees of freedom and was able to handle molten die casting and perform spot welding. General Motors realized the significance of this development and utilized these robots on the car assembly. Manufacturers now had the ability to replace human workers with machines that had no fatigue and the ability to perform tasks with repetitive precision. In 1978, the Programmable Universal Machine for Assembly (PUMA) was invented and utilized electronic motors [4, 5]. This was a smaller version of the Unimate robot with multitasking abilities and more variable usage. The robot was then more utilized in fields outside of large manufacturers including medicine. Unlike manufacturing, robots utilized in medicine have never been automated but rather are used as telemanipulators that obey orders through the voice or hand of the surgeon.

The advancements in surgery in the 1980s allowed for a successful minimally invasive approach. The concept of surgery changed with smaller elongated instruments as extensions of the surgeon's hands becoming normal. Minimally invasive surgery reduced the external trauma of a large access incision leading to faster recovery times. Laparoscopic instruments have limitations without wrist articulation, limited haptic feedback, two dimensional views, and poor ergonomics. Robotic surgery has been developed to overcome these limitations to make minimally invasive surgery to be visually and technically equivalent to open surgery.

The PUMA system was used for surgical purposes for the first time in 1985. Neurosurgeons had been looking for a precise method of brain tumor excision. PUMA was used for a CT-guided brain biopsy with an accuracy of 0.05 mm. The success of this biopsy led to a resection of an astrocytoma of the thalamus. The PUMA system was used in the UK for urologic procedures including transurethral resection of the prostate that was succeeded with the surgeon-assistant robot for prostatectomy or SARP [2]. In the late 1980s the PROBOT used a computer generated 3D model of the prostate to outline area of resection and a 40,000-rpm rotating blade with four axes of movement. The orthopedic surgeons had already been using the Arthrobot in 1983 to assist with orthopedic procedures. This technology advanced to the ROBODOC in 1988 that used the robot to precisely drill the femoral head and insert the hip replacement prosthesis in total hip arthroplasty with 24,000 procedures performed by 2007.

The Automated Endoscopic System for Optimal Positioning (AESOP) was the next breakthrough in robotic surgery in 1994 [6, 7]. This was the first laparoscopic camera holder approved by the FDA with later generations adding voice control and seven degrees of freedom to mimic the human hand with the AESOP 3000 in 1998. This device allowed a more stable camera platform than a surgical assistant with no increase in operative time. The next advancement was seen with the ZEUS system (Computer Motion, Santa Barbara, CA, USA) in 1998 with the idea of telerobotics or telepresence to robotic surgery using a console with a surgeon (master) at a distance from the robot (slave) that operates on the patient. This system has fame for successful first full endoscopic procedure of fallopian tube reanastomosis. This robotic system used three arms with a 3D endoscope viewed and controlled through the surgeon console. In the same year the da Vinci system performed a robot-assisted heart bypass. Telerobotics was research funded by the US Department of Defense to allow for remote surgeries using mobile operating facilities and surgeons able to perform from a distance. In 2000, the da Vinci® robot was FDA approved for use in laparoscopic procedures. Intuitive Surgical, Inc. purchased Computer Motion, Inc. in 2003 and is currently the sole company marketing robotic surgical devices [2].

Intuitive Surgical, Inc. has made impressive and rapid advancements in technology despite less competition. The da Vinci® robot technology consisted of 3D vision, EndoWrist® instrumentation with 7 degrees of freedom, Intuitive motion, ergonomic superiority, and surgical precision. In 2003, a fourth robotic arm was added to the da Vinci® system allowing for greater control of retraction. In 2006, the da Vinci® S system was released with enhanced vision and multi-image display. In 2009 the da Vinci® Si system allowed for dual console capability allowing for collaborative operations and improved training as well as the use of the Single-Site® system. The newest version is the da Vinci® Xi surgical System (2014) has been developed based on surgeon feedback and enhanced engineering. Overhead instrument arm architecture facilitates anatomical access. The endoscope has been designed more compact with improved visual definition and clarity and can now be changed to any arm. The arms have been made smaller and thinner with improved joints for greater range of motion. Longer instrument shafts allow for longer operative reach. This system is designed for easy transitioning to multi-quadrant cases that previously required complicated docking, repositioning and in most cases additional trocars. The system has also been designed compatible with the Firefly® Fluorescence Imaging System. The da Vinci® Sp single port robot-assisted surgical system has been developed to allow multiple flexible instruments and flexible endoscope through a single incision and was designed for urologic procedures.

Single-Site Robotic Surgery

The future of robotic surgery seems limited only to our own imaginations. Minimally invasive surgery has progressed rapidly with the invention of laparoscopy and robotic-assisted surgery. Single-Site® robotic surgery was designed to reduce body wall trauma and improve cosmetic outcomes in patients [8, 9]. Operations through a single incision in the umbilicus to remove the gallbladder or the uterus result in virtually scarless surgery. The single incision was also intended to reduce postoperative pain although this has not been proven compared to multiport laparoscopy. Single-incision laparoscopic surgery had the same intentions but has been criticized for the loss of triangulation and ergonomic difficulties. Single-Site® surgery has permitted more precision and freedom of movement with the robotic system restoring intuitive correlation handedness of the instruments through curved cannulas.

The Single-Site® system is compatible with the da Vinci® Si surgical system. It utilizes a single flexible port consisting of five lumens that provide access for the 8.5 mm 3D high definition endoscope, two 5 mm instruments a 5/10 mm accessory port, and the insufflation adapter. The pliable architecture of the port allows for positioning within a 2.0–2.5 cm incision in the fascia at the umbilicus. The port is marked for accurate placement to ensure remote center. The instrument cannulae are curved to allow crossing within the port to optimize triangulation toward the target anatomy and provide an unobstructed view of the surgical field without camera collisions. The rigid curved cannulae allow for passage of semi-rigid instruments with the flexibility to pass while maintaining enough rigidity for tissue retraction. The software of the robotic system detects and re-associates the user's hands with the instrument tips to create movement and restore handedness. Single-incision laparoscopic surgery that utilizes curved cannulae forces the surgeon to use counterintuitive ergonomics or crossed hands that are resolved with the robotic system [10, 11].

Single-Site® robotic surgery was initially intended for cholecystectomy, removal of the gallbladder. This platform allows for perfect triangulation to display Calot's triangle with a stable three-dimensional high definition view. The robotic system allows for restored dexterity, ease, safety, and precision that is equivalent to the traditional four-trocar laparoscopic cholecystectomy. This technique has also been shown to be significantly faster than single-incision laparoscopic cholecystectomy [12, 13]. No significant difference has been shown in the pain scores between the four-port cholecystectomy and single-incision cholecystectomy [14].

The introduction of Firefly® technology that utilizes infrared fluorescent vision may be able to improve safety of the operation. This system using the Single-Site® platform uses an intravenous injection of indocyanine green preoperatively that is excreted via the biliary system. The surgeon is able to quickly transition between standard high definition 3D view and fluorescence view to obtain a dynamic fluorescent cholangiogram to identify biliary structures. This prevents the need for undocking and the additional equipment and time needed for traditional injected contrast cholangiogram. Studies have shown this to be safe, economical, and equivalent to standard cholangiogram. With larger sample size, this may even be more effective in correctly identifying biliary structures [15, 16].

Although current literature includes only small series of patients who have undergone single-site robotic cholecystectomy, the quantity of procedures that have been performed is rapidly increasing. Konstantinidis et al. reported the largest published experience so far with da Vinci® Single-Site cholecystectomy with 45 patients without conversion to open although in three cases a second trocar was used. Intraoperative blood loss was negligible. Our institution has a series of over 200 patients with no conversion to open or multiport surgery including majority of non-elective cases, most with acute cholecystitis. Most patients were discharged within 24 h of surgery with no major complications and an umbilical hernia rate of 2 % at follow-up.

The possible uses have increased to include gynecologic and colonic surgery. The Single-Site® system has been FDA approved for hysterectomy and cholecystectomy with good feasibility and safety outcomes. Studies have looked at using this technique in low risk endometrial cancer and found it technically feasible [17]. Cases have been performed including appendectomy and right hemicolectomy although these are currently not approved [18].

The advancement of instrumentation to restore instrument flexion with EndoWrist technology and increased degrees of freedom that was initially lost, the single-site system will be able to assist in procedures reserved for multiport cases. Single-Site surgery will expand to additional indications in the years to come.

Robotic-Assisted Abdominal Sacrocolpopexy

Pelvic organ prolapse (POP) is common condition among the female population with resulting symptoms often requiring intervention. In a review of over 10 million women between 2007 and 2011, the lifetime risk of surgery for POP was 12.6 % by the age of 80. The evolution of the management of POP is significant with an increase in minimally invasive techniques coming to the forefront over the last 10 years.

Abdominal sacrocolpopexy has been considered the gold standard for *apical prolapse correction* [19, 20]. One of the largest group of patients that require some type of apical prolapse correction are the patients who have significant vaginal vault prolapse (Fig. 21.1), even progressing toward complete vaginal eversion.

Robotic-Assisted Abdominal Sacrocolpopexy

Though this is an invasive technique, long-term follow-up has demonstrated a failure rate, or recurrent apical prolapse, to be only 5 %. Vaginal techniques for POP correction also exist, however, dyspareunia and other long-term complications

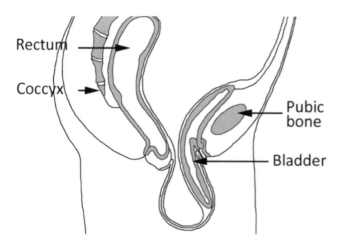

Fig. 21.1   Vaginal vault prolapse

are lower for sacrocolpopexy [21]. Minimally invasive techniques were therefore introduced to improve the morbidity, visualization, and postoperative results of this well-established and durable procedure [22–35]. Laparoscopic or robotic-assisted laparoscopic sacrocolpopexy (RASCP) has the advantage of decreased recovery time, decreased length of stay, decreased blood loss, and equal outcomes to open sacrocolpopexy.

Technique Considerations

In recent years, there has been an expanding use of robot technology. After its FDA approval in 1999, Robotic surgery was formally introduced in the USA. The da Vinci® surgical system was the preferred modality and since its inception at about the same time, it has gained great popularity. The basic principles of laparoscopic surgery apply and the setup is similar. Trocar placement must meet the technical requirements of the da Vinci® itself. Essentially, a 12-mm telescope port is placed midline just superior to the umbilicus at a distance 15 cm from the pubic symphysis. Two 8-mm working arms are placed bilaterally along an imaginary line from the camera port to the anterior superior iliac spine. These ports are placed caudally and should be approximately 8 cm away from the camera trocar to prevent the da Vinci® working arms from colliding.

A fifth port can be placed on the left side in the same fashion if needed for retraction. Typically, the surgeon stands on the patient's left. Newer models have three working surgical arms and a fourth arm for the telescope. Dissection is performed with monopolar scissors and bipolar cautery.

A graft material is selected (e.g., polypropylene mesh) and trimmed to size. A Y-shaped graft is fashioned from two pieces; a long arm placed anteriorly and a shorter posterior arm. The arms are fixed to each other using 2-0 nonabsorbable monofilament suture. The anterior arm is fixed using nonabsorbable 2-0 monofilament sutures through the pores of the mesh and into the vaginal muscularis using robotic needle drivers. One to two are placed at the most distal aspect of the graft and one to two at the most distal aspect of the anterior vaginal cuff. The sutures are placed deep through the muscularis but should not penetrate through the vaginal mucosa itself. Three to four sutures are then placed posteriorly in a similar fashion. Alternatively, bone anchoring devices are available to fix the mesh to the sacral promontory. The third working arm can be set up on the left side and placed approximately 8–9 cm away from the other working port. It should be 5 cm cranial and medial to the anterior superior iliac spine.

Conclusions

Improvements in robotic technology have allowed surgeons without advanced laparoscopic skills to perform minimally invasive surgical techniques. The sacrocolpopexy which requires a significant amount of suturing and dissection within the pelvis highlights some of the benefits of robotic technology which include three-dimensional visualization and improved operative dexterity. The addition of robotics has allowed for a time tested open surgical procedure to be duplicated in the laparoscopic format.

Two important pitfalls regarding the robotic sacrocolpopexy have been operative time and cost. Operative time is significantly affected by surgeon experience and case volume. Intracorporal suturing and knot-tying along with sacral promontory dissection have been identified as critical time-consuming steps for robotic sacrocolpopexy procedures. In an analysis of operative step times as well as overall time for RASCP, it was shown that a significant improvement was seen after 20–60 cases. With this in mind, the idea of robotic training to improve technical skills is highlighted with the overall goal to improve operative efficiency and thus decrease operative time and cost. Simulation training has, therefore, become a focus of many residency training programs. An additional consideration for operative time must include the inclusion of concomitant procedures as more than one third of patients also undergo anti-incontinence procedures. A well-known benefit of any robotic surgery is the opportunity for decreased length of stay. At our institution, robotic sacrocolpopexy has transitioned to an outpatient minimally invasive procedure in many cases. Elliott et al. performed a cost-analysis proving that a robotic approach can be equally or less costly than open if there is sufficient volume and consistent shorter length of stays for patients.

Although the minimally invasive approach to sacrocolpopexy has proven to be beneficial for patients, controversies exist regarding certain aspects of the procedure. Certainly, the controversy regarding the use of mesh has been driven by the Food and Drug Administration's public health notice. Retroperitonealization of the mesh helps to prevent complications that involve mesh interaction with intraabdominal organs. The primary concern regarding mesh has become erosion. Supracervical hysterectomy, after exclusion of cervical disease, has reduced the risk of this to a minimum. In a comparison of patients who underwent sacrocolpopexy with concomitant supracervical or total hysterectomy, erosion rates were found to be 0 vs 14 %, respectively. Often, patients request uterine preservation. This is a reasonable option with proper informed consent preoperative evaluation. Various articles have described techniques for hysteropexy. Hysteropexy is certainly an alternative for women with a normal uterus desiring uterine preservation.

With the first series of patients undergoing a robotic-assisted laparoscopic sacrocolpopexy reported in 2004 by Di Marco et al., significant advancement has been made in this procedure by critical analysis of many patient series. Review of this procedure offers a good example of how robotics has been incorporated to take an effective procedure and allow improvements to now offer this as an outpatient intervention. Future advances will likely be related to robotic technology to continue to improve operative efficiency and materials to continue to decrease operative complications.

References

1. Hockstein NG, Gourin CG, Faust RA, Terris DJ. A history of robots: from science fiction to surgical robotics. J Robot Surg. 2007;1(2):113–8.
2. Bann S, Khan M, Hernandez J, et al. Robotics in surgery. J Am Coll Surg. 2003;196(5):784–95.
3. Yates DR, Vaessen C, Roupret M. From leonardo to da vinci: the history of robot-assisted surgery in urology. BJU Int. 2011;108(11): 1708–13. discussion 1714.
4. Kwoh YS, Hou J, Jonckheere EA, Hayati S. A robot with improved absolute positioning accuracy for CT guided stereotactic brain surgery. IEEE Trans Biomed Eng. 1988;35(2):153–60.
5. Dogangil G, Davies BL, Rodriguez y Baena F. A review of medical robotics for minimally invasive soft tissue surgery. Proc Inst Mech Eng H. 2010;224(5):653–79.
6. Unger SW, Unger HM, Bass RT. AESOP robotic arm. Surg Endosc. 1994;8(9):1131.
7. Paul HA, Bargar WL, Mittlestadt B, et al. Development of a surgical robot for cementless total hip arthroplasty. Clin Orthop Relat Res. 1992;285:57–66.
8. Kroh M, El-Hayek K, Rosenblatt S, et al. First human surgery with a novel single-port robotic system: cholecystectomy using the da vinci single-site platform. Surg Endosc. 2011;25(11): 3566–73.
9. Wren SM, Curet MJ. Single-port robotic cholecystectomy: results from a first human use clinical study of the new da vinci single-site surgical platform. Arch Surg. 2011;146(10):1122–7.
10. Haber GP, White MA, Autorino R, et al. Novel robotic da vinci instruments for laparoendoscopic single-site surgery. Urology. 2010;76(6):1279–82.
11. Pietrabissa A, Sbrana F, Morelli L, et al. Overcoming the challenges of single-incision cholecystectomy with robotic single-site technology. Arch Surg. 2012;147(8):709–14.
12. Spinoglio G, Lenti LM, Maglione V, et al. Single-site robotic cholecystectomy (SSRC) versus single-incision laparoscopic cholecystectomy (SILC): comparison of learning curves. First European experience. Surd Endosc. 2012;26(6):1648–55.
13. Spinoglio G, Lenti LM. Single-port robotically assisted laparoscopic surgery. Br J Surg. 2014;101(2):3–4.
14. Prasad A, Mukherjee KA, Kaul S, Kaur M. Postoperative pain after cholecystectomy: conventional laparoscopy versus single-incision laparoscopic surgery. J Minim Access Surg. 2011;7(1):24–7.
15. Ishizawa T, Tamura S, Masuda K, et al. Intraoperative fluorescent cholangiography using indocyanine green: a biliary road map for safe surgery. J Am Coll Surg. 2009;208(1):e1–4.
16. Osayi SN, Wendling MR, Drosdeck JM, et al. Near-infrared fluorescent cholangiography facilitates identification of biliary anatomy during laparoscopic cholecystectomy. Surg Endosc. 2015; 29(2):368–75.

17. Vizza E, Corrado G, Mancini E, et al. Robotic single-site hysterectomy in low risk endometrial cancer: a pilot study. Ann Surg Oncol. 2013;20(8):2759–64.

18. Ostrowitz MB, Eschete D, Zemon H, DeNoto G. Robotic-assisted single-incision right colectomy: early experience. Int J Med Robot. 2009;5(4):465–70.

19. Nygaard I, Brubaker L, Zycezynski H, et al. Long-term outcomes following abdominal sacrocolpopexy for pelvic organ prolapse. JAMA 2013;309(19):2016–24.

20. Brubaker L, Nygaard I, Richter HE, et al. Two-year outcomes after sacrocolpopexy with and without Burch to prevent stress urinary incontinence. Obstet Gynecol. 2008;112:49–55.

21. Maher C, Feiner B, Baessler K, Adams EJ, Hagen S, Glazener CMA. Surgical management of pelvic organ prolapse in women [update in Cochrane Database Syst Rev. 2013;(4):CD004014]. Cochrane Database Syst Rev. 2010;4:CD004014.

22. Di Biase M, Mearini L, Zucchi A, et al. Abdominal vs laparoscopic sacrocolpopexy: a randomized controlled trial. J Urol. 2015; 193:e1035.

23. Freeman RM, Pantazis K, Thomson A, et al. A randomised controlled trial of abdominal versus laparoscopic sacrocolpopexy for the treatment of post-hysterectomy vaginal vault prolapse: LAS study. Int Urogynecol J. 2013;24:377–84.

24. Serati M, Bogani, G, Sorice P, et al. Robot-assisted sacrocolpopexy for pelvic organ prolapse: a systematic review and meta-analysis of comparative studies. Eur Urol. 2014;66(2):303–18.

25. US Food and Drug Administration. FDA Public Health Notification: serious complications associated with transvaginal placement of surgical mesh in repair of pelvic organ prolapse and stress urinary incontinence. http://www.fda.gov/medicaldevices/safety/alertsand-notices/publichealthnotification/ucm061976.htm.

26. Parkes I, Shveiky D. Sacrocolpopexy for treatment of vaginal apical prolapse: evidence-based surgery. J Minim Invasive Gynecol. 2014;21:546–57.

27. Warner WB, Vora S, Hurtado EA, Welgoss JA, et al. Effect of operative technique on mesh exposure in laparoscopic sacrocolpopexy. Female Pelvic Med Reconstr Surg. 2012;18:113–7.

28. Carey R, Martin C, Pilkington J. Robotic-assisted sacrocolpopexy with uterus preservation: trans-broad ligament anterior and posterior fixation. J Urol. 2013;189(4s):e107.

29. Wu JM, Matthews CA, Conover MM, Pate V, Jonsson Funk M. Lifetime risk of stress urinary incontinence or pelvic organ prolapse surgery. Obstet Gynecol. 2014;123(6):1201–6.

30. Mcdermott CD, Hale DS. Abdominal, laparoscopic, and robotic surgery for pelvic organ prolapse. Obstet Gynecol Clin N Am 2009:36(3);585–614.

31. Osmundsen BC, Clark A, Goldsmith C, Adams K, Denman MA, Edwards R, Gregory WT. Mesh erosion in robotic sacrocolpopexy. Female Pelvic Med Reconstr Surg. 2012;18(2):86–8.

32. Elliott CS, Hsieh MH, Chen B, Comiter, CV, Payne CK, Sokol ER. Can robotic surgery be cost effective? A cost-minimization analysis of robotic-assisted versus open sacrocolpopexy. J Minim Invasive Gynecol. 2011;18(6):S25.

33. Geller EJ, Lin F-C, Matthews CA. Analysis of robotic performance times to improve operative efficiency. J Minim Invasive Gynecol. 2013;20(1);43–8.

34. Di Marco DS, Chow GK, Gettman MT, Elliott DS. Robotic-assisted laparoscopic sacrocolpopexy for treatment of vaginal vault prolapse. Urology 2004;63(2):373–6.

35. Lee RK, Mottrie A, Payne CK, Waltregny D. A review of the current status of laparoscopic and robot-assisted sacrocolpopexy for pelvic organ prolapse. Eur Urol. 2014; 65(6):1128–37.

Okechukwu A. Ibeanu and David A. Gordon

Historical Perspective

Genito-urinary fistulas are abnormal connections between the urinary tract and the vagina which allows for a continuous involuntary drainage of urine into the perineum and excoriating the perineal skin. In addition, the medical complications associated with these fistulae, often have a more profound effect on the patient's emotional well being. The surgical intervention of genito-urinary fistulas is often credited as a modern phenomena, however, in actuality, physicians have been trying to deal with this problem for thousands of years, perhaps as long as women have been baring children. Nevertheless, understanding all of this, it is somewhat surprising that the medical literature is so sparse regarding this clinical issue, relatively speaking.

The earliest evidence that vesicovaginal fistula (VVF) has been a universal plight of women who have had the virtuous opportunity to procreate was actually not uncovered until the twentieth century. It was about 1923 when a medical and archeological tour headed by Dr. Derry uncovered a large VVF in the mummy of Henhenit, who was genealogically traced back to the 11th dynasty of Egypt where she reined as a queen. She lived circa 2050 BC and is the earliest documented case of such a fistulous connection. More importantly, this _

O.A. Ibeanu
Gynecologic Oncology, Johns Hopkins University,
Baltimore, MD, USA

Alvin and Lois Lapidus Cancer Institute, at Sinai Hospital,
Baltimore, MD, USA

Alvin and Lois Lapidus Cancer Institute, at Northwest Hospital,
Randallstown, MD, USA

D.A. Gordon (✉)
Division of Pelvic Neuroscience, Department of Surgery,
The Sinai Hospital of Baltimore, 2401 W. Belvedere Avenue,
Baltimore, MD 21215, USA
e-mail: dgordon@lifebridgehealth.org

discovery started the quest for a *"historical roadmap of VVF"* through the ages. The scientific realization of this medical entity as a clinical complication was not written for another 500 years until circa 1550 BC when it was found on an Egyptian papyrus. However, it was not until Avicenna, a Persian physician, almost 2500 years later in 1037 AD, when the connection between VVF and obstructed labor was formally made in his document "A History of Obstetric VVF."

The first collection of surgical principles outlined for the repair of VVF were described in 1663 by Hedrik von Roonhuyse. Here he talks about specific fundamental maneuvers to be practiced which would give the patient the best chances for clinical cure. In his manuscript he stressed four components. These were (1) placement of the patient in the "dorsolithotomy" position (a novel idea at that time), (2) the use of a vaginal introital spreading apparatus *(a speculum)* to enhance operative exposure and visualization, (3) surgical scraping for denudation of the anomalous "bladder–vaginal connection," and (4) finally mechanical re-approximation of the edges of the fistulous tract with *"freshly cleansed swan quills."* Twelve years later, in 1675, Johann Fatio utilized the above 4 principles that were put forth by von Roonhuyse to perform and document the first successful surgical repair of a VVF. Nevertheless, as innovative and successful as this repair was, the surgical treatment for the correction of VVFs did not become even moderately common until the nineteenth century with the notoriety of Dr. *James Marion Sims*.

Sims was American, born and raised in rural South Carolina, where he spent time with his father often caring for their livestock in a surgical fashion. After entrance into an undergraduate program at the South Carolina College in Columbia, a well-known local surgeon, Dr. Churchill Jones took young Sims under his wing and pushed him to formally study medicine at the Medical College in Charlestown South Carolina. There he became concerned that he would not get the surgical exposure which he longed for, so he transferred to the Jefferson Medical College in Philadelphia Pennsylvania where he graduated in 1835.

© Springer Science+Business Media New York 2017
D.A. Gordon, M.R. Katlic (eds.), *Pelvic Floor Dysfunction and Pelvic Surgery in the Elderly*,
DOI 10.1007/978-1-4939-6554-0_22

After graduation Sims immersed himself into the arena of "female pelvic surgery" in Montgomery, Alabama where he experimented on captive slave women who were outcasts because they suffered from intractable urinary incontinence secondary to large vesicovaginal fistulas. Over the course of the next 5–10 years he successfully repaired fistulas in both slave and Caucasian women. These experiments allowed Sims to perfect his technique as well as develop his instrumentation. Specifically, he devised the Sims' speculum to gain proper exposure, perfected the "rectal position" where a patient is on the left side with the right knee flexed against the abdomen and the left knee slightly flexed is also named after him as "Sims' position." He focused on cleanliness which later gave way to the "concept of sterility" and finally insisted on using "monofilament silver-wire sutures" which he felt decreased his infectious risk and ultimately led to successful repair of the fistula. This was all reported and documented in his 1852 manuscript. The next year (1853), Sims moved north to New York City and was determined to focus on diseases of women. Three years later, in 1855, he founded the first hospital for women in America, The Woman's Hospital of New York City. It was here that he performed operations on indigent women, often in a theater so that others could view it. Interestingly, in 1871, after quarreling with the board of the Woman's Hospital over the admission of cancer patients, Sims went on to found a new hospital, the Memorial Center for Cancer and Allied Diseases, which would later evolve and became The Memorial Sloan–Kettering Cancer Center. The final chapter of his life was spent trying to develop physician organizations in the USA and to that end, he served as president of the upstart American Medical Association from 1876–1877. The remainder of the nineteenth century was studded with names like Trendelenberg, Maisonneuve, and Mackenrodt who were all involved in understanding the subtleties of the pathophysiology of VVF and developing newer techniques to enhance repair. Of these, separating the layers of the fistula and closing each one individually.

At the turn of the twentieth century several additional techniques were developed to improve outcomes in the repair of VVFs. Kelly advocated the use of ureteral catheters to help decrease the risk of ureteral injury. Latzko proposed the technique of partial colpocleisis to repair post hysterectomy VVFs where he promoted the resection of scarred vaginal.

At the turn of the twentieth century several additional techniques were developed to improve outcomes in the repair of VVFs. Kelly advocated the use of ureteral catheters to help decrease the risk of ureteral injury. Latzko proposed the technique of partial colpocleisis to repair post hysterectomy VVFs where he promoted the resection of scarred vaginal mucosa and finish with a layered closure in a horizontal fashion. Latzko's procedure has been cited in many different series' to have success rates that approach 95–100 %. By the midpoint of the century, O'Conor et al. began to popularize a transabdominal approach, which was ideal in patients who had fistulas that were high up in the vagina. In addition, he went on to study smaller VVFs. Specifically, he looked at those less than 4 mm. Here he proposed scraping the tract to attempt to "de-epithelialize" it and then superimposing electrocoagulation at the site, with success rates that range from 70 to 80 %.

The latter half of the twentieth century was spent researching complimentary procedures to enhance fistula closure, more specifically the development of vascularized pedicles or flaps to interpose between individual layers during closure. This list includes Garlock who proposed the Gracilis Muscle Flap with maintenance of its vascular pedicle, Ingelman-Sundberg who proposed utilizing the closet muscle to the fistulous tract where the pedicle can be maintained. His suggestions were to use either the pubococcygeus, bulbocavernosus, gracilis or finally the distal aspects of the rectus abdominis. Kiricuta and Goldstein popularized the use of an Omental Flap based on the pedicle of the right gastroepiploic artery. Finally, and possibly most importantly in these cases are the reconstructive repairs which were proposed by Dr. Martius. He suggested the use of the "*sublabial substance*." This ***sublabial substance*** could be the superficial "fat pad" and its associated vascular pedicle, or if necessary using the associated vascular pedicle and the underlying bulbocavernosus muscle.

The collective discussions regarding the pathology, surgical treatment, and emotional overlay with respect to urogenital fistulae are difficult at best. Many would argue that they are among the most challenging topics that fall within the realm of "Pelvic Surgery." Not only are they difficult to deal with from a clinical perspective, there is a tremendous amount of associated psycho-social and emotional overlay. The technical breakthroughs that have occurred in this arena have often allowed for suffering females who had been cast out of society to be reaccepted. In a final summation, it is important to note that the above historical litany of those who have pushed the reconstructive envelope in this area is by no means complete. As much as it is our desire to be comprehensive, it would be impossible to list all the names of those many creative surgeons who have helped understand, advance, and raise the level of awareness about all aspects of this very difficult problem.

Introduction

Vesicovaginal fistulae stem from two distinct and diverse types of etiology. The first would be neglected obstetrical labor and the second, complications in gynecologic surgery. These are the main etiologic factors for vesicovaginal fistula. Globally, most fistulae are secondary to neglected obstetrical issues surrounding labor. This is especially prominent in sub-Saharan Africa where the numbers are so high that the true incidence is unknown. Some report an incidence of 1 or 2 per 1000 deliveries [1] but recent presentations and discussions at an international fistula meeting at Johns Hopkins in August of 2005 suggest that all estimates are wildly inaccurate such as the estimate of 5 million per year [2].

Interestingly, obstetrically related fistulae have been practically eradicated in more well-developed countries such as the USA, Scandinavia, and Western Europe. The incidence of obstetrical fistulas in these countries has almost hit zero. Today most fistulas seen in the USA are from gynecologic surgery, in particular abdominal hysterectomy [3]. Fistulas from gynecologic malignancy and/or radiation therapy are now more uncommon. The prevalence of obstetrical fistulae still remains a problem in Africa and less developed regions of Asia and Oceania [4]. Until there are improvements in obstetrical care, especially with respect to prolonged obstructed labor, this problem will persist.

We will discuss the gynecologic and obstetric fistula separately as their cause and cure are a bit different. Obstetrical injuries are a "field" injury, often with associated ischemic changes to the bladder and vagina ultimately leading to tissue breakdown from the prolonged pressure of an impacted fetal head against the tissues [5–7]. Finally, it is important to note here that most gynecologic injuries except those related to radiation are a local injury with minimal changes in the adjacent tissues.

Gynecologic Fistulae

Etiology

In modern well-developed countries such as the USA, vesicovaginal fistulae (VVFs) are most commonly associated with hysterectomy. For example, approximately 82% of VVFs seen in the USA are associated with hysterectomy [6]. Urologic procedures account for another 6% while pelvic irradiation, trauma, and malignant disease account for approximately 4% of cases [5]. Gynecologic VVF (Fig. 22.1) are usually secondary to poorly developed dissection planes between the bladder and the cervix in the lower uterine segment. This faulty dissection plane is usually the result of distortion of tissues. Conditions which may predispose to this type of distortion include uterine leiomyoma, previous cesareans, and other pelvic conditions leading to loss of surgical plains such as endometriosis and pelvic inflammatory disease. Tissue trauma leads to local breakdown of tissue. Electrocautery, infection, smoking, radiation, and diabetes contribute to local tissue breakdown and poor wound healing.

It is important to note some of the specifics with respect to wound healing and VVF. Wound healing has 4 phases: (1) coagulation, (2) inflammation, (3) fibroplasia, and (4) remodeling. With respect to gynecologic VVF in the USA, it is during the fibroplasia phase where most of the predisposition toward VVF occurs. Fibroplastic collagen formation peaks at day 7 and continues for 2–3 weeks. It is this time period when hypoxia, ischemia, malnutrition, radiation, or chemotherapy will lead to tissue breakdown. However, Meeks [6] suggests that inadvertent suture in the bladder may or may not contribute to fistula formation. Interestingly, it is the blunt trauma of utilizing a sponge stick to force the dissection of the bladder off the lower uterine segment may also be associated with fistula etiology. In fact, 70–80% of bladder injuries during gynecologic surgery go unrecognized [7]. Radiation fistulae occur with endarteritis and tissue ischemia with necrosis and fibrosis. The lesion may present months to years after radiation treatment [8]. Urologic injury

Fig. 22.1 Gynecologic vesicovaginal fistula

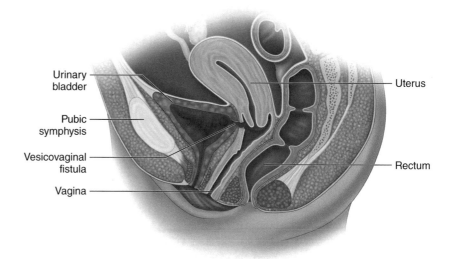

Urinary bladder

Pubic symphysis

Vesicovaginal fistula

Vagina

Uterus

Rectum

Table 22.1 Surgical techniques for minimizing lower urinary tract injuries during gynecologic surgery

1. Proper positioning of the patient to allow abdominal and vaginal access
2. Provide adequate exposure and lighting of the surgical field
3. The surgeon must be familiar with the anatomy of the space being entered
4. Performance of blunt and sharp dissection where appropriate. Blunt dissection is appropriate along certain established spaces in the pelvis (i.e., pubo-cervical space) but sharp dissection is needed to enter the space. When unsure, always use sharp dissection
5. Always be aware of the course of the ureter and protect from injury
6. When encountering bleeding, pressure should be applied while setting up for identifying the source without wild attempts to stop bleeding with a clamp without adequate visualization. Pressure, adequate suction, a deep breath, and then attempt to identify the source of bleeding
7. Avoid large pedicles
8. Continuous bladder drainage for abdominal cases
9. Intraoperative cystoscopy for all hysterectomy and pelvic reconstructive surgery to insure the integrity of the lower urinary tract system[10]
10. Minimize the use of extensive electrocautery in *the area of the bladder in proximity to the vaginal cuff*

is a well-known complication of laparoscopic surgery, and with the increasing use of laparoscopy in gynecologic surgery, such complications will be seen more often. Minimizing the risk of injury at the time of surgery is the goal of the surgeon (Table 22.1).

Presentation

Urinary incontinence is the most common presenting symptom following fistulous injury to the bladder. The loss of urine can be traced to the vagina, not the urethra and although frequently worse with stress or increased Valsalva, it is constant and persistent throughout the voiding cycle. Patients may complain of such symptoms immediately following the procedure once the urethral catheter is removed if there is a gross defect. More commonly the leakage starts in 2–4 weeks after surgery. Other symptoms may include transient hematuria, or fever and chills preceding loss of urine followed by defervescence of fever. Abdominal flank pain may also be present but this association is more common for ureteral vaginal fistula. In most cases, however, patients may remain relatively symptom free and complain of only occasional abnormal vaginal discharge followed by gross leakage. It has been estimated that up to 50 % of post-surgical fistulas may present after 10 days [8]. Signs of peritonitis and ileus may accompany intraperitoneal leakage of urine.

Management

The initial management of heavy leakage of urine from the vagina should be prompted by a high index of suspicion for a vesicovaginal fistula. The fistula may be visualized with a vaginal speculum but very small or high fistulas may be difficult to visualize. Diagnosis will be aided by instilling methylene blue dye into the bladder. If the blue is not seen vaginally, the placement of a tampon may help visualize the small fistula. If still not visualized, an ureterovaginal fistula

must be considered. Either indigo carmine intravenous or phenazopyridine (Pyridium®) orally may be given to determine if the leakage is from an ureterovaginal fistula. Again placing a tampon in the vagina will help to determine if the leakage is from an ureterovaginal fistula. This will also help to distinguish the leakage from intrinsic sphincter deficiency, which may also give continuous leakage. If still unclear, intravenous pyelogram should be performed, especially if suspicion of a compound fistula including the bladder and ureter. If the uterus is still present and the Indigo Carmine test is negative, cystoscopy with retrograde cannulation and injection of a defect may be necessary to rule out a vesicouterine/vesicocervical fistula [9]. Many times there is relative stenosis of the endocervical canal making this diagnosis difficult as urine may spill differentially into the abdominal cavity through the fallopian tubes. The patency of the ureters can also be confirmed by giving the patient intravenous indigo carmine dye just before the cystoscopy. Contrast cystography can also be used as a diagnostic test; however, it is not as sensitive and has a higher false negative rate than other tests. The status of the upper urinary tracts should be investigated with intravenous pyelogram if there is a suspicion of upper tract involvement.

Urinalysis with culture and sensitivity should be performed so that any urinary infection can be aggressively treated. At the time of cystoscopy any foreign bodies such as suture material should be removed from the area of the fistula in order to facilitate clearing inflammation of the area prior to repair.

Treatment

Non-surgical

A small but unknown percentage of vesicovaginal fistulae may heal spontaneously with conservative management involving prolonged bladder drainage using a suprapubic or urethral catheter. While such bladder drainage may increase the risk of infection, very small fistulas involving the poster wall may heal this way. Foley drainage may lessen the perineal irritation while waiting for the inflammatory reaction to resolve. The use of a Foley catheter connected to a birth control diaphragm may also lessen the perineal irritation by diverting the urine flow. Large complicated fistulas will inevitably need to be addressed surgically.

Surgical

Traditionally, an interval of at least 3–6 months was advised before the surgical repair of the vesicovaginal fistula is undertaken. This author only waits for the inflammation to resolve and this has not led to failures of the Latsko colpocleisis procedure in uncomplicated patients who were never radiated has been reported by others. Fistulae associated with radiation therapy should not be immediately repaired as the radiation scarring will continue to affect the tissues for a much longer time. The use of a Foley catheter once the fistula has been diagnosed will allow any associated tissue edema or inflammation to subside and in rare cases will permit spontaneous closure. Prolonged urinary leakage past 2–3 months can be associated with more significant emotional overlay.

Several surgical techniques have been described for closure of VVF. Regardless, any repair must be performed with strict adherence to basic surgical principles in order to maximize the chances of a successful repair. Meticulous tissue dissection should be performed in order to adequately expose the fistula site and all layers of closure should be tension free, watertight, and non-opposing. If deemed necessary, the use of a tissue interposition flaps (Martius) should be employed in order to enhance blood supply and healing and minimize the chances of breakdown. The surgical repair may be approached trans-vaginally or trans-abdominally. Most urogynecological surgeons favor the transvaginal route, with the transabdominal route reserved for fistula involving the ureter or other organs including bowel or a vesicouterine fistula with preservation of the uterus or contraindications to vaginal hysterectomy. The use of specialty vaginal retractors such as the Lonestar® (www.lsmp.com) and/or the use of a generous episiotomy will allow adequate access to most fistulas, including most "high" fistulas. Dr Jack Robertson, considered the father of Urogynecology in the USA, felt that the repair of a vesicovaginal fistula by the abdominal approach was like removing your tonsils through the side of your neck.

Techniques

Latzko Partial Colpocleisis

Latzko's method of partial colpocleisis has been used successfully in the repair of vesicovaginal fistula [11]. It has the advantage of minimal tissue dissection as well as avoiding incision of the bladder. After patient positioning and exposure of the operative site with proper retractors the fistula is again visualized, using methylene blue dye if necessary (Fig. 22.2). Repeat cystoscopy may refresh in the surgeon's mind the location of the fistula in its bladder, especially its relationship to the ureteral orifices. After locating the fistula either the Lonestar retractor or stay sutures are placed between 3 and 4 cm from the fistula at four quadrants at 2, 5, 8, and 11 to delineate the area of epithelium to remove. The principle of the Latzko repair is the colpocleisis of the upper vagina to close the fistula without actually removing the fistula. The removal of the vaginal epithelium allows the underlying fibromuscularis to be sutured from anterior to posterior closing the tissue. All vaginal epithelium must be removed to prevent epithelial inclusion cyst formation or failure of the fibromuscularis tissues to scar together. A generous amount of epithelium removal will increase the success rate of this procedure. The incision is closed in 2 or 3 layers with interrupted 3.0 or 4.0 polyglactin sutures anterior to posterior. If the procedure is a repeat procedure or the tissues are not vascular and you have minimal bleeding, consider the use of a Martius flap to increase vascularity for healing of the closed fistula. The Martius flap utilizes the fat pad overlying the bulbocavernosus muscle. The fat pad is mobilized, usually leaving the posterior pedicle attached and is brought into the vaginal incision though a sub-epithelial tunnel and is sutured to the fibromuscularis prior to closing the vaginal epithelium. Post-operative drainage should be from 10 to 30 days either by indwelling Foley or suprapubic catheter. The method of drainage and length should be individualized to the surgeon's comfort with his/her quality of the closure and the vascularity of the tissues.

Transvaginal Repair of VVF (Excisional Type)

Sometimes the amount of scarring precludes a standard Latzko approach and the fistula tract may be excised (Fig. 22.3). This procedure is also utilized in most obstetric fistula to be discussed later. The fistula is exposed as in the Latzko repair and the fistula tract is excised. If significant scarring Potts scissors with a sharp point are helpful in the dissection. The vaginal epithelium is mobilized away from the underlying fibromuscularis. The fistula is then excised. The margins of the defect in the bladder mucosa and muscularis are identified, insuring they may be closed under no tension. The bladder is closed with 3.0 or 4.0 polyglactin sutures in two layers. Pubo-cervical fibromuscularis is then used to interpose between the bladder and vaginal mucosa if sufficient amount is present. The vaginal mucosa is closed in similar fashion with the same suture. In instances where there is poor tissue quality, or if concerns exist regarding blood supply, a Martius flap can be harvested beneath the labia majora, tunneled beneath the vaginal mucosa, and interposed between the bladder and the vaginal closure. Such a flap does not add any considerable time to the operation and is relatively easy to perform. It should be considered in cases where the risk of breakdown is relatively high. Bladder drainage post-operatively is as described above.

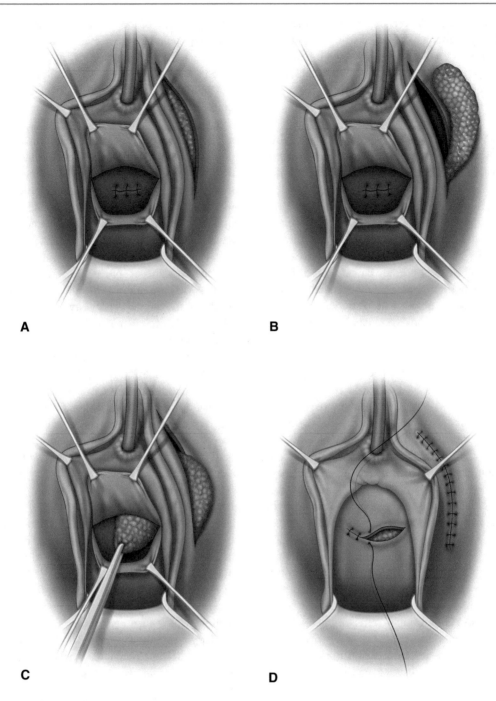

Fig. 22.2 Latzko partial colpocleisis

Transabdominal Repair

This approach may have been more common in past years (Fig. 22.4). Today, most surgeons reserve the transabdominal route for cases of VVF complicated by ureteral injury or radiation, especially when rectovaginal fistulas are involved requiring colonic diversion. It is contraindicated and those cases where uterine preservation is needed. The transabdominal approach affords better access to the retropubic area.

Transvesical Approach

Here the incision is usually made at the anterior bladder wall exposing and identifying the fistula location (Fig. 22.5). Indigo carmine can be given intravenously to help identify the ureteral orifices. However, to be perfectly safe, ureteral catheters should be placed. The fistula is excised and the bladder muscle is dissected off of the anterior vaginal wall, separating both structures. The bladder and vaginal defects

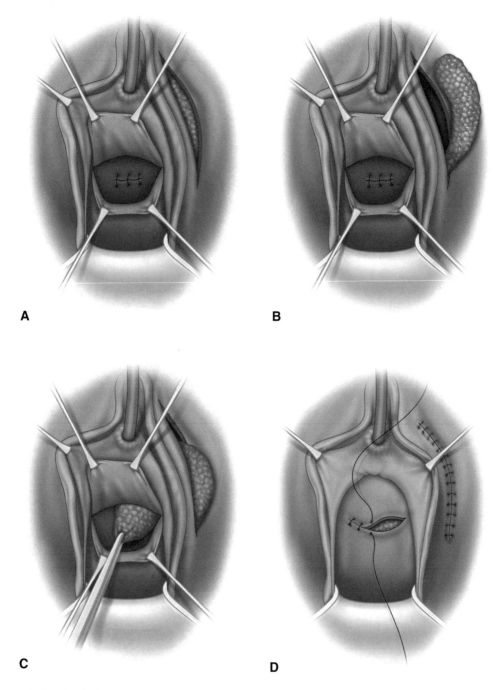

A

B

C

D

Fig. 22.3   Transvaginal repair of VVF (Excisional Type)

are closed in non-opposing fashion using 3.0 or 4.0 absorbable sutures. This approach may be hampered by limited surgical access to the fistula site.

A posterior bladder wall incision offers greater field of view through an incision over the bladder dome extended down to the fistula site. The fistula is excised followed by dissection of the bladder off the vagina, and the defects in the vaginal wall and bladder wall are usually closed with sutures separately.

Tissue interposition may be done using an omental flap and placing it between the bladder and vagina. The use of peritoneal flaps has been described with good results.

Fig. 22.4 Transabdominal repair

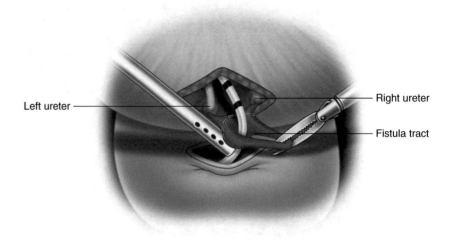

Left ureter ——

—— Right ureter

—— Fistula tract

Fig. 22.5 Transvesical approach

Overhead laparoscopic view

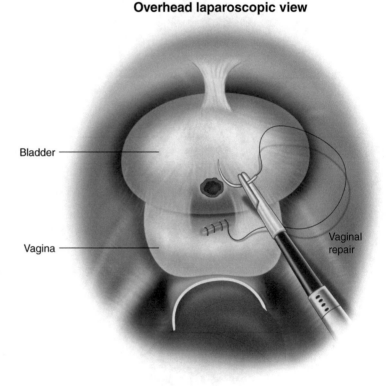

Bladder ——

Vagina ——

Vaginal repair

Omentum is particularly suitable because it has excellent lymphatic drainage and blood supply and also has an intrinsic ability to prevent the spread of inflammation.

Other Techniques

Today the technique that is gaining tremendous popularity is the combined extraperitoneal transvesical/vaginal procedure. Here, two experienced surgeons with VVF repair operate together and are able to separate the layers expediently and efficiently. One surgeon operates from above, utilizing the transvesical approach while the other operates from below at the same time. In that way, after the layers are separated each individual surgeon closes their specific layers. Again, if more, good, well vascularized tissue is needed, a Martius flap or Martius fat pad is easy to mobilize from below (remember, the flap includes the bulbocavernosus muscle, while the fat pad does *not*). The advantage of this technique is that it can dramatically decrease anesthesia time and since the case is done in an entirely "extraperitoneal" fashion, it has minimal associated morbidity.

Various surgeons have reported differing success rates using solutions such as the injection of fibrin sealant into the fistula track to occlude it [12, 13]. Fulguration of the track has also been described [14] but deep fulguration will more likely devitalize tissue and complicate future closure because of tissue destruction of tissue. While these have not undergone rigorous scrutiny, it is not unreasonable to attempt them in well-selected individual cases.

Complications

Success rates as high as 98% have been reported following surgery for simple VVF repair [6]. Heavy cigarette smoking, poor tissue quality, and chronic vascular disease with tissue ischemia, malignancy, and fibrosis following radiation treatment are some factors that can increase the risk of failure and complications.

Radiation-induced fistulae and cancer related fistulas pose a special problem. These can be difficult to repair and are in general associated with a higher recurrence and complication rate. Complications include recurrence of the fistula, infection, tissue breakdown, bladder dysfunction

following prolonged catheterization with urinary urgency especially if large portions of the bladder had to be resected. Other complications include stress urinary incontinence, de novo urge incontinence, and dyspareunia. Fortunately such complications are uncommon and successful closure with resolution of symptoms is the norm when surgical repair is properly performed.

Obstetric Fistula

Obstetrical fistulas are an ancient problem of childbirth. In our introduction we discussed the early work of Sims in the USA. Unfortunately the developing world has medical care centuries behind the developed world. Figure 22.6 shows a fistula treatment algorithm.

In many countries of the developing world, especially sub-Saharan Africa women have a very low socio-economic status. They have few choices in their life. Most have little

Fig. 22.6 Fistula treatment algorithm

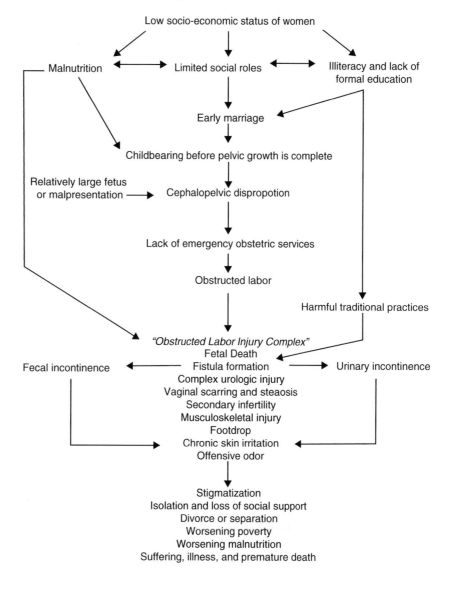

education and are forced to stop school when they are given in marriage at a young age. Childbearing occurs before pelvic growth is completed and there are almost no medical facilities available. Labors are frequently in the hut of the parents or the father for good luck and it is only after 1 or 2 days of second stage that an effort may be made to transport the laboring patient to the nearest facility, usually a day away on a wagon. Help from lay midwives include gishiri, the cutting of the vagina in hope of more space, many times causing the fistula. The stillbirth rate exceeds 75 % and the maternal mortality approaches 1 %. The fistula rate is probably 1 % but good statistics are still unknown. The injury to the pelvic floor depends on where the head impacted in its descent, causing ischemia of the tissues. Bladder base, trigone, urethra, and rectovaginal tissues will breakdown from ischemia and adjacent tissues will have ischemic changes leading to surgical failure from poor healing. The loss of urine is a constant dribble. Poor nutrition, chronic anemia, infections make maintaining hygiene difficult due to a lack of clean water and supplies, accelerating the deterioration of the lesion. The vulva and perineum become constantly exposed to the stream of urine, with subsequent excoriation and maceration of the tissues. Additionally many have a foot drop that has an unclear etiology. Finally, the worst injury is the social isolation of these patients. Most are divorced and even rejected by their family [7, 15, 16]. They have no resources with resultant malnutrition, illness, and premature death.

Epidemiology

The socio-economic conditions of these countries are the main etiology of these fistulas. Most patients with fistula are less than 150 cm tall and less than 44 kg in weight. They are poorly educated and most are divorced prior to their arrival. Most had been in labor for at least 2 days prior to being transported for care. Most had no resources (Sanda et al. Epidemiology and consequences of obstetric fistulas in Niger. Unpublished data). The author has worked with Dr Sanda in Niamey, Niger on obstetrical fistula and has used some of his statistics on his patient population. Dr Sanda also concludes that education will be the key to eradication of the obstetrical fistula in the developing world.

Classification of Fistulae

No universally accepted classification system for VVF is currently in use. The use of size and or location all have limitations regarding the outcomes. Old classifications systems such as the Hamlin's, which refer to an easy fistula or a difficult fistula are not helpful to most surgeons who have not

done thousands of fistulas [17]. Elkins described a classification according to location but again this is not helpful in prediction of the outcome of repair (Table 22.2) [18]. Waaldijk based his classification system on the involvement of the closure mechanism and was able to relate advancing stage to poorer results (Table 22.3) [19].

Roenneburg and Wheeless presented a classification including size and involvement of the closing mechanism that had some correlation to success (International Fistula Conference, July 2005 Johns Hopkins, unpublished data) (Table 22.4). They looked at the statistics of the International Organization for Women and Development, Inc. mission trips to Niamey, Niger since 2003. Table 22.5 shows a summary of their success rates including closure of the fistula and incontinence rates.

Arrowsmith on 229 patients in Jos, Nigeria presented a scoring system that predicted success of repair (International Fistula Conference, July 2005 Johns Hopkins). After analysis of all factors he found that the amount of scarring and the degree of involvement of the urethral closure mechanism was predictive of success of being dry after surgical repair (Table 22.6).

Table 22.2 Elkins classification based on anatomic location

A	Vesicocervical
B	Juxtacervical
C	Midvaginal vesicovaginal fistula (VVF)
D	Suburethral VVF
E	Urethrovaginal

Table 22.3 Waaldijk classification

Type I	Not involving urethral closure mechanism
Type II	Involving the urethral closure mechanism
	A: Without (sub)total urethral involvement
	1. Without circumferential defect
	2. With circumferential defect
	B: With (sub)total urethral involvement
	1. Without circumferential defect
	2. With circumferential defect
Type III	Miscellaneous-ureter/ other fistulas

Table 22.4 Wheeless—based on size of lesion and relation to the bladder trigone

Stage	Description
I	<2 cm size fistula, above the trigone
	Not involving the urethra, trigone, ureteric ridge
II	2–4 cm size fistula, above the trigone
III	4–6 cm size fistula, above the trigone
	Or
	Any size fistula involving the continence mechanism of the proximal urethra, urethrovesical junction, trigone, or ureteric ridge
IV	≥6 cm size fistula

Table 22.5 Staged success of closure and dry—Roenneburg

Stage I (13 patients)	57% dry
	33% incontinence
	10% persistent fistula
Stage II (13 patients)	54% dry
	23% incontinence
	23% persistent fistula
Stage III (32 patients)	75% dry
	10% incontinence
	15% persistent fistula
Stage IV (14 patients)	50% dry
	29% incontinence
	21% persistent fistula

Table 22.6 Arrowsmith fistula scoring system

Scarring	
None	0
Mild	1
Moderate	2
Severe	3
Status of urethra	
Intact	0
Partial damage	2
Complete destruction	3

A score of 3 or less had an 85% DRY; A score of 4 or more had an 41% DRY

The problem with previous classification systems was they were not effective in the prediction of "success." Success must also be defined in that fistula closure is not a "success" if the patient has intrinsic sphincter or intractable urge incontinence. Staging of fistula should probably be a surgical staging. There may be just a pinpoint opening in the vaginal epithelium but once in surgery there may be no viable tissue for repair until the dissection defines the true size of the fistula. There is a need for an internationally agreed upon classification system. This will allow surgeons to compare their data and help to determine the best approach to the repair.

Perioperative Considerations

Evaluation for other Lesions

The presence and anatomic extent of multiple fistulaes must be investigated, understanding that the surgical staging may reveal further lesions.

Nutritional Status

Many patients in sub-Saharan Africa with VVF will have chronic nutritional deprivation. Many will decrease their fluid intake to minimize the drainage. For this reason, nutritional buildup prior to surgery is frequently necessary. This should commence in the weeks before surgery, with nutritional supplements [rich in protein, vitamins, and iron] and in some cases, blood transfusion. They must also increase their hydration as this will be important in their surgical care [20].

HIV

The incidence of HIV infection is highest in sub-Saharan Africa compared to the rest of the world and may affect the success because of chronic immunosuppression.

Timing of Surgery

Controversy currently exists regarding the optimum time at which to operate on patients with VVF. The surgery should be delayed until there is no active infection or necrotic tissue present. Nutritional status may also need to be evaluated prior to surgical repair. A trial of conservative management with catheter drainage of the bladder for small lesions maybe tried but will be unsuccessful in larger fistula. Recent studies have suggested that early repair will have an equal success rate [4, 21–23].

Surgical Route

Most obstetrical fistula may be closed by the transvaginal approach. The need to reimplant a ureter or bowel diversion for a large rectovaginal fistula may require a dual approach. Severe retropubic scarring may also require an abdominal approach for surgical access.

Tissue Flap Interposition

The use of Martius flap (Fig. 22.3) is frequently used in the repair of VVF with poor vascularization of the tissue. An alternative flap is a gracilis muscle flap separating the gracilis muscle from the femoral attachment and then rotating it towards the repair site bringing in vascularity and extra tissue. Limb function is usually not significantly affected. On abdominal cases the use of an omental graft may be utilized.

Ureteral Stent Placement

Ureteral stents are helpful when the trigone is involved in the fistula. The ureter is easy to recognize when the patient is well hydrated or if available indigo carmine. The catheters are brought out per urethra as cystoscopy equipment is frequently not available. The stent will help the surgeon to preserve the ureteral opening during surgery.

Stress Urinary Incontinence

Stress incontinence frequently complicates vesicovaginal fistula, especially when the urethral closure mechanism is compromised. It is unclear whether to place a sling at the time of a urethral reconstruction or after healing. Anecdotally we found in Niamey, Niger that the use of the synthetic mid-urethral slings was not successful and we used fascia lata or abdominal fascia.

Urodynamics

The availability of urodynamic equipment is lacking in most of the developing world. Many of these patients probably additionally have an urge component. Clinically we helped with urge incontinence but the long-term availability of medications is very limited. Fistula centers are now just beginning to perform urodynamics and data may soon be available.

Antibiotics

The use of antibiotics in vesicovaginal patients varies among surgeons. While prophylactic antibiotics are common in the developed world, they may not be available in the developing world and may be replaced by aggressive hydration [22]. Prolonged courses of antibiotics should probably be reserved for complicated cases, especially when bowel surgery has also been performed.

Anesthesia

Spinal anesthesia is commonly used in environments where limited facilities exist. Equipment for general anesthesia is often very old with poor reliability. Intubation is frequently blind without proper lighting and should be avoided when possible. Epidural anesthesia would be an improvement but epidural catheters are generally not available. Complex fistula involving both rectovaginal and vesicovaginal fistula may need to be staged because of the duration of spinal anesthesia, 3–4 h at most.

Treatment

Non-surgical

While Foley catheter drainage may cure gynecologic fistula, it may also be successful in obstetrical fistula [4, 23] in up to 15 % in one study and should be tried initially.

Surgical

Most vesicovaginal fistulae are repaired by the transvaginal approach with the excision of the fistulous tract as described earlier. The use of the Latzko repair (Fig. 22.2) is associated with a higher failure rate and should be avoided in the repair of obstetric fistula [21].

1. Optimization of the patient's medical and psychological condition prior to surgery.
2. Good exposure of the surgical site.
3. Meticulous tissue dissection along any natural tissue planes, taking care to avoid the ureters.
4. Excision of scarred, fibrotic or non-viable tissue, as well as complete excision of the fistula track.
5. Tension free re-approximation of the vaginal and bladder defects.
6. The use of tissue flaps to improve blood supply when necessary.
7. Careful surgical closure of the bladder defect in order to obtain a watertight closure with bladder drainage post-operatively.
8. A staged procedure may be necessary in order to achieve optimal results. Anesthetic time may limit the ability to do all of a complex fistula.
9. The first repair offers the best chance of cure. Subsequent repairs have traditionally been associated with lower success rates.

Surgical Techniques

Simple Closure of Obstetrical VVF

The lithotomy position is favored by most, and affords excellent exposure of the vagina when the lower extremities are well flexed on the hip. The knee-chest position can also be used with good perineal exposure and access to the subpubic area, but is uncomfortable to the patient and usually requires general anesthesia.

Excisional transvaginal repair of vesicovaginal fistula as described earlier is used for most obstetric fistula. Once the patient has been properly positioned and the operative site prepped, the bladder may be catheterized with a urethral catheter if sufficient urethra is present. Ureteral stents are placed if the ureteric ridge is involved. The authors prefer to use a Lone Star™ retractor with self-retaining hooks for tissue retraction and exposure. The Lonestar hooks can bring the fistula to the introital opening as shown by attaching to the cervix, improving exposure. The vaginal epithelium is dissected from the underlying fibromuscularis and the fistula tract is excised until there is fibromuscularis and bladder muscularis tissue that is not scarred. The dissection of the epithelium may extend into the retropubic space in order to allow for a tension free closure of the bladder. Vaginal epithelium may require supplementation from vulva tissue to allow closure. The bladder defect is closed with 3.0 or 4.0 polyglactin suture with either a small RB or SH needle. Access may also dictate the use of a strongly curved needle like a UR needle. It is important to have a tension free closure. Instilling dilute methylene blue dye through the urethral catheter into the bladder tests the integrity of the bladder closure. If possible an addition layer may be used. If the repair has poor vascularity, a Martius flap should be performed as described earlier to improve the chance of healing.

Complex Repairs

Urethral involvement will necessitate the reconstruction of the urethra sometimes with a neourethra sometimes being needed. A flap of anterior or posterior bladder wall may be used as well as vaginal/vulva tissue to reconstruct the urethra. Many of the reconstructed urethras will require an additional sling after the initial surgery is healed to treat the stress incontinence from intrinsic sphincter deficiency. If the repair has poor vascularity, a Martius flap should be performed as described earlier to improve the chance of healing.

Reconstruction of the urethra may require longer drainage than the standard 10–14 days. These neourethrae tend to scar with resultant stenosis and may doom the repair to failure if the urethra is not held open with prolonged drainage.

There is occasional retropubic scarring that extends well into the retropubic space that might be helped by a dual abdominal and vaginal approach. A second team operating from above may be necessary to maximize anesthesia time.

Post-operative Care

The post-operative care of the vesicovaginal fistula patient is just as important as the surgical repair. The main principles of post-operative care include:

1. Maximum bladder drainage post-operatively. This can be at least 14 days. However, a longer period of drainage up to 21 days and even through 28 days may be required taking into account certain technical difficulties and the complexity of the repair. Ureteric stents may be removed the following day if a re-implantation is not involved.
2. Adequate hydration of the patient is necessary in order to maintain a good urine output and keep the urinary catheters patterned. Oral fluids can suffice. This may eliminate the need for antibiotics [4]
3. Perineal hygiene is vital. Sitz baths help to provide cleansing and ease discomfort but facilities are frequently inadequate for adequate care.
4. The avoidance of sexual activity or other vaginal manipulation should be strictly observed until satisfactory healing has taken place.

5. Repeat vaginal exams may be performed periodically for at least the first 3 months in order to detect and manage any tissue breakdown, infection, or recurrent vaginal stenosis. Gentile dilation may help to maintain some caliber to the vaginal opening. Some patients may require reconstruction of their vagina.
6. Recurrent fistulas should be given time to heal spontaneously with continuous bladder drainage if they are small. If drainage does not work, consider reoperation when inflammation has resolved.
7. Urge incontinence should be treated with anticholinergics if available. If the bladder capacity is inadequate because of scarring, an augmentation may be required.
8. Nutritional status post-operatively should continue to be optimized and anemia should be addressed with oral supplements or in severe cases, blood transfusion.
9. Lower limb neuropathy (foot drop) can be better managed with physical therapy if available. Most neuropathies associated with vesicovaginal fistula at least partially resolve spontaneously with time [22].
10. Education, training, and counseling is necessary to help to introduce these patients back into society. Most are divorced and without skills necessary to cope in society.

The Incurable Patient and Urinary Diversion

There are a number of patients with multiple failures of repair or scarring or the vagina with inadequate tissue to reconstruct that may be a candidate for urinary diversion. Ureterosigmoidostomy with extramural serous-lined ureterointestinal anastomosis (Mainz type II) has been used [23]. The ureterosigmoid repair is technically very feasible, even in third world countries. It requires little reconstruction and takes advantage of the intact continence mechanism on the posterior side. It would probably NOT be first choice in a well-developed nation because of other issues. These include serious severe and recurrent episodes of pyelonephritis with its attendant urosepsis. These episodes are decreased when a very competent ureterointestinal anastomosis is created. However, even this does not eradicate the risk. Also, mixing of the fecal and urinary streams can generate a synthetic mechanism that perpetuates the creation of aggressive, invasive "nitrosamines" that lead to malignant degeneration at the anastomotic site. The incidence of this type of degeneration is high and most commonly associated with adenocarcinoma. Wheeless presented his series at an International Fistula Conference at Johns Hopkins July 2004 based on his Niger experience utilizing a Koch pouch using a small bowel reservoir connected to the sigmoid. Surgical complications are common even in developed countries [24]. All of these diversions are associated with metabolic disturbances and need medical follow-up. Furthermore, malabsorption may lead to electrolyte and vitamins [25]. Pyelonephritis without medical care may be fatal. The place of continent diversions is still controversial in the developing world. Post-operative follow-up is difficult and results are unsure. Diversion to the abdominal wall is unsatisfactory because of the lack of access to disposable stoma appliances, especially in the under-developed areas.

Other Fistulas

Other types of fistula may mimic vesicovaginal fistulae or may co-exist with vesicovaginal fistulae. The evaluation of a vesicovaginal fistula must also insure that there is not a coexisting ureterovaginal, vesicocervical, or vesicouterine fistula. Rectovaginal and colovaginal fistulae may also be present as well as enterovesical and colovesical fistulae.

Ureterovaginal Fistulas (UVFs)

Ureterovaginal fistulae occur almost exclusively following injury to the ureters during gynecologic surgery. The incidence is believed to be around 0.5–2.0 % following a simple hysterectomy [26]. Radical hysterectomy is associated with a higher rate, as much as 10–20 % depending on the radicality of the procedure [27]. Recognizing and repairing at the time of the initial repair but the authors believe that prospective cystoscopy is necessary because of up to 1.7 % unrecognized injury rate at the time of hysterectomy [10]. Stenting the ureter at time of injury may prevent the need to reimplant the ureter at a later time. Many patients present in the post-operative period with leakage of urine from the vagina. Actually, these may be the fortunate patients because many of these ureteral injuries are not discovered until much later, often as an incidental finding of a non-functioning kidney. Symptoms of damage may be few with some flank discomfort and possible fever and chills. Urosepsis occurs less frequently. If checked, there is usually a small increase of 0.3 in the serum creatinine. The diagnosis is made when there is leakage of urine from the vagina. The most appropriate initial investigation is intravenous pyelography. At the time of initial evaluation, an immediate attempt should be made to pass a stent, either retrograde through cystoscopy or antegrade through a percutaneous nephrostomy. If stenting is accomplished, the fistula may close without further surgery [28]. If unable to stent the ureter, a nephrostomy will preserve kidney function until surgical repair. Timing of repair is controversial with suggestions of repair within 4 weeks [29–31] to 6 months [29]. Delay in surgical repair will increase the probability of medico-legal issues but attempts prior to resolution of inflammation from the initial surgery may compromise the repair.

The preferred repair is a ureteroneocystostomy sometimes attaching the bladder to the psoas muscle to insure a tension free re-implantation. Alternatively a Boari [31] flap may be used to insure the tension free re-implantation. A Boari flap is a graft of "full thickness" detrusor which is tubularized and used to bridge defects that are usually between 3–5 cm in length. If the injury is above the pelvic brim, it may be necessary to perform an end-to-end anastomosis of the ureter. The use of an end-to-end anastomosis as well as just stenting the injury must be reevaluated later for ureteral strictures. Transureteroureterostomy is a last resort procedure and is rarely used today.

Vesicouterine and Vesicocervical Fistulae

First described by Youssef in 1957 [30], vesicouterine and vesicocervical fistulae were always considered as very rare phenomena. Now, however, especially in first world countries, they are becoming more common with the increasing cesarean delivery rate [31]. It typically occurs as a complication of cesarean section, following the inadvertent placement of sutures in a scarred poorly developed bladder flap or from post cesarean infection. The patient may have symptoms of menouria or urine leakage from the vagina. Because of differential leakage of urine intra-abdominal methylene blue may not be appreciated on vaginal exam. Diagnosis may be confirmed by hysterogram or retrograde injection at the time of cystoscopy [9]. If childbearing is complete hysterectomy at time of repair will facilitate repair. If preservation of the uterus is desired it might be easier to perform surgery from a transabdominal approach, especially if the reason for the cesarean delivery was an inadequate pelvic capacity healing.

Urethrovaginal Fistulae

Urethrovaginal fistulae are relatively uncommon in modern gynecologic practice [32]. They usually occur following surgical procedures such as diverticulectomy, urethropexy, and suburethral sling procedures, as well as procedures involving extensive anterior vaginal wall dissection. Obstetric urethrovaginal fistulae are discussed above in the discussion on obstetrical fistula. The diagnosis may be less than obvious in the evaluation of complaints of incontinence. Distal lesions may have minimal symptoms with vaginal retention of urine that may dribble out on standing. Proximal lesions may have more symptoms, especially if there is funneling of the bladder neck. A zero degree urethroscope may be helpful in diagnosis as well as the use of a small probe passed per urethra. Surgery is usually necessary if symptomatic. Excision of the lesion and a layered closure are the standard therapy. A Martius should be considered for large fistulas and those with poor vascularity. Small asymptomatic lesions may be ignored. Stenting with a urethral catheter for 1–2 weeks is the usual post-operative care. Complications include recurrence, stricture formation, and incontinence.

Rectovaginal Fistulae (RVF) with VVF

Rectovaginal fistulae may also complicate VVFs, especially in obstetrical fistulae and radiation-induced fistulae. While distal rectovaginal fistula associate with obstetrical episiotomy and fourth degree extensions in the developed world may be closed primarily, large proximal fistula and those associated with radiation or Crohn's disease may require fecal diversion to achieve closure [33]. In complex fistulae like this, where VVF is complicated with an RVF, the surgical treatment should be guaged in an appropriate fashion. To this end, the repair of the rectovaginal fistula should be done prior to surgical treatment of the vesicovaginal fistula.

Enterovesical and Colovesical Fistulae

Fistulous connections between the small bowel or colon, and the urinary bladder are also rare, however it should be suspected in patients with Crohn's disease or diverticulitis who complain of dysuria, urinary frequency or urgency and pneumaturia [34–36]. It is generally **more prevalent in males** since the uterus provides a natural tissue interposition between the bowel and bladder. In a review, diverticulitis was the most common cause [41 %] followed by Crohn's disease [17 %] and colorectal cancer [16 %] [36]. Positive urine cultures were obtained in 88 % of the patients, with *E. coli* as the most prevalent organism. Cystoscopy is the most effective diagnostic tool, but even at that, was confirmatory only 67 % of the time in the series by Moss. A barium study was also useful, being generally abnormal 80 % of the time, however it identified the fistula in only 17 % of cases in which it was used. Flexible sigmoidoscopy and CT scan may also be used. The sigmoid colon is the most frequently (53 %) involved segment of the bowel in the series by Moss.

As in colovaginal fistulae, a one-stage procedure in patients without invasive malignancy is the current approach. A multi-stage procedure may be needed in the face of severe intra-abdominal disease. Surgery with resection of the affected bowel segment is probably the standard therapy.

Conclusion

Genito-urinary fistulae are recognized complications of gynecologic surgery and neglected obstetrics. Prevention of these complications is a noble goal but will be difficult to realize. This is especially true in less developed regions anytime in the near future. The care of this problem will continue to be a challenge to the disciplines of both urology and gynecology. So, at least for the foreseeable future, we can expect that GU fistulae will continue to be reported. However, in the final analysis, at least we can be proud to hang our hat on those principles developed over many years that have stood the test of time and changed, for the better, the lives of the afflicted, since the first successful vesicovaginal fistula repair, over a century and a half ago.

References

1. Waaldijk K. The immediate surgical management of fresh obstetric fistulas with catheter and /or early closure. Int J Gynecol Obstet. 1994;45:11–6.
2. Hamson KA. Child bearing, health, and social priorities, a survey of 22,774 consecutive births in Zaire, Northern Nigeria. Br J Obstet Gynaecol. 1985;92:1–19.
3. Lee RA, Symmonds RE, Williams TJ. Current status of genitourinary fistula. Obstet Gynecol. 1988;72:313–9.
4. Wall LL, Arrowsmith SD, Briggs ND, Browning A, Lassey A. The obstetrics vesicovaginal fistula in the developing world. Obstet Gynecol Surv. 2005;60(7):S3–51.
5. Flores-Carreras O, Cabrera JR, Galeano PA, Torres FE. Fistulas of the urinary tract in gynecologic and obstetric surgery. Int Urogynecol J. 2001;12:203–14.
6. Meeks GR, Sams JO, Field W, Fulp KS, Margolis MT. Formation of vesicovaginal fistula: the role of suture placement into the bladder during closure of the vaginal cuff after transabdominal hysterectomy. Am J Obstet Gynecol. 1997;177(6):1298–304.
7. Vakili B, Chesson RR, Kyle BL, Shobeiri SA, Echols KT, Gist R, Zheng YT, Nolan TE. The incidence of urinary tract injury during hysterectomy: a prospective analysis based on universal cystoscopy. Am J Obstet Gynecol. 2005;192(5):1599–604.
8. Angioli, R, Penalver, M, Muzii, L, Mendez, L, Mirhashemi, R. Bellati, F, Croce, C, Panici, PB. Guidelines of how to manage vesicovaginal fistula. Crit Rev Oncol Hematol. 2003;48: 295–304.
9. Shobeiri SA, Chesson RR, Echols KT. Cystoscopic fistulography: a review. Urol Rev J. 2003;1:20–1.
10. Blaivas JG, Heritz DM, Romanzi LJ. Early versus late repair of vesicovaginal fistulas: vaginal and abdominal approaches. J Urol. 1995;153:1110–3.
11. Latzko W. Postoperative vesicovaginal fistulas; genesis and therapy. Am J Surg. 1942;58:211–28.
12. Kanaoka, Y, Hirai, K, Ishiko, O, Ogita S. Vesicovaginal fistula treated with fibrin glue. Int J Gynecol Obstet. 2001;173: 147–9.
13. Sharma SK, Perry KT, Turk TMT. Endoscopic injection of fibrin glue for the treatment of urinary –tract pathology. J Endourol. 2005;19(3):419–23.
14. Stovsky MD, Ignatoff JM, Blum MD, Manmiga JB. Use of electrocoagulation in the management of vesicovaginal fistulas. J Urol. 1994;152:1443–4.
15. Onolemhemhen DO, Ekwempu CC. An investigation of sociomedical risk factors associated with vaginal fistula in northern Nigeria. Women Health. 1999;28(3):103–16.
16. Muleta M. Socio-demographic profile and obstetric experience of fistula patients managed at the Addis Ababa Fistula Hospital. Ethiop Med J. 2004;42:9–16.

17. Hamlin RHJ, Nicholson EC. Reconstruction of urethra totally destroyed in labor. Br Med J . 1969;1:147–50.

18. Elkins TE. surgery for the obstetric vesicovaginal fistula: a review of 100 operations in 82 patients. Am J Obstet Gynecol. 1994;170(4):1108–20.

19. Waaldijk K. Surgical classification of obstetric fistulas. Int J Gynaecol Obstet. 1995;49(2):161–3.

20. Waaldijk K. The immediate management of fresh obstetric fistulas. Am J Obstet Gynecol. 2004;191(3):795–9.

21. Elkins TE, Drescher C, Martey JO, Fort D. Vesicovaginal fistula revisited. Obstet Gynecol. 1988;72(3 Pt 1):307–12.

22. Waaldijk K, Elkins TE. The obstetric fistula and peroneal nerve injury: an analysis of 947 consecutive patients. Int Urogynecol J. 1994;a5:12–4.

23. El-Lamie IK. Preliminary experience with Mainz type II pouch in gynecologic oncology patients. Eur J Gynaec Oncol. 2001; 22(1):77–80.

24. Farnham SB, Cookson MS. Surgical complications of urinary diversion. World J Urol. 2004;22:157–67.

25. Mills RD, Styderm UE. Metabolic consequences of continent urinary diversion. J Urol. 1999;161:1057–66.

26. Everett HS, Mattingly RF. Urinary tract injuries resulting from pelvic surgery. Am J Obstet Gynecol. 1978;71:502–5.

27. Macasaet MA, Lu R, Nwlaon JH. Ureterovaginal fistula as a complication of radical pelvic surgery. Am J Obstet Gynecol. 1976;124:757–60.

28. Elabd S, Ghoniem G, Elsharaby M, Emran M, Elgamasy A, Felfela T, Elshaer A. Use of endoscopy in the management of postoperative ureterovaginal fistulas. Int Urgynecol J. 1997;8:185–90.

29. Macasaet MA, Lu T, Nelson JH. Ureterovaginal fistula as a complication of radical pelvic surgery. Am J Obstet Gynecol. 1076;124:757–60.

30. Youssef AF. Menouria following lower segment caesarean section. Am J Obstet Gynecol. 1957;73:759–67.

31. Tanker ML. Vesicouterine fistula-a review. Obstet Gynecol Surv. 1986;41(12):743–53.

32. Webster GD, Sihelnik SA, Stone AR. Urethrovaginal fistula: a review of the surgical management. J Urol 1984;132:460–2.

33. Saclarides TJ. Rectovaginal fistula. Surg Clin North Am. 2002;82:1261–72.

34. Pollard SG, Macfarlane R, Greatorex R, Everett WG, Hartfall WG. Colovesical fistula. Ann R Coll Surg Engl. 1987;69:163–5.

35. Moss RL, Ryan JA. Management of enterovesical fistulas. Am J Surg. 1990;159:514–7.

36. Pontari MA, McMillen MA, Garvey RH, Ballantyne GH. Diagnosis and treatment of enterovesical fistulae. Am Surg. 1992;58:258–63.

Rectal Prolapse in the Elderly

Susan L. Gearhart

Introduction

Pelvic floor disorders are a challenging and poorly understood clinical entity. These disorders are most commonly found among the elderly. Bharucha et al. demonstrated in a study known as the Women's Health Initiative that nearly 40 % of women 40 years or older suffer from defecatory dysfunction [1]. In fact, 1 out of 10 women by the age of 80 will require surgery for pelvic organ prolapse [1]. An understanding about the treatment of these disorders is especially timely given our aging US population. The purpose of this chapter is to highlight the diagnosis and treatment of rectal prolapse with a focus on the elderly patient.

Rectal prolapse is commonly found in females with a female-to-male ratio that approaches 6:1 in adults. While the incidence of rectal prolapse increases with increasing age in females, males have an equal incidence per decade throughout adult life. Women with rectal prolapse also have a higher incidence of other associated pelvic floor disorders including urinary incontinence, rectocele, cystocele, and enterocele. In a recent study of patients with pelvic floor disorders, rectal prolapse was found more commonly in those patients older than 70 than those younger than 70 (17 vs. 27 %, respectively) [2]. Less common associated conditions include connective tissue disorders such as Ehlers–Danlos syndrome, congenital hypothyroidism, and solitary rectal ulcer.

Rectal prolapse is a circumferential, full-thickness protrusion of the rectal wall through the anal orifice. It is often associated with other anatomical findings such as a redundant sigmoid colon, deep pelvic cul-de-sac (pouch of Douglas), and pelvic laxity. There are three types of rectal prolapse: full-thickness rectal prolapse (procidentia), mucosal prolapse, and internal intussusception. The current theory of why rectal prolapse occurs relates to disorders of defecation that lead to excessive straining. Overtime, this will weaken the supportive structures of the pelvic floor and sphincter complex allowing for herniation of bowel, bladder, or uterus through the pelvic outlet. This weakening may be accelerated as a result of pelvic floor nerve injuries associated with vaginal birth. Longitudinal radiographic studies have demonstrated that the development of prolapse may be a gradual process which begins as internal rectal intussusception and progresses to frank prolapse.

Presentation and Associated Findings

In most instances, patients present after the rectum is noted by a practitioner or the patient to protrude abnormally from the anus. The rectum may spontaneously reduce or require manual reduction. On rare occasions, the rectum may incarcerate requiring a laparotomy to reduce it to its normal location. It is important to differentiate full-thickness prolapse from mucosal prolapse which is 4th degree hemorrhoids. The classic distinction between full-thickness rectal prolapse and mucosal prolapse is the presence on physical exam of circumferential folds seen in full-thickness rectal prolapse and radial folds with mucosal prolapse. Internal prolapse is best seen on imaging studies and is often hard to fully appreciate on physical examination since the rectum does not protrude through the anus.

The symptoms commonly found with all types of rectal prolapse include tenesmus, rectal bleeding, a palpable mass, and fecal soiling. There are several functional pelvic floor disorders associated with rectal prolapse. The most common functional disorders are fecal incontinence and constipation. There is an increased incidence of rectal prolapse among individuals with colonic inertia and obstructed defecation secondary to non-relaxing puborectalis. Defecation occurs through a coordinated effort involving relaxation of the anal

S.L. Gearhart (✉)
Department of Surgery, Johns Hopkins Medical Institution,
600 N Wolfe Street, Baltimore, MD 21287, USA
e-mail: sdemees1@jhmi.edu

© Springer Science+Business Media New York 2017
D.A. Gordon, M.R. Katlic (eds.), *Pelvic Floor Dysfunction and Pelvic Surgery in the Elderly*,
DOI 10.1007/978-1-4939-6554-0_23

sphincter complex as well as the puborectalis muscle. The puborectalis muscle acts like a sling to create an angle between the rectum and the anal canal. Relaxation of this sling obliterates the angle providing a direct passage of stool from the rectum through the anal canal. Paradoxical puborectalis muscle contraction during defecation maintains or exaggerates the anorectal angle resulting in a functional resistance to defecation.

Fecal incontinence occurs in the majority of patients with all types of rectal prolapse and the incidence increases with increasing age and duration of the prolapse. It is thought that fecal incontinence is the result of a combination of an increase in intra-rectal pressure as a result of the prolapse. The increase in the intra-rectal pressure minimizes the normal pressure difference which exists between the rectum and the anal canal resulting in incontinence. Stretch injury to the pudendal nerves may also accelerate symptoms of incontinence. The pudendal nerves innervate the anal sphincter complex and can be injured over time as a result of excessive straining and recurrent herniation of the pelvic floor.

Evaluation

All patients presenting with rectal prolapse should undergo a complete history and physical exam. Associated symptoms such as urinary incontinence, vaginal vault prolapse, fecal incontinence, and constipation should be ascertained. Careful assessment of risk factors for anesthesia and the functional status of the patient should be performed because this information may affect the surgeon's choice of procedure. The physical exam should include careful evaluation of the perineum and prolapsed rectum. With the patient in lithotomy position, the perineum should be inspected in the relaxed position as well as during straining. During straining, the prolapsed rectum can often be seen. If a laxity exists within the rectovaginal septum, a rectocele may be present. A digital rectal exam performed during straining can often demonstrate the lack of fixation of the rectum as well as the presence of internal intussusception. If the prolapse is not easily demonstrated, the use of an enema may help.

Additional investigations in patients with rectal prolapse should include a colonoscopy or barium enema. Both tests provide an evaluation of the colonic mucosa for a lead point causing intussusception or other abnormalities such as diverticular disease or solitary rectal ulcer which may influence the type of procedure performed. Since these patients can manifest with several associated pelvic floor abnormalities, an assessment of pelvic floor anatomy and physiology is required. Depending on associated symptoms, tests may include cinedefecography, pelvic floor dynamic magnetic resonance imaging (MRI), anorectal manometry, endorectal ultrasound, electromyography (EMG), and colon transit studies.

Cinedefecography and dynamic pelvic floor MRI are both useful tests in the evaluation of rectal prolapse. Importantly, these tests can identify associated pelvic floor abnormalities which occur comely with rectal prolapse. Cinedefecography is a test performed by the instillation of contrast into the rectum, vagina, and bladder and allowing the patient to evacuate the contents in the normal sitting position while real time images are obtained. Cinedefecography can detect occult intussusception and rectal prolapse with a sensitivity of 100 % and a specificity of 93 % [3]. Other abnormalities that may be detected include paradoxical puborectalis contraction and pelvic floor weakness such as rectocele, enterocele, and cystocele. In contrast, dynamic pelvic floor MR is performed with the installation of contrast into the rectum and vagina, however, the patient must be kept in the supine position. The patient is asked to bear down to the point of defecation while images are obtained. This test will identify a pelvic floor hernia.

Anorectal manometry and endorectal ultrasound is performed when symptoms of fecal incontinence or obstructed defecation are identified along with internal or external rectal prolapse. Patients with lower resting and maximum squeeze pressures are less likely to recover sphincter control following rectal prolapse repair. However, it is important to note that increasing age is associated with lower anal resting pressure, higher rectal pressure and rectal gradient during simulated evacuation, and a shorter balloon expulsion time in asymptomatic individuals [4]. The balloon expulsion test can be performed at the same time anorectal manometry is performed. The balloon catheter used during this procedure is inflated with 50–100 cc of water and the patient is asked to expel the balloon. Patients without obstructed defecation should easily expel the balloon, whereas patients experiencing obstructed defecation cannot expel the balloon. Endorectal ultrasound may be useful for evaluation of occult sphincter defects especially in older parous women.

Colonic transit studies such as colonic scintigraphy and Sitzmark studies may be necessary in patients with long-standing constipation who have rectal prolapse. Scintigraphy utilizes nuclear medicine principles. This study utilizes 24 radiopaque markers which are ingested by the patient. Sequential daily plain abdominal films are performed to demonstrate the movement of stool throughout the colon. Patients with total colonic inertia will retain at least 80 % of the markers equally distributed throughout the colon at 5 days. Patients with obstructed defecation will have markers concentrated near the rectosigmoid junction. Failure to recognize and treat a dysfunctional colon or obstructed defecation may result in continued straining and ultimately, recurrent prolapse.

Management Options

The goal of treatment is the restoration of normal anatomy and correction of any associated physiologic disorder. Successful treatment results in long-lasting symptom relief and is accomplished best by non-operative and operative techniques.

Non-operative Management

Non-operative therapy should be initiated in all patients with disorders of defecation. Initial treatment should include dietary and lifestyle changes. A review of medications and dietary history will often guide this therapy. It is well known that a high fiber therapy with a total of 40 g of fiber should be consumed daily. Furthermore, patients are instructed to consume more liquids that are not caffeinated. Daily exercise 20 min a day is not only healthy for the cardiovascular system but also healthy for the gastrointestinal system. Biofeedback is the mainstay therapy for obstructed defecation secondary to paradoxical puborectalis contraction and internal intussusception. Biofeedback training is aimed at suppressing the inappropriate contraction of the pelvic floor during defecation. This may result in a reduction in the time spent straining at defecation and prevent recurrence of prolapse.

Operative Management

Operative repair is indicated for full-thickness prolapse and mucosal prolapse. There is a limited role for operative repair for internal intussusception and obstructed defecation. Several types of repairs for rectal prolapse exist and the indication for each type as well as the recurrence rate is listed in Table 23.1. Reported outcomes following repair include recurrence of prolapse and persistent or new symptoms of constipation or fecal incontinence. In general, the literature

supports the use of abdominal procedures rather than perineal procedures for rectal prolapse because of the associated decrease in recurrence rates. The goal of the abdominal approach, whether laparoscopic or open is mobilization and fixation of the anterior or posterior rectum to the presacral fascia. The goal of the perineal procedure is partial or complete removal of the prolapsed rectum through the perineum with minimal operative risk to the patient. Therefore, if a patient's physical condition does not allow for an abdominal procedure, then a perineal procedure is warranted. However, with the advances in anesthetic techniques, nowadays, the physical state of the patient should drive the operative approach. Perineal approaches in active patients are more prone to failure.

Operative Indications

Rectal Prolapse and Constipation

Up to 50 % of patients will present with rectal prolapse without a long-standing history of constipation. Historically, patients who underwent a rectopexy alone for rectal prolapse had an increased rate of postoperative defecatory dysfunction. For this reason, rectopexy and resection was recommended. However, after careful evaluation of the pelvic anatomy, it has been demonstrated that during mobilization of the lateral attachments of the rectum, several nerves important in rectal function can be injured. Recently, several studies have demonstrated that a rectopexy, posterior or ventral, can be performed alone successfully if the lateral attachments of the rectum are preserved preventing denervation of the rectum. Franceschilli et al. demonstrated that in 100 patients with both constipation/obstructed defecation and internal prolapse who underwent a ventral rectopexy, the recurrence rate was 14 % and improvement in constipation occurred in 92 % of patients [4]. Careful evaluation of the patients who did recur demonstrated that severe constipation that persisted following repair was most often associated

Table 23.1 Indications and recurrence rates for perineal vs. abdominal vs. abdominal procedures for full- procedures for full-thickness rectal prolapse

Procedure	Indication	Recurrence (%)
Anal encirclement	Low functional status, high surgical risk	0–60
Delorme	Low functional status, high surgical risk	5–21
Perineal rectosigmoidectomy	High surgical risk	0–44
Ripstein rectopexy (mesh)	Prolapse without constipation,	0–13
Wells rectopexy (mesh)	Prolapse without constipation,	2–10
Suture rectopexy	Prolapse without constipation	0–5
Resection rectopexy	Prolapse WITH constipation, no fecal incontinence	0–6
Anterior resection	Prolapse associated with severe solitary rectal ulcer syndrome	4–9
Ventral rectopexy (mesh)	Internal or external prolapse with constipation or fecal incontinence	4–14

with failure of the repair [4]. In the elderly patient with constipation and rectal prolapse, forgoing a sigmoid colon resection and maintaining the patient on a good bowel regimen decreases the morbidity of this procedure.

Rectal Prolapse with Fecal Incontinence

Up to 70 % of patients may complain of some degree of fecal incontinence. In the presence of severe incontinence, ventral or posterior rectopexy alone should be considered because the combination of a resection and rectopexy may make the symptoms of incontinence worse. In the same study referenced above by Franceschilli et al., fecal incontinence improved in 86 % of patients [4]. In general, a combined approach for sphincter muscle repair at the time of rectopexy is avoided since symptomatic incontinence will improve in most patients.

Mucosal Prolapse

The surgical management of mucosal prolapse is best described by the treatment of hemorrhoids. The goal or repair for mucosal prolapse is to resuspend the mucosa within the anal canal. The surgical options for this repair include conventional hemorrhoidectomy, stapled hemorrhoidectomy, or transhemorrhoidal dearterialization.

Operative Techniques

For all abdominal and perineal procedures including rectopexy without resection, all patients should undergo mechanical bowel prep. Appropriate preoperative antibiotic coverage and anti-thrombotic therapy should be given. A decision regarding the use of a minimally invasive or an open procedure is made based upon the patient's previous surgical history, weight, and known contra-indications to minimally invasive surgery.

Abdominal Approach

Positioning of the patient and port insertion during robotic or a laparoscopic procedure is often based on surgeon preference and is beyond the scope of this chapter. For both open and minimally invasive approaches, the patient is placed in lithotomy and reverse Trendelenburg positions throughout most of the procedure. For both the ventral and posterior rectopexy, the sigmoid colon and the rectum are mobilized so to free the retroperitoneal structures including the left ureter and the hypogastric nerves. The space between the fascia propria of the rectum and the presacral fascia is opened at the sacral promontory and to the level of the third sacral vertebrae. For the posterior rectopexy, this dissection is carried down beyond the coccyx to the levator ani muscle. Care must be taken to avoid mobilization of the lateral

attachments of the rectum which includes the middle hemorrhoidal artery. Preservation of these lateral attachments will prevent injury to the innervation of the rectum and preserve rectal function. For the ventral and posterior rectopexy, the anterior reflection of peritoneum within the pouch of Douglas is opened and the dissection in this pouch is carried down to the level of the levator ani muscle. For the ventral rectopexy, the dissection is then complete and mesh can then be used for fixation of the rectum. The mesh in a ventral rectopexy is generally non-absorbable and attached to the lateral aspect of the rectum and the pelvic floor. There is a concern regarding mesh erosion into the rectum or vagina. Biological mesh has also been used with a low recurrence rate of 14 % at 2 years [5]. However, studies using non-absorbable synthetic mesh have reported minimal complications from the use of this mesh [6]. Once the mesh has been placed, the opposite end will then be attached to the sacrum. For a posterior rectopexy, mesh is attached to the sacrum and the lateral rectal attachments are sewn to the mesh (Wells procedure) using 4 rows of non-absorbable sutures. The peritoneum is then closed over any exposed mesh to limit the risk of adhesions.

Perineal Approach

The perineal approaches used to repair rectal prolapse include the perineal rectosigmoidectomy (Altemeier procedure) and the Delorme. The patient can be positioned in the lithotomy or prone-jackknife position. The perineal rectosigmoidectomy is performed with the rectum fully prolapsed. Anal retracting sutures or the *Lone Star* retractor can be used to assist with exposure. A circumferential full-thickness incision is made 1 cm (handsewn) to 3 cm (stapled anastomosis) above the dentate line. The anterior wall of the hernia sac is identified and opened allowing the rectum to be circumferentially freed from the hernia sac. Once the rectum is mobilized, the mesenteric attachments are freed by careful division with ligation of major vessels. This maneuver will free up the rectum even more. Any laxity in the levator muscles should then be repaired with placation to create a snug fit. Once the correct bowel orientation is confirmed, the redundant bowel is transected. A handsewn anastomosis can be performed reapproximating the proximal and distal ends. Alternatively, a stapled anastomosis can be performed with the use of end-end circular stapler.

The Delorme procedure is best described as a sleeve resection of only rectal mucosa that is removed from the prolapsed rectum. This is facilitated by infiltrating the submucosa with lidocaine and epinephrine (1:100,000). The denuded rectal muscular wall is plicated in four quadrants like an accordion and the remaining mucosal rings are reapproximated. It is recommended that an absorbable suture such as 2-0 Vicryl be used. Further sutures may be needed to complete the mucosal anastomosis.

Surgical Outcomes for the Elderly

Historically, abdominal procedures for the treatment of rectal prolapse were avoided due to high surgical risk. With advances in anesthesia and surgery, particularly the ventral rectopexy, studies have shown improvements in functional outcomes and recurrence rates for the elderly. With an increase in our aging population, these findings are particularly timely. Gultekin et al., using a national database, compared outcomes among patients younger and older than 70 years following a ventral rectopexy for rectal prolapse [2]. The authors demonstrated that minor complications were more common in older patients and that the length of stay was one day longer. However, there was no difference in major complications or mortality in these two groups. The authors concluded that all things considered ventral rectopexy is safe in the elderly and that the increased risk was worth the improvements in quality of life associated with this procedure. This study was the first to incorporate a large number of patients from several centers.

Conclusion

The problems of rectal prolapse remain challenging in the elderly. A key aspect of the care of these patients includes careful preoperative evaluation for identification of any associated functional disorders such as severe constipation that may lead to early failure. Although there are different approaches for these disorders, the best approach is the approach that is tailored to the specific patient.

References

1. Bharucha AE, Zinsmeister AR, Locke GR. Prevalence and burden of fecal incontinence a population-based study in nomen. Gastroenterology. 2005;129:42–9.
2. Gultekin F, Wong M, Podevin J, Barussaud M, Boutami M, Lehur P, Meurette G. Safety of laparoscopic ventral rectopexy in the elderly: results from a nationwide database. Dis Colon Rectum. 2015;58: 339–43.
3. Andromanakos N, Skandalakis P, Troupis T, Filippou D. Constipation of anorectal outlet obstruction: pathophysiology, evaluation, and management. J Gastroenterol Hepatol. 2006;21:638–46.
4. Noelting J, Ratuapli S, Bharucha A, Harvey D, Ravi K, Zinsmeister A. Normal values for high resolution anorectal manometry in healthy women: effects of age and significance of rectoanal gradient. Am J Gastroenterol. 2012;107:1530–6.
5. Franceschilli L, Varvaras D, Capuano I, Ciangola C, Giorgi F, Boehm G, Gaspari A, Sileri P. Laparoscopic ventral rectopexy using biologic mesh for the treatment of obstructed defecation syndrome and/or fecal incontinence in patients with internal rectal prolapse: a critical appraisal of the first 100 cases. Tech Coloproctol. 2015. doi:10.1007/s10151-014-1255-4
6. D'Hoor A, Cadoni R, Penninckx F. Long-term outcome of laparoscopic ventral rectopexy for total rectal prolapse? Br J Surg. 2004;91:1500–5.

Fecal Incontinence

Tisha N. Lunsford, Cari K. Sorrell, and Ha Lam

Introduction

Fecal incontinence (FI), the involuntary passage of stool or the inability to control stool from expulsion, is a common gastrointestinal complaint in patients aged 65 years and older and has an incidental increase with progressive aging [1]. This increase has been shown to be an independent risk factor even after controlling for illness, activity level, and overall health and FI itself may predispose to a greater chance of institutionalization [2]. Prevalence estimates of FI vary widely from 2–36 % in the ambulatory setting to 33–65 % in the nursing home setting. [1] Consequently, direct and indirect costs, patient morbidity, and psychosocial impact are high and it is recommended that a review of this symptom should be a part of any initial or ongoing evaluation of an older patient in both the ambulatory and hospitalized setting. This chapter emphasizes specific age-related colorectal intervention options for FI, including medical, behavioral, and more invasive techniques emphasizing, when available, unique supportive data in the geriatric population. As with any intervention, the patient care team must always be aware of the unique characteristics of the population being treated including age-specific issues (including common diseases of the elderly that may impair continence/functionality), functional status, patient preferences, expectations and goals of therapy.

T.N. Lunsford (✉) • C.K. Sorrell • H. Lam
Department of Internal Medicine, University of Texas Health Science Center at San Antonio, 7703 Floyd Curl Drive, MC 7878, San Antonio, TX 78229, USA
e-mail: lunsfordt@uthscsa.edu

Medical Therapy

Essential to any initial assessment and intervention of fecal incontinence includes appropriate characterization of the incontinence and a subsequent tiered approach to treatment. If possible, it is imperative to classify the underlying pathophysiology of the patient's fecal incontinence as this will direct treatment strategies and may predict outcomes. The differential diagnosis of fecal incontinence is vast and includes central and peripheral nervous system abnormalities including dementia, stroke, and diabetes. Moreover, as the development of fecal incontinence is multifactorial, it is important that the clinician carefully tease out which pathophysiologic factors are responsible for the incontinence, as improvement in any single factor may provide significant clinical improvements.

The four crucial components to maintaining continence include (a) sensory, (b) motor, (c) structural, and (d) cognitive/behavioral mechanisms. Incontinence occurs when one or more of these components are disrupted to an extent that the other components cannot compensate. A practical example would be that of a patient who has suffered from obstetric trauma resulting in damage to the external anal sphincter and pudendal nerve in her early twenties, but did *not* experience incontinence until she developed advanced neuropathy related to poor glycemic control from her diabetes mellitus in her early sixties. While the sphincter defect and nerve injury are consistent with a disruption in sensory and structural mechanisms that are important for maintaining continence, the development of neuropathy of both sensory and motor nerves in addition to diarrhea attributed to her diabetes results in further insult by altering continence control mechanisms. In this case, it is crucial that as soon as an appropriate workup has excluded a luminal, malignant, or infectious cause as the etiology of her diarrhea, antidiarrheal medications should be used to decrease symptoms. Changes in stool consistency coupled with sphincteric dysfunction

© Springer Science+Business Media New York 2017
D.A. Gordon, M.R. Katlic (eds.), *Pelvic Floor Dysfunction and Pelvic Surgery in the Elderly*,
DOI 10.1007/978-1-4939-6554-0_24

and rectal hyposensitivity as a result of diabetic neuropathy can predispose diabetics to FI [1, 3]. Until the diarrhea itself is diagnosed and treated, any intervention to restore an intact sphincter would be unlikely to provide significant relief from incontinence. This case emphasizes the key role that a thorough clinical history and physical examination plays in the development of treatment strategies tailored to meet the specific needs of your incontinent patient. Common etiologies of diarrhea in the older population include adverse effects of medications, bile acid malabsorption (either after cholecystectomy, small intestinal Crohn's disease, or radiation enteropathy), tube feedings, gluten-sensitivity, microscopic colitis, ischemic colitis, radiation proctopathy, small intestinal bacterial overgrowth, carbohydrate (lactose or fructose being the most common) intolerance, and diabetic-associated diarrhea. Further supporting the importance of identifying a possible underlying disordered bowel habit is a Veterans Affairs study of acutely ill patients which found that greater than 30 % of patients reported FI with increased age, illness severity, and liquid stool consistency identified as being the primary risk factors [1, 3]. Conversely, embarrassment or skepticism may lead the patient to focus solely on what they self-report as "diarrhea" as opposed to revelation of the symptom of incontinence. If the practitioner does not carefully ask questions specifically tailored to identify to FI, the fecal impacted patient suffering from overflow incontinence that they are terming "diarrhea" to their family/caregiver/clinician may inadvertently be given more antidiarrheals with obvious risk. However, if the clinician is confident that the patient is suffering from true diarrhea contributing to FI, many medication interventions are available and are outlined below. Special care must be taken when using these medications in the elderly as they may have a higher risk for adverse effects, drug–drug interactions, increased sensitivity to side effects (i.e., anticholinergic effects), and impaired hepatic or renal clearance (Table 24.1).

Table 24.1 Guidelines for use of common antidiarrheal medications in fecal incontinence

Medication	Precautions	Adult dosing	Adverse effects
Fiber supplementation	May interfere with absorption of other medications, therefore very specific dosing guidelines must be outlined for patients May reduce insulin requirement in diabetic patients	Begin 1–2 tablets of preferred formulation BID with *sips* of water only	Flatulence, bloating, abdominal pain, anorexia, asthma reactions, esophageal/intestinal obstruction
Loperamide	Use cautiously in patients with active inflammatory disease of the colon or with infectious diarrhea	Begin prophylactically at 2 mg PO BID Okay to titrate to 4 mg PO QID as needed If larger doses are needed (as they often are in patients with IBS-D, titrate up slowly) May increase resting anal sphincter tone	CNS depression, paralytic ileus, rash, dizziness, fatigue, cramping, constipation, dry mouth, nausea and vomiting
Diphenoxylate/atropine	Use cautiously in patients with active inflammatory disease of the colon or with infectious diarrhea	Begin at dose of diphenoxylate 2.5 mg PO daily Titrate up slowly to a maximum dose diphenoxylate 5 mg PO every 6 h then reduce dose to lowest level needed to maintain solid stool/avoid diarrhea	Toxic megacolon, CNS effects Atropine may cause anticholinergic effects (dry mouth, blurred vision), drowsiness, tachycardia, abdominal pain, pruritis, and urinary retention
Alosetron HCL	Reintroduced/approved by the FDA as unlabeled investigational agent for managing diarrhea in women with severe IBS-D	Prescribing limited to physicians enrolled in Prometheus® prescribing program Begin 0.5 mg PO daily; may be increased slowly up to 1 mg PO BID Discontinue if no improvement at 1 mg BID for 4 weeks	Constipation, ischemic colitis severe enough to be fatal Severe drug–drug interactions detailed in package insert
Clonidine	Use cautiously in patients with coronary artery disease or cerebrovascular disease, patients on other anti-hypertensive agents, impaired liver or renal function	Begin 0.1 mg PO BID May increase to 0.3 mg PO BID. Wean off of medication slowly if ineffective	Severe rebound hypertension, dry mouth, drowsiness, CNS effects, constipation, sedation, orthostatic hypotension, headache, rash, nausea, anorexia, joint pain, impotence, leg cramps, edema, dry eyes

(continued)

Table 24.1 (continued)

Medication	Precautions	Adult dosing	Adverse effects
Cholestyramine	May result in Vitamin K (fat soluble vitamin)/folic acid deficiency May interfere with absorption of other medications, therefore very specific dosing guidelines must be outlined for patients Contraindicated in patients with biliary obstruction	Begin 4 g PO daily Practical dosing is usually 4 g PO BID, however, maximum daily dosing is 24 g	Flatulence, nausea, dyspepsia, abdominal pain, anorexia, sour taste, headache, rash, hematuria, fatigue, bleeding of gums, weight loss
Colestipol	May interfere with fat soluble vitamin absorption May interfere with absorption of other medications, therefore very specific dosing guidelines must be outlined for patients	Begin 2 g (1 g tablets) PO daily Increase to BID or 2–4 g PO every 1–2 months to a maximum of 16 g/day given in divided doses	GI bleeding, abdominal pain, bloating, flatulence, dyspepsia, liver dysfunction, musculoskeletal pain, rash, chest pain, headache, anorexia, dry skin
Probiotics	Avoid using in immuno compromised or septic patients Formulations are highly variable and are not subject to FDA approval	Variable; usually dose is titrated to number of stools patient is having per day Formulations containing *Bifidobacterium* have been shown to be clinically useful in IBS	None currently known
Tincture of opium	Use cautiously in the elderly, patients with seizure disorder, head injury, increased intracranial pressure, asthma, COPD, biliary disease, urethral stricture, prostatic hypertrophy, impaired renal/liver function, Addison's disease and in patients with substance abuse history Care must be taken when prescribing opium tincture as it is 25 times more concentrated than paregoric (anhydrous morphine). The Institute for Safe Medications Practices includes this medication among its list of drugs which have a heightened risk of causing significant patient harm when used in error	Begin 1–2 drops PO BID Slowly titrate up to a maximum dose of 10 drops PO BID (0.5 ml PO BID)	Lightheadedness, dizziness, sedation, nausea, vomiting, sweating, dry mouth, anorexia, urinary hesitancy/retention, weakness, flushing, pruritus, headache, rash, CNS effects/depression, hypotension, bradycardia, syncope, shock, cardiac arrest, increased intracranial pressure, seizures, respiratory depression, abuse/dependency, withdrawal if abrupt discontinuation, dysphoria/euphoria, biliary spasm, anaphylactoid reaction
Amitriptyline	Contraindicated with MAO inhibitor use within past 14 days, recent MI Use caution in the elderly, patients with coronary artery disease, GU obstruction, urinary retention, prostatic hypertrophy, narrow-angle glaucoma, increased intraocular pressure, seizure disorder, thyroid disease, diabetes mellitus, asthma, Parkinson's disease, impaired liver function, schizophrenia, bipolar disorder, history of alcohol abuse or suicide risk	Begin 10 mg PO QHS May increase by 10 mg increments nightly every 7 days if tolerated to a maximum nightly does of 50 mg May give in divided doses	Sedation, nausea, vomiting, increased appetite, weight gain, orthostatic hypotension, hypertension, syncope, severe cardiac effects, CNS effects, increased intraocular pressure, hematologic effects, suicidality, angioedema, anticholinergic effects (dry mouth, blurred vision), urinary retention/frequency, pruritus, libido changes, gynecomastia, galactorrhea, tremor, impotence

Adapted from Scarlett Y. Medical management of fecal incontinence [4]

As noted above, a disordered bowel habit such as diarrhea may be the culprit underlying a patient's complaint of incontinence. Constipation, which is also extremely common in the elderly, may also be a contributing factor to FI. Common etiologies of constipation include IBS, lack of dietary fiber, immobility (sedentary lifestyle), medications, neurological disorders (i.e., Parkinson's disease), metabolic disorders, and pelvic floor dysfunction related to pelvic floor laxity. Constipation may precipitate fecal incontinence by causing fecal impaction with subsequent overflow incontinence. Diminished rectal sensations and increased rectosigmoid compliance can reduce the ability of the rectum to perform its reservoir function and reduce the patient's perception of stool or flatus within the rectum. Altered sensation, coupled with sphincter dysfunction, may result in anal incontinence. As noted above, treatment of the altered bowel habit is crucial to providing symptomatic relief.

Compared to diarrhea, constipation may be more difficult to define but is best divided into three subtypes (a) normal-transit constipation (functional constipation or IBS), (b) slow-transit constipation, and (c) pelvic floor dyssynergia (PFD) [4, 5]. Slow-transit or PFD may precipitate incomplete evacuation, megarectum, and/or decreased rectal sensation. Most cases of fecal incontinence with underlying constipation involve patients who suffer from chronic constipation as opposed to transient bouts of constipation that can be attributed to decreased mobility, decreased fiber or fluid intake, or use of medications such as narcotic analgesics. Constipation is generally defined as three or less bowel movements per week; however, patients may use the term "constipation" to refer to difficult or ineffective defecation. Chronic constipation may predispose a patient to increased rectal capacity and decreased rectal sensitivity, thereby placing the patient at risk for overflow incontinence. As noted above, a patient may actually report that they have diarrhea due to frequent liquid bowel movements and liquid overflow incontinence. It is important for the practitioner to clarify the volume and consistency of incontinent episodes, as overflow incontinence will most likely be associated with small volume, liquid or soft stool loss without a preceding normal bowel movement. This is in opposition to fecal seepage, which usually follows a normal bowel movement although it can certainly also occur in the setting of an abnormal bowel habit. Importantly, constipation may predispose the patient to hemorrhoids or rectal prolapse, which may result in soiling of undergarments with mucus or blood instead of true incontinence; however, the patient may report the staining of undergarments as incontinence. Once constipation has been identified as the underlying etiology for the patient's incontinence, a workup should ensue to define the subtype of constipation. The workup may include endoscopic evaluation, anorectal manometry, defecography, dynamic pelvic floor MRI, and/or a colonic transit studies. Results from the diagnostic evaluation should help guide appropriate intervention strategies. Once the subtype of constipation has been determined, appropriate treatments can be initiated [5]. Dosing guidelines for common pharmacologic therapies used in constipation are outlined below. As with diarrhea, dietary fiber is the first line of therapy in constipation associated with fecal incontinence. However, in patients suffering from constipation or desiccated stool, an adequate water ingestion of at least 64 ounces per day is encouraged. This much water intake may be difficult for patients with urinary frequency/incontinence and limited mobility. Again, caution is advised when initiating fiber therapy in patients who suffer with IBS as abdominal bloating and discomfort may prevent successful use of the supplement. Fiber should always be initiated in low doses and titrated up to 10–15 g of fiber supplementation per day as tolerated. This supplementation is an adjunct to the usual 10–15 g of soluble and insoluble fiber contained in the average Western diet. Pharmacologic agents should be reserved for patients that do not respond to or do not tolerate conservative interventions. However, when using certain laxatives, the practitioner must be careful not to precipitate excess gas production and subsequent incontinence of flatus. Nonabsorbable sugars (lactulose, sorbitol, and glycerin) draw water osmotically into the intestinal lumen, stimulate colonic motility, and may cause initial abdominal discomfort, distention, or flatulence within the first 48 h. These aggravating symptoms usually abate with ongoing treatment. Alternatives to laxatives include pharmacological therapies outlined in Table 24.2.

Patients with Fecal Incontinence and Disordered Defecation with Incomplete Evacuation

The mainstay of treatment in patients who report symptoms of dyssynergic defecation (significant straining, sensation of incomplete evacuation, "want to but can't," excessive toilet time) is pelvic floor rehabilitation with biofeedback therapy and counsel by a skilled professional. Biofeedback therapy (for both pelvic floor dyssynergia and fecal incontinence) will be discussed below. If biofeedback is not indicated or further relief in addition to biofeedback is desired, instruction in clearing the rectal vault of its contents during scheduled intervals may also prove beneficial. Methods for keeping the rectal vault clear include suppositories, retrograde enemas, and the pharmacologic therapies used in chronic constipation. Rectally administered therapies are usually preferred in dyssynergic patients as oral laxation can be both unpredictable and create unwanted abdominal cramping and loose stools with faster colonic transit. Glycerin suppositories are composed of a trihydroxy alcohol, which when placed in direct contact with rectal mucosa, promotes water movement into the distal bowel, stimulates peristalsis, and generally results in a bowel movement within an hour. Tap water enemas are also a very safe alternative, as they contain no irritant chemicals that may result in rectal discomfort, burning, or bleeding. These agents should be used by the dyssynergic patient after an unsatisfactory bowel movement or at scheduled times every day or every other day. For those patients who fail these standard therapies, further evaluation for rare internal hernias with dynamic pelvic floor MRI or referral to a surgeon skilled in the techniques of puborectalis intramuscular injection of botulinum toxin may be necessary. However, most patients will have a marked improvement with instruction in ways to stimulate defecation at scheduled intervals to keep the rectum clear and biofeedback behavioral treatment [6].

Table 24.2 Guidelines for use of medications for constipation in fecal incontinence

Medication	Precaution	Adult Dosing	Adverse effects
Fiber supplementation	May interfere with absorption of other medications, therefore very specific dosing guidelines must be outlined for patients May reduce insulin requirement in diabetic patients	Begin 4 g of preferred preparation daily Titrate up to BID dosing slowly for an optimal daily dose of 16 g of supplemented fiber per day Emphasis on adequate fluid intake is paramount for success of treatment	Flatulence, bloating, abdominal pain, anorexia
Nonabsorbable sugars (lactulose, sorbitol)	Use cautiously in patients with diabetes mellitus, galactosemia	15–30 cc PO daily Maximum dose: 60 cc/daily	Lactic acidosis, hypernatremia, flatulence, bloating, abdominal pain, anorexia, nausea, vomiting, electrolyte disorders
Saline laxatives (sodium phosphate, magnesium sulfate, magnesium citrate, and magnesium hydroxide)	Use cautiously in the elderly Contraindicated in patients with congestive heart failure or renal dysfunction	Variable	Flatulence, bloating, abdominal pain, anorexia, nausea, vomiting, electrolyte disorders
Enemas	Use cautiously in patients with known inflammatory conditions of the rectum	Variable	Hematochezia, rectal burning or stinging
Suppositories (glycerin or bisacodyl)	Use cautiously in patients with known inflammatory conditions of the rectum	Variable	Hematochezia, rectal burning or stinging
Lubiprostone	Use cautiously in pregnant patients or a history of gastrointestinal obstruction	8–24 mcg po BID	Nausea, diarrhea, headache, abdominal pain, flatulence, vomiting, dizziness, fatigue
Linaclotide	Use cautiously in patients with known or suspected mechanical gastrointestinal obstruction	145–290 mcg daily	Diarrhea, abdominal pain, flatulence, abdominal distension

Adapted from Scarlett Y. Medical management of fecal incontinence [4]

Patients with Fecal Seepage

Fecal seepage is distinctly different from fecal incontinence in that it usually involves the loss of small liquid or soft stool after a normal bowel movement [7, 8]. However, patients may report an abnormal bowel habit or may report symptoms more consistent with anal sphincter dysfunction which is not appreciated as a physiologic abnormality on objective anorectal testing. Interestingly, fecal seepage is more prevalent in men and in those patients with preserved anal sphincter function and rectal reservoir capacity. Like patients with disordered defecation, patients with fecal seepage have been shown to demonstrate dyssynergia with impaired balloon expulsion during anorectal manometry testing when compared with other incontinent patients. Similar to patients with dyssynergia, administration of rectal agents and bowel hygiene training (perhaps as a counseling component of biofeedback) are the mainstay of treatment. However, in patients with fecal seepage, clearance of the rectal vault should be performed at a scheduled time each day, regardless of urge to defecate. Ideally, the designated time should be within 30 min after a meal to take advantage of the gastrocolic reflex although any time that the patient has specifically set aside for defecation is likely to be beneficial.

Biofeedback and Cognitive Behavioral Therapy

Biofeedback therapy is a form of operant conditioning or instrumental learning in which information about a physiological process which would otherwise be unconscious is presented to a subject with the aim of having the subject modify that process consciously. For patients with fecal incontinence the process involves brisk external anal sphincter contraction in response to rectal distention, while for patients with dyssynergic defecation, the process focuses on improvement in abdominopelvic coordination. Biofeedback has long been advocated as first-line therapy for patients whose symptoms are mild to moderate due to its safety, affordability, and perceived efficacy. Although often playing a pivotal role in the treatment of fecal incontinence, the Cochrane systematic review of controlled clinical trials on biofeedback has indicated that the combination of a limited number of identified trials and methodological weaknesses would not allow for reliable assessment of the role of biofeedback therapy in the management of patients with fecal incontinence [7, 9–15]. Moreover, a study conducted by leaders in the field suggested that patient–therapist interaction and patient coping strategies may be more important in improving symptoms than performing exercises or receiving physiological feedback on sphincter function [12]. Despite the lack of sound experimental methodology, appropriate control groups and validated outcome measures, reports from centers experienced with the technique suggest that in 60–70 % of a select group of patients, biofeedback may eliminate symptoms in up to one half of patients and decrease symptoms and improve quality of life in up to two thirds. Excellent results can be anticipated if the correct subsets of patients are chosen for treatment. Although there is insufficient evidence with which to select patients suitable for anorectal biofeedback training, most experts agree that the appropriate patient for referral should have physiological evidence of anal dysfunction, be able to cooperate, be well motivated and possess some degree of perception of rectal distention and the ability to contract the external anal sphincter [16]. The presence of severe fecal incontinence, pudendal neuropathy, and underlying neurologic problems has been associated with a suboptimal prognosis. This may be an issue in the elderly population where critical factors for success of biofeedback may be compromised. These factors include cognitive status, vision, gait, and any comorbidity that may limit mobility [1]. Interestingly however, studies with predominantly elderly population have supported the use of biofeedback with a skilled practitioner, particularly for female patients, more severe FI and the absence of a prolonged history of constipation as noted above [17, 18].

Cognitive behavioral therapy (CBT) is an action-oriented form of psychosocial therapy that assumes that maladaptive, or faulty, thinking patterns evoke maladaptive behavior and negative emotions. Maladaptive behavior is defined as behavior that is counter-productive or interferes with everyday living. CBT focuses on redirecting an individual's maladaptive or negative thoughts (cognitive patterns) in order to change his or her behavior and emotional state. Although CBT has less systematic support than biofeedback therapy, some leaders in the field believe that it may improve outcomes [19]. Its use is based on evidence that it is helpful in patients who suffer from functional gastrointestinal disorders such as IBS, rumination syndrome, and functional fecal incontinence. Currently, there are no recommendations as to which patients would most benefit from CBT. The success of CBT is highly dependent upon the availability of CBT therapy and the patient's openness to therapy. Patients who are candidates for CBT should be referred to a certified specialist in this area [16].

Types of Biofeedback Therapy

The goals of all types of biofeedback therapy are essentially the same and include: (a) improvement in anal sphincter muscle strength, (b) improvement in abdominopelvic coordination during voluntary squeeze and following rectal perception, and (c) improvement of anorectal sensory discrimination. However, despite these common goals, each individual treatment protocol should be customized for each patient based upon the underlying pathophysiological mechanism(s) of their incontinence. In order to achieve the goal of continence, two main modalities of biofeedback therapy have been described: (a) use of an intra-anal electromyographic (EMG) sensor, a probe to measure intra-anal pressure, or perianal surface EMG electrodes to teach the patient how to exercise the anal sphincter, and (b) use of a rectal balloon with manometric sensors in the anal canal for sensory discrimination training, usually with the aim of enabling the patient to discriminate and respond to smaller rectal volumes. Manometric probes are also used to teach Kegel exercises aimed at increasing anal muscle strength. These modalities utilize immediate visual and auditory cues to provide feedback for subconscious body processes and to evaluate the level of performance and verbal reinforcement is simultaneously provided by the therapist during each session. The therapist also plays a crucial role in a biofeedback program by reviewing symptom diaries and questionnaires, providing patient education in lifestyle modification and current medical regimens, providing emotional support and reassurance and instruction in practical management of incontinence, anal sphincter exercises and instruction in clinic or home-based biofeedback units [7, 16].

Elements of Biofeedback Therapy

Aside from the pivotal role of the therapist, the remaining elements of biofeedback therapy for each of the modalities outlined above are as follows:

1. Biofeedback methods utilize an intra-anal EMG sensor, perianal surface EMG sensors, or anal manometry probes. All use auditory and visual cues to assist in instructing the patient in how to correctly perform Kegel exercises with the objective of improving anal sphincter strength. While some practitioners use this method to instruct the patient in correct technique to facilitate home exercises and to monitor progress, some have used this method to show correct isolation and use of anal squeeze in response to rectal filling. Although early studies tended to focus on the maximum squeeze increment (mmHg), more recent study results have suggested that the strength and endurance of the squeeze is more important in maintaining continence [16].

2. In most labs, sensory discrimination training is usually performed along with strengthening methods. Sensory discrimination training involves the use of a rectal balloon to retrain the rectal sensory threshold. The initial

distention is usually high and is progressively decreased to diminishing volumes in an effort to teach incontinent patients to respond quickly to lower volumes of stool that present to the rectal vault with the same intensity as they had felt earlier with a higher volume. Appropriate external sphincter contraction in response to rectal distention is rewarded verbally during each repeated effort. As perception and response improve, the audio or visual cue is gradually eliminated in order to assess the threshold for conscious perception (of a once subconscious behavior) of rectal distention [7, 15].

Invasive Therapy

Several intervention options are available to patients who suffer with FI. These procedures depend on the anatomic defect documented after judicious testing with anal manometry, anal ultrasound by an experienced practitioner and, if indicated, endoscopic and radiographic evaluation. Surgical treatments and implantation of associated devices should be reserved for those with medically refractory FI [1].

Perianal Injectable Bulking Agents

The majority of resting continence is maintained by the internal anal sphincter [20]. This sphincter is often not repairable by surgical means. One intervention that has shown some promise in the improvement of passive fecal incontinence due to sphincter dysfunction is the use of injectable bulking agents to improve continence. These agents have been studied since the 1990s as an alternative to their use for urinary incontinence and have included a varying number of different substances [21]. The theory behind the injectable agents is to increase the pressure inside the anal canal to prevent fecal incontinence by bulking the tissue around the anal canal, specifically the anal cushions, with material injected into the space between the two anal sphincters (Fig. 24.1) [22, 23]. Over the last 20 years, some of the materials used include autologous fat, Teflon, carbon-coated zirconium oxide beads (Duraphere®), cross-linked collagen (Contigen®), porcine dermal collagen (Permacol®), synthetic calcium microspheres in aqueous based gel carrier (Coaptite®), silicon biomaterial (PTQ™), and dextranomer microspheres in non-animal stabilized sodium hyaluronate (Solesta®) [22, 23]. Some substances have worked better than others with varying complication rates. The materials are usually injected under endoanal ultrasound or digital (finger) guidance [22]. There has been some evidence that the use of an ultrasound may lead to a greater efficacy of the intervention [22]. The approach taken to inject varies from intersphincteric, trans-sphincteric, or transanal with some

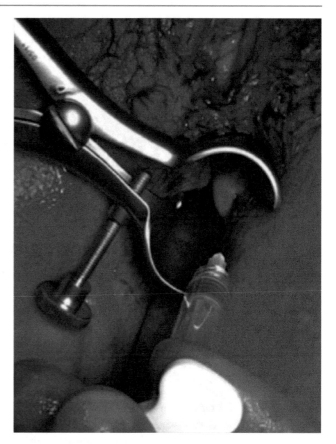

Fig. 24.1 Injection of bulking agent with visible bulge. With permission from Watson NF, Koshy A, Sagar PM. Anal bulking agents for faecal incontinence. Colorectal Dis 2012 Dec;14(3):29–33. © 2012 John Wiley and Sons [23]

data showing the intersphincteric approach leading to a lower complication rate [23]. All of the procedures can take place under local, regional, or general anesthesia after some form of a bowel preparation [23]. Most studies shows the procedure could be done in an outpatient setting, even in the elderly population, except in the setting of a complication [21].

Currently the only FDA approved agent for fecal incontinence, outside of a research setting, is Solesta® which was approved in 2011 for the treatment of fecal incontinence in patients 18 years and older who have failed conservative therapy (Fig. 24.2).

However, a systematic review completed in 2010 determined that a definitive conclusion could not be drawn regarding the effectiveness of perianal injection of bulking agents for fecal incontinence due to the lack of trials that have occurred up to that time. [22] In addition, they also determined that there was no reliable evidence for the effectiveness of one substance over another although there may be a safety benefit in the use of silicon over carbon-coated zirconium oxide beads [22]. There have been several trials since that time, including many randomized trials for Solesta®, suggesting there be a re-evaluation of the use of injectable

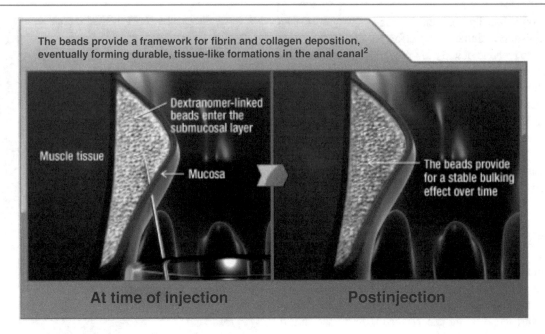

Fig. 24.2 Solesta bulking agent. Courtesy of Salix Pharmaceuticals, downloaded from http://www.solestainfo.com/hcp/about_solesta.aspx on 05/27/2013, with permission

bulking agents outside of a research setting. Much of the long-term data for up to 2 years after injection has shown that there could be a quality of life improvement for those patients with mild–moderate symptoms, who experienced at least a 50–75 % reduction in their fecal incontinence episodes, although re-treatment may be needed to obtain this improvement and long-term efficacy has yet to be defined [21, 23]. The most common adverse side effects seen with most of the injectable material are slight pain or discomfort, urgency, diarrhea, tenderness all of which usually resolve within 1 week. Expulsion of the bulking agent via the insertion needle tract can also be seen [23]. During the first 3 months, a small number of patients may experience mild pain or discomfort with defecation from time to time or the feeling of obstruction at defecation [21]. There have been reports of sepsis in the form of perianal abscess up to years later but it seems to be a rare occurrence [23, 24]. The current consensus is that injectable therapy seems to be safe and with the available data, efficacious for patients with non-severe fecal incontinence symptoms [23]. Current studies with older patients specifically demonstrate acceptable safety profiles [1, 25]. Hopefully, these interventions will become more widely available and affordable in the near future.

Sacral Nerve Stimulation

Sacral nerve stimulation for fecal incontinence has been approved in Europe since 1994, and in the USA since 1997 and is considered the first-line surgical therapy for FI [26].

Sacral nerve stimulation is considered minimally invasive and completely reversible. Sacral nerve stimulation has a low mortality rate and a high efficacy rate [27]. It is recommended in patients with idiopathic fecal incontinence, neurogenic incontinence, small anal sphincter defects, and those with history of complicated vaginal delivery. Women with fecal incontinence tend to have a more complex etiology, making them good candidates for sacral nerve stimulation. Those with history of complicated childbirth likely have a combination of a structural defect of the anal sphincter, rectal hypersensitivity, and sphincter weakness [28]. Sacral nerve stimulation works on the lower bowel and pelvic floor, resulting in an increase in the function of the external anal sphincter. Function of the internal anal sphincter and rectal sensation has been reported as well, but less consistently. In addition, sacral nerve stimulation does not affect gastric emptying or colonic transit time [29].

Prior to the procedure, the physiology of the pelvic floor is evaluated by several modalities including manometry with assessment of anal sphincter function (strength) by pull-back technique and rectal sensation to volumetric distension, endoanal ultrasonography, pudendal nerve terminal motor latency, and defecating proctography or dynamic pelvic floor MRI.

Prior to any permanent forms of stimulation patients undergo peripheral nerve evaluation. A stimulating electrode is inserted percutaneously into the sacral foramen in the bilateral S3 foramina under general or local anesthesia, and positioning is confirmed by fluoroscopy and observation of motor responses. The side with best response is chosen and subsequently connected to an external pulse generator. Parameters are usually set at 210 µs pulse width, 15 Hz frequency, and subsensory amplitude ranging between 0.5 and 10 V with the amplitude being patient controlled. Perineal sensation is documented throughout the test period. The temporary implant will be left in place for 14 days. The electrode is removed in the outpatient setting. If the patient has a 50 % reduction in episodes of fecal incontinence, this is considered a successful result, and the patient can then be offered permanent stimulation [30].

The therapeutic effects of sacral nerve stimulation are mediated through sensory pathways rather than motor pathways. Peripheral neuromodulation has been showed to have direct effect on the cerebral cortex. A study by Griffin et al. evaluated the effect of sacral nerve stimulation on the primary somatosensory cortex in rats. Polysialylated neural cell adhesion molecules (PSA-NCAM) in the cerebral cortex were measured to indicate neuroplasticity. PSA-NCAM is a molecular marker of plasticity. Anal canal stimulation leads to an increase in density of PSA-NCAM cells in the somatosensory cortex. This study also showed no involvement of C-fibers or change in blood pressure or respiratory rate, indicating that nociception was not affected by sacral nerve stimulation [31].

For those who elect to pursue permanent stimulation, a unilateral tined lead and pulse generator are implanted under general anesthesia. The same sacral foramen originally chosen for the trial period is preferred for permanent usage. The pulse generator is placed into the subcutaneous pocket of the ipsilateral buttock of the implanted electrode. Similar stimulation parameters are set at a subsensory threshold [30].

Device and therapy related adverse events included implant site pain, paresthesias, change in sensation, infection, urinary incontinence, neurostimulator battery depletion, diarrhea, pain in extremity, buttock pain, and migration of implant. Most of these were able to be alleviated noninvasively with medication or reprogramming. In a study by Hull et al., 47 out of 120 patients had to have at least 1 device revision, replacement, or explant [32]. Other interventions, while not ideal, included formation of colostomy, explantation or cessation of use of the stimulator, conservative management (although not defined), reprogramming, sphincter repair, change to bilateral stimulation, revision of the implant, and injection of silicone biomaterial [33]. One noteworthy case report demonstrated a severe complication leading to explantation of a sacral nerve stimulator. A patient that required MRI to evaluate lumbar pain required electrode removal prior to the imaging study. The tine electrode was subsequently removed under general anesthesia through the third sacral foramen. During the removal by gentle traction, sudden hemorrhage was observed through the anterior part of the sacral foramen. The original surgery turned into a more complex procedure, requiring enlargement of the wound to enable compression of the bleeding. The patient ultimately required hospitalization for over 1 month, including ICU level of care for hemorrhagic shock. The patient required several units of blood transfusion and vasopressors. The hospitalization was also complicated by infection requiring a 14-day course of antibiotics [34].

Since sacral nerve stimulation was first approved in Europe, most of the studies on cost effectiveness of sacral nerve stimulation were not analyzed in American dollars. In a study by Hetzer et al., sacral nerve stimulation was shown to be most effective in the short term. The patient selection process, which requires an initial 2-week trial period prior to the implantation of a permanent implant also rules out patients who are less likely to find relief from sacral nerve stimulation. The procedure is even less expensive in an outpatient setting and without the aid of general anesthesia. Other more invasive measures usually require an inpatient hospitalization of about a week, thus incurring more cost for the patient. In addition, less complications mean less expense for the patient [28]. Pain as a complication may mean more cost for the patient, but newer models such as Interstim II by Medtronic are associated with decreased pain for the patient [35].

A meta-analysis by Tan et al. in 2011 examined a total of 34 studies on outcome measures of sacral nerve stimulation showed that the procedure increased the quality of life. Patients had an increase in both anal resting and squeeze pressure. Increase in muscle hypertrophy and recruitment of atrophic muscle units could also play a role. The studies in the meta-analysis also showed that rectal sensation improved. It was noted that patients had a decreased threshold for balloon distension (improved sensory discrimination) in addition to decreased urge and maximal tolerable volumes (improved ability to defer defecation). Improved sensation would indicate that the patient would sense rectal content earlier, and therefore defer defecation and decrease episodes of incontinence. Overall patients reported increased quality of life, decreased depression and embarrassment [36]. The majority of patients who underwent sacral nerve stimulation reported improvement of their fecal incontinence after 5 years. Improvement of symptoms was defined as at least 50 % decrease in episodes of incontinent episodes. Using the Fecal Incontinence Quality of Life (FIQOL) and the Fecal Incontinence Severity Index (FISI) questionnaires to evaluate quality of life, sacral nerve stimulation seemed to have a statistically significant impact. FIQOL measures the patient's perception of their own quality of life, whereas the FISI score rates both patient and physician perception of fecal incontinence severity. Patients also notably reported decreased use of protective undergarments such as pads or pantiliners [32].

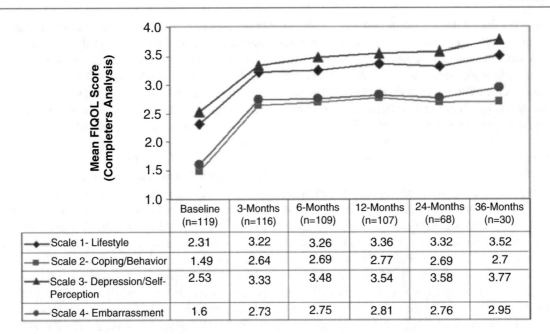

	Baseline (n=119)	3-Months (n=116)	6-Months (n=109)	12-Months (n=107)	24-Months (n=68)	36-Months (n=30)
Scale 1- Lifestyle	2.31	3.22	3.26	3.36	3.32	3.52
Scale 2- Coping/Behavior	1.49	2.64	2.69	2.77	2.69	2.7
Scale 3- Depression/Self-Perception	2.53	3.33	3.48	3.54	3.58	3.77
Scale 4- Embarrassment	1.6	2.73	2.75	2.81	2.76	2.95

Fig. 24.3 Mean FIQoL scores after sacral nerve stimulation. With permission from Wexner S, Coller J, Devroede G, et al. Sacral Nerve Stimulation for Fecal Incontinence: Results of a 120-Patient Prospective Multicenter Study. Ann Surg 2010;251:441. © 2010 Wolters Kluwer [26]

Fig. 24.4 Improvement in weekly incontinence episodes. With permission from Wexner S, Coller J, Devroede G, et al. Sacral Nerve Stimulation for Fecal Incontinence: Results of a 120-Patient Prospective Multicenter Study. Ann Surg 2010;251:441. © 2010 Wolters Kluwer [26]

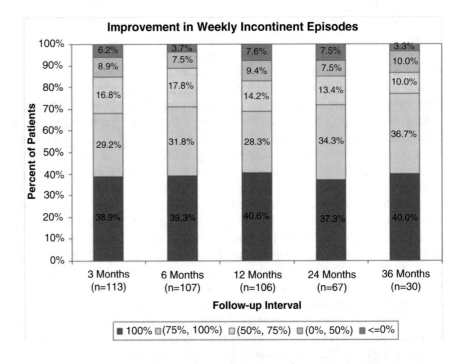

In Figs. 24.3 and 24.4, the Wexner study demonstrated a high efficacy rate of sacral nerve stimulation. In Fig. 24.4, 40 % of patients had 100 % improvement in weekly incontinence episodes, while 37 % had a 75 % improvement 36 months after implantation. Sacral nerve stimulation had similar quality of life scores compared to mechanical barriers such as artificial bowel sphincter and gracioplasty. Being non-mechanical, it also is less likely to worsen antecedent constipation. The Wexner study showed that sacral nerve stimulation had a high efficacy rate with low complication rate, and is completely reversible, making it more appealing to patients [26]. Moreover, a recent trial of 23 patients over the age of 65 showed promising and comparable results to those outcomes found with SNS in younger patients. The number of FI episodes per 2-week period decreased from baseline to an end follow-up of almost 4 years leading to the conclusion that this may be of benefit in the elderly. Of note in this population, SNS may hold most promise for those who do not respond to biofeedback [37].

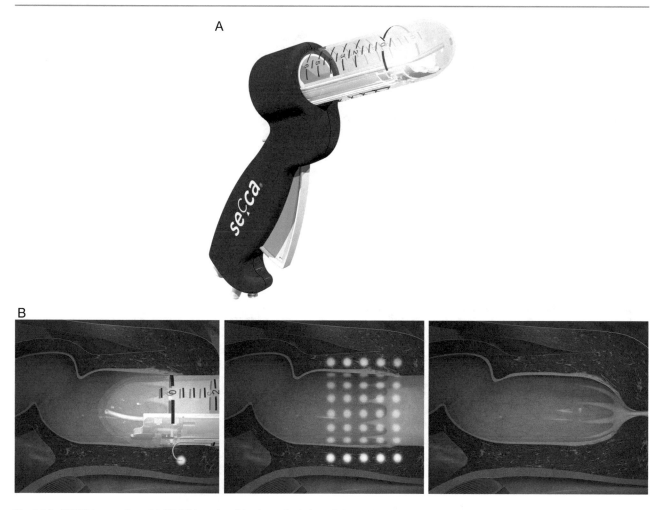

Fig. 24.5 SECCA procedure. (**a**) SECCA probe; (**b**) schematic design of the probe in the anal canal. With permission from Mederi Therapeutics

Radiofrequency Energy

The use of radio frequency energy has been investigated in multiple areas of medicine including gastroenterology. It is a well-established treatment in the use of LES dysfunction in the esophagus but has more recently been under investigation, since its first use in 1999, as a treatment for anal sphincter dysfunction causing moderate fecal incontinence in the form of SECCA procedure (Fig. 24.5a, b) [20, 38]. This procedure is usually reserved for patients who have failed conservative management [38]. During this minimally invasive procedure, temperature-controlled radio frequency energy is delivered to the anal canal muscle. The premise is that the heat from the energy causes collagen contraction, focal wound healing, remodeling, and tissue compliance reduction improving the function of the sphincter [20, 39]. The procedure takes around 30–40 min in an outpatient setting after a form of bowel prep with sedation and local anesthesia [38]. Complications include minimal bleeding, pain, and rarely diarrhea or constipation. Some patients have reported improvement in quality of life up to 1–2 years afterwards, or longer, with some improvement in fecal severity scores as well, although this has been mostly in younger patients with a shorter mean duration of fecal incontinence which may not translate to improved FI scores in the elderly population [38–41]. Long-term studies are still underway and required to ascertain the long-term effects of radiofrequency ablation in the use of moderate fecal incontinence [20].

Artificial Bowel Sphincter

The artificial bowel sphincter was first used in 1996 for patients with fecal incontinence after being modified from an artificial sphincter being used at the time for urinary incontinence. Since then, over 500 have been implanted for patients with severe fecal incontinence who have failed conservative therapy, with varying results [42]. The name of the current device in use is the Action™ Neosphincter (Fig. 24.6a, b) and is solid silicone with three parts: an occlusive anal cuff,

Fig. 24.6 (**a**) Action™
Neosphincter. (**b**) Action™
Neosphincter in a female. With
permission from American Medical
Systems

A

B

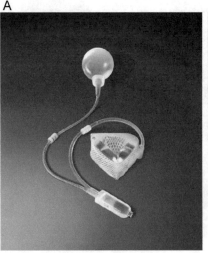
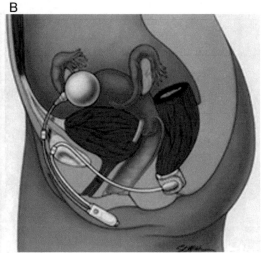

a pressure regulating balloon, and a control pump. The cuff is implanted around the anal canal and uses pressure to occlude the anal canal. The balloon is placed into the space of Retzius with the control pump in either the labia or scrotum [20]. The patient will deflate the cuff using the control pump, which leads to evacuation of the rectum and then the cuff will passively refill over the next few minutes [20]. Many patients go from being completely incontinent to both liquid and solid stool to only minor seepage and have improvement in the fecal continence and quality of life. Unfortunately, some evidence have shown a failure rate as high as 30 % with a high complication rate [20]. The procedure would require a form of bowel prep, general anesthesia, and possible hospital stay. Complications vary from infections, surgical revision, and erosion of the cuff and/or pump, pain with activation, constipation, or fecal impaction. After prolonged wear and tear some cuffs may begin to leak and require repair or re-implantation. Up to a third of patients eventually have their device removed or re-implanted due to complications leading to a recent systematic review deeming it experimental. One study cited a risk for revision at 1 year at around 7 % and up to 88 % after 10 years [42]. Despite this information, the device still remains a non-surgical option for severe fecal incontinence when nerve stimulation has failed or not an option [20, 42].

New research is underway is new types of artificial bowel sphincters that will not require manipulation by the patient to evacuate including one powered by a hydraulic-electric mechanism [43]. These technologies are not in use yet but may be the wave of the future for artificial bowel sphincters.

Magnetic Bowel Sphincter

A novel non-surgical approach to severe fecal incontinence that has failed conservative therapy is the magnetic bowel sphincter. The magnetic sphincter uses magnetic forces to

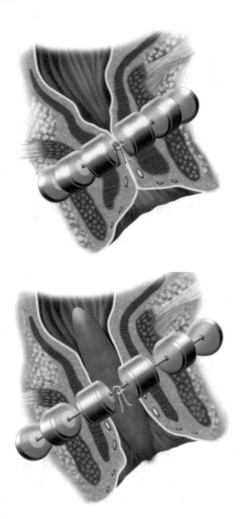

Fig. 24.7 Magnetic bowel sphincter. Courtesy of Torax Medical, Shoreview, MN

augment the native anal sphincter (Fig. 24.7) [42]. An advantage of this technology is that once it has been implanted it, there is usually no need for further augmentation [42].

The beads have magnetic cores and form a flexible ring that rests around the external anal sphincter in a circular fashion. The length of the magnetic strand can be altered to fit the size of the native sphincter. Prior to the procedure, patients must undergo a form of bowel preparation and will require general anesthesia with possible need for hospital admission. Complications include mild rectal bleeding, and passing of the device out the rectum. Most patients have some improvement in fecal incontinence scores as well as quality of life despite anal manometry evidence that there is not an increase in anal pressure with the magnetic sphincter. Some data show this may not have the same efficacy as the artificial bowel sphincter but given the ease of insertion, the need for no further manipulation and low complication rates, this could be considered therapy for severe fecal incontinence in patients who have failed conservative therapy but do not desire surgical intervention [42].

Overlapping Sphincteroplasty

The use of overlapping sphincteroplasty (Fig. 24.8) for sphincter injury dates back to the 1970s when it was first used to repair any obstetric sphincter injury. It has been a cornerstone for moderate to severe fecal incontinence due to sphincter injury since that time [44–46]. It is universally available and deemed a possible intervention in the elderly population, making it an option when electrical stimulation, injectable bulking agents, or other interventions are not available or when patients are not candidates for these other interventions. Short-term data shows improvement for most

patients in regard to their quality of life as well as a reduction in the frequency of fecal incontinence, however, most of the long-term data about the efficacy of the procedure to decrease fecal incontinent episodes have not been encouraging [45, 46]. One review article showed that by 10 years post-procedure many patients had substantial decline in their fecal continence even if some maintain an improvement in quality of life [46]. There are multiple techniques and approaches (bulk repair vs. repair of individual muscles with or without levatorplasty) but there does not seem to be a general consensus as to the preferred technique and how this relates to outcomes. In the past few years there has also been research into the use of biological grafts in sphincter augmentation to increase reinforcement to the native tissue after the procedure [46]. The most recent data shows this may increase patient satisfaction and time until decline in fecal continence post-procedure but more long-term data is needed to assess the true benefit of using the grafts [46]. Side effects include many commonly seen in any surgical procedure such as wound infection or hematoma development [47]. Until a minimally invasive procedure is available to improve fecal continence in patients with severe symptoms, overlapping sphincteroplasty will continue to be cornerstone in the treatment of these patients [46].

Dynamic Gracioplasty

Gracioplasty presents as a surgical option for severe fecal incontinence. A neosphincter is created around the anal canal with the gracilis muscle (Fig. 24.9) [48, 49]. The gracilis

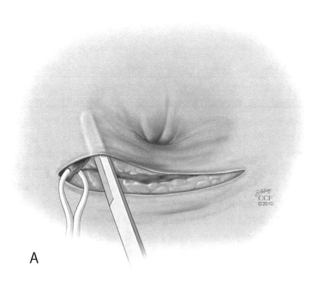

A

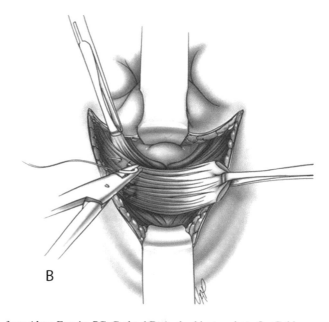

B

Fig. 24.8 Schematic drawing for overlapping sphincteroplasty. (**a**) The external sphincter is identified and grasped with the Allis clamp; (**b**) The external sphincter is overlapped and sutured into place. With permission from Alves-Ferreira PC, Gurland B. Anal sphincteroplasty. In: Goldman HB. Complications of Female Incontinence and Pelvic Reconstructive Surgery. Springer, New York 2013; pp:189–195. © 2013 Springer [54]

Fig. 24.9 Configuration of the anal dynamic graciloplasty. Showing the transposed gracilis muscle, the electrodes, the neurostimulator, and the external magnet

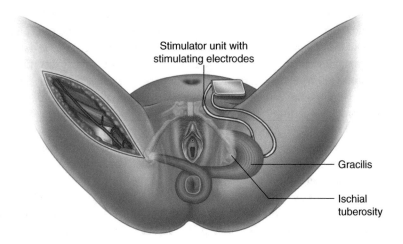

muscle was chosen due to its constant innervation by the obturator nerve and vascular supply from the profunda femoris [50]. Initially the results of graciloplasty were unfavorable, as the muscle was not able to sustain a contraction. The gracilis muscle contains mostly type II muscle fibers, leading to earlier muscle fatigue and therefore only enabling short bursts of muscle contraction. The procedure was improved with electrical stimulation; the implantation of electrodes and a pulse generator enables a sustained contraction. Type II muscle fibers are turned into type I fatigue-resistant fibers. With the assistance of a stimulator, the gracilis can function as a neosphincter.

Resting manometry pressures after nonstimulated graciloplasty increased by 4.1 mmHg and with stimulation increased by 20.9 mmHg in a 2001 multicenter study by Wexner et al. However neither of these was statistically significant. In the same study, enema retention time was improved after dynamic graciloplasty, however again was not statistically significant. Despite the lack of statistical significance in the above measurements, quality of life had improved significantly for these patients. In addition, the manometry results could be utilized to adjust the stimulator [50].

Malone Antegrade Continence Enema

Since 1989, antegrade continence enemas have been used in pediatric patients with a history of neurological abnormality or structural defect, such as spina bifida or imperforate anus, respectively. These pathologies have led to an increased likelihood of fecal incontinence. Malone developed a procedure where a stoma is creating using the appendix implanted into the cecum, creating a non-refluxing channel to enable the use of antegrade washouts to clear the colon and therefore prevent episodes of fecal incontinence. This method was utilized as the last-line attempt at treating fecal incontinence before colostomy was considered. The antegrade continence enema was a more aesthetic option than the formation of a permanent colostomy [51].

The Malone antegrade continence enema has been shown to be effective in children, however not as ideal in the adult population. The patient is required to have time, be highly motivated, and physically able to perform the enemas. The enemas require a high compliance rate in order to be effective. The procedure in adults is more ideal for those with neurogenic disorders rather than structural abnormalities. Even those with neurogenic disorders can lack the ability to relax their anal sphincter, making it difficult to perform the enema. Adult anatomy tends to be more complex and is longer than children's anatomy, making the antegrade enemas more difficult in the adult population. Overall the antegrade enema is more psychologically and physically difficult for the adult patient to cope with the long-term usage [52].

Colostomy

If patients have failed the above option, colostomy formation remains an option. However, it is aesthetically less appealing to most patients. It would be considered curative and less likely to fail in regard to fecal incontinence [7]. Colostomy does require more day-to-day care than the other options and could present some of the same issues for patients as fecal incontinence. For example, patients may still experience anxiety regarding the nearest bathroom or fear of accidents. Overall, patients who undergo colostomy formation for fecal incontinence experience improved quality of life [53]. For patients who are immobile, colostomy is ideal as it would function as a diversion of fecal matter to prevent skin breakdown and further medical complications [7]. Specifically, it is an option in the elderly because it would offer a more scheduled bowel care regimen for caregivers as well as an overall ease of defecation for the elderly patient who may be at high risk for complications from poor stool hygiene (Table 24.3) [1].

Table 24.3 Comparison of invasive treatments for fecal incontinence

Type of intervention	Indications	Advantages	Disadvantages	Contraindications/Precautions
Injectable bulking agents	Mild–moderate FI	Outpatient procedure, ease of administration, lack of general anesthesia	Expensive, considered experimental, infection risk, need of repeat procedure to maintain effect	Children, patients who currently have a rectal infection or bleeding, anal fissures, hemorrhoids, IBD, HIV/AIDS, undergoing chemotherapy or organ transplant, previous pelvic radiation, or current anal device in place, allergy to agent [Solesta® insert]
Sacral nerve stimulation	Mod–Severe	Minimally invasive, can be done outpatient, reversible	Expensive, risk of infection, failure of stim device	Diathermy, patients who failed initial temporary testing, patients who are unable to operate device
MACE	Severe	Good for pediatric patients and those with neurogenic bowel	Requires general anesthesia, not ideal for adults	Not typically intended for the adult population
Radiofrequency ablation	Mild–moderate FI	Outpatient procedure, low risk procedure, lack of general anesthesia	No long-term data on efficacy	Children, patients who currently have rectal infection or bleeding, anal fissures/fistulas, chronic constipation, abnormal blood coagulation or use of anticoagulant other than aspirin, collagen vascular disease, IBD, previous pelvic radiation, pregnancy, history of laxative abuse or unstable psychiatric disorder [Mederi Therap.]
Artificial bowel sphincter	Moderate–severe FI	Low risk procedure	Need of general anesthesia, inpatient procedure, variable success rates, decline in efficacy over years, patient manipulation required	Children, IBD, pelvic sepsis, pregnancy, or patients who practice anal-receptive intercourse [42], poor candidate for a surgical procedure or anesthesia, irreversible obstructed bowel [American medical systems insert]
Magnetic bowel sphincter	Moderate–severe FI	No need for patient manipulation after fitted, low risk procedure	Need of general anesthesia, inpatient procedure, variable success rates	IBD, pelvic sepsis, previous rectal surgery, poor candidate for a surgical procedure or anesthesia, anal fistula, current rectal or vaginal prolapse, previous pelvic radiation, recent colon cancer, nearby metallic implants, pregnancy, patients who practice anal-receptive intercourse [42]
Overlapping sphincteroplasty	Severe FI	Short-term improvement for severe FI, widely available with long-term success data available	Need of general anesthesia, inpatient procedure with recovery time, infection risk, decline in efficacy after 5–10 years	Pelvic sepsis, poor candidate for a surgical procedure or anesthesia, IBD [46]
Stimulated graciloplasty	Severe FI	Good for patients with structural abnormality, controlled by the patient	Major surgery requiring general anesthesia and inpatient admission, risk of requiring revision, expensive	Not ideal for poor surgical candidates
Colostomy	Severe FI	Preferred in patients that are bed-bound or at high risk for decubitus ulcers	Aesthetically displeasing, requires daily care, major surgery requiring general anesthesia and inpatient admission, expensive	Not ideal for poor surgical candidates

FI fecal incontinence

Key Points

- Fecal incontinence (FI) is a common complaint among older patients that is frequently not addressed by clinicians
- Patients with FI may inaccurately report diarrhea as the presenting problem

- Evaluation of older patients in both ambulatory and inpatient care settings should prompt review of any FI symptoms
- In addition to behavioral changes, empiric symptomatic treatment of a disordered bowel habit (diarrhea or constipation) is often helpful in treating FI
- Biofeedback with skilled practitioners may be an appropriate initial therapy for some patients with FI who have

failed conservative treatment and who are motivated and ambulatory

• Referral for more invasive interventions should be based on objective testing and demonstration of promising results in older patients.

References

1. Shah BJ, Chokhavatia S, Rose S. Fecal incontinence in the elderly: FAQ. Am J Gastroenterol. 2012;107:1635–46.
2. AlAmeel T, Andrew MK, MacKnight C. The association of fecal incontinence with institutionalization and mortality in older adults. Am J Gastroenterol. 2012;105(8):1830–4.
3. Wald A. Fecal incontinence: three steps to successful management. Geriatrics. 1997;52(7):49–52.
4. Scarlett Y. Medical management of fecal incontinence. Gastroenterology. 2004;126(1):S55–63.
5. Prather CM. Subtypes of constipation: sorting out the confusion. Rev Gastroenterol Disord. 2004;4 Suppl 2:S11–6.
6. Crowell MD. Pathogenesis of slow transit and pelvic floor dysfunction: from bench to bedside. Rev Gastroenterol Disord. 2004;4 Suppl 2:S17–27.
7. Rao SSC. Diagnosis and management of fecal incontinence. Am J Gastroenterol. 2004;1585–1604.
8. Rao SS, Ozturk R, Stessman M. Investigation of the pathophysiology of fecal seepage. Am J Gastroenterol. 2004;99(11): 2204–9.
9. Enck P. Biofeedback training in disordered defecation: a critical review. Dig Dis Sci. 1993;38:1953–60.
10. Glia A, Gylin M, Akerlund JE. Biofeedback training in patients with fecal incontinence. Dis Colon Rectum. 1998;41(3):359–64.
11. Miner PB, Donnelly TC, Read NW. Investigation of the mode of action of biofeedback in treatment of fecal incontinence. Dig Dis Sci. 1990;35:1291–8.
12. Norton C, Hosker G, Brazzelli M. Effectiveness of biofeedback and/or sphincter exercises for the treatment of fecal incontinence in adults. Cochrane Electron Libr. 2003;1.
13. Wald A. Biofeedback therapy for fecal incontinence. Ann Intern Med. 1981;146–9.
14. Whitehead WE, Burgio KL, Engel BT. Biofeedback treatment of fecal incontinence in geriatric patients. J Am Geriatr Soc. 1985;33:320–4.
15. Norton C. Behavioral management of fecal incontinence in adults. Gastroenterology. 2004;126:S64–70.
16. Lunsford TEJ. Fecal incontinence: office-based management. In: Sands LR, Sands DR, editors. Ambulatory colorectal surgery. 1st ed. Informa Healthcare; 2008. p. 121–34.
17. Byrne CM, Solomon MJ, Young JM, Rex J, Merlino CL. Biofeedback for fecal incontinence: short-term outcomes of 513 consecutive patients and predictors of successful treatment. Dis Colon Rectum. 2007;50(4):417–27.
18. Heymen S, Scarlett Y, Jones K, Ringel Y, Drossman D, Whitehead WE. Randomized controlled trial shows biofeedback to be superior to pelvic floor exercises for fecal incontinence. Dis Colon Rectum. 2009;52(10):1730–7.
19. Drossman DA, Toner BB, Whitehead WE, Diamant NE, et al. Cognitive-behavioral therapy versus education and desipramine versus placebo for moderate to severe functional bowel disorders. Gastroenterology. 2003;125:19–31.
20. Margolin DA. New options for the treatment of fecal incontinence. Ochsner J. 2008;8(1):18–24.
21. Danielson J, Karlbom U, Sonesson AC, Wester T, Graf W. Submucosal injection of stabilized nonanimal hyaluronic acid with dextranomer: a new treatment option for fecal incontinence. Dis Colon Rectum. 2009;52(6):1101–6.
22. Maeda Y, Laurberg S, Norton C. Perianal injectable bulking agents as treatment for faecal incontinence in adults. Cochrane Datab Syst Rev. 2010;12(5).
23. Watson NF, Koshy A, Sagar PM. Anal bulking agents for faecal incontinence. Colorectal Dis. 2012;14(3):29–33.
24. Berger MBMD. Delayed presentation of pseudoabscess secondary to injection of pyrolytic carbon-coated beads bulking agent. Female Pelvic Med Reconstr Surg. 2012;18(5):303–5.
25. Dodi G, Jongen J, de la Portilla F, Raval M, Altomare DF, Lehur PA. An open-label, noncomparative, multicenter study to evaluate efficacy and safety of NASHA/DxGel as a bulking agent for the treatment of fecal in continence. Gastroenterol Res Pract. 2010;467136.
26. Wexner S, Coller J, Devroede G, et al. Sacral nerve stimulation for fecal incontinence: results of a 120-patient prospective multicenter study. Ann Surg. 2010;251:441.
27. Devroede G. Quality of life is markedly improved in patients with fecal incontinence after sacral nerve stimulation. Female Pelvic Med Reconstr Surg. 2012;18:103.
28. Hetzer FH. Outcome and cost analysis of sacral nerve stimulation for faecal incontinence. Br J Surg. 2006;93:1411.
29. Damgaard M. The influence of sacral nerve stimulation on gastrointestinal motor function in patients with fecal incontinence. Neurogastroenterol Motil. 2011;23:556.
30. Boyle D. Efficacy of sacral nerve stimulation for the treatment of fecal incontinence. Dis Colon Rectum. 2011;54:1271.
31. Griffin K. Sacral nerve stimulation increases activation of the primary somatosensory cortex by anal canal stimulation in an experimental model. Ir J Med Sci. 2010;179:S284.
32. Hull T. Long-term durability of sacral nerve stimulation therapy for chronic fecal incontinence. Dis Colon Rectum. 2013;56:234.
33. Maeda Y. Postoperative issues of sacral nerve stimulation for fecal incontinence and constipation: a systematic literature review and treatment guideline. Dis Colon Rectum. 2011;54:1443.
34. Faucheron J. Life threatening haemorrhage after electrode removal: a severe complication following sacral nerve stimulation procedure for the treatment of faecal incontinence. Colorectal Dis. 2011; 14:e133.
35. Leroi A. Outcome and cost analysis of sacral nerve modulation for treating urinary and/or fecal incontinence. Ann Surg. 2011; 253(4):720.
36. Tan E. Meta-analysis: sacral nerve stimulation versus conservative therapy in the treatment of faecal incontinence. Int J Colorectal Dis. 2011;26:275.
37. George AT, Kalmar K, Goncalves J, Nicholls RJ, Vaizey CJ. Sacral nerve stimulation in the elderly. Colorectal Dis. 2012;14(2):200–4.
38. Ruiz D, Pinto RA, Hull TL, Efron JE, Wexner SD. Does the radiofrequency procedure for fecal incontinence improve quality of life and incontinence at 1-year follow-up? Dis Colon Rectum. 2010;53(7):1041–6.
39. Lefebure B, Tuech JJ, Bridoux V, Gallas S, Leroi AM, Denis P, Michot F. Temperature-controlled radio frequency energy delivery (Secca procedure) for the treatment of fecal incontinence: results of a prospective study. Int J Colorectal Dis. 2008;23(10):993–7.
40. Takahashi-Monroy T, Morales M, Garcia-Osogobio S. SECCA procedure for te treatment of fecal incontinence: results of five-year follow-up. Dis Colon Rectum. 2008;51:355–9.
41. Felt-Bersma RJ, Szojda MM, Mulder CJ. Temperature-controlled radiofrequency energy (SECCA) to the anal canal for the treatment of faecal incontinence offers moderate improvement. Eur J Gastroenterol Hepatol. 2007;19(7):575–80.
42. Wong MT, Meurette G, Wyart V, Glemain P, Lehur PA. The artificial bowel sphincter: a single institution experience over a decade. Ann Surg. 2011;254(6):951–6.

43. Zan P, Yang B, Zhang JY, Shao Y. Research on a novel artificial anal sphincter for human incontinence. J Med Eng Technol. 2010;34(7–8):386–92.
44. Wong MT, Meurette G, Stangherlin P, Lehur PA. The magnetic anal sphincter versus the artificial bowel sphincter: a comparison of 2 treatments for fecal incontinence. Dis Colon Rectum. 2011;54(7):773–9.
45. El-Gazzaz G, Zutshi M, Hannaway C, Gurland B, Hull T. Overlapping sphincter repair: does age matter? Dis Colon Rectum. 2012;55(3):256–61.
46. Zutshi M, Ferreira P, Hull T, Gurland B. Biological implants in sphincter augmentation offer a good short-term outcome after a sphincter repair. Colorectal Dis. 2012;14(7):866–71.
47. Johnson E, Carlsen E, Steen TB, Backer Hjorthaug JO, Eriksen MT, Johannessen HO. Short- and long-term results of secondary anterior sphincteroplasty in 33 patients with obstetric injury. Acta Obstet Gynecol Scand. 2010;89(11):1466–72.
48. Briel JW, de Boer LM, Hop WC, Schouten WR. Clinical outcome of anterior overlapping external anal sphincter repair with internal anal sphincter imbrication. Dis Colon Rectum 1998;41(2):209–14.
49. Baeten C. Anal dynamic graciloplasty in the treatment of intractable fecal incontinence. NEJM. 1995;332:1600.
50. Wexner S. Long-term efficacy of dynamic graciloplasty for fecal incontinence. Dis Colon Rectum. 2002;45:809.
51. Malone PS. Preliminary report: the antegrade continence enema. Lancet. 1990;336:1217.
52. Gerharz EW. The value of the MACE (Malone Antegrade Colonic Enema) procedure in adult patients. J Am Coll Surg. 1997;185:544.
53. Sjodahl R. Long-term quality of life in patients with permanent sigmoid colostomy. Colorectal Dis. 2012;14, e335.
54. Alves-Ferreira PC, Gurland B. Anal sphincteroplasty. In: Goldman HB. editor. Complications of female incontinence and pelvic reconstructive surgery. Springer, New York 2013; p. 189–95.

Chronic Constipation

Erica N. Roberson and Arnold Wald

Introduction

Chronic constipation is a common disorder in adults older than 60 years, and is a frequent reason for their seeking medical care. Clinically, constipation may be defined as unsatisfactory defecation resulting from infrequent stools, difficult stool passage, hardness of stool, or feeling of incomplete evacuation [1]. Although constipation is rarely a life-threatening disorder, it can impair quality of life and carries a significant economic burden [2]. Treatment is usually empiric, using dietary changes and laxatives. Only if conservative measures fail should specialized testing be considered to define pathophysiologic subgroups, as this will influence treatment [3].

Definition and Classification

Although physicians frequently define constipation on the basis of frequency alone (less than 3 stools per week), patients are more likely to complain of unsatisfactory defecation and this is often influenced by cultural and social customs [4]. Symptoms include the type of stool (hard/lumpy), and subjective feelings such as excessive straining, feeling of incomplete evacuation, sense of difficulty passing stool, and the need for manual maneuvers during defecation [1, 3]. Chronic constipation is clinically distinguished from acute or intermittent constipation by the presence of symptoms for greater than 3 months [1]. The Rome Criteria have been used to attempt to identify homogeneous groups of patients for clinical trials investigating treatments for constipation (Table 25.1) but are less suitable for routine clinical use [5]. Constipation predominant IBS (IBS-C) should be considered in constipated patients with significant abdominal discomfort or pain although there is an overlap with functional constipation in clinical practice (Table 25.1). Potentially treatable conditions which cause or exacerbate constipation should be considered in all patients with chronic *constipation* (Table 25.2).

Classifying chronic constipation into three major groups (normal transit constipation, pelvic floor dysfunction, and slow transit constipation) is clinically useful for patients who do not respond to conservative measures and empiric laxatives. Pelvic floor dysfunction, also called functional defecation disorder, may be associated with inadequate propulsive forces and/or increased resistance to evacuation caused by incoordination of abdominal, rectal, and anal muscles resulting in inadequate or difficult emptying of rectum (Table 25.3) [6]. Dyssynergic defecation, for example, is associated with inappropriate contraction of the puborectalis muscle and the external anal sphincter (Type 1) or incomplete relaxation of the anal canal (Type 2) during defecation attempts [6, 7]. This disorder may occur with normal or slow colonic transit. Pelvic floor dysfunction can result in secondary delayed colon transit which reverses with successful treatment of the defecatory disorder. The term slow transit constipation should be reserved for patients with slow transit of the colon and normal rectal evacuation, a distinction which is of considerable clinical importance.

Epidemiology

As many as one-fifth of all persons will experience chronic constipation during their lifetime [2, 8]. Prevalence and incidence data vary according to survey methods; for example, rates of self-reported constipation are higher compared to

E.N. Roberson
Oregon Health and Science University, Portland, OR, USA

A. Wald (✉)
Division of Gastroenterology and Hepatology, University of Wisconsin School of Medicine and Public Health,
Centennial Building, Suite 4000, 1685 Highland Avenue, Madison, WI, USA
e-mail: axw@medicine.wisc.edu

© Springer Science+Business Media New York 2017
D.A. Gordon, M.R. Katlic (eds.), *Pelvic Floor Dysfunction and Pelvic Surgery in the Elderly*,
DOI 10.1007/978-1-4939-6554-0_25

Table 25.1 Definitions of constipation by various gastroenterology society and groups

	Constipation	Constipation predominant IBS
AGA [3]	Syndrome of bowel symptoms including difficult or infrequent passage of stool, hardness of stool, or a feeling of incomplete evacuation that may occur either in isolation or secondary to another underlying disorder (e.g., Parkinson's disease)	Abdominal discomfort that is temporally associated with 2 of the following 3 symptoms: relief of discomfort after defecation, hard stools, or less frequent stools
ACG [1]	Difficult stool passage that includes straining, a sense of difficulty passing stool, incomplete evacuation, hard/lumpy stools, prolonged time to stool, or need for manual maneuvers to pass stool. Chronic constipation is defined as the presence of these symptoms for at least 3 months	Abdominal pain or discomfort that occurs in association with altered bowel habits over a period of at least 3 months
Rome III [5]	1. Must include *two or more* of the following: (a) Straining during at least 25 % of defecations, (b) Lumpy or hard stools at least 25 % of defecations (c) Sensation of incomplete evacuation at least 25 % of defecations (d) Sensation of anorectal obstruction/blockage at least 25 % of defecations (e) Manual maneuvers to facilitate at least 25 % of defecations (e.g., digital evacuation, support of the pelvic floor) (f) Fewer than 3 defecations per week 2. Loose stools are rarely present without the use of laxatives 3. Insufficient criteria for IBS 4. Symptoms present for 6 months	1. Recurrent abdominal pain or discomfort at least 3 days per month in the past 3 months associated with 2 or more of the following: (a) Improvement with defecation (b) Onset associated with change in frequency of stool (c) Onset associated with change in form (appearance) of stool 2. Hard or lumpy stools 25 % and loose (mushy) or watery stools <25 % of bowel movements

Table 25.2 Secondary causes of constipation in the elderly

Mechanical
Colorectal cancer
Anal fissure
Rectal/anal stricture
Rectocele (some)
Pseudo obstruction
Megacolon
Neurologic disease
Spinal cord lesion
Stroke
Parkinson's disease
Multiple sclerosis
Metabolic disturbances
Hypercalcemia
Hypokalemia
Hypomagnesemia
Hypothyroidism
Uremia
Medications
Opiates
Anticholinergics
Calcium channel blockers
Anticonvulsants
Antidepressants
Antispasmodics
Antihistamines Non-steroidal anti-inflammatory drugs
Miscellaneous
Amyloidosis
Scleroderma
Heavy metal poisoning

Table 25.3 Functional defecation disorder definitions [7]

Functional defecation disorders
1. The patient must satisfy diagnostic criteria for functional constipation (Table 25.1)
2. During repeated attempts to defecate must have at least 2 of the following:
(a) Evidence of impaired evacuation, based on balloon expulsion test or imaging
(b) Inappropriate contraction of the pelvic floor muscles (i.e., anal sphincter or puborectalis) or less than 20 % relaxation of basal resting sphincter pressure by manometry, imaging, or EMG
(c) Inadequate propulsive forces assessed by manometry or imaging
3. Criteria fulfilled for the last 3 months with symptom onset at least 6 months prior to diagnosis
Dyssynergic defecation
Inappropriate contraction of the pelvic floor or less than 20 % relaxation of basal resting sphincter pressure with adequate propulsive forces during attempted defecation
Inadequate defecatory propulsion
Inadequate propulsive forces with or without inappropriate contraction or less than 20 % relaxation of the anal sphincter during attempted defecation

rates assessed using Rome Criteria. Worldwide, the prevalence of constipation in adults approximates 16 % with some differences among countries [9]. Constipation is more prevalent in elderly populations in all surveys [9]. Persons older than age 60 in community based populations are 1.4 times more likely to report constipation than adults less than 29 years old [10]. Of these, 24 % fulfill criteria for functional constipation and 21 % for outlet delay defined as structural or pelvic floor muscle abnormalities resulting in difficulties with defecation [11]. Older patients are more likely to associate constipation with difficulty passing stools and hard stools and are more likely to use laxatives [12, 13]. Among nursing home residents, the prevalence of constipation is as high as 70 % [14].

Chronic constipation is twice as prevalent in women as men, although this difference is somewhat attenuated as age increases [8, 15]. Dyssynergic defecation is more common in women, who also are more likely to have slow transit constipation in addition to dyssynergic defecation [16]. Other factors reported to be associated with constipation include nonwhite race, low income, low education, and physical inactivity [17].

Burden of Disease

Constipation has a negative impact on quality of life [18]. Patients with constipation are more likely to visit their health care provider, have more emergency room visits, are more likely to miss work, and are less productive at work [19]. From 2001–2004, there were almost 8 million ambulatory visits for constipation in the USA, with an estimated 1.12 million visits to a gastroenterologist [3, 20]. The annual direct cost of constipation per patient was calculated to be $7522, with average out of pocket expenses of $390; the figures were based on administrative claims from patients seen in primary care and gastroenterology clinics in a health maintenance organization [21]. Colonoscopy is responsible for more than one-third of the cost of evaluating constipation [6]. More than $800 million dollars is spent on laxatives annually in the USA, although an exact estimate is difficult as many patients use over-the-counter laxatives [4].

Physiology of Colonic Transit and Defecation

The primary function of the colon is to absorb water and electrolytes, store fecal waste until defecation, and periodically propel contents toward the anus. Segmental and retrograde propulsive contractions slow movement of stool and enhance absorption. High amplitude propagated contractions (HAPCs) are migrating motor complexes that propel large quantities of fecal matter into the sigmoid colon and rectum. Colonic motility has a circadian rhythm with maximum activity occurring upon awakening and minimal activity during sleep. Eating results in increased colonic motility for several hours, the magnitude of which varies with the amount and composition of food. Colonic transit is also controlled by the vagus and pelvic nerves, which carry parasympathetic innervations while the sympathetic innervation comes from the superior and inferior mesenteric ganglia. Intrinsic motor activity is regulated by the enteric nervous system located in the myenteric (Auerbach) and submucosal (Meissner) plexuses [22].

Normal defecation involves neuromuscular coordination of the muscles of the pelvic floor and anal sphincters. The former consist of the levator ani and puborectalis muscles (Fig. 25.1) whereas the latter include the internal (involuntary) and external (voluntary) anal sphincters. A mechanical barrier to stool movement is created by the anorectal angulation created by the puborectalis which receives innervation through the pudendal and perineal nerves; the pudendal nerve alone innervates the external anal sphincter. When defecation is initiated, intraabdominal pressures increase while the anal sphincters and puborectalis muscle relax. Consequently, the anorectal angle widens, the perineum descends, and anal canal pressure decreases to allow expulsion of stool [23].

Pathophysiology of Constipation

Since patients with constipation are frequently treated empirically with conservative measures and over-the counter laxatives and do not undergo diagnostic testing, the precise pathophysiology of functional constipation in most patients is unknown. However, patients who are refractory to such measures should be evaluated for a pelvic floor disorder or slow transit constipation. Patients with pelvic floor disorders are a diverse group with a common final pathway: they are unable to generate sufficient propulsive forces to overcome the resistance of the anorectal complex (Table 25.3). In addition and importantly, such patients may also have slow colon transit, either secondary to and/or in addition to a pelvic floor disorder. These distinctions become important for management because biofeedback retraining is highly effective for pelvic floor disorders such as dyssynergic defecation.

Slow transit constipation is defined as chronic constipation associated with prolonged stool transit through the colon as established with diagnostic testing [6]. Some patients with slow transit constipation have altered colon motility which impedes propulsive movement. Colectomy specimens from patients with slow transit constipation have revealed decreased interstitial cells of Cajal, the pacemaker cells electrically coupled to smooth muscles that generate and propagate slow waves in the colon. In the absence of these cells, contractile activity of the colon is reduced, resulting in decreased intestinal transit [24, 25]. Colonic manometry shows few or absent HAPCs in patients with slow transit constipation although this is not a universal finding. These patients frequently have a decreased response to a meal or to pharmacologic stimuli such as bisacodyl or neostigmine [26].

Although colon response to feeding and colonic motility is not affected by healthy aging, there may be physiologic changes affecting colonic physiology and anorectal function

Fig. 25.1 At rest, the anorectal mechanics function to store fecal waste by the angle created by the puborectalis muscles and contraction of the anal sphincters. During defecation, the angle decreases and puborectalis muscle relaxes allowing expulsion of stool [23]

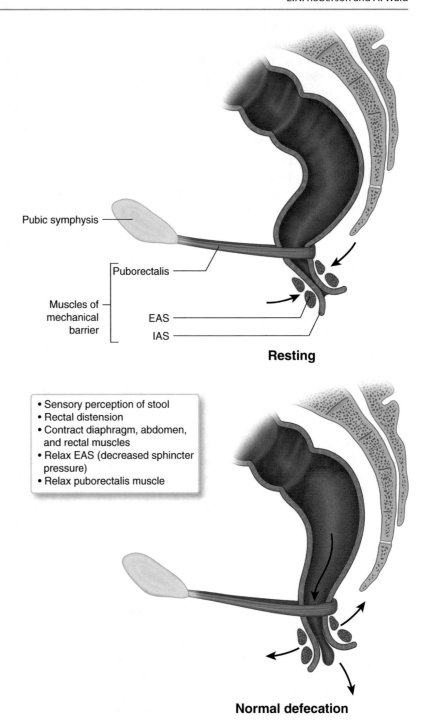

Pubic symphysis

Puborectalis

Muscles of mechanical barrier

EAS

IAS

Resting

- Sensory perception of stool
- Rectal distension
- Contract diaphragm, abdomen, and rectal muscles
- Relax EAS (decreased sphincter pressure)
- Relax puborectalis muscle

Normal defecation

in the elderly that may predispose to the development of constipation in this population [27]. Additional contributors to constipation in an elderly population include impaired mobility, poor oral intake, cognitive disorders such as dementia, neurologic disorders including Parkinson's disease and stroke, and medications. Medications associated with constipation and frequently used by elderly persons include anticholinergic drugs, calcium supplements, calcium channel blockers, non-steroidal anti-inflammatory drugs (NSAIDs), and opioid analgesics [2, 17].

Clinical Aspects

History and Physical Exam

Duration of symptoms, frequency of stools, and consistency of stools should be documented, as well as excessive straining, feeling of incomplete evacuation, sense of difficulty passing stool, and the need for manual maneuvers during defecation. The Bristol Stool Scale (Fig. 25.2) is a useful

Fig. 25.2 Bristol stool scale

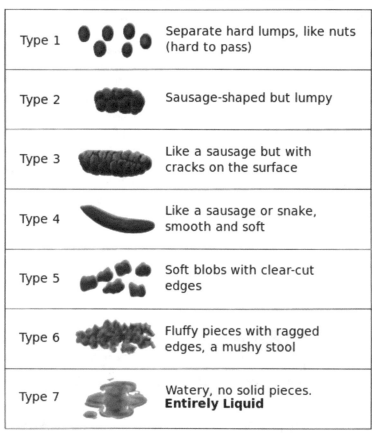

Bristol Stool Chart

Type 1		Separate hard lumps, like nuts (hard to pass)
Type 2		Sausage-shaped but lumpy
Type 3		Like a sausage but with cracks on the surface
Type 4		Like a sausage or snake, smooth and soft
Type 5		Soft blobs with clear-cut edges
Type 6		Fluffy pieces with ragged edges, a mushy stool
Type 7		Watery, no solid pieces. **Entirely Liquid**

visual representation of stool forms and correlates well with colon transit [28]. Other important clinical information includes calorie and fiber intake, exercise, onset during childhood, and obstetric events. Prior and current use of over-the-counter and prescription laxatives should be assessed [3].

Clinical evaluation should also focus on excluding organic causes (Table 25.2) and the presence of so-called alarm symptoms. Alarm symptoms include hematochezia, sudden change in bowel habits, unexpected weight loss, family history of colon cancer or inflammatory bowel disease, anemia, and positive fecal occult blood test (Table 25.4). Pelvic floor disorders do not respond well to empiric laxatives and thus are important to identify. Excessive straining even with soft stools or use of an enema is a symptom that may indicate a pelvic floor disorder. Use of perineal or vaginal digital pressure may also suggest a pelvic floor disorder or a clinically significant rectocele. Although such history can indicate pathophysiology, absence of these symptoms does not exclude a pelvic floor disorder [1].

A digital rectal exam (DRE) including simulation of evacuation is a key component of the physical examination, although it is underutilized in clinical practice because of inadequate training and little confidence in performing the exam by health care providers [29]. Although a normal exam does not exclude dyssynergic defecation, the positive predictive

Table 25.4 Alarm symptoms for chronic constipation

History & physical
Hematochezia
Unexpected weight loss >10 lb
Sudden change in bowel habits after the age of 50
Family history
Colon cancer
Inflammatory bowel disease
Evaluation
Positive fecal occult blood test
Iron deficiency anemia

value of a DRE in identifying dyssynergic defecation in patients with chronic constipation was reported to be 97 % by experienced examiners [30]. A DRE is usually, but not necessarily, performed in the left lateral position. Inspection of the perianal area should evaluate for skin tags, fissures, fistulas, hemorrhoids, or anal cancers. Stricture, mass, tenderness, blood, or fecal impaction may be noted as the examining finger enters the anal canal. After resting tone is noted, the patient should be asked to bear down. Relaxation of the external anal sphincter and puborectalis muscle (above the anal canal) in conjunction with the descent of the perineum is normal [23].

Diagnostic Testing

Patients who present with constipation without alarm symptoms may be treated empirically with limited diagnostic evaluation. Recent guidelines recommend obtaining a complete blood cell count whereas thyroid-stimulating hormone, glucose, creatinine, and calcium should be obtained selectively in patients with a relevant history or physical findings [3]. Diagnostic colonoscopy should be performed only in patients who require colorectal cancer screening and/or any patient with alarm symptoms (see Chap. 12 on colonoscopy for details). This recommendation is endorsed by all three of the major GI societies and is based, in part, on data that the prevalence of colon cancer or polyps is no higher in persons with chronic constipation than in those without constipation [1, 3, 31].

A pelvic floor disorder should be suspected when constipation responds poorly to laxatives, with reports of excessive straining even with soft stools, if digital pressure is routinely employed to facilitate evacuation, and/or when DRE is suggestive (Fig. 25.3). In this situation, a balloon expulsion test in conjunction with anorectal manometry should be obtained in a center experienced with these studies. Balloon expulsion assesses the ability to expel a balloon filled with 50 mL warm water or air while the subject is sitting on a commode in a private setting; the balloon should be expelled within 1 min according to most studies [32]. In one study, this simple test had a negative predictive value of 97 %, with a sensitivity of 88 % and specificity of 89 % [33]. However, balloon expulsion by itself cannot be used to confirm or refute a defecation disorder. Therefore, anorectal manometry should be performed in conjunction with balloon expulsion [34]. During manometry, a small catheter is positioned in the rectum and anal canal to measure pressure changes at rest and during simulated defecation; other important parameters are rectal sensation, rectal pressure volume ratios, and recto-anal reflexes [35]. New high-resolution catheters have evenly distributed sensors that straddle the anal canal allowing

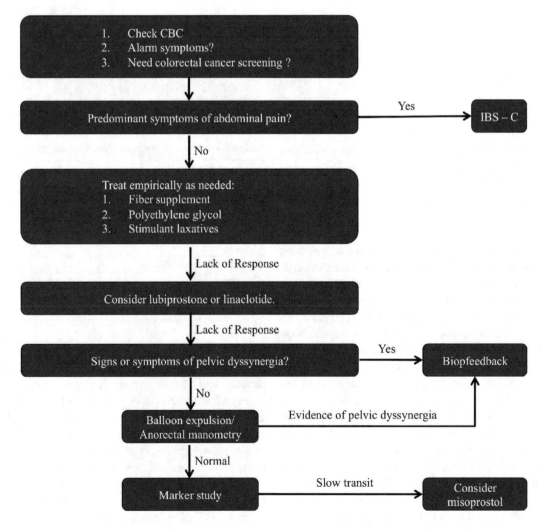

Fig. 25.3 Algorithm for management of constipation

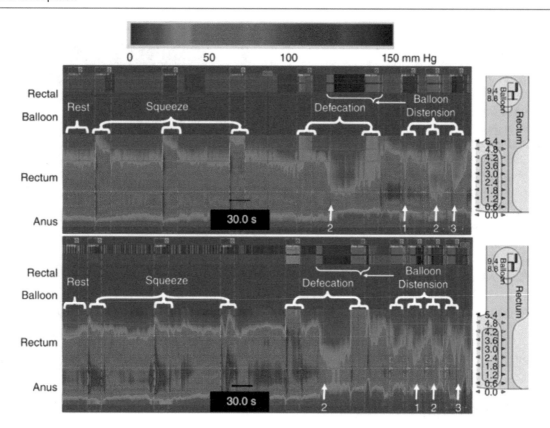

Fig. 25.4 Examples of high-resolution manometry in an asymptomatic woman (*upper panel*) and woman with dyssynergic defecation (*lower panel*). The lower panel shows a higher resting pressure, higher squeeze pressure, and higher anal pressure during simulated evacuation before rectal distension. Rectal sensory thresholds for first sensation (1), urgency (2), and maximum discomfort (3) were recorded during rectal balloon distention up to 60 ml (*upper panel*) and 90 ml (*lower panel*). Asymptomatic older women compared to younger women may have lower anal resting pressure, shorter high-pressure zone was shorter, but maintained squeeze response [57]

pressures to be topographically mapped along a time continuum in much greater detail (Fig. 25.4). Patients with dyssynergia are unable to generate sufficient propulsive force in concert with relaxation of sphincter and puborectalis muscle; several patterns have been identified [35].

Defecography is a technique in which contrast thickened to simulate soft stool is injected into the rectum and the patient is asked to expel the contrast while sitting on a commode. It can suggest dyssynergic defecation using various criteria if findings on manometry and balloon expulsion are inconsistent. It is also useful to detect structural causes of defecation difficulty such as a rectocele or enterocele which are not identified by other tests. Disadvantages of defecography include radiation exposure and the performance of the test in a public venue; this may be particularly problematic in women and lead to inhibited defecation [34, 36].

If dyssynergic defecation is excluded as a cause of chronic constipation, radiopaque markers, wireless capsule, or scintigraphy can be used to assess colon transit. These studies may be useful to educate and reassure patients about their symptoms and occasionally to assess response to therapy [3]. A marker study is a non-invasive way to measure colonic transit. Patients swallow a capsule containing 24 radiopaque markers (Sitzmarks, Konsyl Pharmaceuticals, Fort Worth, TX) and a plain abdominal X-ray (110 keV) is obtained five days (120 h) later. Normally, greater than 80 % of markers will pass by day 5; greater than 6 markers on the X-ray can indicate slow transit. A more sophisticated approach is to have a patient swallow a Sitzmarks capsule on days 1, 2, and 3. A plain abdominal X-ray is obtained on day 4 and (if greater than 35 markers are present) on day 7. More than 68 markers on both X-rays (number of markers on day 4 X-ray plus number of markers on the day 7 X-ray) indicate slow transit [37]. However, since more than half of patients with dyssynergic defecation have slow transit that improves with correction of the defecation disorder, slow transit constipation can be diagnosed only in the absence (and successful treatment if present) of dyssynergia. Because the presence of slow transit does not avoid the need for anorectal manometry/balloon expulsion, treatment of pelvic floor disorders is with pelvic floor retraining, and initial treatment for slow transit constipation is no different than normal transit constipation (i.e., laxatives), recent guidelines recommend that anorectal manometry and/or balloon expulsion be performed before a colon transit study [6].

A wireless pH motility capsule (SmartPill, Given, Yoqneam, Israel) can provide a radiation-free estimate of colonic transit time, gastric emptying, and small bowel transit in addition to pH and pressure along the gastrointestinal tract. Although approved by the Food and Drug Administration to evaluate patients for chronic constipation, it may be most appropriate to investigate whole gut transit in patients with suspected diffuse motility issues [38, 39]. Alternatively, colonic transit scintigraphy can be used to assess colonic transit as well as gastric emptying and small bowel transit. This technique is commonly used in clinical trials to assess responsiveness of medications, but is not widely available clinically [35].

Magnetic resonance imaging (MRI) defecography is a novel method to assess global pelvic floor anatomy and dynamic motion without radiation exposure. If available, images should be obtained with the patient in a sitting position using an open-configuration MRI to be more physiologic. MRI is limited by high cost and lack of availability and therefore has a role primarily in identifying structural abnormalities [40].

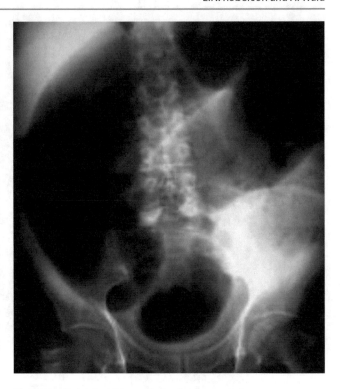

Fig. 25.5 Abdominal X-ray of volvulus

Special Considerations in the Elderly

Special considerations arise in the elderly with medical illnesses. Although these situations are not unique to the elderly, they are more common in older individuals. The elderly have more illnesses that can affect bowel function directly or indirectly though medications, immobility, and/or institutionalization [1]. Limited mobilization and constipating medications can lead to fecal impaction. Fecal impaction is defined as a large mass of stool in the rectum that develops in the setting of chronic constipation. In addition to obstipation, it may present with overflow pseudodiarrhea and fecal incontinence. Because of this contradictory presentation, fecal impaction is often overlooked and under diagnosed, although it is a significant source of morbidity, especially in hospitalized elderly patients. Fecal impaction should be suspected in elderly patients with a history of chronic constipation who present with abdominal pain, nausea, poor appetite, and even weight loss. Abdominal exam may show a tubular mass indicating stool in the rectosigmoid; hard stool may be palpable with rectal exam. Fecal impaction can be easily diagnosed on a plain abdominal X-ray once the diagnosis is considered [41].

Chronic megacolon and megarectum refer to dilation of the colon and rectum, respectfully and are usually associated with enteric abnormalities and weakening of the connective tissue elements of the bowel leading to dilation and thinning of the circular smooth muscle of the colon. Megacolon can occur chronically in patients with a long history of constipation. Acquired chronic megacolon may be seen in patients

with chronic neurologic disorders (spine injury, myotonic dystrophy, Parkinson's disease) and systemic diseases including amyloidosis, dermatomyositis, lupus, and scleroderma. Patients usually present with increasing constipation or fecal impaction. Abdominal X-rays confirm diffuse colonic distension with feces or air throughout the colon. Megacolon can predispose to a volvulus, or twisting of the colon at the mesenteric attachment, producing acute intestinal obstruction. A volvulus most often occurs in the sigmoid colon or cecum and can often be diagnosed on abdominal X-ray (Fig. 25.5). Sigmoid volvulus is initially treated with endoscopic decompression, although more than 80 % will recur and will require surgery; cecal volvulus is treated initially with surgery [42].

Treatment

In elderly patients who are healthy, constipation should be treated in a manner similar to the general population. Specifically, after appropriate tests are done, and if pelvic dyssynergia is not suspected based on clinical presentation or exam, an empiric and conservative approach should be taken. These empiric measures are safe and recommended by experts [43]. Management should begin with discontinuation of constipating medications if possible, exercise, establishment of a bowel routine, and a gradual increase in dietary or supplemental fiber. Patients should be advised to heed the call to stool, especially in the morning, and set a routine time each day to have a bowel movement [2, 23]. Except in the case of dehydration, there is no merit to increasing fluid intake beyond normal requirements, as it will serve only to increase urination [6]. An osmotic laxative such as polyethylene glycol (17 g daily, adjusted as needed) is an effective, inexpensive addition. If needed, a stimulant laxative or suppository (bisacodyl) can be added several times a week or daily. Newer, more expensive prescription agents (lubiprostone, linaclotide) could be considered if response to non-prescription agents is unsatisfactory. Treatment failure should lead to consideration of a defecation disorder and obtaining appropriate diagnostic tests (see above).

Treatment of fecal impaction entails manual disimpaction, enemas, and perhaps oral laxatives, usually polyethylene glycol. In contrast to chronic constipation, treatment of chronic megacolon includes a low fiber diet in addition to aggressive laxative use to prevent fecal impactions. If symptoms of megacolon are intractable and disabling, if sigmoid volvulus is not responsive to attempts to untwist the bowel or recurs, or if there is a cecal volvulus, surgery should be performed. If anal sphincter function is intact, this entails a sub subtotal colectomy with ileorectal anastomosis; alternatively, a Hartmann's pouch could be performed.

Medical Treatment of Functional Constipation

Bulking Agents

Bulking agents are organic polymers that increase stool bulk and consistency, thereby increasing colon motility and shortening colon transit time. Included in this category are natural soluble fiber (psyllium, ispaghula), insoluble fiber (bran), and synthetic fibers such as methylcellulose and calcium polycarbophil. Fiber-rich foods include fruits, vegetables, nuts, bran, and beans. Published studies of fiber in chronic constipation have generally been small, poorly designed, assessed for relatively short periods of time, and have not used rigorous definitions such as Rome criteria to select patients. However, fiber is recommended as a first line therapy for constipation because of its good safety profile, low cost, and other potential health benefits [1]. Prunes (50 g prunes/6 g fiber once to twice daily), which improve stool frequency and consistency and decrease straining, are a good alternative to fiber for those who like them [36, 44]. Common side effects include bloating and flatulence, which occur more often with insoluble fiber and may be less common with synthetic fiber. Bowel obstruction occurs rarely [1]. The effect of fiber supplementation is gradual and may take several weeks. Patients should also be warned about the side effects of increased bloating and flatulence although these may subside after several days to weeks; alternatively,

patients can try a different fiber supplement. To minimize side effects, fiber should be increased slowly, about 5 g daily every 1–2 weeks according to tolerance and improved symptoms [2]. Bulking agents are ineffective in patients with slow transit constipation and dyssynergic defecation and often make symptoms worse.

Stool Softeners and Probiotics

Stool softeners (docusate) act as detergents to allow water to permeate stool, thereby softening it. Although FDA approved for treatment of occasional constipation, there is insufficient evidence for use in chronic constipation [1]. Preliminary data suggest that *Bifidobacterium lactis*, *Lactobacillus casei*, and *Escherichia coli* Nissle may improve stool frequency and consistency in constipation, but data and safety profiles are limited and probiotics should be considered investigational at the present time [45].

Stimulant Laxatives

Stimulant laxatives increase intestinal motility by inhibiting water absorption and stimulating the myenteric plexus. Bisacodyl is included in this category, as are castor oil and anthraquinones (senna, cascara sagrada, rhubarb, frangula, and aloe). Sodium picosulfate is a diphenylmethane laxative closely related to bisacodyl. It is available in the USA only in a combined form with magnesium oxide marketed as a colonoscopy prep (Prepopik, Ferring Pharmaceuticals Inc., Parsippany, NJ) and is currently available only in Europe. Although older studies were poorly designed by today's standards, several high quality recent clinical trials of bisacodyl and picosulfate have demonstrated improved stool frequency and quality of life [46, 47]. Stimulant laxatives may be used up to but not more than once daily, in addition to or instead of a daily osmotic laxative [48]. Side effects of stimulant laxatives include abdominal cramps, diarrhea, and, very infrequently, electrolyte abnormalities. Hepatotoxicity has been reported with senna and cascara sagrada, although this may be dose related [49, 50]. Melanosis coli is a dark brown pigmentation of the colon mucosa seen in patients who chronically use anthraquinones, and is more prominent in the proximal colon. Colonic bacteria convert these laxatives to compounds that induce apoptosis of colon epithelial cells. Macrophages ingest and convert the compound to a black pigment called lipofuscin. Melanosis coli is functionally inconsequential; it occurs after months of use and may take months to resolve after discontinuation. It is not associated with the development of colon cancer. There is no evidence that stimulant laxatives cause permanent damage to either the colonic musculature or enteric nervous system [48].

Osmotic Laxatives

Osmotic laxatives contain poorly absorbed compounds that retain luminal water and result in increased stool water content, softer stools, and enhanced propulsion of stool through the colon. This class includes sorbitol, magnesium salts, lactulose, and polyethylene glycol (PEG) [10]. The efficacy and safety of PEG is extensively documented in the literature and it is available without prescription [43]. Side effects of all osmotic laxatives include abdominal cramping, nausea, bloating, and flatulence. High doses of PEG in elderly nursing home patients have been associated with diarrhea and excessive stool frequency but this is easily modulated with dose adjustments. Lactulose is also effective but is not as well tolerated, as it causes gas and is more expensive than PEG. Electrolyte abnormalities (hypermagnesemia, hyperphosphatemia, hypercalcemia, hyponatremia, hypokalemia) are more likely to occur with magnesium compounds, which should be used cautiously in older persons who often have renal impairment [1].

Intestinal Secretagogues

When constipation is refractory to non-prescription laxatives, newer prescription-based pharmacologic agents should be considered. Lubiprostone is a selective chloride channel-2 activator which stimulates active secretion of chloride into the intestinal lumen followed by passive diffusion of sodium and water, thus accelerating small intestine and colon transit and facilitating defecation [6]. Lubiprostone 24 mcg twice daily improves stool frequency in short-term studies of chronic constipation [51, 52] and is also approved for IBS-C at a dose of 8 μg twice daily. Commonly reported side effects include nausea, diarrhea, and headache. Interestingly, fewer side effects have been reported in patients older than 65 years [2]. Linaclotide is a gut-selective guanylate cyclase-C receptor agonist which also increases chloride secretion in the intestinal lumen using the CFTR channel. Studies showed linaclotide improves stool frequency and consistency and also quality of life in patients with constipation. Diarrhea is the predominant side effect. Linaclotide has recently been approved and is now available for both IBS-C and chronic constipation (dosage: 290 μg and 145 μg, respectively) [23].

Treatment of Defecation Disorders

Pelvic floor retraining using biofeedback is the treatment of choice in patients with disordered defecation. Biofeedback therapy trains patients to use their abdominal muscles to make a propulsive force while simultaneously relaxing the pelvic floor muscles, thus promoting defecation. This is done with electromyographic sensors or pressure transducers in conjunction with visual or auditory feedback to retrain these muscles. Rectal sensory retraining can also be performed, which improves patient recognition of rectal filling. In many patients with dyssynergic defecation and slow colon transit, correction of dyssynergia is associated with improved colon transit, suggesting that colon dysmotility was not the primary reason for slow transit. Clinical trials have shown improved symptoms of defecation in more than 70 % of patients who fulfill diagnostic criteria for a defecation disorder [53, 54]. Biofeedback has been shown to be more effective than sham biofeedback or PEG and has minimal side effects [55]. A typical training program consists of 6 training sessions lasting 30–60 min every 1–2 weeks. Crucial to the success of biofeedback is the patient's cognition, receptiveness and motivation to the therapy, as well as the therapist's experience [6]. Cognitive disturbances, such as may be found in elderly or institutionalized individuals, limit usefulness of biofeedback in these populations. Biofeedback therapy at home may be an effective and alternative option. This consists of patients placing a disposable two-sensor probe that is attached to a display box into the rectum and gives visual input regarding patient's performance. Cost may limit use, as home biofeedback is not currently covered by insurance plans [23].

Treatment of Slow Transit Constipation

In a very selective patient population with slow transit constipation, a subtotal colectomy with ileorectal anastomosis may be an effective alternative. Critical to success are normal continence mechanisms. Patients must have failed aggressive therapy of laxative agents. Dyssynergic defecation should be absent or, if present, treated successfully. Additionally, a more diffuse motility disorder should be ruled out with gastric and small intestine motility studies. Patient's expectations should include improvement of constipation only, because bloating and abdominal pain are often not improved [6]. Given these strict criteria, it is unusual to pursue a subtotal colectomy in elderly patients. An alternative medical management would include misoprostol in addition to polyethylene glycol. Misoprostol should be dosed once a day to minimize side effects of cramping [56, 57].

Key Points

- Constipation is defined as unsatisfactory defecation consisting of a variable combination of infrequent stools (less than 3 per week), hard or lumpy stools, and symptoms such as excessive straining, feeling of incomplete evacuation, sense of difficulty passing stool, or the need for manual maneuvers during defecation.

- Chronic constipation is defined as constipation for more than 3 months and may be distinguished from constipation predominant IBS (IBS – C) by the lack of significant abdominal discomfort or pain.
- Constipation is common in patients older than 65 years, especially in nursing home settings, and is twice as common in women as men.
- A defecation disorder may result from inadequate propulsive forces and/or increased resistance to evacuation caused by incoordination of abdominal, rectal, and anal muscles; it is best treated with pelvic floor retraining using biofeedback.
- Defecation disorders frequently cause secondary slow transit, and need to be ruled out or adequately treated before a diagnosis of slow transit constipation is made.
- All patients with chronic constipation should have a complete blood cell count, but further laboratory evaluation is needed only if clinical suspicion exists.
- Colonoscopy should be performed in individuals needing colon cancer screening or manifesting "alarm symptoms."
- Although not unique to the elderly, constipating medications, immobility, and medical conditions should be considered in evaluating and treating elderly patients.
- Constipation in otherwise healthy elderly patients should be treated with empiric conservative measures including discontinuation of constipating medications if possible, exercise, bowel routine, and gradual increase in dietary or supplemental fiber; an osmotic laxative such as polyethylene glycol or a stimulant may be added as necessary.

References

1. An evidence-based approach to the management of chronic constipation in North America. Am J Gastroenterol. 2005;100 Suppl 1:S1–4.
2. Gallegos-Orozco JF, Foxx-Orenstein AE, Sterler SM, Stoa JM. Chronic constipation in the elderly. Am J Gastroenterol. 2012;107(1):18–25. quiz 6.
3. Bharucha AE, Dorn SD, Lembo A, Pressman A. American gastroenterological association medical position statement on constipation. Gastroenterology. 2013;144(1):211–7.
4. Sanchez MI, Bercik P. Epidemiology and burden of chronic constipation. Can J Gastroenterol. 2011;25 Suppl B:11B–5B.
5. Longstreth GF, Thompson WG, Chey WD, Houghton LA, Mearin F, Spiller RC. Functional bowel disorders. Gastroenterology. 2006;130(5):1480–91.
6. Bharucha AE, Pemberton JH, Locke 3rd GR. American gastroenterological association technical review on constipation. Gastroenterology. 2013;144(1):218–38.
7. Bharucha AE, Wald A, Enck P, Rao S. Functional anorectal disorders. Gastroenterology. 2006;130(5):1510–8.
8. Choung RS, Locke 3rd GR, Schleck CD, Zinsmeister AR, Talley NJ. Cumulative incidence of chronic constipation: a population-based study 1988–2003. Aliment Pharmacol Ther. 2007;26(11–12):1521–8.
9. Mugie SM, Benninga MA, Di Lorenzo C. Epidemiology of constipation in children and adults: a systematic review. Best Pract Res Clin Gastroenterol. 2011;25(1):3–18.
10. Ford AC, Suares NC. Effect of laxatives and pharmacological therapies in chronic idiopathic constipation: systematic review and meta-analysis. Gut. 2011;60(2):209–18.
11. Talley NJ, Fleming KC, Evans JM, O'Keefe EA, Weaver AL, Zinsmeister AR, et al. Constipation in an elderly community: a study of prevalence and potential risk factors. Am J Gastroenterol. 1996;91(1):19–25.
12. Crane SJ, Talley NJ. Chronic gastrointestinal symptoms in the elderly. Clin Geriatr Med. 2007;23(4):721–34.
13. Harari D, Gurwitz JH, Avorn J, Bohn R, Minaker KL. Bowel habit in relation to age and gender. Findings from the National Health Interview Survey and clinical implications. Arch Intern Med. 1996;156(3):315–20.
14. Fosnes GS, Lydersen S, Farup PG. Drugs and constipation in elderly in nursing homes: what is the relation? Gastroenterol Res Pract. 2012;2012:290231.
15. Higgins PD, Johanson JF. Epidemiology of constipation in North America: a systematic review. Am J Gastroenterol. 2004;99(4):750–9.
16. Shin A, Camilleri M, Nadeau A, Nullens S, Rhee JC, Jeong ID, et al. Interpretation of overall colonic transit in defecation disorders in males and females. Neurogastroenterol Motil. 2013;25(6):502–8.
17. Bouras EP, Tangalos EG. Chronic constipation in the elderly. Gastroenterol Clin North Am. 2009;38(3):463–80.
18. Wald A, Scarpignato C, Kamm MA, Mueller-Lissner S, Helfrich I, Schuijt C, et al. The burden of constipation on quality of life: results of a multinational survey. Aliment Pharmacol Ther. 2007;26(2):227–36.
19. Sun SX, Dibonaventura M, Purayidathil FW, Wagner JS, Dabbous O, Mody R. Impact of chronic constipation on health-related quality of life, work productivity, and healthcare resource use: an analysis of the National Health and Wellness Survey. Dig Dis Sci. 2011;56(9):2688–95.
20. Shah ND, Chitkara DK, Locke GR, Meek PD, Talley NJ. Ambulatory care for constipation in the United States, 1993–2004. Am J Gastroenterol. 2008;103(7):1746–53.
21. Nyrop KA, Palsson OS, Levy RL, Korff MV, Feld AD, Turner MJ, et al. Costs of health care for irritable bowel syndrome, chronic constipation, functional diarrhoea and functional abdominal pain. Aliment Pharmacol Ther. 2007;26(2):237–48.
22. Sleisenger MH, Feldman M, Friedman LS, Brandt LJ. Sleisenger and Fordtran's gastrointestinal and liver disease: pathophysiology, diagnosis, management. 9th ed. Philadelphia, PA: Saunders/Elsevier; 2010.
23. Schey R, Cromwell J, Rao SS. Medical and surgical management of pelvic floor disorders affecting defecation. Am J Gastroenterol. 2012;107(11):1624–33; quiz p 34.
24. He CL, Burgart L, Wang L, Pemberton J, Young-Fadok T, Szurszewski J, et al. Decreased interstitial cell of cajal volume in patients with slow-transit constipation. Gastroenterology. 2000;118(1):14–21.
25. Sanders KM, Koh SD, Ward SM. Interstitial cells of cajal as pacemakers in the gastrointestinal tract. Annu Rev Physiol. 2006;68:307–43.
26. Ravi K, Bharucha AE, Camilleri M, Rhoten D, Bakken T, Zinsmeister AR. Phenotypic variation of colonic motor functions in chronic constipation. Gastroenterology. 2010;138(1):89–97.
27. Camilleri M, Lee JS, Viramontes B, Bharucha AE, Tangalos EG. Insights into the pathophysiology and mechanisms of constipation, irritable bowel syndrome, and diverticulosis in older people. J Am Geriatr Soc. 2000;48(9):1142–50.
28. Lewis SJ, Heaton KW. Stool form scale as a useful guide to intestinal transit time. Scand J Gastroenterol. 1997;32(9):920–4.
29. Wong RK, Drossman DA, Bharucha AE, Rao SS, Wald A, Morris CB, et al. The digital rectal examination: a multicenter survey of physicians' and students' perceptions and practice patterns. Am J Gastroenterol. 2012;107(8):1157–63.

30. Tantiphlachiva K, Rao P, Attaluri A, Rao SS. Digital rectal examination is a useful tool for identifying patients with dyssynergia. Clin Gastroenterol Hepatol. 2010;8(11):955–60.

31. Qureshi W, Adler DG, Davila RE, Egan J, Hirota WK, Jacobson BC, et al. ASGE guideline: guideline on the use of endoscopy in the management of constipation. Gastrointest Endosc. 2005;62(2):199–201.

32. Bharucha AE. Difficult defecation: difficult problem assessment and management; what really helps? Gastroenterol Clin North Am. 2011;40(4):837–44.

33. Minguez M, Herreros B, Sanchiz V, Hernandez V, Almela P, Anon R, et al. Predictive value of the balloon expulsion test for excluding the diagnosis of pelvic floor dyssynergia in constipation. Gastroenterology. 2004;126(1):57–62.

34. Videlock EJ, Lembo A, Cremonini F. Diagnostic testing for dyssynergic defecation in chronic constipation: meta-analysis. Neurogastroenterol Motil. 2013

35. Rao SS, Camilleri M, Hasler WL, Maurer AH, Parkman HP, Saad R, et al. Evaluation of gastrointestinal transit in clinical practice: position paper of the American and European neurogastroenterology and motility societies. Neurogastroenterol Motil. 2011;23(1):8–23.

36. Attaluri A, Donahoe R, Valestin J, Brown K, Rao SS. Randomised clinical trial: dried plums (prunes) vs. psyllium for constipation. Aliment Pharmacol Ther. 2011;33(7):822–8.

37. Metcalf AM, Phillips SF, Zinsmeister AR, MacCarty RL, Beart RW, Wolff BG. Simplified assessment of segmental colonic transit. Gastroenterology. 1987;92(1):40–7.

38. Tran K, Brun R, Kuo B. Evaluation of regional and whole gut motility using the wireless motility capsule: relevance in clinical practice. Therap Adv Gastroenterol. 2012;5(4):249–60.

39. Rao SS, Kuo B, McCallum RW, Chey WD, DiBaise JK, Hasler WL, et al. Investigation of colonic and whole-gut transit with wireless motility capsule and radiopaque markers in constipation. Clin Gastroenterol Hepatol. 2009;7(5):537–44.

40. Reiner CS, Tutuian R, Solopova AE, Pohl D, Marincek B, Weishaupt D. MR defecography in patients with dyssynergic defecation: spectrum of imaging findings and diagnostic value. Br J Radiol. 2011;84(998):136–44.

41. Araghizadeh F. Fecal impaction. Clin Colon Rectal Surg. 2005;18(2):116–9.

42. Larkin JO, Thekiso TB, Waldron R, Barry K, Eustace PW. Recurrent sigmoid volvulus - early resection may obviate later emergency surgery and reduce morbidity and mortality. Ann R Coll Surg Engl. 2009;91(3):205–9.

43. Ramkumar D, Rao SS. Efficacy and safety of traditional medical therapies for chronic constipation: systematic review. Am J Gastroenterol. 2005;100(4):936–71.

44. Hull MA, McIntire DD, Atnip SD, Dreadin J, Nihira MA, Drewes PG, et al. Randomized trial comparing 2 fiber regimens for the reduction of symptoms of constipation. Female Pelvic Med Reconstr Surg. 2011;17(3):128–33.

45. Chmielewska A, Szajewska H. Systematic review of randomised controlled trials: probiotics for functional constipation. World J Gastroenterol. 2010;16(1):69–75.

46. Mueller-Lissner S, Kamm MA, Wald A, Hinkel U, Koehler U, Richter E, et al. Multicenter, 4-week, double-blind, randomized, placebo-controlled trial of sodium picosulfate in patients with chronic constipation. Am J Gastroenterol. 2010;105(4): 897–903.

47. Kamm MA, Mueller-Lissner S, Wald A, Richter E, Swallow R, Gessner U. Oral bisacodyl is effective and well-tolerated in patients with chronic constipation. Clin Gastroenterol Hepatol. 2011; 9(7):577–83.

48. Wald A. Is chronic use of stimulant laxatives harmful to the colon? J Clin Gastroenterol. 2003;36(5):386–9.

49. Nadir A, Reddy D, Van Thiel DH. Cascara sagrada-induced intrahepatic cholestasis causing portal hypertension: case report and review of herbal hepatotoxicity. Am J Gastroenterol. 2000;95(12):3634–7.

50. Vanderperren B, Rizzo M, Angenot L, Haufroid V, Jadoul M, Hantson P. Acute liver failure with renal impairment related to the abuse of senna anthraquinone glycosides. Ann Pharmacother. 2005;39(7–8):1353–7.

51. Johanson JF, Morton D, Geenen J, Ueno R. Multicenter, 4-week, double-blind, randomized, placebo-controlled trial of lubiprostone, a locally-acting type-2 chloride channel activator, in patients with chronic constipation. Am J Gastroenterol. 2008;103(1):170–7.

52. Barish CF, Drossman D, Johanson JF, Ueno R. Efficacy and safety of lubiprostone in patients with chronic constipation. Dig Dis Sci. 2010;55(4):1090–7.

53. Rao SS, Seaton K, Miller M, Brown K, Nygaard I, Stumbo P, et al. Randomized controlled trial of biofeedback, sham feedback, and standard therapy for dyssynergic defecation. Clin Gastroenterol Hepatol. 2007;5(3):331–8.

54. Rao SS, Valestin J, Brown CK, Zimmerman B, Schulze K. Long-term efficacy of biofeedback therapy for dyssynergic defecation: randomized controlled trial. Am J Gastroenterol. 2010; 105(4):890–6.

55. Chiarioni G, Whitehead WE, Pezza V, Morelli A, Bassotti G. Biofeedback is superior to laxatives for normal transit constipation due to pelvic floor dyssynergia. Gastroenterology. 2006; 130(3):657–64.

56. Wald A. Slow transit constipation. Curr Treat Options Gastroenterol. 2002;5(4):279–83.

57. Noelting J, Ratuapli SK, Bharucha AE, Harvey DM, Ravi K, Zinsmeister AR. Normal values for high-resolution anorectal manometry in healthy women: effects of age and significance of rectoanal gradient. Am J Gastroenterol. 2012;107(10):1530–6.

Fecal Diversion and Ostomies

Jennifer L. Bennett and Elizabeth C. Wick

Introduction

Surgeons create an ostomy as a means to connect a patient's internal organ to the skin surface [1]. The terms ostomy and stoma are frequently used interchangeably, but the two terms originate from unique terms. Ostomy is derived from the Latin word ostium, meaning mouth or opening. Stoma originates from the Greek word denoting mouth [1]. In abdominal surgery, ostomies are usually constructed from the small or large bowel. Jejunostomy refers to an ostomy created using the jejunum, ileostomy from the ileum, and colostomy from the colon. Other intestinal sites such as the appendix and cecum have limited indications, and will not be discussed in this chapter [2]. Colostomies and ileostomies are the most common intestinal stomas and will be the focus of this chapter [2].

Preoperative Preparation

It is essential that patients be counseled preoperatively about the potential creation of an ostomy. For many patients, having an ostomy can initially be a traumatic experience, and ample preparation and education can improve the experience. If available, patients who might have an ostomy created should meet with an enterostomal therapist or ostomy nurse in advance of the procedure [1]. This meeting should include basic information as well as selection of a site on the skin for the stoma. The decision to create a stoma should not be taken lightly, and including the patient in the decision making process is important to their future adjustment to the stoma [3, 4].

Indications for Ostomies

Indications for ostomy creation are varied. General indications for ostomies are to bypass an area of obstruction, control severe incontinence or dysmotility, or protect an anastomosis or area of the bowel distal to the ostomy [5]. Ostomies are created as part of the surgical treatment of a wide range of diseases including GI trauma, diverticulitis, perforation, fecal incontinence, constipation, intestinal obstruction, infectious colitis, ischemic colitis, radiation colitis, colorectal cancer, fistulas, abscesses, or inflammatory bowel disease (Crohn's disease and ulcerative colitis) all may require the creation of an ostomy (Table 26.1).

The definition of pelvic floor disorders varies but generally refers to urinary or anal incontinence, symptoms of prolapse, constipation, obstructed defecation, and any type of vaginal or bladder repair [8, 9]. Pelvic floor disorders are associated with the female gender, advancing age and parity [8, 9]. Overall prevalence of pelvic floor dysfunction among women ranges from 37 to 67.7 % [8–10]. The leading indications for a stoma related to pelvic floor dysfunction are constipation, fecal incontinence, or general pelvic floor dysfunction.

Fecal incontinence is a common problem for elderly patients affecting 3–21 % of community dwelling elderly, with increased prevalence in hospitalized elderly patients [11]. Creating an ostomy should not always be looked at as the last resort or a failure for fecal incontinence patients [12]. Patients with fecal incontinence fear that a stoma will lead to deterioration in their quality of life but are frequently pleasantly surprised with the improvement in lifestyle post-surgery

J.L. Bennett
Johns Hopkins University, School of Medicine,
Baltimore, MD, USA

E.C. Wick (✉)
Department of Surgery, Johns Hopkins Hospital,
600 N. Wolfe Street, Blalock #618, Baltimore, MD 21287, USA
e-mail: ewick1@jhmi.edu

© Springer Science+Business Media New York 2017
D.A. Gordon, M.R. Katlic (eds.), *Pelvic Floor Dysfunction and Pelvic Surgery in the Elderly*,
DOI 10.1007/978-1-4939-6554-0_26

Table 26.1 Indications for ostomy construction [5–7]

- Fecal Incontinence—aging, central or peripheral nerve damage, internal and external sphincter damage, weak sphincter muscles, changes in rectal capacity or sensation
- Constipation or obstructed defecation
- Diverticular disease
- Obstruction
- Abdominal or perineal trauma
- Rectal injury
- Perforation
- Infectious or infectious colitis
- Radiation enteritis
- Colorectal cancer resections
- Inflammatory bowel disease—ulcerative colitis, Crohn's disease
- Motility or functional disorders—idiopathic megarectum and megacolon
- Congenital disorders—imperforate anus, Hirschsprungs, necrotizing enterocolitis, intestinal atresias
- Complex anorectal disease
- Fecal stream diversion—protecting a low colorectal or ileoanal anastomosis, complex fistula, abscess, treatment of anastomotic leak

[13]. A colostomy for incontinence helps create a manageable abdominal stoma in the place of a previously unmanageable perineal stoma [14]. On average after surgery, patients report high social function, and higher scores in coping, embarrassment, lifestyle and depression scales than those living with fecal incontinence. The quality of the stoma is the most important indicator of patient satisfaction after surgery [11, 13, 14].

Temporary vs. Permanent

A stoma can be constructed under the pretense of being either temporary or permanent. The surgical indication drives the decision as to whether the stoma should be permanent or not. A temporary stoma is typically created to divert the fecal stream in order to protect a distal anastomosis while it heals and prevent fecal contamination in the event of an anastomotic leak. In considering a de-functioning ostomy, the benefits of stoma formation (and risk of anastomotic leak from the primary anastomosis) must be weighed against the risk of additional surgery for ostomy closure. Anastomotic leakage from a primary colorectal anastomosis varies depending on the location of the anastomosis and the surgical indication, but has been reported for low anastomosis to range between 2.6 and 26.2 % [15, 16]. Diversion of the fecal stream in high-risk patients will prevent fecal contamination and peritonitis in the event of anastomotic leak [16–19]. The morbidity rate of elective stoma closure is up to 36.5 % and carries a mortality rate of 1–4 % [16, 20]. Preoperatively, it is important to counsel patients that temporary ostomies may become permanent. At least 15 % of temporary ostomies are not closed [21, 22].

A permanent stoma may be necessary when there is no distal intestine to restore bowel continuity, for example in abdominoperineal resections where the anorectum is removed due to cancer. A permanent stoma may also be indicated to treat severe fecal incontinence. Complications of the underlying disease state or treatments may prevent restoration of intestinal continuity [1]. In general, permanent stomas are created as end ostomies, and temporary ostomies are created as loop ostomies [23].

Fecal Diversion: Loop Colostomy vs. Loop Ileostomy

A loop colostomy or a loop ileostomy may be used for the creation of a de-functioning temporary stoma. In general, loop ileostomies are preferred over loop colostomies. Typically, loop ileostomies are easier to care for due to their accessibility and smaller size [17]. Ileostomies have fewer stoma management problems and require less appliance changes [24]. Loop ileostomies have a lower risk of sepsis and stoma prolapse, and the procedure is associated with a lower wound infection and incisional hernia rate [18, 25]. For the most part, reversal of a loop ileostomy is more straightforward, and associated with a shorter length of stay and lower rate of postoperative morbidity [6, 26, 27].

Ostomy Site Selection

It is important to determine the optimal site for a stoma prior to surgery. Site selection is best done with the ostomy nurse or enterostomal therapist, surgeon, and patient. The site should be assessed with the patient sitting, standing, and lying down. First, it is essential to find a spot that is flat and where there are few skin folds to allow the appliance adhesive to fix properly to the abdominal wall [28]. Second, the patient must be able to see and manipulate the stoma. Some patients prefer the stoma to be located below the beltline, if possible, to conceal the stoma and bag. Finding a good site can be particularly challenging in patients who are obese, have excess abdominal skin, or a history of multiple abdominal surgeries/scars. In obese or wheelchair bound patients, stoma placement in the upper abdominal quadrants is an option to allow for better visualization and self-care. Ostomies are usually placed overlying the right or left rectus muscle—generally ileostomies are on the right side and colostomies are on the left side [2, 6, 22, 28, 29]. Poor site selection can have a devastating impact on patient quality of life with failure of the appliance to adhere leading to excessive leakage and skin excoriation. Studies have demonstrated an association of failure to have a patient preoperatively marked for a stoma and an increase in stoma related complications, particularly skin excoriation (Fig. 26.1) [28–30].

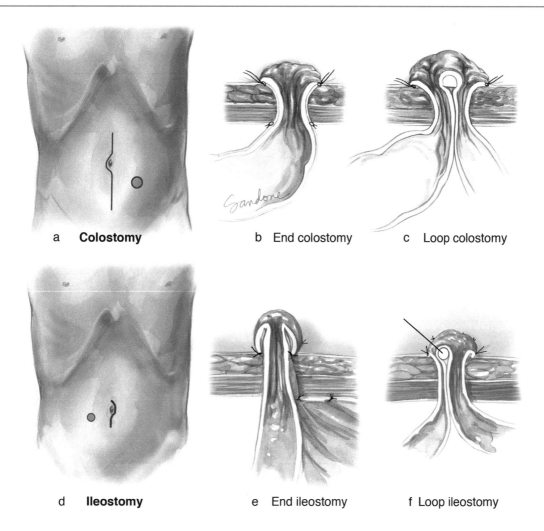

a **Colostomy**   b End colostomy   c Loop colostomy

d **Ileostomy**   e End ileostomy   f Loop ileostomy

Fig. 26.1 Head depicted towards the *right* in above images (**a–c**). (**a**) Laparotomy incision and colostomy site. Note the incision is taken to patient's right around the umbilicus, away from the colostomy. (**b**) End colostomy. (**c**) Loop colostomy. Head depicted towards the *left* in above images (**d–f**). (**d**) Laparotomy incision and ileostomy site. Note the incision is taken to patient's left around the umbilicus, away from the ileostomy. (**e**) End ileostomy. (**f**) Loop ileostomy. Illustration from John L. Cameron and Corinne Sandone, Atlas of Gastrointestinal Surgery, 2nd edition, Vol. II; used with permission from People's Medical Publishing House—USA, Shelton, CT

Operative Approach

Creation of Stoma Aperture

Ostomy creation is usually done at the end of an operation. The operative principles of ostomy creation are similar in laparoscopic and open cases. The appropriate segment of bowel is identified and adequately mobilized to allow it to reach the anterior abdominal wall without any tension on the mesentery. Then a circular skin incision (2–4 cm in diameter) is made at the site of the preoperative marking and the disc of skin is excised. Although there is variation in surgeon practice, leaving some of the subcutaneous fat behind may help prevent stoma retraction. The anterior rectus sheath is then identified and a vertical or cruciate incision is made (surgeon preference). The underlying rectus muscle is split

in the direction of the muscle fibers with simple retraction or the tips of heavy scissors. Electrocautery is used to divide the posterior fascia and peritoneum with care to protect the abdominal viscera. A general rule is the fascial defect should be two fingerbreadths width to prevent a functional narrowing in the ostomy (Fig. 26.2) [2, 6, 31].

A Babcock clamp is passed through the skin opening into the peritoneal cavity and placed on a segment of bowel. In an end ostomy, the bowel is gently brought through the fascial opening with a Babcock. With a loop stoma, a Penrose drain or umbilical tape is placed through the mesentery below the site of the planned ostomy opening. The drain or tape is grasped with the Babcock and the bowel is gently brought through the abdominal wall. The bowel should protrude 2–5 cm above the skin once passed through the skin opening. Once the bowel has been passed through the fascial defect, the primary abdominal

Fig. 26.2 Opening of the abdominal wall. (**a**) Disc of skin and fatty tissue excised. (**b**) Rectus muscle, posterior fascia, and peritoneum incised longitudinally. (**c**) Widening of the fascial defect to approximately two fingerbreadths. Illustration from John L. Cameron and Corinne Sandone, Atlas of Gastrointestinal Surgery, 2nd edition, Vol. II; used with permission from People's Medical Publishing House— USA, Shelton, CT

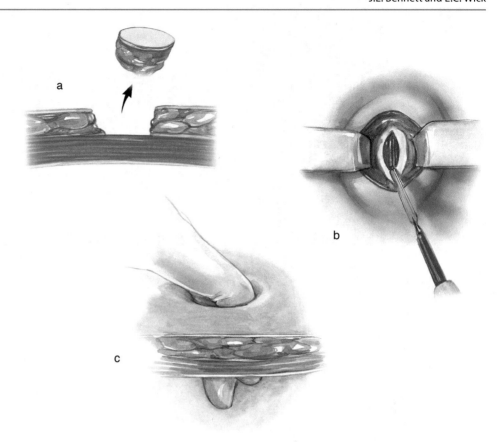

incision is closed to prevent contamination from opening the bowel while maturing the ostomy [2, 6, 31].

Maturation of the Stoma

Maturing the ostomy involves everting the edges of the bowel to create a spout to direct the ostomy output into the appliance and allow the appliance to seal around the stoma edge. Eversion also prevents stricture formation. In end ostomies, the previous staple line is excised. For an end colostomy, the bowel should protrude about 2–3 cm above the abdominal skin while an end ileostomy should protrude about 5 cm above the skin. The exteriorized bowel is then everted. With eversion, an end colostomy should protrude 1–1.5 cm, and an end ileostomy should protrude about 2.5 cm to ensure a sufficient spout for the output to drain into the pouch without causing leakage onto the skin. Four interrupted absorbable sutures are placed in each quadrant to mature an end stoma. These are full-thickness bites at the end of the colon, then a seromuscular bite of the emerging colon at the skin layer, and lastly a bite through the subepidermal layer of the skin opening. In between the four sutures are interrupted sutures that are full-thickness bites of the end of

the colon and subepidermal bites of the skin edge (Figs. 26.3 and 26.4) [2, 6, 31].

In loop colostomies, a transverse incision is made in the apex of the bowel loop on the anti-mesenteric side. The Penrose drain or umbilical tape is replaced with a bridge or rod to support the loop at the level of the skin. The cut edges of the bowel are everted, and sutured to the skin with full-thickness bites through the colon and subepidermal bites of the skin. In creating a loop ileostomy, a semilunar incision in the distal limb of the ileal loop is made, preserving the mesentery. The cut edge in the proximal limb of the bowel loop is everted to create a spout. Absorbable sutures take bites through the cut edge of the ileum and the subepidermal skin layer. On the proximal limb side some sutures also should take bites through the serosa of the emerging ileum at skin level. The distal limb is sutured flush to the skin level (Figs. 26.5 and 26.6) [2, 6, 31].

Ostomy Management

Patient education on ostomy management starts preoperatively once the decision for surgery has been made. Education before surgery helps to reduce anxiety and

Fig. 26.3 Maturation of an end colostomy. (**a**) Excision of the staple line. (**b**) Eversion of the bowel and suturing of the everted mucosa to the skin. Head is depicted towards the *left* in above images. Illustration from John L. Cameron and Corinne Sandone, Atlas of Gastrointestinal Surgery, 2nd edition, Vol. II; used with permission from People's Medical Publishing House—USA, Shelton, CT

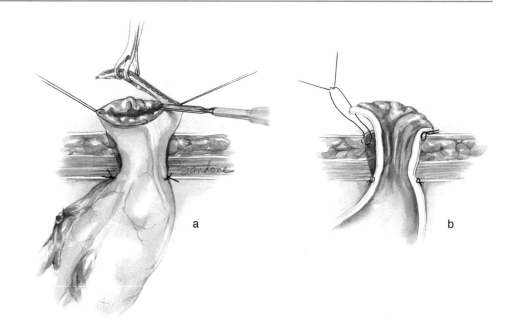

Fig. 26.4 Maturation of an end ileostomy. (**a**) Babcock clamp used to guide the bowel through the abdominal defect. (**b–c**) Eversion of the bowel and suturing of the everted mucosa to the skin. Head is depicted towards the *right* in above images. Illustration from John L. Cameron and Corinne Sandone, Atlas of Gastrointestinal Surgery, 2nd edition, Vol. II; used with permission from People's Medical Publishing House—USA, Shelton, CT

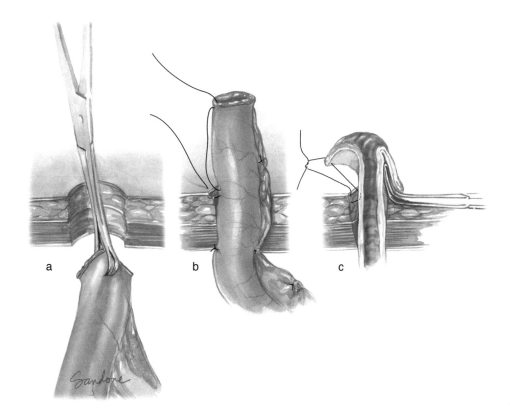

Fig. 26.5 Maturation of a loop colostomy. (**a**) Umbilical tape or Penrose drain used to guide the bowel loop through the abdominal defect. (**b**) Umbilical tape or Penrose drain replaced with a support bridge or rod under bowel loop. Incision in the apex of the bowel loop. (**c**) Eversion of the bowel and suturing of the everted bowel to the skin. Illustration from John L. Cameron and Corinne Sandone, Atlas of Gastrointestinal Surgery, 2nd edition, Vol. II; used with permission from People's Medical Publishing House—USA, Shelton, CT

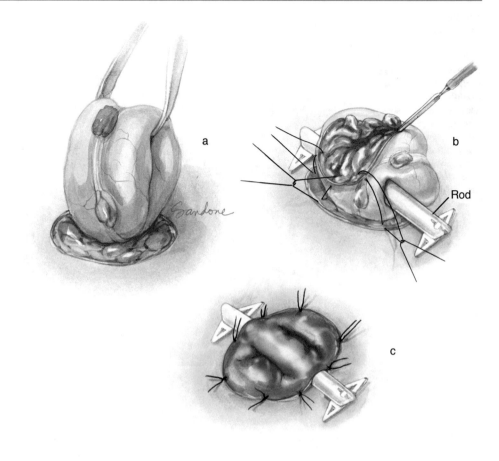

Fig. 26.6 Maturation of a loop ileostomy. (**a**) Umbilical tape or Penrose drain used to guide the loop of bowel through the abdominal defect. (**b**) Umbilical tape or Penrose drain replaced with a support bridge or rod under bowel loop. Incision in the apex of the bowel loop. (**c**) Eversion of the bowel and suturing of the everted mucosa to the skin. Head is depicted to the *right* in above images. Illustration from John L. Cameron and Corinne Sandone, *Atlas of Gastrointestinal Surgery*, 2nd edition, Vol. II; used with permission from People's Medical Publishing House—USA, Shelton, CT

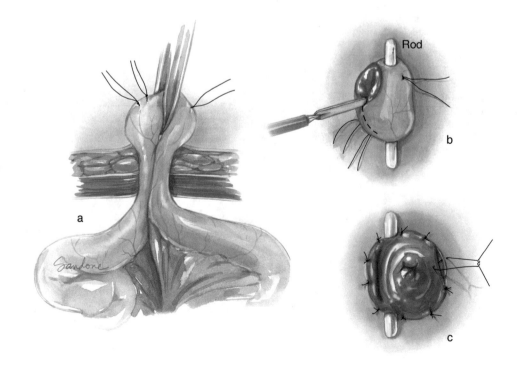

stress related to a new ostomy, and eases the postoperative recovery process [5]. Following surgery, it is best practice for an enterostomal nurse to educate patients on appliance use, emptying and changing pouches, and caring for the peristomal skin. This should be done prior to hospital discharge [22].

Stoma Appearance

In the operating room, a clear pouch is usually applied to the peristomal skin to allow for visualization of the stoma and the ostomy output. The stoma tissue will appear pink or red and moist. A stoma should be watched carefully, if it appears brown, black, grey or flaccid, all signs concerning for ischemia [5]. Most stomas will be edematous after surgery having a taut, shiny appearance. The stoma typically shrinks over the next 6–8 weeks—the changing stoma size will require refitting of the ostomy appliance [5, 32]. Some minor bleeding may occur with the stoma during cleaning or trauma to the stoma, this is usually self-limited [32].

Appliance Products

Pouching systems provide a secure sealed system to collect ostomy output and protect the peristomal skin. In addition to the pouching system itself, many products are used to ensure a well-sealed system including sealants, barriers, cleansers, and adhesives [32]. Pouches are available in one- or two-piece systems and may be reusable or disposable. One-piece pouches have an attached adhesive skin barrier, whereas two-piece pouches must be snapped onto a separate adhesive skin barrier [32]. Two-piece pouches allow the pouch portion to be changed independently of the adhesive skin barrier portion. Most pouches require patients to measure the size of their stoma in order to cut the skin barrier opening to appropriately fit the stoma with a 2–3 mm margin [1]. Given the vast variety of pouching systems and ostomy products available, the enterostomal nurse and patient should discuss the best option for the patient's needs [32].

Ostomy Output

Ostomy output varies depending on the location of the stoma in the intestine. The more proximal the stoma, the less surface area available for water and electrolyte absorption, therefore proximal stomas have a more liquid ostomy output. Ileostomy output in the immediate postoperative period tends to be liquid bilious green that thickens over the week following surgery to a more yellow-brown watery porridge consistency. Right-sided colostomies have a high volume output that is malodorous from the colonic bacteria—these ostomies should be avoided whenever possible. In contrast, left sided colostomies have formed output similar to the stool passed from the anorectum and are very manageable [6].

Patients with long-term ileostomies usually have about 500 ml of effluent per day, but this can increase to 1000–1500 ml/day depending on dietary intake and underlying conditions. In the postoperative period, an ileostomy usually produces a higher volume of up to 1000–3000 ml a day. In this case, the risk of dehydration is greater [6, 33]. Ileostomy output peaks on postoperative day 4 and then, in most cases, the output will thicken and have lower total daily volume [34]. Due to the liquid nature of ileostomy output, typically 500 ml of water is lost daily along with an average of 60 mmol of sodium per day, 2–3 times the normal amount of fecal sodium. Therefore, ileostomy patients are in a state of chronic sodium depletion, dehydration, and hyperaldosteronism. Most patients are able to drink sufficient fluid to compensate for their extra loses. In the immediate postoperative period when the output is higher, this may not be possible despite the use of antidiarrheal medications like Imodium, loperamide, and dilute tincture of opium. Ideally the patient will not be discharged until the ileostomy output is less than 1000 ml/day. Dehydration is a leading cause of hospital readmission in ileostomy patients. Evidence is emerging that increased education and aggressive use of antidiarrheal medications may help avoid readmission in this patient group. In the event that the patient's ostomy output is refractory to medicinal and dietary management, consideration should be made for placement of an intravenous line to be used at home for resuscitative fluid therapy [23, 26].

It is increasingly recognized that Clostridium difficile infection can be a cause of high output ileostomies. Evidence suggests that C. difficile can act pathologically similar in the small bowel as in the colon causing pseudomembranous enteritis and may be responsible for some high output ileostomies [35]. Ileostomy output cultures for C. difficile toxins, PCR assays, or enzyme immunoassay should be performed to evaluate for C. difficile infection, especially in the setting of recent antibiotic therapy, recent hospitalization, gastrointestinal manipulation, or older age [36–38]. Delaying diagnosis due to the rarity Clostridium difficile enteritis should be avoided, as delaying treatment is largely responsible for the high mortality rate in these high output ileostomy patients [35].

Postoperative Complications

Stomal-related complications are fairly common and can negatively impact a patient's ability to adapt to their ostomy [39]. The complication rate for ostomies has been reported anywhere between 21 and 70 % depending on ostomy type. In end colostomies up to 51 % of patients developed complications [40]. Among ileostomy patients, reported complication rates vary by surgical indication—in ulcerative colitis complication rates approach 76 % whereas in Crohn's disease the incidence of complications is about 59 % [26, 41, 42]. Many patient related factors such as advancing patient age, body-mass index greater than 30 kg/m^2, diabetes, ASA class, emergency procedures, and musculoskeletal co-morbidities are associated with increased incidence of stoma related complications. An association between stoma complications and mortality has been identified [30, 39, 43–46]. Although not all risk factors are modifiable, preoperative counseling regarding stomal-related risks and a visit with an enterostomal therapist may prevent some postoperative complications. The majority of complications can be treated conservatively [44, 47]. The first choice in operative treatment of stomal complications is to restore intestinal continuity, if feasible.

Vascular Compromise

It is essential that ostomies have excellent vascular supply. In the event that the vascular supply is compromised, anything from mild ischemia to frank necrosis may occur. During surgery damage to the mucosa or mesentery may either disrupt the blood supply or result in vasospasm, which could compromise the blood supply and cause the stoma to turn dusky or dark. If this happens, the mucosa will slough off with time, and stenosis and/or retraction may occur. Tension on the mesentery or poor collateral arterial supply may also compromise stoma viability and lead to necrosis. Especially in obese patients with thick abdominal walls, it is essential to have excellent mobility on the bowel to prevent devascularization. If the mesentery is fatty, the stoma orifice in the fascia and skin may need to be enlarged [28]. A needle may be used to scratch the serosa, if the serosa bleeds that is an encouraging sign that the vascular supple is sufficient. Ischemia noted in the operating room should be immediately revised. If it is noted postoperatively, superficial necrosis can be watched as it often improves on its own, but if the necrosis extends into the abdominal cavity, then urgent reoperation is necessary to prevent intraperitoneal contamination [28].

Retraction

Stoma retraction is defined as the stoma sitting half a centimeter or more below the skin surface within 6 weeks of surgery and requires surgical intervention [23]. Retraction may occur when there is too much tension on the bowel or mesentery from insufficient mobilization. Risk factors for retraction are compromised wound healing (diabetic or malnourished patients) and obesity. Acute retraction with mucocutaneous separation can cause subcutaneous or subfascial contamination, peritonitis, and sepsis—necessitating immediate laparotomy. Retraction without mucocutaneous separation makes appliance fitting challenging, which in turn leads to fecal leakage and skin irritation. Definitive treatment for retraction is stoma revision. In some cases, minor issues may be addressed by revising the stoma with a small incision around the orifice, but frequently revision requires a laparotomy incision and complete revision of the ostomy [26, 28].

Prolapse

Stoma prolapse occurs when the proximal bowel intussuscepts and the full thickness of the bowel protrudes through the stomal opening increasing the length of the stoma [23, 26, 43]. Prolapse results from redundancy in the bowel near the stoma, and/or failure of the bowel to adhere to the abdominal wall close to the stoma site. Prolapse is most common in patients with loop colostomies but prolapse may occur with all stoma types. Usually patients with stoma prolapse have discomfort or difficulty fitting their appliance. If a patient has symptoms of obstruction, incarceration, or strangulation, these are absolute indications for repair. A higher incidence of prolapse is seen in patients with obesity, bowel obstruction at the time of stoma construction, no preoperative stoma site marking by an enterostomal nurse, and older patients [26].

In the acute setting of a prolapsed stoma, granulated sugar can be applied topically to the edematous stoma to decrease the mucosal edema and allow for manual reduction. If there is any change in the color of the stoma, signs of ischemia, or gangrene surgical consultation should be sought. Surgical options are resection, revision, or relocation. Resection is normally used with end ostomies where the redundant bowel segment is resected followed by rematuration of the stoma. A loop stoma may be revised into an end or end-loop stoma. Stoma relocation is also an option, especially a consideration in cases with poor stoma location or a concurrent parastomal hernia. When bowel continuity can be restored that is the best treatment option [2, 23, 26].

Parastomal Herniation

A parastomal hernia is defined as an incisional hernia associated with the incision for the stoma opening [48]. Hernias often become more apparent with increased intra-abdominal pressure (Valsalva maneuver) [26]. The hernia rate after colostomy construction is higher than following ileostomy construction [49]. The location of where to the mature the stoma and its relation to herniation risk remains debated.

Traditionally, it has been recommended to bring the stoma through the body of the abdominis rectus muscle, although reports are conflicting on the relationship between the transrectus approach and the risk of herniation [41, 49]. The size of the fascial abdominal opening is crucial as making the aperture too small can constrict the bowel or obstruct blood flow whereas an aperture too large may allow for extra bowel loops to pass through resulting in a parastomal hernia. It is best to create the smallest opening possible for a stoma without causing ischemia [26, 28, 48]. Increasing aperture size is predictive of hernia development with each 1-millimeter increase there is a 10 % increase in the risk of developing a hernia [26]. Also with increasing age, the risk of hernia development increases 4 % per each additional year. Obesity, postoperative weight gain, poor nutritional status, immunosuppressive medications, emergent creation, wound sepsis, disseminated malignancy, and chronic elevation of intra-abdominal pressure, like chronic obstructive pulmonary disease, all are associated with increased likelihood of a hernia [23, 26, 34, 49].

Most parastomal hernias are asymptomatic for patients. These patients can be managed with reassurance, use of an abdominal support belt, and avoidance of heavy lifting. About 10–30 % of patients are symptomatic enough to seek surgical management, such as those patients with symptoms of incarceration, strangulation, obstruction, pain, complaints related to cosmesis, and poor appliance fitting. Also when the hernia occurs simultaneously with other stomal complications requiring operative repair, it may be sensible to repair the hernia as well [26, 48, 50]. Surgical management options are: primary fascial defect repair, stoma relocation, and mesh repairs. Local suture repair of the fascial defect is attractive as it avoids the risks of laparotomy, but the risk of hernia recurrence is high [26, 48]. Stomal relocation is another option with lower recurrence rate than local repair, yet still carries the risk of a high re-herniation rate along with the potential need for re-laparotomy. Better results are seen with re-siting the stoma to the contralateral side of the abdomen [26, 48, 51]. Prosthetic mesh hernia repair has a lower rate of hernia recurrence, although using mesh for hernia repair adds complications related to the mesh including adhesions, infection, erosion, and fistulization. Intraperitoneal, preperitoneal, and on lay mesh repair techniques have all been described with a recurrence rate of 7–33 % [23]. A laparoscopic approach for mesh repair has also been reported with varying success of 8–44 % recurrence rates [52, 53].

Stricture/Stenosis

Stoma stenosis is a rare complication resulting from postoperative ischemia or infection [26]. Inadequate blood supply

to the stoma edges can cause retraction and circumferential scar formation around the stoma [54]. Stenosis usually develops within 5 years of stoma formation [40, 41]. It may also occur in the acute postoperative period if the surgical opening in the skin or fascia is too tight, thereby constricting the bowel. This usually resolves with time as the edema decreases. Strictures can result in periods of low ostomy output followed by high volume output and loud flatus, which for patients can be particularly bothersome [23, 26]. In Crohn's disease patients, stenosis occurs more frequently due to the thickened foreshortened mesentery. When a patient presents with symptoms of stenosis, all potential causes should be investigated including recurrent Crohn's disease, malignancy, ischemic necrosis, or tension. Treatment of stenosis depends on the cause. Initially, dilatation can be tried. Local revision with excision of the stenotic stoma and rematuration is often adequate. Laparotomy may be required when tension, poor blood supply, or Crohn's disease are the underlying cause [22, 23, 26, 34].

Peristomal Skin Irritation

Peristomal skin irritation is a common early complication reported in up to 42 % of patients [54]. It can range from peristomal dermatitis to necrosis and ulceration. Skin irritation is usually from improper stoma placement, poor appliance fit, or stoma neglect. Chemical dermatitis from stoma leakage occurs more often with ileostomies due to the more liquid caustic nature of the bilious output compared to the more formed colostomy output, which contains less bile acid. Proper stoma appliance fitting is crucial to prevent leakage and irritation. The proper fit of an appliance should be measured to fit the stoma diameter without any skin exposed between the mucocutaneous junction of the stoma and the appliance. Normally appliances should be changed every 3–7 days, but in retracted or skin level stomas more frequent appliance changes may be needed. Frequent appliance changes can exacerbate skin irritation by causing desquamation. It becomes difficult to treat irritation as ointments and anti-inflammatory creams make adhesion of appliance products difficult leading to more leakage, ultimately worsening irritation. Any signs of irritation should be aggressively treated to prevent a cycle of irritation from developing [23, 26, 28, 54].

Contact dermatitis from allergies to stoma appliance products can cause symptoms from mild erythema and itching to skin breakdown with blisters, burning, and pain. A key in diagnosing contact dermatitis is the pattern of irritation which will resemble the shape and size of the stoma appliance products. It is best treated with identifying the appliance product causing the allergy and stopping use of that product. Topical steroids and oral antihistamines may be used to supplement the treatment [26]. Commonly Candida albicans can cause fungal infection of the peristomal skin due to the warm, moist environment. Miconazole nitrate 2 % anti-fungal powder can help to treat the infection [26, 28]. Peristomal pyoderma gangrenosum can also affect ostomy patients, most often in those with inflammatory bowel disease. After surgery, time to onset of pyoderma gangrenosum ranges from 2 months to 25 years. In patients with active inflammatory bowel disease, treatment should be targeted with systemic therapy for the underlying disease as well as local topical corticosteroids while those with inactive disease may try local therapy first [26, 55]. Patient education on stoma management is imperative to the prevention and treatment of skin complications.

Small Bowel Obstruction

Obstruction related to stoma surgery is possible from many causes. Volvulus or internal herniation around the bowel exiting through the stoma can be devastating, and if there is concern early operation should be considered. Intra-abdominal adhesions from past operations, stomal stenosis, parastomal hernias, and recurrent disease may all also lead to obstruction and management decisions are dependent on the underlying cause of obstruction and the condition of the patient [2, 34].

Peristomal Abscess, Infection, and Fistula

Acutely peristomal abscesses may occur with stomal reconstruction or revision from preoperative colonization of the peristomal skin or from perioperative seeding of the stoma site. Also, an infected suture granuloma or hematoma can lead to an abscess. In mature stomas, an abscess may form as a consequence of folliculitis or recurrent inflammatory bowel disease. With a colostomy, a paracolostomy abscess may result from colon perforation, often the result of an incarcerated parastomal hernia. Fistulas may be seen if fascial-seromuscular sutures used to tack the stoma to the anterior abdominal wall erode or enter the bowel lumen. A fistula in a Crohn's disease patient may indicate recurrent disease [28, 34, 54].

Quality of Life

Stomas can have a considerably impact on a patient's lifestyle and patients have many concerns related to their stoma. The majority of patients reported a change in their lifestyle after stoma surgery; about 40 % of patients have a hard time adjusting to their stoma and many significant others also struggle with adjusting. About half of patients commented that their ostomy changed how they felt about themselves and their self-image. Most patients report their ostomy care is apart of their normal daily toilet, but some patients feel their ostomy care takes too much time [3, 56–58].

Sexuality is a major area of concern for patients in the long term. Patients have reported that intercourse is physically and psychologically more difficult with a stoma. Many patients feel less sexually desirable and many of their concerns about sexual intercourse are related to an altered body image [59]. Despite concerns related to sexual intercourse, a third of females of childbearing age with a stoma were able to become pregnant and have normal deliveries [58].

Although ostomy patients report many changes in their lives after surgery, the majority of patients are able to return to their previous work. Most patients reported an increase in their physical and mental health, and their social lives improved following their stoma construction. Most patients are able to return to a normal diet without restrictions while those that have some restrictions are only minor like avoiding popcorn or certain high fiber fruits and vegetables. About half of ostomy patients reported their lives improved after surgery while the other half of patients felt their surgery did not change their lives [3, 56–58].

Adapting to a new life with a stoma can be difficult, but patients tend to adapt more easily if they do not have problems related to their stoma care. Ostomy symptoms are a negative predictor of quality of life [60]. Patients with problematic stomas have more domestic problems and increased psychological distress. Many report anxiety and shame related to their ostomy, largely due to ostomy leakage and improper sealing of ostomy appliances [39, 57]. Poor psychosocial adaption to stomas correlates to depression and is a predictor of death later on [4]. Counseling and educating patients throughout the entire process is the best care we can provide for patients to help them continue to have happy and productive lives.

Key Points

- Understand the general indications for ostomy construction.
- Preoperative planning for ostomy creation.
- Overview of the operative technique for constructing colostomies and ileostomies.
- Summary of the daily care and management of ostomies.
- Assessment and management of postoperative stomal-related complications.
- Appreciation of the quality of life concerns for patients with ostomies.

References

1. Wexner SD, Beck DE, Roberts PL, Rombeau J, Stamos MJ. The ASCRS manual of colon and rectal surgery. New York: Springer; 2009.
2. Souba WW, American College of Surgeons. ACS surgery: principles & practice 2006. New York: WebMD Professional Pub.; 2006.
3. Silva MA, Ratnayake G, Deen KI. Quality of life of stoma patients: temporary ileostomy versus colostomy. World J Surg. 2003;27(4):421–4.
4. Brown H, Randle J. Living with a stoma: a review of the literature. J Clin Nurs. 2005;14(1):74–81.
5. Colwell JC, Goldberg MT, Carmel JE. Fecal & urinary diversions: management principles. St. Louis: Mosby; 2004.
6. Wolff BG, Beck DE, Church JM, Fleshman JW, Garcia-Aguilar J, Pemberton JH, et al. The ASCRS textbook of colon and rectal surgery. New York: Springer; 2007.
7. Beck DE, Roberts PL, Saclarides TJ, Senagore AJ, Stamos MJ, Wexner SD, et al. The ASCRS textbook of colon and rectal surgery. New York: Springer; 2011.
8. MacLennan AH, Taylor AW, Wilson DH, Wilson D. The prevalence of pelvic floor disorders and their relationship to gender, age, parity and mode of delivery. BJOG. 2000;107(12):1460–70.
9. Kepenekci I, Keskinkilic B, Akinsu F, Cakir P, Elhan AH, Erkek AB, et al. Prevalence of pelvic floor disorders in the female population and the impact of age, mode of delivery, and parity. Dis Colon Rectum. 2011;54(1):85–94.
10. Lukacz ES, Lawrence JM, Contreras R, Nager CW, Luber KM. Parity, mode of delivery, and pelvic floor disorders. Obstet Gynecol. 2006;107(6):1253–60.
11. Tariq SH. Fecal incontinence in older adults. Clin Geriatr Med. 2007;23(4):857–69. vii.
12. Rotholtz NA, Wexner SD. Surgical treatment of constipation and fecal incontinence. Gastroenterol Clin North Am. 2001;30(1):131–66.
13. Colquhoun P, Kaiser Jr R, Efron J, Weiss EG, Nogueras JJ, Vernava 3rd AM, et al. Is the quality of life better in patients with colostomy than patients with fecal incontinence? World J Surg. 2006;30(10):1925–8.
14. Madoff RD, Williams JG, Caushaj PF. Fecal incontinence. N Engl J Med. 1992;326(15):1002–7.
15. Lipska MA, Bissett IP, Parry BR, Merrie AE. Anastomotic leakage after lower gastrointestinal anastomosis: men are at a higher risk. ANZ J Surg. 2006;76(7):579–85.
16. Tan WS, Tang CL, Shi L, Eu KW. Meta-analysis of defunctioning stomas in low anterior resection for rectal cancer. Br J Surg. 2009;96(5):462–72.
17. Khoo RE, Cohen MM, Chapman GM, Jenken DA, Langevin JM. Loop ileostomy for temporary fecal diversion. Am J Surg. 1994;167(5):519–22.
18. Rondelli F, Reboldi P, Rulli A, Barberini F, Guerrisi A, Izzo L, et al. Loop ileostomy versus loop colostomy for fecal diversion after colorectal or coloanal anastomosis: a meta-analysis. Int J Colorectal Dis. 2009;24(5):479–88.
19. Gastinger I, Marusch F, Steinert R, Wolff S, Koeckerling F, Lippert H, et al. Protective defunctioning stoma in low anterior resection for rectal carcinoma. Br J Surg. 2005;92(9):1137–42.
20. Kaiser AM, Israelit S, Klaristenfeld D, Selvindoss P, Vukasin P, Ault G, et al. Morbidity of ostomy takedown. J Gastrointest Surg. 2008;12(3):437–41.
21. Gooszen AW, Geelkerken RH, Hermans J, Lagaay MB, Gooszen HG. Temporary decompression after colorectal surgery: randomized comparison of loop ileostomy and loop colostomy. Br J Surg. 1998;85(1):76–9.
22. Kaidar-Person O, Person B, Wexner SD. Complications of construction and closure of temporary loop ileostomy. J Am Coll Surg. 2005;201(5):759–73.
23. Shabbir J, Britton DC. Stoma complications: a literature overview. Colorectal Dis. 2010;12(10):958–64.
24. Williams NS, Nasmyth DG, Jones D, Smith AH. De-functioning stomas: a prospective controlled trial comparing loop ileostomy with loop transverse colostomy. Br J Surg. 1986;73(7):566–70.
25. Tilney HS, Sains PS, Lovegrove RE, Reese GE, Heriot AG, Tekkis PP. Comparison of outcomes following ileostomy versus colostomy for defunctioning colorectal anastomoses. World J Surg. 2007;31(5):1142–51.
26. Bafford AC, Irani JL. Management and complications of stomas. Surg Clin North Am. 2013;93(1):145–66.
27. Klink CD, Lioupis K, Binnebosel M, Kaemmer D, Kozubek I, Grommes J, et al. Diversion stoma after colorectal surgery: loop colostomy or ileostomy? Int J Colorectal Dis. 2011;26(4):431–6.
28. Kann BR. Early stomal complications. Clin Colon Rectal Surg. 2008;21(1):23–30.
29. Bass EM, Del Pino A, Tan A, Pearl RK, Orsay CP, Abcarian H. Does preoperative stoma marking and education by the enterostomal therapist affect outcome? Dis Colon Rectum. 1997;40(4):440–2.
30. Park JJ, Del Pino A, Orsay CP, Nelson RL, Pearl RK, Cintron JR, et al. Stoma complications: the Cook County Hospital experience. Dis Colon Rectum. 1999;42(12):1575–80.
31. Chen H. Illustrative Handbook of General Surgery. New York: Springer; 2010.
32. Hampton BG, Bryant RA. International Association for Enterostomal Therapy. Ostomies and continent diversions: nursing management. St. Louis: Mosby Year Book; 1992.
33. Brooke BN. Ileostomy. surgery, physiology and management. Graham L. Hill. 225×155mm. Pp. 187+xiv. Illustrated. 1976. New York: Grune & Stratton. $15.75: John Wiley & Sons Ltd.; 1977.
34. Shellito PC. Complications of abdominal stoma surgery. Dis Colon Rectum. 1998;41(12):1562–72.
35. Kim KA, Wry P, Hughes Jr E, Butcher J, Barbot D. Clostridium difficile small-bowel enteritis after total proctocolectomy: a rare but fatal, easily missed diagnosis. Report of a case. Dis Colon Rectum. 2007;50(6):920–3.
36. Williams RN, Hemingway D, Miller AS. Enteral Clostridium difficile, an emerging cause for high-output ileostomy. J Clin Pathol. 2009;62(10):951–3.
37. El Muhtaseb MS, Apollos JK, Dreyer JS. Clostridium difficile enteritis: a cause for high ileostomy output. ANZ J Surg. 2008;78(5):416. doi:10.1111/j.416-2197.2008.04494.x.
38. Freiler JF, Durning SJ, Ender PT. Clostridium difficile small bowel enteritis occurring after total colectomy. Clin Infect Dis. 2001;33(8):1429–31. discussion 1432.
39. Cottam J, Richards K, Hasted A, Blackman A. Results of a nationwide prospective audit of stoma complications within 3 weeks of surgery. Colorectal Dis. 2007;9(9):834–8.
40. Londono-Schimmer EE, Leong AP, Phillips RK. Life table analysis of stomal complications following colostomy. Dis Colon Rectum. 1994;37(9):916–20.
41. Leong AP, Londono-Schimmer EE, Phillips RK. Life-table analysis of stomal complications following ileostomy. Br J Surg. 1994;81(5):727–9.
42. Miles RM, Greene RS. Review of colostomy in a community hospital. Am Surg. 1983;49(4):182–6.
43. Arumugam PJ, Bevan L, Macdonald L, Watkins AJ, Morgan AR, Beynon J, et al. A prospective audit of stomas--analysis of risk factors and complications and their management. Colorectal Dis. 2003;5(1):49–52.
44. Nastro P, Knowles CH, McGrath A, Heyman B, Porrett TR, Lunniss PJ. Complications of intestinal stomas. Br J Surg. 2010;97(12):1885–9.

45. Harris DA, Egbeare D, Jones S, Benjamin H, Woodward A, Foster ME. Complications and mortality following stoma formation. Ann R Coll Surg Engl. 2005;87(6):427–31.

46. Leenen LP, Kuypers JH. Some factors influencing the outcome of stoma surgery. Dis Colon Rectum. 1989;32(6):500–4.

47. Phillips R, Pringle W, Evans C, Keighley MR. Analysis of a hospital-based stomatherapy service. Ann R Coll Surg Engl. 1985;67(1):37–40.

48. Carne PW, Robertson GM, Frizelle FA. Parastomal hernia. Br J Surg. 2003;90(7):784–93.

49. Pilgrim CH, McIntyre R, Bailey M. Prospective audit of parastomal hernia: prevalence and associated comorbidities. Dis Colon Rectum. 2010;53(1):71–6.

50. Martin L, Foster G. Parastomal hernia. Ann R Coll Surg Engl. 1996;78(2):81–4.

51. Allen-Mersh TG, Thomson JP. Surgical treatment of colostomy complications. Br J Surg. 1988;75(5):416–8.

52. LeBlanc KA, Bellanger DE, Whitaker JM, Hausmann MG. Laparoscopic parastomal hernia repair. Hernia. 2005;9(2):140–4.

53. Safadi B. Laparoscopic repair of parastomal hernias: early results. Surg Endosc. 2004;18(4):676–80.

54. Pearl RK, Prasad ML, Orsay CP, Abcarian H, Tan AB, Melzl MT. Early local complications from intestinal stomas. Arch Surg. 1985;120(10):1145–7.

55. Hughes AP, Jackson JM, Callen JP. Clinical features and treatment of peristomal pyoderma gangrenosum. JAMA. 2000;284(12):1546–8.

56. Erwin-Toth P, Spencer M. A survey of patient perception of quality of care. J ET Nurs. 1991;18(4):122–5.

57. Nugent KP, Daniels P, Stewart B, Patankar R, Johnson CD. Quality of life in stoma patients. Dis Colon Rectum. 1999;42(12):1569–74.

58. Roy PH, Sauer WG, Beahrs OH, Farrow GM. Experience with ileostomies. Evaluation of long-term rehabilitation in 497 patients. Am J Surg. 1970;119(1):77–86.

59. Rolstad BS, Wilson G, Rothenberger DA. Sexual concerns in the patient with an ileostomy. Dis Colon Rectum. 1983;26(3):170–1.

60. Smith DM, Loewenstein G, Jankovic A, Ubel PA. Happily hopeless: adaptation to a permanent, but not to a temporary, disability. Health Psychol. 2009;28(6):787–91.

Pelvic Hernias

Veerabhadram Garimella and John R.T. Monson

Introduction

Pelvic hernias are relatively rare among all hernias. They are more commonly seen in older patients. They present both diagnostic and therapeutic dilemma due to their relative infrequency as well as their location deep in the pelvis. The three major hernias which come under this heading are obturator, perineal, and sciatic hernia.

Obturator Hernia

Anatomy

Obturator hernia constitutes only 0.05–1.4 % of all hernias but remains the most frequently encountered pelvic hernias [1, 2]. This hernia passes through the obturator canal, an opening in the superior part of the obturator foramen. The obturator foramen is formed by the union of the pubic bone and ischium and is covered by the obturator membrane (Fig. 27.1). The defect is usually located anterior and medial to the obturator neurovascular bundle [3]. The hernia sac is deep within the thigh between the pectineus and adductor longus muscles.

Development

Developmentally an obturator hernia goes through three stages [4]. The first stage is characterized by the entry of preperitoneal fat into the obturator canal. This is followed by the formation of a true sac containing the peritoneal lining. Subsequent progress leads to herniation of the viscera into the sac (Fig. 27.2). This stage is characterized by clinical symptoms. The contents of the sac could include small intestine, bladder, uterus, or adnexa. According to cadaveric studies, obturator hernias are anatomically divided into three types [5]. Type 1 or anterior branch type hernia, the sac passes along the anterior division of the obturator nerve. In type 2 or posterior branch type, the sac passes along the posterior branch of the obturator nerve. The more rare type 3, the sac passes in the space between the internal and external obturator membranes. More recently, Karasaki et al. have used multi-detector-row CT examination of patients with obturator hernias to confirm the anatomical types (type 1 and 2) [6].

Clinical Features

These hernias have a female predisposition (6-9:1) due to their larger and wider pelvis and horizontally oriented triangular obturator openings. Other predisposing factors include advanced age, weight loss causing loss of preperitoneal fat, multiparity, and increased intra-abdominal pressure from conditions such as chronic constipation, COPD, ascites, and kyphoscoliosis.

Obturator hernias characteristically occur on the right side as presence of sigmoid colon usually prevents left sided hernias. However, they can still occur bilaterally or in association with another hernia, most often a femoral hernia [3]. Preoperative diagnosis is difficult due to the small incidence, vague, nonspecific symptoms and hence high index of suspicion is required. The hernia is often found at laparotomy performed for obstruction or peritonitis.

V. Garimella
Royal Stoke University Hospital, Stoke on Trent, ST4 6QG, UK

Center for Colon and Rectal Surgery,
Florida Hospital Medical Group, Orlando, FL, USA

J.R.T. Monson (✉)
Center for Colon and Rectal Surgery,
Florida Hospital Medical Group, Orlando, FL, USA
e-mail: john.monson.md@flhosp.org

© Springer Science+Business Media New York 2017
D.A. Gordon, M.R. Katlic (eds.), *Pelvic Floor Dysfunction and Pelvic Surgery in the Elderly*,
DOI 10.1007/978-1-4939-6554-0_27

Fig. 27.1 Anatomy of the pelvis showing the obturator canal in the superior aspect of the obturator foramen. This area is not covered by the obturator membrane and is the potential site for obturator hernia

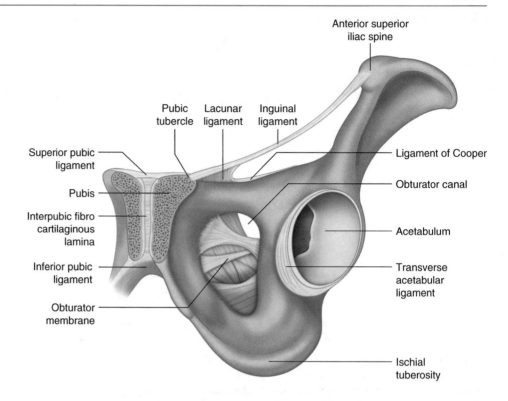

Fig. 27.2 CT scan of the pelvis showing an obturator hernia in the left side. *Source*: With permission from Sze Li S, Kenneth Kher Ti V. Two Different Surgical Approaches for Strangulated Obturator Hernias. Malays J Med Sci. 2012 Jan-Mar;19(1):69–72. Copyright © Penerbit Universiti Sains Malaysia, 2012

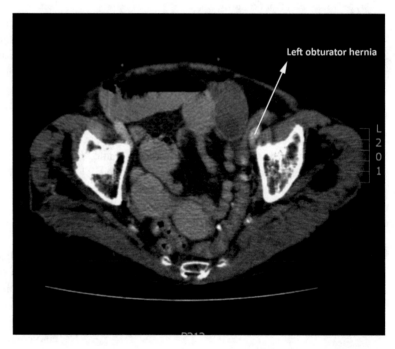

Symptoms and Signs

The classic symptom attributed to this hernia is groin pain radiating down the medial aspect of the thigh to the knee in the distribution of the obturator nerve. Howship–Romberg sign is present in 37–50 % of patients and is described ipsilateral pain along the inner thigh exacerbated by extension, adduction, or medial rotation of the hip, and relieved by flexion [7]. It is considered to be pathognomonic of an obturator hernia but the sensitivity of the test is low and specificity varies considerably [8–10]. Both the symptoms of pain in the groin and HR sign could be misinterpreted in this elderly patient population as being osteoarthritis. The Hannington–Kiff sign is the absence of the adductor reflex of the thigh with an intact patellar tendon reflex and is more specific than the Howship–Romberg [11]. This sign is elicited by percussing on the index finger placed on the adductor muscle above the knee. The contraction of the muscle either seen or felt rules out an obturator hernia. Comparison with the opposite side is helpful to discern this reflex. Palpationof a mass in the upper medial thigh is difficult as the hernia is covered by the pectineus however, a tender mass may be palpable on vaginal or rectal exam. A recent correlation of the clinical signs with CT scan showed that the HR sign was seen more often in type 1 OH and Hannington–Kiff sign in type 2 OH [6].

Investigations and Diagnosis

Up to 90 % of cases present as intestinal obstruction (Fig. 27.3) and strangulation, usually involving the small bowel, which is an indication for operative management [12]. When acutely incarcerated, mortality rates for obturator hernias can reach 70 % [13]. However, if the clinical status of the patient allows, imaging modalities have become crucial in the management of obturator hernias and have been suggested to be the standard of care. CT scan has been used to aid diagnosis and has been reported to reduce the rate of intestinal resection and surgical mortality and hence a recent review advocates early imaging with CT (Fig. 27.3) [1, 14]. Diagnostic accuracy can be improved up to 90 % with the use of CT in suspected patients [2]. Other investigative modalities that have been used are ultrasound scan and MRI [8, 15]. Patients with chronic pain after inguinal surgery should also have obturator hernia on their list of differential diagnoses, after ruling out other causes such as recurrent inguinal hernias, nerve entrapment, or meshoma [12].

Surgical Repair

The high rate of intestinal obstruction and bowel strangulation as the presenting symptom of an obturator hernia means that midline laparotomy and primary repair remains the most common approach, with up to 50 % of cases requiring bowel resection [2]. In the absence of acute and complete intestinal obstruction, it has been advocated that laparoscopy (Fig. 27.3) may serve as a method of diagnosis and treatment of obturator hernias. Other operative approaches include an extraperitoneal technique using an inguinal or thigh incision but these can only be used in elective situations where preoperative diagnosis has been made and bowel resection is not required. Reduction of the hernia may require incision of the obturator membrane posteromedially and parallel to the neurovascular bundle with care to avoid its injury.

Mesh based repairs are particularly beneficial in circumstances where the boundaries of the hernia are rigid and difficult to approximate. The preferred repair technique consists of placing a large flat synthetic mesh in the preperitoneal space to cover the obturator orifice, femoral, and inguinal areas. Therefore, a thorough examination for coexisting groin hernias with concurrent repair if possible is recommended [2]. In the case of strangulation, the abdominal approach is favored, with entry into the parietal peritoneum. A biologic mesh, periosteal flap, bladder wall, uterine fundus, or ligaments may be mobilized and used in cases of gross contamination, where use of synthetic mesh may be precluded.

The totally extraperitoneal approach (TEP) to hernia repair has been employed for obturator hernias and is not different from the direct, indirect, or femoral repair [16]. The obturator space is exposed by sweeping away the preperitoneal fat overlying the Cooper ligament, visualizing the obturator

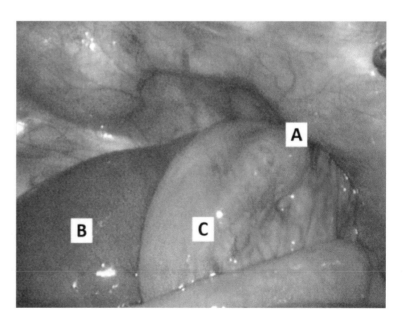

Fig. 27.3 Laparoscopic appearance of an incarcerated obturator hernia. (*A*) Small bowel loop and omentum incarcerated in hernia. (*B*) Distended proximal bowel loop. (*C*) collapsed distal bowel. With permission from Lynch NP, Corrigan MA, Kearney DE, Andrews EJ. Successful laparoscopic management of an incarcerated obturator hernia. J Surg Case Rep. 2013 July; 2013(7): rjt050. doi:10.1093/jscr/rjt050. © Oxford University Press

Fig. 27.4 Anatomy of the pelvis demonstrating the greater and lesser sciatic foramina, the sites for sciatic hernia

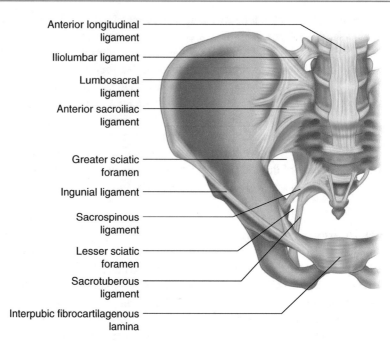

Anterior longitudinal ligament

Iliolumbar ligament

Lumbosacral ligament

Anterior sacroiliac ligament

Greater sciatic foramen

Ingunial ligament

Sacrospinous ligament

Lesser sciatic foramen

Sacrotuberous ligament

Interpubic fibrocartilagenous lamina

artery and vein leading to the obturator fossa along with the nerve. The endopelvic fascia and obturator defect are exposed by retracting the bladder medially [16]. Recurrence is rare, possibly because most patients with obturator hernias are elderly and die of unrelated causes before their hernias might otherwise have recurred. As in lumbar hernias, long-term studies comparing the different techniques of repair for durability are absent in the literature. The usual philosophy of tension-free hernia repair applies in these cases. Peritoneal closure of the defect and patching the defect with adjacent structures such as ovary, round ligament, or uterus seem to be viable options in the face of peritonitis. The use of prosthetic materials overcomes the lack of suitable local tissue, which is relatively immobile in an obturator hernia, constituting a rigid membrane spanning most of the bony obturator foramen. A larger prosthesis can also encompass multiple defects if they are present. Even elective single-incision laparoscopic hernioplasty has been successfully performed [17].

Sciatic Hernia

Sciatic hernias are the most infrequent of hernias of the pelvic floor, occurring through either the greater or lesser sciatic foramen A recent review of the literature on sciatic hernia over the last century reveals the rarity of this entity, with a total of 99 patients reported [18].

Anatomy

Sciatic hernias can be classified into two varieties depending on the anatomic spaces they arise from, i.e. the greater or lesser sciatic foramen (Fig. 27.4). The piriformis muscle divides the greater sciatic foramen further into the suprapiriform and infrapiriform spaces (Fig. 27.5). The lesser sciatic foramen hernia lies between the sacrospinous and sacrotuberous ligaments or the spinotuberous space (Fig. 27.5). Sciatic hernias are difficult to identify clinically until they are large as they are typically covered by the gluteus maximus muscle (Fig. 27.5).

Clinical Features

The review by Losanoff et al. noted that 46 % of patients had significant comorbidities or predisposing conditions such as neoplasms, coexisting hernias, congenital anomalies, disorders of the pelvic bones, metabolic problems, multiparity or pregnancy (female predominance), and malnutrition. Other factor that has been recognized from several reports has been the attenuation or atrophy of the piriformis muscle [18].

Symptoms and Diagnosis

Similar to other pelvic hernias the onset of symptoms is insidious with abdominal pain being the presenting symptom in around 50 % of patients [18]. Others present with urinary infection, gluteal sepsis, or mass. In a series of 20 women, chronic pelvic pain was the presenting symptom and diagnostic laparoscopy facilitated the diagnosis [19]. The common clinical signs of sciatic hernia pertain to intestinal obstruction. A less frequent presentation is of sciatica type pain due to sciatic nerve compression. A recent case report described a chronic sciatic hernia with nerve entrapment that resulted in atrophy of the gluteal muscles [20]. Digital rectal or vaginal examination may reveal a mass in the sciatic

Fig. 27.5 Anatomy of the pelvis showing the piriformis muscle that divides the greater sciatic foramen into supra and infra piriform spaces. Also showing the cut end of gluteus maximus that makes clinical diagnosis of the sciatic herniae difficult

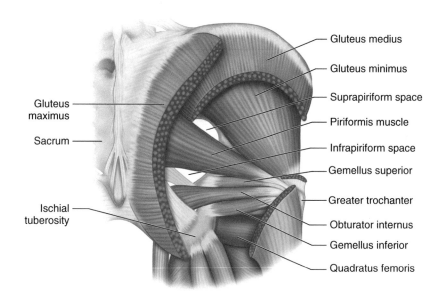

region but other diagnoses like a gluteal lipoma, gluteal artery aneurysm, and an abscess need to be ruled out [21].

An unusual variant of the sciatic hernia is the ureterosciatic hernia. The urinary bladder or the ureter is involved in the hernia causing symptoms of obstructive uropathy. Patient could present with intermittent crampy abdominal pain, chronic renal insufficiency, hydronephrosis, hydroureter, or rarely pyonephrosis [22]. Diagnosis of this variant can be made by the retrograde pyelogram, classically showing the pathognomonic "curlicue ureter" [23] or with contrast-enhanced CT.

The contents of the hernial sac in sciatic hernia vary and include ovary, ureter, small intestine, colon, neoplasm, omentum, or urinary bladder [18]. Resection has been rarely needed but has included small bowel, ureter, or a neoplasm in the retroperitoneum contained in the hernia. However, hernias involving retroperitoneal structures have no peritoneal sac [24].

A palpable mass in the gluteal region with associated symptoms such as pain or obstruction is diagnostic of a sciatic hernia but because of the rarity of these hernias and the wide spectrum of presentation, preoperative clinical diagnosis is difficult. A CT scan can reliably diagnose the hernia emerging through the sciatic foramen, with the sac beneath the gluteus maximus muscle, as well as diagnose coexistent hernias, if present. MRI and MR neurography may be adjunctive tool in preoperative evaluation of patients presenting with sciatica to best evaluate the location of the nerve to prevent iatrogenic injury [20].

Surgical Repair

Several approaches to repair the sciatic hernia have been described. Of these, the trans-peritoneal approach has been the most frequently used. In the trans-peritoneal approach, the hernia defect is identified posterolateral to the rectum in men and in the ovarian fossa in women [18]. After reduction of the contents the defect may be repaired by positioning the mesh in the extraperitoneal space, anchoring to the periosteum of the inner side of the pubis and posteriorly to the periosteum of the sacrum. Large or recurrent hernias need extensive reconstruction of the pelvic floor using mesh while allowing for the rectum, iliac vessels, and ureters to descend alongside the prosthesis to the pelvis.

The transgluteal approach can be used in elective cases where preoperative diagnosis is made and there is no bowel compromise in the hernia. The gluteal approach involves splitting the gluteus maximus muscle along a line that connects the greater trochanter and the middle portion of the sacrum, corresponding to the course of the piriformis muscle [18]. In a large hernia where there is an increased risk of neurovascular injury a combined abdomino-gluteal approach may be more useful. A preperitoneal approach may be used if the diagnosis of ureteric sciatic hernia is established preoperatively. More recent studies have shown successful treatment of uretero-sciatic hernia by stent placement or percutaneous reduction [25, 26].

Laparoscopic techniques have also been used to repair these hernias. Bernard et al. described a laparoscopic plug and patch extraperitoneal repair which aimed at reducing the risk of injury to neurovascular structures [21]. The authors note that the techniques required for laparoscopic sciatic hernia repair are the same as a laparoscopic extraperitoneal inguinal hernia repair. Various methods of repair have been reported to include a variety of endogenous tissue and prosthetic meshes. More recently, robot assisted laparoscopic repair of sciatic hernia has been reported [27]. A recurrence rate of 4% is reported but absence of long-term follow-up and the very small number of patients precludes any accurate assessment of true recurrence.

Perineal Hernia

Anatomy

Weakness of endopelvic fascia and muscles that form the pelvic diaphragm may result in a perineal hernia. The levator ani, consisting of the puborectalis, iliococcygeus and pubococcygeus muscles and the coccygeus muscles make up the pelvic diaphragm (Fig. 27.6). These hernias are rare and can be further classified according to their location into anterior

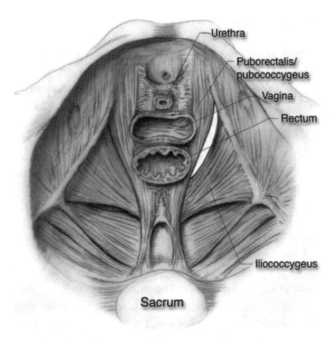

Fig. 27.6 Laparoscopic repair of perineal hernia. *Source*: Rayhanabad J, Sassani P, Abbas MA. Laparoscopic repair of perineal hernia. Pelvic floor musculature with potential spaces for perineal herniae. JSLS. 2009 Apr-Jun;13(2):237–41. Copyright © 2009 by JSLS, Journal of the Society of Laparoendoscopic Surgeons. This is an Open Access article distributed under the terms of the Creative Commons Attribution Non-Commercial No Derivatives License (http://creativecommons.org/licenses/by-nc-nd/3.0/), which permits for non-commercial use, distribution, and reproduction in any medium, provided the original work is properly cited and is not altered in any way

and posterior varieties. Anterior hernias are seen in women only, present as a mass in the labium majus and are due to protrusion through the urogenital diaphragm. On the other hand, posterior hernias are seen in both men and women and present as a mass below the lower margin of the gluteus maximus or protruding through the lateral part of the levator ani (between ischial tuberosities).

Clinical Features

According to clinical presentation, perineal hernias can be classified into congenital or acquired. Acquired perineal hernias are further classified into primary and secondary types. The primary acquired variety is attributed to increased intra-abdominal pressure, such as vaginal birth, aging, obesity, or chronic constipation. Neurogenic atrophy of the pelvic floor is another plausible etiology of some of the cases of primary perineal hernia [28].

To date only nine cases of congenital perineal hernias have been reported in the literature [29]. Primary acquired perineal hernias are also rare, with 100 reported cases [3].

Pelvic exenteration and abdominoperineal excision of rectum result in secondary acquired hernias in 3% and 0.6% patients, respectively [29]. A recent case series of 245 patients treated with abdominoperineal excision for T3-4 rectal cancer showed a symptomatic perineal hernia rate of 11.8% (29/245) [30]. There is renewed interest as well as increased incidence of perineal hernias after the advent of extralevator abdominoperineal excision for low rectal cancer. This procedure leads to greater tissue loss and bigger cavity when compared to traditional APR. Primary reconstruction of the perineum is performed either with autologous tissue or biological mesh [31]. Other surgical procedures associated with postoperative hernias are coccygectomy and sacrectomy, perineal prostatectomy, and cystoureterectomy [32]. Pelvic irradiation, non-healing perineal wounds, tobacco use, and hysterectomy may increase the risk of hernia development [32, 33]. These hernias usually present with symptoms within 1 year or the original surgery and are 4 times more common in women than men attributable to the larger female pelvic outlet. The contents of the hernia are usually bowel and omentum but leiomyoma and bladder diverticulum have been reported [34].

Symptoms and Diagnosis

Swellings in the perineum need to be differentiated from other conditions that present similarly, such as Bartholin cysts, lipoma, epidermoid cysts, and sciatic hernias [35]. Common symptoms from perineal hernia include discomfort

Fig. 27.7 CT scan appearances of a perineal hernia after abdominoperineal excision of rectum. *Source*: Rayhanabad J, Sassani P, Abbas MA. Laparoscopic repair of perineal hernia. Pelvic floor musculature with potential spaces for perineal herniae. JSLS. 2009 Apr–Jun;13(2):237–41. This is an Open Access article distributed under the terms of the Creative Commons Attribution Non-Commercial No Derivatives License (http://creativecommons.org/licenses/by-nc-nd/3.0/), which permits for non-commercial use, distribution, and reproduction in any medium, provided the original work is properly cited and is not altered in any way

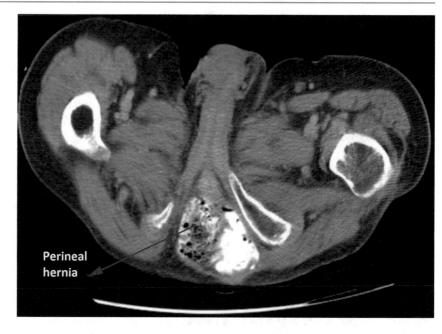

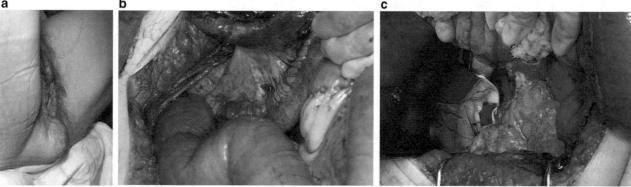

a   b   c

Fig. 27.8 (**a**) Perineal hernia following Abdominoperineal excision of rectum. (**b**) Pelvic view of the perineal hernia after the small bowel loops have been dissected free. (**c**) Mesh repair of the hernia defect with Strattice™ mesh (biological). *Source*: Fallis SA, Taylor LH, Tiramularaju RM. Biological mesh repair of a strangulated perineal hernia following abdominoperineal resection. J Surg Case Rep. 2013 Apr 8;2013(4). Copyright Published by Oxford University Press and JSCR Publishing Ltd. All rights reserved. © The Author 2013. This is an Open Access article distributed under the terms of the Creative Commons Attribution License (http://creativecommons.org/licenses/by-nc/3.0/), which permits non-commercial use, distribution, and reproduction in any medium, provided the original work is properly cited. For commercial re-use, please contact journals.permissions@oup.com

and pain, difficulty with micturition from bladder herniation or ulceration and ischemic changes of the sac. Due to the laxity of the surrounding tissues symptoms of bowel obstruction are unusual. Overall prevalence may be higher than reported numbers due to the rarity of symptoms.

Dynamic mode of imaging may enhance the ability for clinicians to diagnose pelvic floor disorders and thus impact treatment planning (Fig. 27.7). Araki et al. reported the use of fluoroscopic cystocolpoproctography in 46 consecutive women with the primary complaint of sensation of perineal prolapse and were able to diagnose coexisting female pelvic organ prolapse [36].

Surgical Repair

Surgical repair of pelvic hernias can be performed through the perineal, abdominal, or a combined abdominoperineal approach. The abdominal repair can be performed either open or laparoscopically (Fig. 27.8a–c). Congenital pelvic hernias and symptomatic acquired hernias are the indication for surgical repair [29]. Primary repair with native tissues can be performed in congenital cases due to the proximity of pelvic organs [28]. Pelvic floor reconstruction has been achieved with the mobilization of the uterus [37] or bladder, for reconstruction with muscle flaps of the fascia lata, gracilis, rectus abdominis, and gluteus maximus [38]. Use of synthetic material may be necessitated in postoperative hernia that is particularly large. However, there are no direct comparative studies confirming superiority of either the synthetic or biologic meshes.

The transabdominal approach through a lower midline incision provides excellent exposure of pelvic structures for safe reconstruction of the pelvic floor. Trendelenburg positioning allows for structures to fall out of the pelvis for optimal visualization. After the sac is ligated and excised, native tissue like uterosacral ligaments can be re-approximated in women. Alternatively, the sac may be eliminated by suturing the posterior wall of the cervix to the anterior wall of the rectum. More commonly composite or biological mesh or autologous tissue such as muscle flaps can be used to fill the defect (Fig. 27.8a–c) [28, 39].

The perineal approach affords less exposure as compared to the transabdominal technique but is less morbid. This procedure can be performed with patient in Lloyd Davis position or prone jackknife position. The sac is opened, the contents reduced, the sac excised, and the hernia ring closed. Although this approach may be attractive for its limited invasiveness and avoidance of entering the abdominal cavity, limited exposure may pose difficulties for mesh fixation. Earlier studies showed good results with simple closure or mesh repair (13/19) in most cases but overall recurrence rate was 16 % [40]. A recent study showed that perineal repair with absorbable and composite meshes (PTFE, Vypro) led to 100 % (eight cases) recurrence whereas high-tension repair using a non-absorbable mesh resulted in very low recurrence rates of 5 % (1/21) [30]. A further pooled analysis of cases published in 2010 showed that perineal approach to repair was more successful if mesh or muscle flap was used rather than primary closure [41].

The combined approach is advantageous of being able to reconstruct the pelvic floor from both aspects, however there is higher morbidity. A successful combined laparoscopic and perineal approach to repair a symptomatic post-APR perineal hernia was reported [42].

Variable techniques in managing these hernias have recently been reported. Hultman et al. reported on 70 patients who underwent pelvic floor reconstruction after APR or pelvic exenteration and found that omental flaps used as a primary flap or in concert with a myocutaneous flap decreased postoperative pelvic complications such as abscess, urinoma, DVT, flap dehiscence, hernia, bowel obstruction, or fistula [43]. A subsequent recent study has shown that perineal hernia occurred in 21 % of patients who had primary reconstruction with gluteal flap but 0 % recurrence in those that underwent reconstruction with biological mesh [44]. However, a pooled analysis of data from studies has shown no major difference in pelvic hernias after flap reconstruction or biologic mesh repair [31]. Laparoscopic repair, as in other hernias, has been successfully performed on small series of patients to repair postoperative hernias with the use of synthetic mesh to cover the defect in the pelvic outlet [38]. Other novel techniques to repair perineal hernias have been reported and include using a de-epithelialized gracilis myocutaneous flap and insertion of tissue expander in the pelvis [45, 46].

Key Points

- Pelvic hernias are unusual and are seen predominantly in elderly patients. The clinical diagnosis of these herniae is difficult due to their location
- CT scan and MRI of the pelvis are useful investigations in the diagnosis of these herniae
- Obturator hernias are the most common variety of pelvic hernia and can be primarily repaired after reduction of contents
- Sciatic hernias are very rare and can present with chronic pelvic pain
- The most common cause of secondary acquired perineal hernias are extralevator abdominoperineal excision (ELAPE), abdominoperineal excision (APER), and pelvic exenteration
- The incidence of perineal herniae secondary to ELAPE for low rectal cancer is on the rise with renewed interest in primary perineal reconstruction as well as repair of recurrent herniae
- Mesh repair (biological/ synthetic) of perineal is superior to primary repair by approximation of tissues

References

1. Chang S et al. A review of obturator hernia and a proposed algorithm for its diagnosis and treatment. World J Surg. 2005;29:450–4.
2. Losanoff JE, Richman BW, Jones JW. Preoperative diagnosis of obturator hernia. J Emerg Med. 2002;23(1):87–8.
3. Salameh JR. Primary and unusual abdominal wall hernias. Surg Clin North Am. 2008;88:45–60.
4. Skandalakis JL, Androulakis J, Colborn GL. Obturator hernia. Embryology, anatomy, and surgical applications. Surg Clin North Am. 2000;80(1):71–84.
5. Gray's anatomy: the anatomical basis of clinical practice. 40th ed. Elsevier, Churchill-Livingstone; 2008. p. 1371–83.
6. Karasaki T, Nakagawa T, Tanaka N. Obturator hernia: the relationship between anatomical classification and the Howship-Romberg sign. Hernia. 2014;18:413–6.
7. Nasir BS et al. Obturator hernia: the Mayo Clinic experience. Hernia. 2012;16(3):315–9.
8. Yokoyama Y et al. Thirty-six cases of obturator hernia: does computed tomography contribute to postoperative outcome? World J Surg. 1999;23(2):214–6. discussion 217.
9. Rodriguez-Hermosa JI et al. Obturator hernia: clinical analysis of 16 cases and algorithm for its diagnosis and treatment. Hernia. 2008;12(3):289–97.

10. Petrie A et al. Obturator hernia: anatomy, embryology, diagnosis, and treatment. Clin Anat. 2011;24(5):562–9.
11. Hannington-Kiff JG. Absent thigh adductor reflex in obturator hernia. Lancet. 1980;1(8161):180.
12. Moreno-Egea A et al. Obturator hernia as a cause of chronic pain after inguinal hernioplasty: elective management using tomography and ambulatroy total extraperitoneal laparoscopy. Surg Laparosc Endosc Percutan Tech. 2006;16:54–7.
13. Ramshaw B et al. Laparoscopic inguinal hernia repair: lessons learned after 1,224 consecutive cases. Surg Endosc. 2001;15:50–4.
14. Kammori M et al. Forty-three cases of obturator hernia. Am J Surg. 2004;187(4):549–52.
15. Mantoo SK, Mak K, Tan TJ. Obturator hernia: diagnosis and treatment in the modern era. Singapore Med J. 2009;50(9):866–70.
16. Shapiro K et al. Totally extraperitoneal repair of obturator hernia. Surg Endosc. 2004;18:954–6.
17. Hirano Y et al. Single-incision laparoscopic hernioplasty for obturator hernia. Surg Laparosc Endosc Percutan Tech. 2010;20(3):144–5.
18. Losanoff JE et al. Sciatic hernia: a comprehensive review of the world literature (1900–2008). Am J Surg. 2010;199(1):52–9.
19. Miklos JR, O'Reilly MJ, Saye WB. Sciatic hernia as a cause of chronic pelvic pain in women. Obstet Gynecol. 1998;91:998–1001.
20. Chitranjan, Kandpal H, Madhusudhan KS. Sciatic hernia causing sciatica: MRI and MR neurography showing entrapment of the sciatic nerve. Br J Radiol. 2010;83:e65–6.
21. Bernard AC et al. Sciatic hernia: laparoscopic transabdominal extraperitoneal repair with plug and patch. Hernia. 2010; 14:97–100.
22. Stockle M, Muller SC, Riedmiller H. Ureterosciatic hernia. A rare cause of pyonephrosis. Eur Urol. 1989;16(6):463–5.
23. Beck WC, Baurys W, Brochu J. Herniation of the ureter into the sciatic foramen ('curlicue ureter'). JAMA. 1952;179:441–2.
24. Speeg JS et al. An unusual presentation of a sciatic hernia. Am Surg. 2009;75(11):1139–41.
25. Sugimoto M et al. Ureterosciatic hernia successfully treated by ureteral stent placement. Int J Urol. 2011;18(10):716–7.
26. Weintraub JL et al. Percutaneous reduction of ureterosciatic hernia. AJR Am J Roentgenol. 2000;175(1):181–2.
27. Singh I et al. Robot assisted laparoscopic repair of sciatic hernia (RASH): a case report. Indian J Surg. 2011;73(6):467–9.
28. Rayhanabad J, Sassani P, Abbas MA. Laparoscopic repair of perineal hernia. JSLS. 2009;13:237–41.
29. Stamatiou D et al. Perineal hernia: surgical anatomy, embryology, and technique of repair. Am Surg. 2010;76:475–9.
30. Martijnse IS et al. Perineal hernia repair after abdominoperineal rectal excision. Dis Colon Rectum. 2012;55(1):90–5.
31. Foster JD et al. Reconstruction of the perineum following extralevator abdominoperineal excision for carcinoma of the lower rectum: a systematic review. Colorectal Dis. 2012;14(9):1052–9.
32. Veenhof AA, van der Peet DL, Cuesta MA. Perineal hernia after laparoscopic abdominoperineal resection for rectal cancer: report of two cases. Dis Colon Rectum. 2007;50(8):1271–4.
33. Aboian E et al. Perineal hernia after proctectomy: prevalence, risks, and management. Dis Colon Rectum. 2006;49(10):1564–8.
34. Skipworth RJE, Smith GHM, Anderson DN. Secondary perineal hernia following open abdominoperneal excision of the rectum: report of a case and review of the literature. Hernia. 2007; 11:541–5.
35. Sistla SC et al. Pelvic leiomyoma presenting as perineal hernia. Hernia. 2009;13(2):213–5.
36. Araki Y et al. Perineal hernia in women: assessment with evacuation fluoroscopic cystocolpoproctography. Kurume Med J. 2007; 54:51–5.
37. Washiro M et al. Using the uterus to close a pelvic defect after primary perineal posterior hernia repair: report of a case. Surg Today. 2010;40(3):277–80.
38. Dulucq JL, Wintringer P, Mahajna A. Laparoscopic repair of postoperative perineal hernia. Surg Endosc. 2006;20:414–8.
39. Conner CA, Noblett K, Lane FL. Repairing perineal hernia. Am J Obstet Gyn. 2007;197:554.e1-e2.
40. So JB, Palmer MT, Shellito PC. Postoperative perineal hernia. Dis Colon Rectum. 1997;40:954–7.
41. Mjoli M et al. Perineal hernia repair after abdominoperineal resection: a pooled analysis. Colorectal Dis. 2012;14(7):e400–6.
42. Gomez Portilla A et al. Giant perineal hernia: laparoscopic mesh repair complemented by a perineal cutaneous approach. Hernia. 2010;13(2):199–201.
43. Hultman CS et al. Utility of the omentum in pelvic floor recnstruction following resection of anorectal malignancy: patient selection, technical caveats, clinical outcomes. Ann Plast Surg. 2010;64(5):559–62.
44. Christensen HK et al. Perineal repair after extralevator abdominoperineal excision for low rectal cancer. Dis Colon Rectum. 2011;54(6):711–7.
45. Ali JM et al. Tissue expanders: early experience of a novel treatment option for perineal herniation. Hernia. 2013;17:545–9.
46. Douglas SR, Longo WE, Narayan D. A novel technique for perineal hernia repair. BMJ Case Rep. 2013;2013, bcr2013008936.

Caitlin W. Hicks and Jonathan E. Efron

Definition and Classification

Rectovaginal fistulas are abnormal communications between the rectum and the vagina (Fig. 28.1). The communication allows for the passage of rectal contents, including stool, gas, and in some cases pus, into the vagina. In addition to severely compromising the quality of life of affected patients, rectovaginal fistulas can also cause serious infectious morbidities of the vagina and urinary tract.

"Rectovaginal fistula" is a term that is frequently used to describe any fistulous communication between the rectum and the vagina. However, a more precise classification based on the anatomic location, size, or etiology of the defect allows for greater accuracy when describing fistulas which is required for selection of appropriate medical and surgical interventions [1]. Fistulas that manifest themselves between the vagina and the rectum proximal to the dentate line are considered true rectovaginal fistulas. In contrast, fistulas that occur within the first 3 cm of the anus below the dentate line are classified as "anovaginal fistulas," while fistulas that occur between the colon and the vagina are classified as "colovaginal fistulas." This distinction is important because anovaginal fistulas almost always involve the sphincter complex. In addition, the location of the fistula in the vagina—low if close to the vaginal introitus, high if close to the cervix, and intermediate anywhere in between—is also important. The size of fistulas may be described as small (<0.5 cm), medium (0.5–2.5 cm), and large (>2.5 cm), and

classification as it relates to etiology is frequently divided into congenital, traumatic, inflammatory bowel disease, infectious, radiation damage, or neoplastic.

A more commonly used classification, and one that takes all of the above factors into account, is to divide fistulas as either "simple" or "complex." Simple fistulas are benign, located in the low- or mid-vaginal septum, measure less than 2.5 cm in diameter, and secondary to trauma or infection. Complex fistulas are greater than 2.5 cm in diameter, persist after one or more attempts at repair, and are caused by other factors such as Crohn's disease, radiation damage, or malignancy [2]. The surgical approach to simple versus complex fistulas is different, so this method of classification becomes important for operative planning.

Epidemiology and Etiology

Rectovaginal fistulas, which can be congenital or acquired, account for approximately 5 % of all anorectal fistulas [3]. Although rectovaginal fistulas are relatively infrequent complication of vaginal delivery (the incidence is approximately 0.1 % of all vaginal births [4]), nearly 90 % of all rectovaginal fistula occur as a result of obstetric trauma [5]. The stretching and laceration of the perineum and rectovaginal septum during childbirth can result in an unwanted open tract between the vagina and rectum [6]. In developed countries, this is most commonly seen after the unsuccessful or unrecognized need for repair of perineal lacerations, or as a complication of episiotomy infection. Inflammatory bowel disease (specifically Crohn's disease), radiation injury, operative trauma (specifically hysterectomies, low anterior resections, hemorrhoidectomy, and pelvic floor surgery), and infection are generally considered to account for the remaining 10–15 % of cases [7]. In elderly patients, the etiology of rectovaginal fistulas is somewhat different because obstetric trauma is a nonissue. The most common causes of rectovaginal fistulas in this population are diverticulitis causing a

C.W. Hicks
Department of Surgery, The Johns Hopkins University, Baltimore, MD, USA

J.E. Efron (✉)
Ravitch Division, Department of Surgery, Johns Hopkins University, 600 N Wolfe Street, Blalock 655, Baltimore, MD 21287, USA
e-mail: jefron1@jhmi.edu

© Springer Science+Business Media New York 2017
D.A. Gordon, M.R. Katlic (eds.), *Pelvic Floor Dysfunction and Pelvic Surgery in the Elderly*,
DOI 10.1007/978-1-4939-6554-0_28

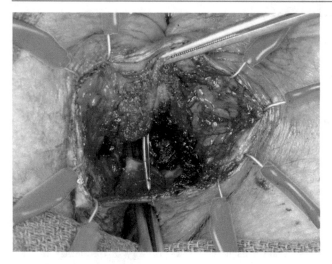

Fig. 28.1 Rectovaginal fistula. Rectovaginal fistulas are abnormal communications between the rectum and the vagina that allows for the passage of rectal contents, including stool, gas, and in some cases pus, into the vagina

colovaginal fistula, colon cancer, radiation injury, fecal impaction causing necrosis of the rectovaginal septum, or cryptoglandular disease resulting in an anovaginal fistula.

Clinical Presentation and Evaluation

Initial Presentation

Women with rectovaginal fistulas may be asymptomatic in cases with small defects, but generally present with a primary complaint of discharge and malodorous gas from the vagina. The quantity of discharge increases with soft or liquid bowel movement, thereby worsening symptoms. Vaginal flatus and recurrent vaginitis are common, and such complaints should be raise immediate suspicion for an enteric-vaginal fistulous connection.

When examining a patient for suspected rectovaginal fistula, a careful history is important to identify possible etiologies of the disease. Physical examination should include both digital rectal and vaginal examinations, which may reveal defects in the rectovaginal septum ranging from a small pit to an obvious open tract. Three quarters of rectovaginal fistulas arise within 1 cm of the dentate line [8], so it is important to take particular notice of this area. In contrast to the discomfort associated with fistula-in-ano, manual palpation of a rectovaginal fistula is generally painless, and patients tend to tolerate digital examination well.

When examining a patient with suspected rectovaginal fistula, it is imperative that a clinician also examines her anal sphincter mechanism. This is particularly true when the rectovaginal defect occurs within 3 cm of the dentate line, which is the normal length of the sphincter complex. Concomitant anal sphincter injury has been reported in as many as one third of women with rectovaginal fistulas [9, 10], and may frequently contribute to symptoms of incontinence. Failure to recognize the presence of a coexisting sphincter injury may lead to continued complaints of incontinence and discharge following successful fistula repair.

Advanced Examination

In addition to physical examination, visualization with a sigmoidoscope or speculum may be helpful to localize and characterize larger rectovaginal defects. Probing the tract with lacrimal duct or silver wire probes can be used to pinpoint the location of a fistula tract and assess its course from the rectum through the vagina.

In cases where the presence of a rectovaginal fistula is in question, a methylene blue dye test can be used. To perform this test, the patient is asked to insert a tampon into her vagina, and an enema with a few drops of methylene blue dye is introduced into the rectum via a genitourinary syringe. The anus is plugged for 15–20 min, after which the tampon is removed and inspected. The presence of blue dye on the tampon indicates a positive test confirming a fistula. Specula examination can allow for visualization of the tract by looking for dye extravasation. If a peroxidase solution is used, tissue staining can be minimized making the tract easier to identify.

Alternatively, a patient can be taken to the operating room for an examination under anesthesia. After positioning in lithotomy, the vagina should be filled with water until the posterior wall is completely covered. The rectum is gently insufflated with air, and the water covering the vaginal wall is observed for the presence of bubbles, indicating the presence of a rectovaginal fistula. Lacrimal duct or silver wire probes can also be used in this setting for more extensive probing of the defect. In general, an intra-operative examination is reserved for cases with severe symptoms but inconclusive physical examination and imaging findings, and for instances where surgical intervention is being considered and precise mapping of the defect is necessary for operative planning. When sepsis is identified, drainage with seton placement is performed to allow for resolution of any cavities and fibrosis of the tract.

Radiographic Imaging

Traditional imaging modalities to visualize fistulas have become mostly obsolete in favor of an extensive physical exam, with or without use of magnetic resonance imaging (MRI). Defecography, which visualizes the anatomy and mechanics of a patient defecating in real-time using fluoroscopy, is unreliable because the fistula tract is often collapsed; thus, the sensitivity of the study is low at 34 % [11, 12]. Vaginography has been shown to be more effective at diagnosing vaginal fistulas (sensitivity approximately 78 % [13]), but is a poor examination for low fistulas that may be tamponaded by the balloon used to occlude the vaginal opening. In addition, vaginography does not allow for evaluation of the anal sphincters, which is important when planning surgical interventions. Fistulography, which was once standard-of-care for diagnosing all fistulas, has become obsolete in the diagnosis of rectovaginal fistula; its sensitivity for low anal fistula is only 16 %, making any negative test unhelpful in making a diagnosis [14].

MRI is becoming increasingly popular for diagnosing and mapping out rectovaginal fistulas. The efficacy of high-resolution imaging can be variable due to the thin-walled nature of the tracts; they are often much shorter, collapsed, and without chronic inflammation, making diagnosis based on the presence of fluid or edema and stranding unreliable. However, the presence of gas in the rectovaginal septum as seen on MRI is an important positive predictive finding [15]. The sensitivity of MRI performed with an endoluminal coil has been reported to be as high as 92 % when evaluating the presence of a rectovaginal fistula [16]. Endoluminal ultrasound is similarly sensitive, and both modalities can be used to successfully identify concomitant sphincter injuries [16–18]. Endoluminal imaging in general is useful because it allows for evaluation and diagnosis not only of the rectovaginal fistula in question, but also for additional abnormalities including sphincter damage, abscesses within the rectovaginal septum, and secondary perianal fistula tracts, which may be identified in as many of 35 % of cases. Therefore depending on a patient's fistula etiology, severity of symptoms, and the operative approaches under consideration, proceeding with pre-operative endoluminal imaging may or may not be a helpful component in the workup of a rectovaginal fistula.

In patients with suspected concomitant fecal incontinence and sphincter disruption, incontinence assessment tools such as the Fecal Incontinence Severity Index (FISI) [19], the Fecal Incontinence Quality of Life (FIQL) [20], or the Cleveland Clinic Fecal Incontinence Score [21] may be helpful in establishing a patient's pre-operative baseline continence score so that improvements (or lack therefore) after surgical repair can be objectively assessed [22]. Anal manometry may also provide objective evidence of decreased sphincter function those patients suspected of have fecal incontinence.

Medical Management

Rectovaginal fistulas rarely heal with medical management alone [23], but symptoms can be significantly improved with some simple lifestyle and dietary modifications.

This is particularly relevant in elderly patients who may not be amenable to operative repair, and in patients who for a variety of reasons require a delay in their repair. Patients should be advised to use Sitz baths at least daily to keep the vaginal area clean and to bulk the stool to prevent leakage. This can be accomplished with fiber supplementation and loperamide if diarrhea or stool frequency is in excess. Bulking is often beneficial in colovaginal fistulas, as the defects tend to be small. These same interventions also help improve overall continence in patients with concomitant sphincter dysfunction.

In fistulas induced by inflammatory bowel disease, optimization of medical therapy to alleviate proctitis and attempt to induce healing of the fistula is required. It is essential that all inflammation be resolved prior to attempting surgical repair. Conventional therapy with antimetabolites (i.e., azothiaprine, 6-mercaptopurine) and infliximab are first-line approaches after induction therapy with oral or topical steroids. In a post-hoc analysis of data from the landmark ACCENT II study, a randomized controlled trial evaluating the efficacy of infliximab maintenance therapy in 306 adult patients with fistulizing Crohn's disease [24], 44.9 % of women with rectovaginal fistulas achieved closure of their fistula within 14 weeks of induction infliximab treatment (5 mg/kg infliximab given intravenously at weeks 0, 2, and 6) [25]. Infliximab maintenance therapy (infliximab 5 mg/kg given intravenously every 8 weeks) also prolonged fistula exposure better than placebo among the initial responders. Unfortunately, cessation of treatment is associated with a recurrence rate of more than 50 % [26]. The incidence of abscess development was not increased with increasing infliximab exposure in the ACCENT II study [27], refuting the concern that infliximab treatment may be associated with abscess formation due to early closure of the external portion of the fistula tract [28]. There is some evidence that oral tacrolimus may also provide symptomatic relief in some patients when conventional therapy fails [29], although data from randomized controlled trials on this subject is currently lacking.

Surgical Management

While surgical repair is often required to definitively heal most rectovaginal fistulas, success rates vary. Most medical interventions can help to minimize symptoms and improve quality of life, but once a communicating tract between the rectum and vagina is formed the most effective way to close it is to do so mechanically. Surgical repairs of rectovaginal fistulas vary, with techniques including local, muscle interposition, and transabdominal approaches. The majority of data available in the literature consists of case reports and case series, so the "best" way to treat any given patient is based on the surgeon's discretion. The intervention of choice is largely patient-dependent, and the decision of which approach to use should involve consideration of disease severity, location of the defect, sphincter involvement, etiology of disease, patient comorbidities, and patient preference. Benign fistulas can often be managed with local procedures, whereas those caused by radiation damage or malignancy may require more extensive intervention. All patients who have a history of a prior malignancy in the area of the fistula or who have findings on physical exam or imaging suspicious for malignancy require biopsy of the fistula. If cancer is documented, then appropriate management with possible neoadjuvant therapy and surgical resection is required.

No matter what approach is used, there are four major principles that are essential to achieving successful surgical repair of a rectovaginal fistula. These include:

1. Appropriate timing of repair
2. Wide mobilization of tissue planes adjacent to the fistula tract
3. Complete excision of the fistula tract
4. A tension-free, multilayered closure

Timing of Surgery

Rectovaginal fistula repairs should be delayed until any infection, acute inflammation, induration, or cellulitis is cleared. Patients with evidence of infection, including pustular discharge and/or the presence of abscess, should undergo incision and drainage, aggressive use of Sitz baths, and a 10- to 14-day course of broad-spectrum oral antibiotics. A seton may be placed and repair delayed until the infection and inflammation has completely resolved. In acutely inflamed tracks, the tissues should be allowed to heal for at least 6 weeks before operative intervention is attempted; however, longer periods of time are often needed.

Pre-Operative Management

A mechanical bowel preparation regimen is appropriate in patients undergoing both local and transabdominal rectovaginal fistula repairs. Starting 48 h prior to surgery, patients should be restricted to a clear liquid diet and magnesium citrate or Golytely should be prescribed to achieve clear rectal output. A fleet or tap water enema should be given immediately before surgery to complete the cleanse. The goal of this pre-operative prep is to prevent continuous fecal seeding of the fistula tract during repair, thereby theoretically reducing the risk of postoperative infection, complication, and fistula recurrence. In addition, peri-operative antibiotics (e.g., cefotetan, or clindamycin and gentamycin in patients with

penicillin allergies) should be given 30 min prior to surgery, but are not indicated post-operatively unless there is evidence of infection.

Local Repairs

Simple Fistulotomy

Small, simple rectovaginal fistulas can be repaired by simple fistulotomy via either a transvaginal or transrectal approach. Simple fistulotomy involves division of the tissue above the fistulous tract. This procedure is usually reserved for simple subcutaneous fistulas with minimal muscle involvement. Great care is taken not to divide a significant portion of the perineal body as this procedure allows for secondary healing of the fistula tract.

Simple fistulotomy should be reserved for low rectovaginal fistulas that are completely free of sphincteric involvement. Partial or total fecal incontinence is a frequent complication, and thus should be avoided in patients with any pre-operative incontinence or suspected sphincter disruption.

Transsphincteric and Transperineal Repairs

Transsphincteric repairs involve wide mobilization of the posterior vaginal wall followed by a multilayer closure. A midline perineal incision is made and the rectovaginal septum is mobilized, crossing the fistula. The defect in the posterior vaginal wall is closed with a multilayered closure similar to that used for chronic third- or fourth-degree perineal tears. Sphincteroplasty is performed during the repair if a sphincter defect is present. The sphincter is often used as a muscle bridge. This approach is indicated in patients with low rectovaginal or anovaginal fistulas resulting from obstetric trauma, most of who have both anal sphincter and perineal body damage.

A transperineal repair consists of separating the rectum from the vagina through a transverse perineal incision, followed by reinforcement of the rectovaginal septum and multilayer closure. This technique is indicated in patients with intact anal sphincters, as the approach allows the surgeon to dissect between the rectum and posterior vaginal wall while avoiding the sphincter complex [30]. Following mobilization, the fistula tract is fully excised and then the rectal mucosa, perirectal fascia, vaginal mucosa, and perineal body are each closed longitudinally to avoid shortening of the anal canal and narrowing of the vaginal introitus. Alternatively, the rectal wall layers can be closed transversely and the vaginal layers longitudinally to avoid overlapping suture lines. No matter whether a parallel or perpendicular closure technique is utilized, closure of the defect must be multilayered to ensure obliteration of all potential space; a 4-layered approach is ideal. Depending on the etiology and the number of previous repairs, the addition of a Martius or gracilis flap is easily accommodated with this approach.

Success rates of the transsphincteric and transperineal approaches are varied and range from 35 to 100 % [31–33]. The main disadvantage of these techniques is the creation of a perineal incision, which can be prone to infection and poor wound healing. These risks are of particular concern in patients who are immunocompromised, malnourished, or have poor tissue quality to begin with. In elderly women, the transsphincteric and transperineal techniques should be approached with caution.

Transvaginal Approaches

Transvaginal approaches are generally avoided in rectovaginal fistula repair, largely because there is minimal data on the outcomes, and the pressure difference between the rectum and the vagina makes vaginal repairs prone to failure. Occasionally, gynecologists will perform local advancement flaps via a transvaginal approach, and combined laparoscopic-transvaginal repairs have been described [34, 35]. Infrequently a transvaginal inversion repair, which involves primary repair of the vaginal opening of the fistula tract via purse-string inversion of the vaginal mucosa, may be employed [36]. However, this approach is only appropriate in patients with small, low fistulas in the setting of surrounding healthy tissue, and thus would rarely be indicated in an elderly patient no matter size or location of her fistula.

Setons, Fibrin Glue, and Fistula Plugs

Use of a seton in the management of a rectovaginal fistula is really a temporizing measure before more definitive treatment can be performed [37]. Seton placement is appropriate in patients with actively draining fistulas and/or frank abscesses, who would likely experience failure with definitive repair but who require more than medical management alone for symptom control. Similarly, fibrin glue and fistula plugs have been used with some success [38, 39], although results have varied and the techniques are not well documented for rectovaginal fistulas.

Endorectal Advancement Flap

The most commonly utilized approach for rectovaginal fistula repair is an endorectal advancement flap, which has a reported success rate ranging anywhere from 43 to 100 % [2, 8, 40–44]. The technique involves the interposition of local tissue—with or without circular muscle depending on surgeon preference—between the rectal and vaginal walls. Using local, regional, or general anesthesia, patients are positioned in the prone position and the buttocks separated and secured with tape or a retractor to ensure adequate exposure (Fig. 28.2A, B). Once the fistula is located, usually via anoscopy, it is gently curetted to remove any epithelial tissue that may prevent closure of the tract. Local epinephrine-containing anesthesia is injected to help raise the flap and

minimize bleeding, and a flamed-shaped flap consisting of mucosa, submucosa, and sometimes circular muscle adjacent to the fistula is created (Fig. 28.2C). The flap is then advanced over the tract opening and sutured in place with simple interrupted absorbable sutures (Fig. 28.2D). This closes off the rectal end of the tract, forcing drainage of the fistula exclusively into the vagina. In theory, the high pressure within the rectum helps to secure the flap against the defect, and is the reason why transvaginal repairs are infrequently used amongst colorectal specialists [37].

In general, we recommend use of the endorectal advancement flap technique as the first-line approach to managing simple rectovaginal fistulas (Fig. 28.3). The use of concomitant sphincteroplasty will depend on the presence of a sphincter deficit. Endorectal advancement repairs that are performed with concomitant sphincteroplasty appear to demonstrate a trend toward better overall outcomes [2, 8], although available data on the subject is limited. Endorectal advancement flaps are not recommended in patients with complex or recurrent rectovaginal fistulas due to a risk of recurrence [45, 46]. The use of a rectal advancement flap is technically difficult in those patients in whom the technique has been performed previously. When the patient has undergone a prior repair, it is often difficult to mobilize a repeat flap without significant tension on the flap, setting the procedure up for failure. The key to a successful endorectal flap is a wide-based, well-vascularized flap that is tension-free when secured to the anal musculature.

Muscle Interposition

Rectovaginal fistula repair with muscle interposition most commonly involves use of the gracilis, rectus abdominus, or bulbocavernosus muscle (also known as the Martius graft). Muscle interposition is most appropriate in patients with large fistulas or fistulas located in the middle to upper third of the vaginal vault, where the local tissue supply may not sufficient to cover the defect. It is also appropriate in patients with fistulous etiologies of inflammatory bowel disease and radiation injury, and patient with previous failed surgical repairs.

Gracilis Interposition

Gracilis interposition is probably the most commonly used pedicled muscular flap in cases of complex and recurrent rectovaginal fistulas. Success rates range between 75 and 92 % [47, 48], including both Crohn's disease and non-Crohn's disease patients. The success of the procedure is thought to be a reflection of improved healing of the excised fistula tract in the setting of the healthy, well-vascularized tissue that is provided from the flap. However, fistula recurrence rates may be as high as 20 % in non-Crohn's patients and 66 % in Crohn's patients [37], so success of the procedure is by no means perfect.

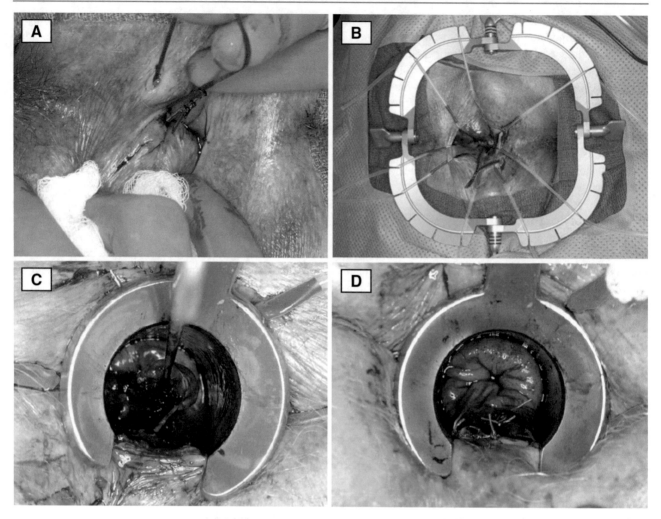

Fig. 28.2 Endorectal advancement flap. With the patient in a prone position, the fistula is identified (Panel **a**) and exposed (Panel **b**). Following injection of local epinephrine-containing anesthesia, a flamed-shaped flap consisting of mucosa, submucosa, and sometimes circular muscle adjacent to the fistula is created (Panel **c**). The flap is then advanced over the tract opening and sutured in place with simple interrupted absorbable sutures to close off the rectal end of the tract (Panel **d**)

The fistula is usually approached through a perineal incision as described above. When the fistula has been divided and repaired, the gracilis muscle is mobilized through several small incisions on the medial aspect of the thigh (Fig. 28.4). During mobilization the neurovascular bundle, which is located at the junction between the proximal and middle thirds of the muscle, should be identified and carefully preserved. The muscle is then released from its insertion on the tibial tuberosity, and the flap is carefully rotated through a subcutaneous tunnel connecting the thigh to the perineal incision. At this point care must be taken to identify and avoid twisting (and thereby obstructing) the gracilis vascular pedicle. Once properly oriented in the perineal wound, the flap should be sutured in place to the apex of the mobilized rectovaginal dissection plane on the vaginal side [49]. It may be helpful to place the securing suture prior to rotating the flap in order to facilitate optimal positioning of the muscle over the defect. The perineum is then closed in a multilayer fashion in the same manner as is used for a transperineal repair.

Martius Graft

A modified Martius graft involves transposition of healthy vascularized tissue from the bulbocavernosus muscle or labial fat pad to the rectovaginal fistula repair site (Fig. 28.5a) [50]. An incision is made over the labia majora (Fig. 28.5b), and the graft is mobilized with sharp dissection to maintain adequate blood supply via a vascular pedicle (Fig. 28.5c, d). The graft is rotated medially around this pedicle (Fig. 28.5e) and then tunneled beneath the vaginal mucosa and labia minor to cover the excised fistula tract (Fig. 28.5f). Similar to the gracilis interposition graft, the Martius graft promotes neovascularization and improved granulation by providing strong blood supply and healthy surrounding tissue.

Fig. 28.3 Muscle interposition. After identification and exposure of the rectovaginal fistula (Panel **a**), a muscular flap (in this case, the gracilis muscle) can be mobilized at its distal end and rotated around a well-vascularized pedicle down toward the fistula site (Panel **b**). The muscle graft is transposed between the rectum and vagina where the local tissue supply may not be sufficient to cover the defect, and then the defect is closed using a 4-layered closure (Panel **c**)

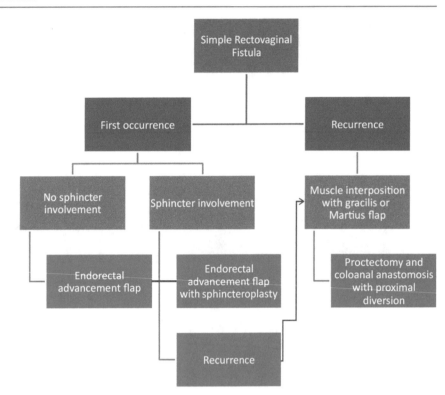

The graft also helps obliterate any dead space, thereby preventing early tract recurrence. This technique is gaining popularity due to its reported success among patients with recurrent rectovaginal fistulas [51] and less invasive nature compared to the gracilis interposition procedure.

Bioprosthetic Repairs

Bioprosthetic interposition grafts (Fig. 28.6) have been used with promising results in certain cases where muscular interposition was not possible [39]. Existing literature consists only of case reports, and success rates vary between 0 and 100 % [7]. The use of bioprosthetic materials in a potentially dirty field carries a real risk of infectious complications, but more experience is necessary before the risks and benefits of this technique can be fully ascertained.

Transabdominal Approaches

High rectovaginal fistulas near the apex of the vaginal vault are often not amenable to local or transrectal repair approaches due to poor visualization and access. Commonly affected patients include those with inflammatory bowel disease, malignancy- or radiation injury-related fistulas, and fistulas with diverticular etiology. Elderly patients will often fall into this category, as episodic diverticulitis is frequently the cause of rectovaginal fistulas in the older population. In these cases, a transabdominal approach, either through laparotomy or laparoscopy, may be necessary [52]. Transabdominal repair options include an omental J-flap, rectus abdominus interposition, proctectomy, abdominal perineal resection, and colpocleisis [37].

The omental J-flap technique involves dissection of the omentum off the transverse colon and creation of a J-shaped incision 4 cm inside the lateral border that extends from adjacent to the stomach past the distal termination of the mesenteric vessels. The resulting omental flap is then rotated down to the excised fistula site, where it is secured in place to provide reinforcement between the posterior vaginal wall and the anterior rectum. Initial experiences with this technique have demonstrated positive results, but long-term data is lacking [53].

Rectus abdominus interposition follows a similar principle; the rectus muscle is mobilized at its distal end, and the resulting flap is rotated around a well-vascularized pedicle down toward the fistula site (Fig. 28.7). The muscle graft is transposed between the rectum and vagina and serves as a course of blood supply and healthy host tissue that promotes wound healing and provides reinforcement of the fistula repair. This technique has been employed successfully in a small series of patients with both Crohn's disease and recurrent rectovaginal fistula with minimal postoperative morbidity [54].

Colpocleisis, which is an obliterative procedure that closes off the vaginal canal completely, is a more extreme alternative approach to fistula repair [55]. It is appropriately offered to patients who cannot tolerate extensive transabdominal surgery, or who have severe pelvic organ prolapse in

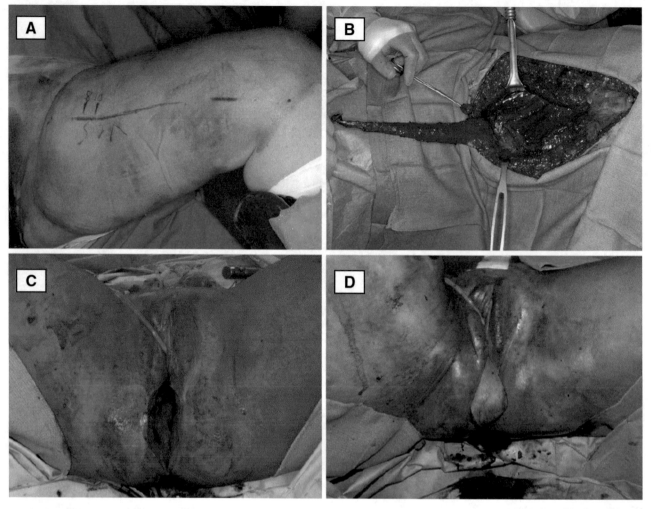

Fig. 28.4 Gracilis interposition. For a gracilis interposition flap, the gracilis muscle is mobilized through several small incisions on the medial aspect of the thigh (Panel **a**) and then released from its insertion on the tibial tuberosity (Panel **b**). The flap is then carefully rotated through a subcutaneous tunnel connecting the thigh to the perineal inci- sion and sutured in place to the apex of the mobilized rectovaginal dis- section plane on the vaginal side (Panel **c**, **d**). Mobilization of the muscle should occur after the fistula has been divided and repaired through a perineal incision

addition to their rectovaginal fistula. Although many elderly women may fall into this category, it is important to communicate that sexual intercourse will no longer be possible following colpocleisis. Thus this option is not to be recommended lightly, and should be reserved for patients with extreme symptomatic complaints and no desire to preserve coital function. It is rarely used in 2013.

Diversion

The utility of a diverting stoma for treating rectovaginal fistulas is controversial. In general, there is little data to support routine use of this approach. Fistula recurrence rates in patients with diverting stomas may be as high as 49 %, and have been shown to be comparable to those in patients with bowel continuity [37, 46, 56–61]. However, diversion may be indicated in specific groups of patients, such as those with

rectovaginal fistulas caused by radiation injury, defects greater than 4 cm in diameter, and recurrent fistulas in patients with poorly controlled inflammatory bowel disease [62]. In instances where a diverting stoma is employed, definitive repair of the fistula should be delayed until any peri-fistular tissue inflammation resolves (approximately 8–12 weeks). Ostomy reversal should be delayed until approximately 3–4 months following fistula repair.

Special Considerations

Crohn's Disease

Surgical failure rates following rectovaginal fistula repair have been reported to be twice as high in Crohn's patients as compared to non-Crohn's patients (50 % versus 24 %) [63]. Even in studies with slightly better overall success rates,

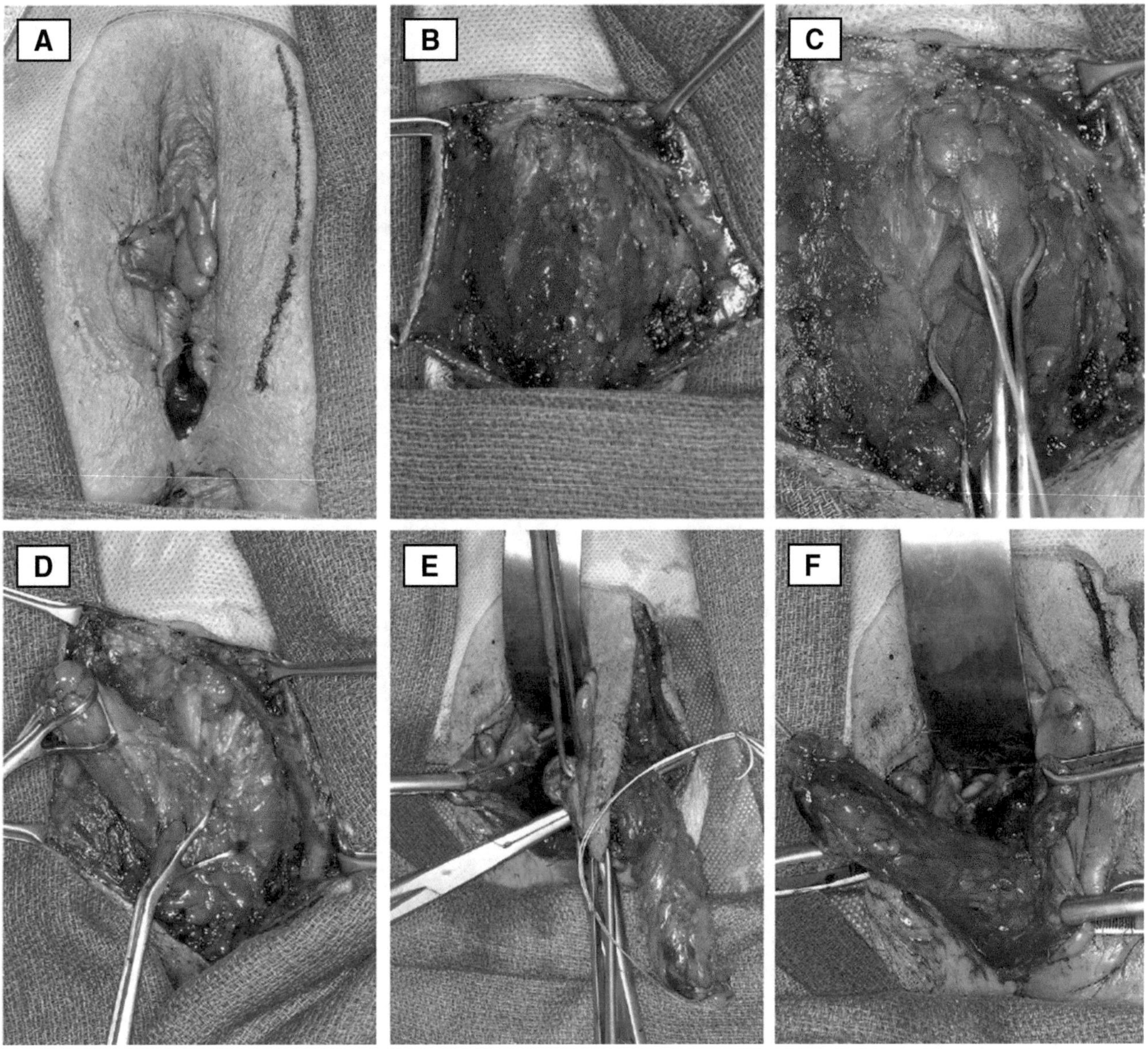

Fig. 28.5 Martius graft. A modified Martius graft involves transposition of healthy vascularized tissue from the bulbocavernosus muscle or labial fat pad (Panel **a**) to the rectovaginal fistula repair site. An incision is made over the labia majora (Panel **b**), and the graft is mobilized with sharp dissection to maintain adequate blood supply via a vascular pedicle (Panels **c**, **d**). The graft is rotated medially around this pedicle (Panel **e**) and then tunneled beneath the vaginal mucosa and labia minor to cover the excised fistula tract (Panel **f**)

Crohn's disease is associated with high rates of fistula recurrence [48, 56]. Successful repair of rectovaginal fistulas in patients with Crohn's disease is completely dependent on disease control and operative timing, which ideally should be in a period of remission, if possible (Fig. 28.8). Patients with active rectal disease should not undergo operative repair because of a high risk of tract recurrence and/or new tract formation. Patients using steroids and with a history of cigarette use are also at high risk for operative failure [57]. Transabdominal repairs should be avoided to prevent unnecessary adhesion formation, since Crohn's patients are highly likely to require laparotomy at some point in their disease course. Instead, a transperineal or Martius graft approach should be utilized. The transperineal technique is appropriate because the likelihood of sphincteric involvement in patients with inflammatory bowel disease is rare. The Martius graft is promoted because it can be used to fill in the large defects that may result from resection of the extensive fistula tracts that are common in this population.

Radiation Injury

The appropriate management for complex rectovaginal fistulas is complicated (Fig. 28.9). Rectovaginal fistulas caused by radiation injury are frequently large, located high on the

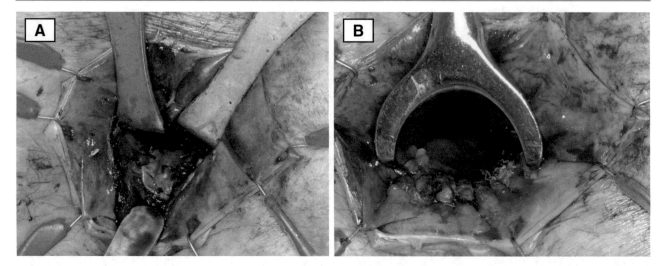

Fig. 28.6 Bioprosthetic interposition grafts. Bioprosthetic materials to close a rectovaginal fistula have been used with promising results in certain cases where muscular interposition was not possible, but may increase the risk of infectious complications. In panel **a**, a biologic implant is shown sutured over the fistula defect (*arrow*). In panel **b**, an Alloderm implant is used for a similar purpose (*arrow*)

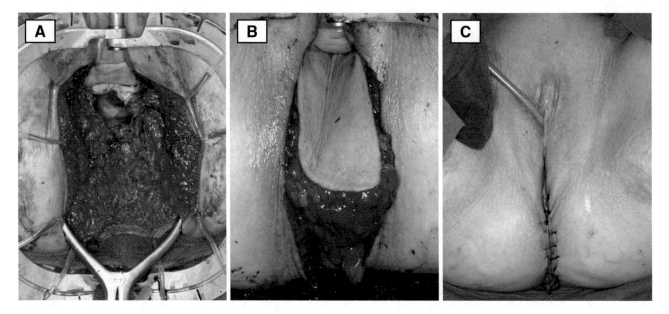

Fig. 28.7 Rectus abdominus interposition. After identification and exposure of rectovaginal fistula (panel **a**), the rectus abdominus muscle is mobilized at its distal end and rotated around a well-vascularized pedicle down toward the fistula site (panel **b**). The muscle flap is transposed between the rectum and vagina where the local tissue supply may not be sufficient to cover the defect, and then the defect is closed using a 4-layered closure (panel **c**)

posterior vaginal wall, and associated with extensive fibrosis of surrounding tissues. Patients will often have concomitant rectal strictures as a result of tissue scarring as well, leading to increased intrarectal pressures that make any surgical repair of a rectovaginal fistula more tenuous. As mentioned previously, a diverting stoma may be appropriate in many of these cases. Radiation-related fistulas may heal spontaneously with diversion alone in 17 % of cases [62]. Alternatively, the Martius flap with temporary diversion has been described

with some success in a small series of ten patients [64], although recurrence rates tend to be high [65]. In cases of extensive radiation injury, laparotomy with extensive excision of both scar and fistula tract may be the best approach, since it allows for complete resection of the involved rectum. If appropriate with respect to comorbidities, an abdominal approach with proctectomy and coloanal anastomosis and proximal diversion is the best approach for fistulas secondary to radiation therapy.

Fig. 28.8 Algorithm for surgical management of rectovaginal fistulas in Crohn's disease

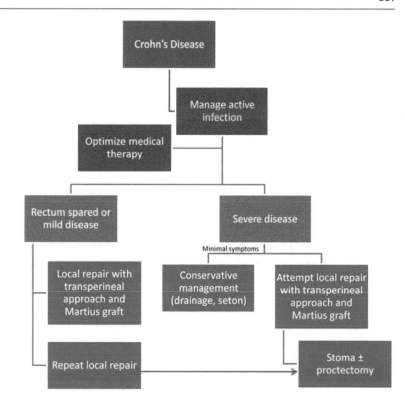

Fig. 28.9 Algorithm for surgical management of complex rectovaginal fistulas associated with radiation injury or malignancy

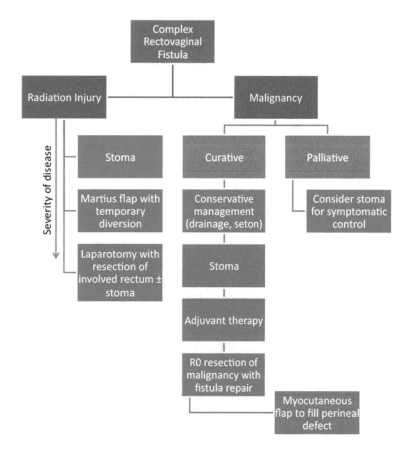

Malignancy

The majority of malignancy-associated rectovaginal fistulas occur as a result of radiation-induced injury, and should be approached as outline above. Repair of rectovaginal fistulas associated with a current malignancy should be deferred until after appropriate treatment of the malignancy (Fig. 28.9). Seton drainage or other temporizing procedures can be used for symptomatic control in the interim time period. Rectal and gynecologic cancers are the most common malignancies associated with rectovaginal fistulas [66], both of which may require treatment with chemoradiation therapy before or after surgical resection. In patients with a new malignancy, a complete R0 resection of the disease should involve en bloc resection of the offending fistula tract along with the primary specimen [67]. In patients with recurrent malignancy, radiation therapy is common and thus fistula repair should be delayed until the resulting tissue inflammation resolves. Delaying surgical repair in these patients will also allow for identification of any new fistula tracts that might form as a result of radiation injury, thereby allowing for multiple repairs during a single trip to the operating room.

R0 resection of these cancers often requires an abdominoperineal resection with posterior vaginal wall resection. Filling the perineal defect requires rotation of a myocutaneous flap into the space. These flaps can be used to close the defect and reconstruct the vagina. The rectus abdominus flap is most commonly used. Bilateral gracilis muscles flaps may also be used, but do not provide adequate tissue bulk for many of the defects created. An alternative that has been recently described is the free anterolateral thigh flap, which has adequate tissue bulk for large reconstructions [68, 69]. The decision to use a myocutaneous flap in elderly patients should be based on the patient's underlying medical condition and not age. The procedures are extensive and at times can be associated with significant blood loss, so those patients with multiple comorbid medical conditions may not be good candidates for resection.

Recurrence

Unfortunately, fistula recurrence following surgical repair is common. Traditionally it was thought that patient age, body mass index, diabetes, steroid use, and immunosuppression were associated with worse surgical outcomes following rectovaginal fistula repair. However, recent studies suggest that there is no significant association between these factors and postoperative failure or recurrence rates [37, 70]. Likewise, the size and duration of the fistula and the presence of a concomitant sphincter injury are not associated with worse outcomes [70]. The only demographic factor that has been shown to reliably predict fistula recurrence is cigarette use [37].

The pathophysiology of this association is thought to be decreased tissue perfusion resulting from catecholamine-induced vasoconstriction and microvascular occlusion from increased platelet adhesiveness [71–73]. The lack of consistent demographic risk factors other than cigarettes suggests that rectovaginal fistula repairs can and should be attempted in elderly women with defects that are appropriate for surgery, provided of course that their other comorbidities and overall health allows for operative intervention.

In addition to cigarette use, prior failed attempts at rectovaginal repair are also associated with progressively worse outcomes; there appears to be a correlation between the number of prior surgical attempts and failure rates [2, 37, 63]. Extending the amount of time between repairs may improve outcomes, with one study demonstrating an improvement from 45 % success to 71 % success after implementing a time interval of at least 3 months between repairs [63]. Although this benchmark was chosen based on mostly arbitrary criteria, it allows for resolution of inflammation and should be considered a guideline for operative planning.

Summary and Recommendations

Rectovaginal fistulas are relatively rare epithelial-lined defects involving a communicating tract between the vagina and rectum. Patients' main presenting complaints are usually malodorous vaginal discharge and gas, with fecal incontinence in cases with concomitant anal sphincter injury. Although most rectovaginal fistulas are formed as complications following obstetric trauma, alternative etiologies such as diverticular disease, malignancy, radiation injury, fecal impaction, inflammatory bowel disease, and surgical trauma are more common in the elderly population.

The diagnosis of a rectovaginal fistula is based primarily on physical exam, either in the office or in the operating as an exam under anesthesia. High-resolution imaging with endoluminal MRI can be helpful in diagnosing concomitant anal sphincter defects, which are common, as well as other associated abnormalities.

Medical management is rarely effective for the definitive management of rectovaginal fistulas, but should serve as a first-line approach for symptom control. This is particularly true in patients with inflammatory bowel disease, who should delay surgery until a period of disease remission, and in patients suffering from radiation therapy, who may experience limited success with surgical repair.

The surgical options for repair of a rectovaginal fistula are varied and range from local procedures to muscle flaps to transabdominal approaches. There is no single "right" way to approach a rectovaginal fistula; rather, operative technique should be based on a combination of the fistula's characteristics, patient factors, and patient preferences.

Endorectal advancement flaps are the mainstay of treatment for simple fistulas, and are associated with success rates ranging from 43 to 100 %. Gracilis interposition and the Martius graft appear to be the most effective treatments for complex or recurrent fistulas, with success rates ranging from 75 to 92 %. Other approaches including simple fistulotomy, seton placement, transsphincteric and transperineal repairs, bioprosthetic repairs, and transabdominal techniques have been utilized with success in specific patient groups. In particular, special considerations need to be made in patients with inflammatory bowel disease, radiation injury, and malignancy.

Despite medical optimization and targeted surgical intervention, fistula recurrence is common and largely unpredictable. Cigarette smoking, prior fistula repairs, and inflammatory bowel disease are associated with increased failure rates, but no other patient or fistula-specific characteristics have been reliably shown to predict recurrence. Elderly patients appear to have outcomes that are just as good as those of younger patients, so age alone should not be a deterrent to surgical repair. However, patient comorbidities and overall health should be taken into consideration before surgical intervention is recommended.

Key Points

- Rectovaginal fistulas are relatively rare epithelial-lined tracts between the vagina and rectum
- Patients' main presenting complaints are vaginal discharge and passage of flatus per vagina with or without fecal incontinence
- Most rectovaginal fistulas result from obstetric trauma, but inflammatory bowel disease, radiation injury, malignancy, surgical trauma, and diverticular disease are more common etiologies in the elderly population
- Surgical repair is the mainstay of treatment; medical management is rarely effective
- The techniques of choice for single and complex/recurrent rectovaginal fistulas are the endorectal advancement flap and gracilis interposition, respectively
- Patients with inflammatory bowel disease, radiation injury, or malignancy require special consideration, and may benefit from a diverting stoma
- Fistula recurrence is common, especially among patients with a history of cigarette use and among those with prior failed attempts at fistula repair
- Surgical outcomes are similar in elderly and younger patients, so age alone should not be a deterrent to surgical repair

References

1. Rosenshein NB, Genadry RR, Woodruff JD. An anatomic classification of rectovaginal septal defects. Am J Obstet Gynecol. 1980;137(4):439–42.
2. Lowry AC, Thorson AG, Rothenberger DA, Goldberg SM. Repair of simple rectovaginal fistulas. Influence of previous repairs. Dis Colon Rectum. 1988;31(9):676–8.
3. Rothenberger DA, Goldberg SM. The management of rectovaginal fistulae. Surg Clin North Am. 1983;63(1):61–79.
4. Homsi R, Daikoku NH, Littlejohn J, Wheeless Jr CR. Episiotomy: risks of dehiscence and rectovaginal fistula. Obstet Gynecol Surv. 1994;49(12):803–8.
5. Senatore Jr PJ. Anovaginal fistulae. Surg Clin North Am. 1994; 74(6):1361–75.
6. Genadry RR, Creanga AA, Roenneburg ML, Wheeless CR. Complex obstetric fistulas. Int J Gynaecol Obstet. 2007;99 Suppl 1:S51–6.
7. Ommer A, Herold A, Berg E, Furst A, Schiedeck T, Sailer M. German S3-guideline: Rectovaginal fistula. Ger Med Sci. 2012; 10:Doc15.
8. Baig MK, Zhao RH, Yuen CH, Nogueras JJ, Singh JJ, Weiss EG, et al. Simple rectovaginal fistulas. Int J Colorectal Dis. 2000; 15(5-6):323–7.
9. Corman ML. Anal incontinence following obstetrical injury. Dis Colon Rectum. 1985;28(2):86–9.
10. Hibbard LT. Surgical management of rectovaginal fistulas and complete perineal tears. Am J Obstet Gynecol. 1978;130(2):139–41.
11. Stoker J, Rociu E, Wiersma TG, Lameris JS. Imaging of anorectal disease. Br J Surg. 2000;87(1):10–27.
12. Bird D, Taylor D, Lee P. Vaginography: the investigation of choice for vaginal fistulae? Aust N Z J Surg. 1993;63(11):894–6.
13. Giordano P, Drew PJ, Taylor D, Duthie G, Lee PW, Monson JR. Vaginography--investigation of choice for clinically suspected vaginal fistulas. Dis Colon Rectum. 1996;39(5):568–72.
14. Kuijpers HC, Schulpen T. Fistulography for fistula-in-ano. Is it useful? Dis Colon Rectum. 1985;28(2):103–4.
15. Stoker J, Rociu E, Zwamborn AW, Schouten WR, Lameris JS. Endoluminal MR imaging of the rectum and anus: technique, applications, and pitfalls. Radiographics. 1999;19(2):383–98.
16. Stoker J, Rociu E, Schouten WR, Lameris JS. Anovaginal and rectovaginal fistulas: endoluminal sonography versus endoluminal MR imaging. AJR Am J Roentgenol. 2002;178(3):737–41.
17. Yee LF, Birnbaum EH, Read TE, Kodner IJ, Fleshman JW. Use of endoanal ultrasound in patients with rectovaginal fistulas. Dis Colon Rectum. 1999;42(8):1057–64.
18. Dwarkasing S, Hussain SM, Hop WC, Krestin GP. Anovaginal fistulas: evaluation with endoanal MR imaging. Radiology. 2004; 231(1):123–8.
19. Rockwood TH, Church JM, Fleshman JW, Kane RL, Mavrantonis C, Thorson AG, et al. Patient and surgeon ranking of the severity of symptoms associated with fecal incontinence: the fecal incontinence severity index. Dis Colon Rectum. 1999;42(12):1525–32.
20. Rockwood TH, Church JM, Fleshman JW, Kane RL, Mavrantonis C, Thorson AG, et al. Fecal incontinence quality of life scale: quality of life instrument for patients with fecal incontinence. Dis Colon Rectum. 2000;43(1):9–16. discussion 16-7.
21. Jorge JM, Wexner SD. Etiology and management of fecal incontinence. Dis Colon Rectum. 1993;36(1):77–97.
22. Cavanaugh M, Hyman N, Osler T. Fecal incontinence severity index after fistulotomy: a predictor of quality of life. Dis Colon Rectum. 2002;45(3):349–53.

23. Nyam DC, Pemberton JH. Management of iatrogenic rectourethral fistula. Dis Colon Rectum. 1999;42(8):994–7. discussion 997-9.

24. Sands BE, Anderson FH, Bernstein CN, Chey WY, Feagan BG, Fedorak RN, et al. Infliximab maintenance therapy for fistulizing crohn's disease. N Engl J Med. 2004;350(9):876–85.

25. Sands BE, Blank MA, Patel K, van Deventer SJ, ACCENT II. Study. Long-term treatment of rectovaginal fistulas in crohn's disease: response to infliximab in the ACCENT II study. Clin Gastroenterol Hepatol. 2004;2(10):912–20.

26. Tozer P, Ng SC, Siddiqui MR, Plamondon S, Burling D, Gupta A, et al. Long-term MRI-guided combined anti-TNF-alpha and thiopurine therapy for crohn's perianal fistulas. Inflamm Bowel Dis. 2012;18(10):1825–34.

27. Sands BE, Blank MA, Diamond RH, Barrett JP, Van Deventer SJ. Maintenance infliximab does not result in increased abscess development in fistulizing crohn's disease: results from the ACCENT II study. Aliment Pharmacol Ther. 2006;23(8):1127–36.

28. van Bodegraven AA, Sloots CE, Felt-Bersma RJ, Meuwissen SG. Endosonographic evidence of persistence of crohn's disease-associated fistulas after infliximab treatment, irrespective of clinical response. Dis Colon Rectum. 2002;45(1):39–45. discussion 45-6.

29. Gonzalez-Lama Y, Abreu L, Vera MI, Pastrana M, Tabernero S, Revilla J, et al. Long-term oral tacrolimus therapy in refractory to infliximab fistulizing crohn's disease: a pilot study. Inflamm Bowel Dis. 2005;11(1):8–15.

30. Wiskind AK, Thompson JD. Transverse transperineal repair of rectovaginal fistulas in the lower vagina. Am J Obstet Gynecol. 1992;167(3):694–9.

31. Tsang CB, Madoff RD, Wong WD, Rothenberger DA, Finne CO, Singer D, et al. Anal sphincter integrity and function influences outcome in rectovaginal fistula repair. Dis Colon Rectum. 1998;41(9): 1141–6.

32. Russell TR, Gallagher DM. Low rectovaginal fistulas. approach and treatment. Am J Surg. 1977;134(1):13–8.

33. MENGERT WF, FISH SA. Anterior rectal wall advancement; technic for repair of complete perineal laceration and recto-vaginal fistula. Obstet Gynecol. 1955;5(3):262–7.

34. Pelosi 3rd MA, Pelosi MA. Transvaginal repair of recurrent rectovaginal fistula with laparoscopic-assisted rectovaginal mobilization. J Laparoendosc Adv Surg Tech A. 1997;7(6):379–83.

35. Herbst F, Jakesz R. Method for treatment of large high rectovaginal fistula. Br J Surg. 1994;81(10):1534–5.

36. Rahman MS, Al-Suleiman SA, El-Yahia AR, Rahman J. Surgical treatment of rectovaginal fistula of obstetric origin: a review of 15 years' experience in a teaching hospital. J Obstet Gynaecol. 2003; 23(6):607–10.

37. Pinto RA, Peterson TV, Shawki S, Davila GW, Wexner SD. Are there predictors of outcome following rectovaginal fistula repair? Dis Colon Rectum. 2010;53(9):1240–7.

38. Lindsey I, Smilgin-Humphreys MM, Cunningham C, Mortensen NJ, George BD. A randomized, controlled trial of fibrin glue vs. conventional treatment for anal fistula. Dis Colon Rectum. 2002; 45(12):1608–15.

39. Ellis CN. Bioprosthetic plugs for complex anal fistulas: an early experience. J Surg Educ. 2007;64(1):36–40.

40. Zimmerman DD, Gosselink MP, Briel JW, Schouten WR. The outcome of transanal advancement flap repair of rectovaginal fistulas is not improved by an additional labial fat flap transposition. Tech Coloproctol. 2002;6(1):37–42.

41. Sonoda T, Hull T, Piedmonte MR, Fazio VW. Outcomes of primary repair of anorectal and rectovaginal fistulas using the endorectal advancement flap. Dis Colon Rectum. 2002;45(12):1622–8.

42. Venkatesh KS, Ramanujam PS, Larson DM, Haywood MA. Anorectal complications of vaginal delivery. Dis Colon Rectum. 1989;32(12):1039–41.

43. Hoexter B, Labow SB, Moseson MD. Transanal rectovaginal fistula repair. Dis Colon Rectum. 1985;28(8):572–5.

44. Kodner IJ, Mazor A, Shemesh EI, Fry RD, Fleshman JW, Birnbaum EH. Endorectal advancement flap repair of rectovaginal and other complicated anorectal fistulas. Surgery. 1993;114(4):682–9. discussion 689-90.

45. Ozuner G, Hull TL, Cartmill J, Fazio VW. Long-term analysis of the use of transanal rectal advancement flaps for complicated anorectal/vaginal fistulas. Dis Colon Rectum. 1996;39(1):10–4.

46. MacRae HM, McLeod RS, Cohen Z, Stern H, Reznick R. Treatment of rectovaginal fistulas that has failed previous repair attempts. Dis Colon Rectum. 1995;38(9):921–5.

47. Furst A, Schmidbauer C, Swol-Ben J, Iesalnieks I, Schwandner O, Agha A. Gracilis transposition for repair of recurrent anovaginal and rectovaginal fistulas in crohn's disease. Int J Colorectal Dis. 2008;23(4):349–53.

48. Wexner SD, Ruiz DE, Genua J, Nogueras JJ, Weiss EG, Zmora O. Gracilis muscle interposition for the treatment of rectourethral, rectovaginal, and pouch-vaginal fistulas: results in 53 patients. Ann Surg. 2008;248(1):39–43.

49. Bailey HR, Snyder MJ. Ambulatory anorectal surgery. New York: Springer; 2003.

50. Seow-Choen F, Seow-En I. Martius flap for ano-vaginal fistula: a photographic step by step guide. Tech Coloproctol. 2013;17: 467–8.

51. McNevin MS, Lee PY, Bax TW. Martius flap: an adjunct for repair of complex, low rectovaginal fistula. Am J Surg. 2007;193(5):597–9. discussion 599.

52. van der Hagen SJ, Soeters PB, Baeten CG, van Gemert WG. Laparoscopic fistula excision and omentoplasty for high rectovaginal fistulas: a prospective study of 40 patients. Int J Colorectal Dis. 2011;26(11):1463–7.

53. Schloericke E, Hoffmann M, Zimmermann M, Kraus M, Bouchard R, Roblick UJ, et al. Transperineal omentum flap for the anatomic reconstruction of the rectovaginal space in the therapy of rectovaginal fistulas. Colorectal Dis. 2012;14(5):604–10.

54. Tran KT, Kuijpers HC, van Nieuwenhoven EJ, van Goor H, Spauwen PH. Transposition of the rectus abdominis muscle for complicated pouch and rectal fistulas. Dis Colon Rectum. 1999; 42(4):486–9.

55. BLAIKLEY JB. Colpocleisis for difficult vaginal fistulae of bladder and rectum. Proc R Soc Med. 1965;58:581–6.

56. Penninckx F, Moneghini D, D'Hoore A, Wyndaele J, Coremans G, Rutgeerts P. Success and failure after repair of rectovaginal fistula in crohn's disease: analysis of prognostic factors. Colorectal Dis. 2001;3(6):406–11.

57. El-Gazzaz G, Hull T, Mignanelli E, Hammel J, Gurland B, Zutshi M. Analysis of function and predictors of failure in women undergoing repair of crohn's related rectovaginal fistula. J Gastrointest Surg. 2010;14(5):824–9.

58. Buchmann P, Keighley MR, Allan RN, Thompson H, Alexander-Williams J. Natural history of perianal crohn's disease. ten year follow-up: a plea for conservatism. Am J Surg. 1980;140(5): 642–4.

59. Marchesa P, Hull TL, Fazio VW. Advancement sleeve flaps for treatment of severe perianal crohn's disease. Br J Surg. 1998; 85(12):1695–8.

60. Lee PY, Fazio VW, Church JM, Hull TL, Eu KW, Lavery IC. Vaginal fistula following restorative proctocolectomy. Dis Colon Rectum. 1997;40(7):752–9.

61. Soriano D, Lemoine A, Laplace C, Deval B, Dessolle L, Darai E, et al. Results of recto-vaginal fistula repair: retrospective analysis of 48 cases. Eur J Obstet Gynecol Reprod Biol. 2001;96(1):75–9.

62. Piekarski JH, Jereczek-Fossa BA, Nejc D, Pluta P, Szymczak W, Sek P, et al. Does fecal diversion offer any chance for spontaneous

closure of the radiation-induced rectovaginal fistula? Int J Gynecol Cancer. 2008;18(1):66–70.

63. Halverson AL, Hull TL, Fazio VW, Church J, Hammel J, Floruta C. Repair of recurrent rectovaginal fistulas. Surgery. 2001;130(4): 753–7. discussion 757-8.

64. Boronow RC. Repair of the radiation-induced vaginal fistula utilizing the martius technique. World J Surg. 1986;10(2):237–48.

65. Aartsen EJ, Sindram IS. Repair of the radiation induced rectovaginal fistulas without or with interposition of the bulbocavernosus muscle (martius procedure). Eur J Surg Oncol. 1988;14(2):171–7.

66. Narayanan P, Nobbenhuis M, Reynolds KM, Sahdev A, Reznek RH, Rockall AG. Fistulas in malignant gynecologic disease: etiology, imaging, and management. Radiographics. 2009;29(4):1073–83.

67. Peiretti M, Bristow RE, Zapardiel I, Gerardi M, Zanagnolo V, Biffi R, et al. Rectosigmoid resection at the time of primary cytoreduction for advanced ovarian cancer. A multi-center analysis of surgical and oncological outcomes. Gynecol Oncol. 2012;126(2): 220–3.

68. Maxhimer JB, Hui-Chou HG, Rodriguez ED. Clinical applications of the pedicled anterolateral thigh flap in complex abdominal-pelvic reconstruction. Ann Plast Surg. 2011;66(3):285–91.

69. Neligan PC, Lannon DA. Versatility of the pedicled anterolateral thigh flap. Clin Plast Surg. 2010;37(4):677–81. vii.

70. Tozer PPJ, Balmforth D, Kayani B, Rahbour G, Hart AL, Phillips RK. Surgical management of rectovaginal fistula in a tertiary referral centre: many techniques are needed. Colorectal Dis. 2013; 15:871–7.

71. Al-Belasy FA. The relationship of "shisha" (water pipe) smoking to postextraction dry socket. J Oral Maxillofac Surg. 2004;62(1): 10–4.

72. Balaji SM. Tobacco smoking and surgical healing of oral tissues: a review. Indian J Dent Res. 2008;19(4):344–8.

73. Mayfield L, Soderholm G, Hallstrom H, Kullendorff B, Edwardsson S, Bratthall G, et al. Guided tissue regeneration for the treatment of intraosseous defects using a biabsorbable membrane. A controlled clinical study. J Clin Periodontol. 1998;25(7):585–95.

Andrea Chao Bafford and Thai Lan Tran

Pruritis Ani

Epidemiology and Classification

Pruritus ani is a dermatologic condition characterized by intense chronic itching affecting the perianal region. It affects 1–5 % of the general population, and is most common between the fourth and sixth decades of life. Men are more commonly affected than women by a 4:1 ratio [1, 2]. Pruritus ani is classified into primary and secondary. The primary form, also known as idiopathic pruritus ani, has no demonstrable cause and accounts for 50–90 % of cases [2]. Secondary pruritis ani results from an identifiable co-existing pathology. The spectrum of causes of secondary pruritis ani varies widely and can be divided into several broad categories as shown in Table 29.1.

Etiology and Management

The Latin term pruritus ani simply means itchy anus. Itch is a phenomenon mediated by pain fibers. Because itch receptors are superficially located, even innocuous and light mechanical stimuli can induce the symptom. The elderly may have a lower threshold for the perception of itch due to decreased skin hydration and increased awareness due to inactivity [3, 4]. Causes of pruritis ani can be divided into five categories: Infectious, dermatologic, systemic disease and psychological factors, anorectal causes, and neoplasm.

A.C. Bafford (✉)
Department of Surgery, University of Maryland Medical Center, 29 S. Greene St., Suite 600, Baltimore, MD 21201, USA
e-mail: abafford@smail.umaryland.edu

T.L. Tran
Department of Surgery, University of California, Irvine, Irvine, CA, USA

Infectious

Infectious sources are rarely the cause of pruritus ani. Perianal infection can be bacterial, fungal, viral, or parasitic in origin. Non-sexually transmitted bacterial causes include Beta-hemolytic streptococci, *Staphylococcus aureus*, and *Corynebacterium minutissimum* [1, 5–7]. The typical presentation is a moist, well-defined, erythematous rash without satellite lesions, often long-standing, which fails to respond to topical steroids. Treatment of pruritis ani due to these bacterial infections is with topical erythromycin, clindamycin, or dicloxacillin [5, 8, 9]. Although rare, perianal tuberculosis can also cause pruritus. Perianal tuberculosis can present as an ulcer with a grayish, granular base, or as extensive perianal inflammation. Diagnosis is proven with acid-fast organisms in scrapings from the lesion [10]. Exudates from the chancre or condyloma latum of perineal *Treponema pallidum* (syphilis) infection can also lead to pruritis ani [2].

Large, scaly, patches of skin, initially pink in color and subsequently turning brown, characterize erythrasma, caused by *C. minutissimum*. It accounts for 1–18 % of cases of pruritis ani and classically affects additional intertriginous areas of the body [11–14].

Fungal infections account for 10–15 % of pruritis ani [1, 2]. Although *Candida albicans* is commonly cultured from the perianal region, it is commensal, only becoming pathogenic in patients who are diabetic, immunosuppressed, or exposed to prolonged antibiotics [1]. Dodi et al. found that only 26 % of patients whom cultured positive for *C. albicans* were affected by pruritis ani [15]. Lesions of *C. albicans* appear moist, red, and macerated, with poorly defined margins and satellite lesions. Mycelian forms and spores can be seen under microscope examination of the scrapings. Treatment includes nystatin powder or ointment in addition to eliminating the precipitating cause [10]. In contrast to *C. albicans*, dermatophytes (*Epidermophyton floccosum*, *Trichophyton mentagrophytes*, and *Trichophyton rubrum*) are always associated with pruritus, and should be considered pathogenic [15].

© Springer Science+Business Media New York 2017
D.A. Gordon, M.R. Katlic (eds.), *Pelvic Floor Dysfunction and Pelvic Surgery in the Elderly*,
DOI 10.1007/978-1-4939-6554-0_29

Table 29.1 Etiologies of pruritus ani

Primary	Idiopathic	
Secondary	Infectious	Bacterial, fungal, viral, parasitic
	Dermatologic	Psoriasis, lichen planus, lichen simplex chronicus, lichen sclerosis, contact dermatitis, atopic dermatitis, local malignancy (Bowen's disease, extramammary Paget's)
	Systemic and psychological factors	Diabetes, leukemia, lymphoma, hepatic diseases, thyroid disorders, chronic renal failure, polycythemia vera, psychogenic, anxiety, stress, neuropathy
	Colorectal and anal causes	Prolapse, anal fistula, fissures, diarrhea, skin tags, deep gluteal clefts, hirsutism
	Neoplasm	Paget's disease, Bowen's disease

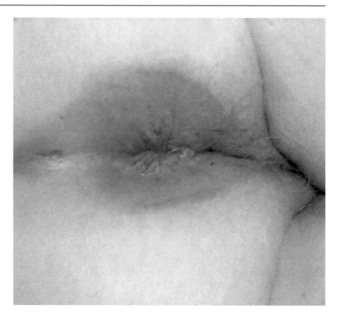

Fig. 29.1 Pruritis ani due to contact dermatitis

Dermatophyte lesions appear as erythematous patches with central clearing, giving a ringworm appearance. Diagnosis is made by potassium hydroxide examination of scales scraped from the lesion, which will show the characteristic segmented hyphae and arthrospores. Treatment consists of fungicidal preparations such as tolnaftate topical or topical imidazoles [10].

Several viral infections can present with pruritus ani, including condyloma acuminatum, herpes simplex virus, and herpes zoster. Parasitic infections can also be the cause of pruritus ani. Some common parasites are *Enterobius vermicularis* (pinworms), *Sarcoptes scabiei* (scabies), and *Pediculosis pubis* (pubic lice) [2].

Dermatologic

Dermatologic conditions associated with pruritus ani include psoriasis, seborrheic dermatitis, contact dermatitis, lichen planus, lichen sclerosis, and lichen simplex chronicus. Many of these conditions do not show the classic appearance in the perianal region; therefore, when dermatologic condition is suspected, the patient's entire body must be examined [2].

Psoriasis is found in 5–55 % of patients with pruritus ani [1]. The clinical presentation of well-demarcated, erythematous lesions with thick silvery scales over the scalp and extensor surfaces is diagnostic. Lesions in the perianal area do not share this typical appearance, due to the moisture in the intergluteal region. Rather, poorly demarcated, paler, and nonscaling lesions are seen. Psoriasis is not curable, but symptoms can be controlled with topical therapies, such as 1 % hydrocortisone cream, fluocinolone acetonide 0.025 % cream, flurandrenolide, or fluocinolone cream in a coal tar base [2, 16].

Perianal seborrheic dermatitis is characterized by moisture and erythema. A thorough examination of the scalp, chest, ears, suprapubic area, and beard will help make the diagnosis. The treatment is 2 % sulfur with 1 % hydrocortisone or miconazole lotion [2].

Contact dermatitis results in erythematous, macerated skin with vesicle formation (Fig. 29.1). Many inciting agents can be found in cleansing and therapeutic preparations, such as lanolin, neomycin, parabens, topical anesthetics, topical antihistamines, and moistened toilet paper containing methyldibromoglutaronitrile [10, 17]. Certain medications, such as quinidine, colchicine, mineral oil, and antibiotics can also irritate the skin [18]. Treatment is with avoidance of local irritants, tight clothing, and perianal moisture. Warm sitz baths and emollient creams should be used to cleanse the skin. Topical steroids such as 1 % hydrocortisone or 0.05 % flurandrenolide lotion may also be useful unless secondary infection is present [2, 10].

Lichen planus begins on the genitals and perianal region and eventually spreads to other regions. This condition may have an immunologic basis. Lesions are characterized by shiny, flat-topped papules that are more darkly pigmented than the surrounding skin. Plaques are often found on the volar aspects of the wrists and forearms. Wickham's striae, small intersecting gray lines that can be seen when mineral oil is applied to the plaques, can help establish the diagnosis. This is a self-limited disease that resolves within 8–12 months. Symptoms are treated with low potency topical steroids. Severe eruptions can be treated with short courses of systemic steroids [10].

Lichen sclerosis is a lymphocyte-mediated skin condition that can affect any part of the body, but is most commonly found in the anogenital region of both sexes. This condition is more common in women, especially postmenopausal women, than men with a ratio of 5:1 [19]. Patients present with ivory-colored, atrophic papules that eventually break down, leaving a raw edematous surface that can be extremely pruritic and painful. As the area heals, the edema is replaced by sclerosis and chronic inflammation. The white patches around the vulva and anus are commonly described as having a "figure-of-8" appearance. Diagnosis is made via skin biopsy. Lichen sclerosis is associated with a risk of invasive squamous cell carcinoma; therefore, all patients should be monitored closely for any suspicious skin changes [1]. There is no known effective cure. Symptoms can be controlled with topical corticosteroids, pimecrolimus, or tacrolimus [19–21]. In severe, nonresponsive cases, systemic therapies such as retinoids, cyclosporine, stanozolol, hydroxychloroquine, potassium aminobenzoate, and calcitriol have been used. Surgery may be required for the release of scarring and fusion, most commonly to relieve urinary obstruction in the geriatric population [20].

Lichen simplex chronicus, or neurodermatitis, is a localized variant of atopic dermatitis. This condition develops when repetitive mechanical trauma, such as from frequent and vigorous cleansing or scratching, leads to lichenification. Lichenification is a thickening and scaling of the epidermis. The itch-scratch-itch cycle leads to a well-demarcated, erythematous, thickened lesion. Diagnosis is confirmed by skin biopsy. Symptom can be controlled with topical steroids and antihistamines [2].

Systemic Disease and Psychological Factors
Several systemic diseases are associated with pruritus ani, including diabetes mellitus, liver disease, lymphoma, leukemia, pellagra, vitamin A and D deficiencies, renal failure, iron-deficiency anemia, and hyperthyroidism. Psychological disturbances, including depression, anxiety, and stress, can exacerbate the symptoms of pruritus ani [2, 3, 22].

Anorectal Causes
Prolonged perianal moisture and fecal contact can cause local skin irritation and pruritus [1, 23, 24]. This can be especially troublesome in the elderly, in whom anal sphincter muscle weakness is common. Anorectal problems that can cause excessive moisture and fecal contamination in the perianal region include hemorrhoids, anal fissures, anal fistulae, rectal prolapse, chronic diarrhea, fecal incontinence, and polyps/cancer [2]. Correcting the underlying pathology is crucial in the management of pruritus ani [25].

Neoplasm
More than half of patients with perianal Paget's disease and Bowen's disease experience pruritus ani [1]. Extramammary Paget's disease (cutaneous adenocarcinoma in situ) is rare and typically occurs in the seventh decade of life [2]. Bowen's disease (intraepithelial squamous cell carcinoma in situ) is also most common in the elderly. Extragenital lesions have a 3–5 % risk of progression into invasive squamous carcinoma, while genital lesions have an approximately 10 % risk. Wide local excision to negative margins is the treatment of choice for both diseases [10].

Diagnosis

A thorough search for causes of secondary pruritis ani should be undertaken before classifying the disease as primary or idiopathic.

History and Physical Examination
During the first initial visit, it is important to take a detailed history including frequency and consistency of bowel movements, anal hygiene, and any co-existing skin diseases. Inquiries about allergic conditions, previous patch testing, history of over-the-counter topical therapy usage, along with a detailed past medical history to look for systemic diseases that can cause pruritus are essential.

In addition to a careful anorectal examination, the physical exam should also survey the entire skin [2]. Skin lesions with sharp, distinct borders usually suggest tinea, psoriasis, or neoplastic changes. Hyperpigmentation in intertriginous areas indicates chronic inflammatory conditions, such as infection or chronic discharge. Erythema is often seen with chronic steroid use, whereas bright erythema suggests perianal candidiasis. Idiopathic inflammation has borders that are indistinct and nondescript. Groin adenopathy points to neoplasia and infection [1].

Laboratory Examination
Cultures and histology can aid in the diagnosis of infectious or dermatologic causes. Fungal and bacterial specimens should be placed in the appropriate bacterial transport medium and refrigerated, while anaerobic specimens should be placed in a specific anaerobic medium and stored at room temperature. Vesicles should be unroofed and exudates placed in a viral culture medium. Skin scraping can be sent for fungal culture and microscopy. Skin biopsies should include an area of adjacent normal skin. Swabs should be taken before internal examination since conventional water-soluble lubricant is bactericidal [1, 10].

Treatment

The management of pruritus ani includes identifying and treating specific causes and reestablishing clean, dry, and intact perianal skin. Three facets of treatment are: Elimination of irritants, general control measures, and active treatment measures. Irritants such as soaps, perfumes, lotions, baby wipes, witch hazel products, dyes in clothes, and certain foods must be eliminated. Foods that have been associated with pruritus ani are coffee, tea, chocolate, beer, citrus fruits, alcohol, dairy products, and tomatoes [1, 22].

General control measures that help relieve symptoms include the use of detachable showerheads for cleansing the perianal region and eliminating soap residues, followed by hair dryers to eliminate moisture without abrading the tissue. Application of a barrier cream, such as calmoseptine or butt paste, will protect the perianal skin from local irritants [10]. Wearing loose-fitting clothing allows air circulation and promotes dryness. Acute itch may indicate fecal seepage, and immediate cleansing is advisable. If washing is not immediately available, oil-based preparations (Balneol) or aqueous creams can be squeezed onto cotton tissue and used to gently cleanse the perianal area. Burow's solution is another useful cleanser. Fecal seepage can be reduced by adding fiber to the diet, avoiding excessive fluid intake, and employing antidiarrheal agents judiciously.

Patients with mild to moderate symptoms and minimal skin changes can be treated with a weak topical steroid, such as 1 % hydrocortisone cream. This can be combined with topical antibiotics or antifungals. Once symptoms improve, the frequency of application should be reduced with the goal of substituting to a barrier cream. Patients with severe symptoms respond well to a short duration (less than 8 weeks) of a high potency steroid, such as 0.05 % betamethasone dipropionate or 0.05 % clobetasol propionate [1]. The prolonged use of potent steroids can cause skin atrophy, systemic absorption with adrenal suppression, allergic contact dermatitis, and rebound worsening after withdrawal.

Topical capsaicin produces a short, intense, burning sensation, which often eliminates the urge to scratch. A randomized, cross-over study showed topical capsaicin to be superior to placebo in a group of patients with chronic pruritus ani [26]. For intractable pruritus ani, intradermal injection of methylene blue has shown good results in some studies [1, 27].

Hemorrhoids

Anatomy

The term "hemorrhoids" refers to the normal submucosal cushions of highly vascular tissue within the anal canal. These anal cushions contain blood vessels, smooth muscle, and elastic connective tissue [28]. They are located from the dentate line to the anorectal ring, and are classically found in the right anterior, right posterior, and left lateral positions. Hemorrhoids are thought to contribute to anal continence by providing complete closure of the anus. They may also act as a compressible lining that protects the underlying anal sphincters [27].

The superior hemorrhoidal artery provides the main blood supply to hemorrhoids, with branches of the middle hemorrhoidal arteries also contributing. Venous drainage is via the superior, middle, and inferior hemorrhoidal veins, which connect the portal and systemic circulations in the region of the dentate line [10].

Etiology

Factors thought to contribute to hemorrhoidal disease include constipation, pregnancy, chronic straining, diarrhea, obstruction of venous return due to increased intraabdominal pressure, and aging [10, 29]. The muscular fibers within the anal cushions arise from both the internal sphincter and the conjoined longitudinal muscle. These help maintain adherence of the hemorrhoidal tissues to the underlying internal sphincter. With aging, the supporting muscular fibers can deteriorate or weaken, leading to distal displacement of the vascular cushions. Thomson's theory of the "sliding anal cushion" is the most widely accepted.

Epidemiology

The true prevalence of symptomatic hemorrhoids is almost impossible to assess due to patients' tendency to self-medicate rather than seek proper medical care [30]. In addition, patients often attribute other anorectal problems such as pruritus ani, anal fissures, fistulas, and skin tags to hemorrhoids. According to the National Center for Health Statistics, the reported prevalence of hemorrhoids in the USA is 4.4 % [31]. The peak incidence of the disease occurs in between the ages of 45 and 65, and its presence prior to the age of 20 is unusual [30, 31].

Classification

Hemorrhoids are classified based on their location and degree of prolapse. Internal hemorrhoids are located proximal to the dentate line, and are covered by columnar epithelium. The overlying tissue is viscerally innervated, and therefore is not sensitive to touch, pain, or temperature. Internal hemorrhoids are further divided into categories based on appearance and degree of prolapse (Table 29.2). Grade 1 internal hemorrhoids contain anal cushions that bleed but do not prolapse. Grade 2 internal hemorrhoids are those that prolapse past the dentate line and can be seen at the anal verge during straining, but reduce spontaneously. Grade 3 internal hemorrhoids protrude beyond the anal verge and require manual reduction. Grade 4 internal hemorrhoids lie permanently outside the anal verge and are irreducible.

Table 29.2 Classification and management of internal hemorrhoids

Grading	Findings	Treatments
Grade 1	Anal cushions bulge into lumen of anal canal with painless bleeding	Dietary and lifestyle modification, medical treatment, RBL
Grade 2	Cushions protrude past dentate line during straining, but can reduce spontaneously	Dietary and lifestyle modification, medical treatment, RBL, sclerotherapy, IRC
Grade 3	Cushions protrude beyond anal verge spontaneously or with straining, and require manual reduction	Dietary and lifestyle modification, RBL, sclerotherapy, IRC, PPH, hemorrhoidectomy
Grade 4	Cushions are permanently prolapsed and irreducible	Dietary and lifestyle modification, PPH, hemorrhoidectomy

RBL rubber band ligation, *IRC* infrared coagulation, *PPH* procedure for prolapse and hemorrhoids

External hemorrhoids are located distal to the dentate line, and are covered by modified squamous epithelium. They are somatically innervated and are sensitive to touch, pain, stretch, and temperature. Mixed hemorrhoids consist of both internal and external hemorrhoids [32].

Diagnosis and Examination

Bright red, painless rectal bleeding occurring at the end of defecation is the classic symptom of internal hemorrhoids. Bleeding can also be occult, which may result in guaiac-positive stools or anemia. Other causes of anemia must be ruled out prior to attributing it to hemorrhoids, especially in the elderly population. The prolapsing columnar epithelial tissue of internal hemorrhoids can lead to mucous deposition on the perianal skin, which can cause itching and irritation [30]. In addition, the prolapsed cushions can prevent a tight seal of the anal verge, causing fecal seepage. This is particularly troublesome in the elderly population, in whom decreased sphincter tone often causes concomitant fecal incontinence [33]. Internal hemorrhoids rarely cause pain, unless they become incarcerated or strangulated. Symptoms from external hemorrhoids usually stem from acute thrombosis. Thrombosed external hemorrhoids are characterized by severe pain; bleeding may also occur due to pressure necrosis. External skin tags at the anal verge may be the end result of thrombosed external hemorrhoids.

The definitive diagnosis of hemorrhoids relies on a precise history and careful physical examination. Rectal prolapse, anorectal cancer, anal fissure, and cryptoglandular disease are in the differential diagnosis of hemorrhoids [10]. History should include characterization of pain, bleeding, protrusion, and bowel patterns, along with assessment of preexisting bleeding disorders or liver disease with portal hypertension. The perianal area should be inspected for skin tags, external hemorrhoids, protrusion of rectal tissue (both at rest and with Valsalva), perianal dermatitis, anal fistula, and anal fissure. Digital examination should be performed to rule out low-lying anorectal neoplasms and to assess sphincter tone. Anoscopy is often used to assess the extent of disease, including hemorrhoid size, location, and presence of bleeding. At a minimum, patients with bright red rectal bleeding should be evaluated with both anoscopy and flexible sigmoidoscopy. In the elderly population, full colonoscopy is indicated due to the significant risk for colonic neoplasia. Colonoscopy should also be performed in patients with unusual symptoms and in those with a strong family history of colorectal cancer [10].

Treatment

Treatment of symptomatic hemorrhoids ranges from dietary and lifestyle modification to hemorrhoidectomy, depending on the severity of the symptoms. In general, grade 1 and 2 hemorrhoids can be treated with nonoperative management, while grade 3 and 4 hemorrhoids often require operative intervention (Table 29.2).

Nonoperative Treatment

The goal of dietary and lifestyle modification is to minimize straining during defecation. Increasing intake of fiber, fluid, and adding psyllium may resolve symptoms [32]. Lifestyle modification can be used for treatment and also as a preventative measure. Patients are advised to exercise regularly, improve anal hygiene, avoid straining and reading on the toilet, and reduce consumption of fat [30].

Oral flavonoids are used for the treatment of hemorrhoids, particularly in Europe and Asia. These compounds appear to work by increasing vascular tone, reducing venous capacity, decreasing capillary permeability, and facilitating lymphatic drainage [34]. Oral calcium dobesilate is also used to treat the acute symptoms of hemorrhoids. The beneficial effects relate to its ability to decrease capillary permeability, inhibit platelet aggregation, and improve blood viscosity; therefore reducing tissue edema [35]. Topical medications lack the rigorous levels of evidence to support their efficacy.

Minor Office Procedures

Rubber Band Ligation

The goals of nonsurgical hemorrhoid treatments are to decrease hemorrhoid vascularity, reduce redundant tissue, and promote hemorrhoid fixation to the rectal wall. Rubber band ligation (RBL) is a quick and effective means of treating grade 1 and 2 and selected cases of grade 3 hemorrhoids [36, 37]. RBL causes ischemic necrosis of the banded mucosa, which in turn induces an inflammatory reaction, which fixes the tissues to the underlying anal sphincter [30]. This technique has been widely used for the outpatient treatment of hemorrhoids. Short-term success rate of RBL ranges from 80 to 89 %; however, recurrence rate can be as high as 68 % within 4–5 years follow-up [38]. The complication rate is low, ranging from <1 to 3 %. Minor complications include pain, bleeding, vasovagal symptoms, band slippage, mucosal ulceration, and priapism. Bat et al. studied 512 patients who underwent hemorrhoid banding. Major complications occurred in 2.5 % of patients [39]. These included massive hemorrhage, severe pain, urinary retention, and perianal sepsis [30, 39, 40]. Even though pelvic sepsis is rare, it requires immediate medical attention. The classic triad of symptoms that indicates perianal infection is fever, worsening pain, and urinary dysfunction. RBL is not recommended in immunocompromised patients due to risk of necrotizing infection [32, 41].

Sclerotherapy

Sclerotherapy is another office procedure that works best for first and second-degree hemorrhoids. It involves injection of chemical agents into hemorrhoids, creating fibrosis, scarring, shrinkage, and fixation. Sclerotherapy can be used for patients on anticoagulation. It is not recommended for patients with anorectal infection or with prolapsed thrombosed hemorrhoids [27].

Infrared Coagulation, Bipolar Diathermy, Direct-Current Electrotherapy

The infrared coagulator causes inflammation, scarring, and fixation of hemorrhoidal tissue using infrared radiation. It has been reported to cause less pain than RBL. It is useful in treating small bleeding hemorrhoids (grade 1 or 2), but is not effective in larger, bulkier hemorrhoids that require tissue destruction. Complications are infrequent and maximal discomfort usually occurs during the procedure [27].

Bipolar diathermy devices generate heat to coagulate tissue. Success rates for grade 1–3 hemorrhoids have been reported to be in the range of 88–100 %. Complications include pain, bleeding, fissure, and sphincter spasm [38]. Jutabha et al. showed that bipolar coagulation required more treatment sessions and had more failures than rubber band ligation [42].

Direct-current electrotherapy causes tissue destruction by producing sodium hydroxide at the negative electrode of the device. This technique is not widely used due to lengthy treatment time required and poor control of higher-degree hemorrhoids [38].

Operative Treatment

Only 5–10 % of patients require surgical hemorrhoidectomy. Surgical options for the treatment of hemorrhoids are typically reserved for grade 3 hemorrhoids unresponsive to other less invasive approaches, grade 4 hemorrhoids, large external hemorrhoids, mixed hemorrhoids, and concomitant anorectal pathology [32].

Hemorrhoidectomy

Excisional hemorrhoidectomy is highly effective with low recurrence rates. The operation can be performed using scissors, diathermy, or vascular-sealing device such as Ligasure or Harmonic scalpel. The aim of surgical hemorrhoidectomy is to restore the anal canal to normal or near normal function and anatomic status. The Milligan-Morgan (open) and Ferguson (closed) hemorrhoidectomy techniques are commonly used worldwide [43]. The major drawbacks of hemorrhoidectomy are significant postoperative pain and prolonged recovery period. Other postoperative complications include acute urinary retention (2–36 %), bleeding (0.03–6 %), bacteremia and septic complications (0.5–5.5 %), anal stenosis (0–6 %), and fecal incontinence (2–12 %) [30]. A majority of the randomized prospective studies comparing open versus closed hemorrhoidectomy did not show any significant difference in pain, analgesic use, hospital stay, and complications [38].

Stapled Hemorrhoidectomy

To minimize postoperative pain, Longo proposed stapled hemorrhoidopexy, also known as procedure for prolapse and hemorrhoids (PPH), to treat hemorrhoids [44]. This technique involves the use of a circular stapling device to perform a circumferential resection of distal rectal mucosa. A systemic review by Chen et al. comparing PPH to conventional hemorrhoidectomy showed that PPH had shorter operation time, less postoperative pain, less postoperative urinary retention, and a quicker return to normal activity. However, serious complications have been reported, including rectal perforation, pelvic sepsis, rectovaginal fistula, intraabdominal bleeding, and Fournier's gangrene [45]. Further, PPH does not address external hemorrhoids or skin tags.

Special Cases

Thrombosed External Hemorrhoids

Thrombosed external hemorrhoids typically present as an abrupt onset of a painful perianal mass. Pain peaks between 48 and 72 h and subsides after the fourth day as the thrombus shrinks and dissolves within the next few weeks. Since the disease is self-limited, therapy is guided by the severity and duration of symptoms. Excision is recommended if the patient presents early in the disease course with intense pain. Otherwise, treatment is nonoperative, and includes sitz baths, stool softeners, non-constipating analgesics, and proper anal hygiene [32].

Strangulated Hemorrhoids

A hemorrhoidal crisis occurs when prolapsed grade 3 or 4 hemorrhoids become strangulated. Urgent excisional hemorrhoidectomy is required. The open technique should be performed in cases where necrotic tissues are present. Another method of treatment is reduction after perianal block, with deferred, less invasive therapy.

Anorectal Abscess and Fistula-in-Ano

Anorectal abscess and anal fistula are different stages of the same disease process. Abscess is the acute manifestation, while fistula represents the chronic condition. The majority of anorectal abscesses are due to cryptoglandular infection. Other causes include Crohn's disease, tuberculosis, actinomycosis, malignancy, trauma, and radiation. The disease is most common between the ages of 20–60, with a 2:1 male to female ratio [46].

Anatomy and Classification of Anorectal Abscess

Anorectal abscesses are classified based on their location: perianal, ischioanal, intersphincteric, and supralevator (Fig. 29.2) [47]. The anal glands are concentrated in the posterior anal canal and empty into crypts located at the level of the dentate line. When these become obstructed, infection and abscess develop. Perianal abscesses located close to the anal verge are most common. Supralevator abscesses are least common and most difficult to identify. Infection can also spread circumferentially through the intersphincteric, ischiorectal, or ischioanal spaces, resulting in a horseshoe abscess.

Diagnosis

The classic symptoms of an anorectal abscess are pain, swelling, and fever. Physical exam reveals a tender, erythematous, fluctuant mass at the anal verge (Fig. 29.3). Intersphincteric abscesses can present as severe rectal pain and urinary symptoms, without any external findings. Supralevator abscesses often present with less dramatic cutaneous findings. Placing the patient under anesthesia for a thorough examination is advisable in these latter two scenarios. Endorectal ultrasound and MRI can also be used to locate hidden abscesses.

Treatment

Abscesses in the perineum share the same treatment principle as abscesses in other parts of the body; that is, they must be adequately drained. Many perianal and ischiorectal abscesses can be drained under local anesthesia in the outpatient setting. An elliptical or cruciate incision, excising the skin edges, is recommended to allow for free drainage. Packing is avoided as it impedes the drainage of pus and causes more pain for the patient [46]. Suspicion of an intersphincteric abscess should be high for patients presenting with pain out of proportion to the physical findings. When the diagnosis is confirmed by physical examination, the treatment consists of dividing the fibers of the internal sphincter along the length of the abscess cavity. When a supralevator abscess is found, it is important to determine its origin, as this will dictate drainage technique [48]. Adequate drainage of a horseshoe abscess requires a posterior midline incision between the coccyx and anus, separating the superficial

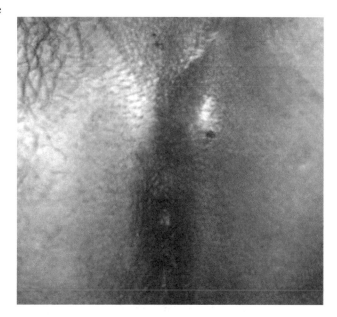

Fig. 29.3 Acute anorectal abscess

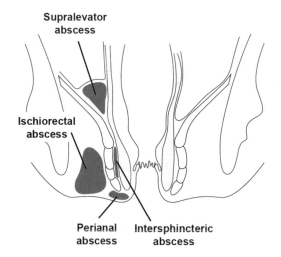

Fig. 29.2 Classification of anorectal abscesses

external sphincter muscle, to drain the deep postanal space, as well as counter-incisions over each ischioanal fossa to drain the anterior extensions of the abscess.

Abscesses resolve after drainage alone in the majority of the patients. The use of adjunctive antibiotics may be indicated in patients who have rheumatic or acquired valvular heart disease, immunosuppression, extensive cellulitis, diabetes, or prosthetic devices [46]. Recurrence of disease may occur due to missed infection in adjacent spaces, incomplete drainage, and undiagnosed fistula.

Postoperative care includes sitz baths, stool softeners, and analgesics. Follow-up examination is required to ensure complete healing.

Fistula-in-Ano

A fistula-in-ano is an abnormal cavity communicating with the rectum or anal canal. Anal fistula occurs after 34–66 % of all anorectal abscesses [49]. Drainage for more than 2–3 months after abscess drainage should raise suspicion of an anal fistula.

Classification

Fistulae are classified based on their relation to the sphincter complex. Parks and Thomson provided a classification system of anorectal fistulae that is widely used today. Parks divided anal fistulae into the following: intersphincteric, transsphincteric, suprasphincteric, and extrasphincteric [50]. Approximately 45 % of fistulae are intersphincteric, 30 % transsphincteric, 20 % suprasphincteric, and 5 % extrasphincteric [47]. An intersphincteric fistula results from a perianal abscess that has tracked within the intersphincteric plane. Ischioanal abscesses that tract through both the internal and external sphincters result in transsphincteric fistulae. Suprasphincteric fistulae occur after supralevator abscesses. The tract originates at the dentate line, extends above the puborectalis, then curves downward lateral to the external sphincter to the perianal skin. Extrasphincteric fistulae transverse through the levator ani and ischioanal fossa to reach the perianal skin [47]. They result from trauma, Crohn's disease, and carcinoma.

Diagnosis

Fistula-in-ano typically presents as cyclical pain, swelling, and purulent drainage. A thorough history often reveals a prior anal abscess that was drained either surgically or spontaneously. On examination, the external opening may be seen as an elevation of granulation tissue with purulent dis-

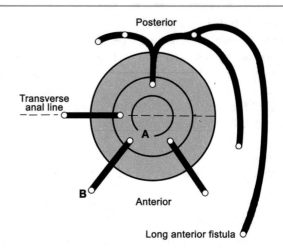

Fig. 29.4 Goodsall's rule

charge on compression. The further away the external opening is from the anal verge, the higher the likelihood of a complicated tract. The fistula tract can be palpated as a cord-like structure connecting the external opening and the anal canal. In most cases, the internal opening may not be apparent. Goodsall's rule states that posteriorly located external openings curve to enter the anorectum in the posterior midline, while anteriorly located external openings tract radially to the nearest crypt (Fig. 29.4) [48].

Treatment

The main objective of fistula surgery is to eliminate the fistula while preserving anal sphincter function. Spontaneous healing of fistula-in-ano is rare, so the presence of a symptomatic anal fistula is an indication for surgery. Anoscopy and proctoscopy will help locate the internal opening and exclude underlying pathology, such as neoplasia.

Colonoscopy is indicated in patients with symptoms of inflammatory bowel disease, and in patients with multiple or recurrent fistulae. Anal manometry may be useful in planning the operative approach, especially in the elderly, in whom incontinence is more prevalent. Endoanal ultrasound and MRI are useful tools for the preoperative evaluation of complicated or recurrent fistulae.

Traditionally, intersphincteric and low-lying transsphincteric fistulae are treated with simple fistulotomy, which involves laying open the fistula tract in its entirety [49]. Sphincter-sparing procedures are often employed for anterior fistulae, especially in women, and for fistulae that traverse longer distances of the anal sphincter, such as high transsphincteric and suprasphincteric fistulae. They should also be considered in the elderly, in whom division of any portion of the sphincter mechanism may result in worsened incontinence. Correcting their underlying etiology treats extrasphincteric fistulae.

Operative Techniques

The use of synthetic biological "fillers" is an attractive, non-cutting option. However, despite promising early results, repeated studies evaluating a variety of fibrin-based glues and bioprosthetic plugs demonstrated low success rates of only 14–40 % [49] and 30–50 % [46, 49], respectively. For patients with complex fistulae, the endorectal advancement flap is a useful technique for eliminating the fistula while preserving fecal continence. This procedure involves elevating a flap of mucosa, submucosa, and some internal sphincter muscle, to cover the internal fistula opening [49]. A meta-analysis of 35 studies by Soltani and Kaiser showed a healing rate of >80 % for fistulas of cryptoglandular origin, and an incontinence rate of 13 % [51]. Endorectal advancement flaps are relatively contraindicated in patients with anal stenosis, active proctitis, and Crohn's disease due to high complication and failure rates. The most recently developed surgical treatment for anal fistulae is the ligation of the internal fistula tract (LIFT) procedure, originally described by Rojanasakul et al. [52]. In this technique, all infected cryptoglandular tissue in the intersphincteric plane is removed and the internal fistula opening is sutured closed. A recent retrospective study reported a healing rate of 62 % at 12 months with no reports of incontinence [53]. Staging repairs of complex fistulae by employing setons, loops of nonabsorbable suture material which promote drainage and fibrosis, for 6–8 weeks prior to definitive repair results in higher rates of success [54].

Postoperative Care

After fistula repair, patients are placed on bulking agents and non-codeine analgesics. Frequent sitz baths aid with perianal hygiene. Regular evaluations are recommended to ensure adequate wound healing. For patients' status post fistula plug placement, rigorous activity should be avoided to minimize the risk of plug dislodgement.

Anal Fissure

Etiology and Pathophysiology

Anal fissure is a longitudinal tear in the anoderm distal to the dentate line. It can be classified as acute or chronic. The majority of acute fissures heal spontaneously or with conservative management within 4–6 weeks. If symptoms persist beyond 6 weeks and secondary changes develop, the condition is considered chronic. Features of chronic anal fissure include indurated edges, hypertrophied anal papilla, distal sentinel pile, and exposed transverse internal sphincter fibers at the fissure base (Fig. 29.5) [55]. About 74 % of anal

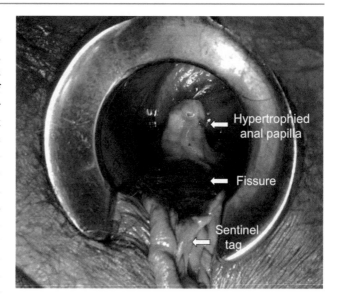

Fig. 29.5 Chronic anal fissure

fissures are found in the posterior midline and 16 % in the anterior midline [56]. Fissures located off midline or synchronous fissures should raise suspicion for disease processes such as Crohn's disease, HIV, syphilis, herpes, tuberculosis, or anal cancer [55].

The exact etiology of anal fissure remains unknown. The initiating factor is thought to be trauma from the passage of a hard and painful bowel movement; however, some patients do not report constipation or may even have watery diarrhea [57]. Studies from the 1970s and 1980s suggested internal sphincter hypertonia as the cause. By performing postmortem angiography of the inferior rectal artery, Klosterhalfen et al. demonstrated that the posterior commissure of the anal canal is poorly perfused compared to the other portion of the anal canal in 85 % of the cases [58]. This finding implicated the role of ischemia in the pathogenesis of anal fissure. Using Doppler laser flowmetry, Schouten et al. showed higher mean maximum anal resting pressure and lower anodermal blood flow at the fissure site compared to the posterior commissure of the controls [59]. These authors were able to demonstrate that internal sphincterotomy decreases internal sphincter pressures and improves anodermal blood flow at the posterior midline.

Epidemiology

Anal fissure is one of the most common anorectal problems. It can occur at any age, but is most common in younger and middle-aged adults. Both genders are affected equally. Anterior fissures are more common in women than in men [56, 60].

Diagnosis

The hallmark symptom of anal fissure is anal pain during and after defecation. Rectal bleeding is common. Blood is bright red in appearance and usually scant in amount. Patients describe fissure pain as sharp and cutting, with discomfort lasting from a few minutes to several hours. A detailed history may reveal constipation, dysuria, and sometimes dyspareunia as accompanying symptoms. Usually, the diagnosis can be made by careful inspection after gentle separation of the buttocks. Further evaluation with digital and endoscopic examination is not necessary and should be avoided, as it is associated severe pain. Nonhealing fissures should be biopsied. The differential diagnosis of anal fissure includes anorectal abscess in particular intersphincteric abscess, anal fistula, pruritus ani, Crohn's disease, sexually transmitted disease, tuberculosis, leukemia, and anal cancer [27].

Treatment

Conservative Management

Initial therapy for acute anal fissure is with conservative measures, including warm sitz baths, increased fluid intake, and fiber supplementation. Warm baths help relieve sphincter spasm via a somatoanal reflex that results in relaxation of the internal anal sphincter. Bulk-forming foods may be helpful as large bulky stool may result in physiologic dilatation of the sphincter mechanism [55].

Medical Management

The aim of medical therapy for nonhealing fissures is to reduce sphincter tone without permanent sphincter injury. The conventional pharmacologic therapy involves the use of topical muscle relaxants, including nitrates, glyceryl trinitrate (GTN), calcium channel blockers, and botulinum toxin. Cholinergic agonists, muscarinic agonists, and adrenergic antagonists have been used to a lesser degree.

In a Cochrane Review of 75 randomized controlled trials of nonsurgical therapies, GTN was found to be better than placebo in healing anal fissures; however, late recurrence rate was about 50 %. Topical calcium channel blockers were equally effective with fewer side effects [61]. The major drawback of GTN is the side effect of headache, which has been reported at a rate of 29–72 % [62, 63].

Botulinum toxin, produced by the bacterium *Clostridium botulinum*, binds to the presynaptic nerve terminal and prevents the release of acetylcholine, resulting in relaxation of both internal and external anal sphincters [55]. In a double-blinded study of botulinum toxin versus placebo in the treatment of chronic anal fissure, botulinum toxin injection led to higher healing rates at 2-month follow-up [64]. A meta-analysis of 180 patients comparing botulinum toxin injection

with GTN showed that both methods shared equal healing rates; however, GTN had higher side effects [65]. The main complaint of botulinum toxin is mild incontinence with flatus and stool lasting up to 3 weeks. When compared to lateral internal sphincterotomy, botulinum toxin injection has lower healing rates and higher recurrence, but a lower chance of long-term incontinence [66].

Operative Treatment

Surgical intervention is indicated in nonhealing fissures after failure of medical treatment. The primary goal of surgical treatment for chronic anal fissure is to decrease the maximum resting anal pressures. The primary operative techniques used to treat chronic anal fissure are lateral internal sphincterotomy and advancement flap anoplasty.

Lateral internal sphincterotomy was first described by Eisenhammer in 1951 for the management of anal fissure [67]. This technique involves a radial incision through the distal internal sphincter muscle, classically the same length as the fissure itself. A lateral incision avoids the keyhole deformity often seen after posterior internal sphincterotomy.

Complications after lateral internal sphincterotomy include hematoma, wound infection, perianal abscess, anal fistula, prolapsed hemorrhoids, and incontinence. Recurrence rates range from 0 to 3.3 % [68]. Sphincterotomy should generally be avoided in individuals with inflammatory bowel disease, anterior fissures, in women with obstetric injuries, and in the elderly, as these patients are at high risk for incontinence. Anorectal manometry and endoanal ultrasound may be beneficial in planning the surgical approach.

Advancement flap anoplasty is used to treat low-pressure fissures. This procedure involves using a subcutaneous flap to cover the fissure site [69]. More recent studies showed healing rates up to 98 % for the treatment of chronic anal fissure [55, 70].

Sexually Transmitted Diseases

Persons aged 50 or older account for approximately 15 % of new HIV/AIDS diagnoses and 24 % of persons living with HIV/AIDS [71]. A recent study out of the UK revealed that in the past 10 years, many common sexually transmitted infections have more than doubled in 50- to 90-year-olds [72]. Postmenopausal physiologic changes, such as thinning of the vaginal mucosa and decreased lubrication, may lead to minor genital injuries and microabrasions that facilitate the entry of pathogens in older women [73]. Jena et al. showed that men who use erectile dysfunction drugs have higher rates of sexually transmitted diseases (STD), particularly HIV infection [74]. The increasing availability of these medications may be contributing to the rising rate of STD among seniors. STD has a wide range of clinical presentations, including involvement of the anorectal region. Although infection of the anal canal and perianal skin often results from anal receptive intercourse, contiguous spread from the infected genital region can also occur.

Epidemiology

Among the most common STDs in the USA, human papillomavirus (HPV) accounts for the majority of new cases, followed by chlamydia, trichomoniasis, gonorrhea, herpes simplex virus type 2 (HSV-2), syphilis, HIV, and hepatitis B [75].

Diagnosis

A detailed history, including a sexual history, is important for successful treatment. Patients may present with proctitis or perianal ulceration. Perianal ulceration can be seen in syphilis, HSV, HIV, chancroid, and granuloma inguinale. Proctitis is associated with anal pain and discharge, and is often caused by *Neisseria gonorrhoeae*, *Chlamydia trachomatis*, *Treponema pallidum*, and herpes virus [76].

A thorough physical examination along with diagnostic tools such as anoscopy, proctoscopy, serologic tests, biopsy, and culture will aid in narrowing down the correct diagnosis. Patients should be advised that partners must also be examined.

Etiology and Management

Bacterial Pathogens

Neisseria Gonorrhea

Gonorrhea is caused by *Neisseria gonorrhoeae,* a gram-negative diplococcus. The organism can cause urogenital, anorectal, conjunctival, and pharyngeal infections. It is the second most commonly reported notifiable disease in the USA [77]. Gonococcal proctitis occurs as a result of anal receptive intercourse with a partner inflicted with urethral gonorrhea. Patients often report mucopurulent discharge, tenesmus, pruritus, and anal pain. Systemic spread may cause unilateral migratory suppurative arthritis, perihepatitis, pericarditis, endocarditis, and meningitis [78]. On anoscopic examination, the mucosa of the anal canal and lower rectum is reddened and friable. Gentle pressure on the anal crypts will produce purulent discharge. Diagnosis is confirmed by Gram's stain of the discharge or culture on Thayer-Martin or Stuart's media [79]. Rectal gonorrhea is more resistant to treatment than at other sites due to the presence of antibiotic-activating enzymes in the rectal flora. The current treatment consists of a single dose of ceftriaxone 250 mg IM.

Given the frequency of co-infection with *Chlamydia trachomatis*, empiric treatment with doxycycline, 100 mg orally twice a day for 7 days is also recommended.

Chlamydia Trachomatis

Chlamydial species are obligate intracellular parasites that cause a similar clinical presentation as *N. gonorrhoeae*. There are 15 immunotypes. Serotypes D through K are responsible for most cases of proctitis. Serotypes L1, L2, and L3 cause lymphogranuloma venereum (LGV), a more severe disease form [76, 80]. Chlamydia is the most commonly reported notifiable disease in the USA [77]. Anorectal chlamydial infection is transmitted through anoreceptive intercourse. Symptoms include rectal pain, bleeding, mucus discharge, and diarrhea. Inguinal lymph nodes may be enlarged and matted. Proctoscopy reveals friable, erythematous, and edematous mucosa. Diagnosis is made via tissue culture of biopsies from the anal lesions. Chlamydia proctitis can be treated with doxycycline 100 mg twice a day for 7 days, or erythromycin 500 mg four times a day for 1–2 weeks. LGV proctitis is treated with a 3-week course of doxycycline. Empiric treatment of gonorrhea is recommended due to high rates of co-infection [76].

Syphilis

The causative organism of syphilis is the spirochete *Treponema pallidum*. The disease is spread by anal receptive intercourse and oral–anal contact. Primary anal syphilis appears within 2–10 weeks of infection with lymphadenopathy, proctitis, and chancre at the anal verge. Over time, the chancre becomes ulcerated and causes significant pain. Anal ulcers may be multiple, irregular, and eccentrically located. Untreated syphilis will progress to a secondary stage, which appears about 2–3 months after initial infection. Symptoms of secondary syphilis include a maculopapular rash over the trunk and extremities, lymphadenopathy, and condyloma lata in the perianal region. Approximately one third of untreated patients will have spontaneous cure, one third will remain latent, and one third will progress to tertiary syphilis [10]. Tertiary syphilis manifests with neurologic, cardiovascular, renal, hepatic, and ocular symptoms. Diagnosis can be made by dark field microscopic examination of scrapings from the chancre or biopsy specimens from the anal ulcer. Treponemal and non-treponemal serologic tests are used to evaluate for prior infection and to follow response to treatment, respectively [27]. Treatment of primary or secondary syphilis consists of a single intramuscular injection of 2.4 million U of benzathine penicillin. Penicillin-allergic patients are treated with doxycycline 100 mg twice a day for 14 days. Tertiary syphilis is treated with 2.4 million U of benzathine penicillin given IM weekly over 3 consecutive weeks. Penicillin-allergic patients are given doxycycline for 28 days [76]. Follow-up serology should be used to monitor patients after treatment [27].

Viral Pathogens

Herpes Simplex Virus

Herpes simplex virus is a DNA virus that belongs to the *Herpesviridae* family. Its transmission is through mucosal surfaces or breaks in the skin. The majority of anogenital infection is due to HSV-2, acquired through anorectal intercourse [79]. Infection is life-long and shedding can occur at any time. Further, is not isolated to symptomatic outbreaks. Primary infection is characterized by fever, malaise, and lymphadenopathy. Subsequent infections manifest with local symptoms, including anal pain, pruritus, tenesmus, rectal discharge. Perianal lesions range from small vesicles to large ruptured vesicles that ulcerate and eventually coalesce into an aphthous ulcer. Herpetic proctitis is usually limited to the distal 10 cm of the rectum [76]. Anoscopy reveals friable mucosa, diffuse ulcerations, vesicles, and pustules. Cultures from ulcer scrapings, rectal swabs, or biopsies confirm the diagnosis. Tzank prep can reveal multinucleated giant cells, but it is less sensitive than viral culture. There is no cure for herpetic infections; therefore, treatment is directed towards symptom relief. Acute anorectal symptoms are managed with analgesics, sitz baths, and stool softeners as needed. Herpes proctitis responds to acyclovir 400 mg, given orally 5 times a day for 10 days [76, 81]. Other treatment options include famciclovir, valacyclovir, and foscarnet [82, 83]. If left untreated, herpetic proctitis is self-limited and usually resolves within 3 weeks.

Human Immunodeficiency Virus

The colon, rectum, and anus are the most common sites requiring surgery in HIV patients [84]. A major concern in treating common anorectal disorders, such as anal fissures, symptomatic hemorrhoids, and perianal abscesses in HIV patients is poor wound healing [85]. Management principles include utilizing conservative measures whenever possible, avoidance of large wounds, and more liberal use of antibiotics in this patient population.

Anal ulcers occur in HIV patients and must be distinguished from idiopathic anal fissure. HIV-related ulcers are typically deeper, wider, and more proximal. They may occur anywhere within the anal canal, are sometimes multiple, and are often associated with anal hypotonia. Biopsies should be obtained to rule out other pathologies. Surgical debridement and intralesional steroid injection can be performed [79].

Human Papillomavirus

HPV is the most prevalent STD in the USA. Besides having a strong association with cervical cancer, there is a growing body of evidence linking HPV with anogenital cancers. Over 100 different HPV genotypes have been characterized and about 40 of them can infect the anogenital tract [86, 87]. HPV genotypes 6, 11, 42, 43, and 44 are associated with anogenital condylomata and low-grade dysplasia, whereas

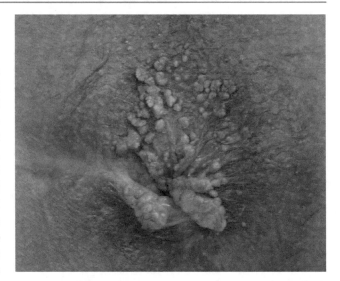

Fig. 29.6 Anal condyloma

HPV-16, 18, 31, 35, 58 are linked with high-grade dysplasia and carcinoma [76]. The virus is acquired through sexual intercourse with an infected partner. The majority of HPV infections are asymptomatic and 90 % regress within 2 years [88]. Anogenital warts or condyloma acuminata are the most common clinical manifestation of HPV. These lesions are located in the perianal region, the anal canal, and the urogenital area. Patients often complain of pruritis, pain, bleeding, and malodorous discharge.

Diagnosis can be made by gross appearance alone. Upon inspection, fleshy cauliflower-like masses are seen surrounding the anal verge (Fig. 29.6). Anoscopy is required for the detection of intraanal lesions. The differential diagnosis includes skin tags, condyloma lata, molluscum contagiosum, and carcinoma.

The goals of treatment are the removal of gross disease and the amelioration of symptoms. Treatment does not eradicate the underlying HPV infection. Current therapy includes topical application of caustic agents and physical ablation. Topical agents such as podophyllin, bichloroacetic acid (BCA), trichloroacetic acid (TCA), 5-fluorouracil (5-FU), and imiquimod are useful for mild to moderate disease. Ablative therapies including cryotherapy, surgical excision, electrocautery, and laser treatment have the highest success and lowest recurrence rates [89]. These are used to treat moderate to severe disease and recurrences. BCA, TCA, and all of the ablative methods can be used inside the anal canal.

Conclusions

Benign anorectal disorders are common in the geriatric population. Treatment in this patient group is unique due to higher rates of fecal incontinence and soilage. Neoplastic conditions must always be ruled out. Finally, sexually transmitted diseases are on the rise in older Americans and therefore, care providers must maintain a high index of suspicion for these conditions.

Key Points

- Patients at high risk for fecal incontinence should be evaluated with anorectal manometry prior to offering surgery.
- At a minimum, anoscopy and flexible sigmoidoscopy should be performed for bright red rectal bleeding. Full colonoscopy is recommended for geriatric patients.
- Pruritis ani is typically idiopathic. Once specific causes are ruled out treatment is aimed at eliminating irritants and reestablishing clean, dry, and intact perianal skin.
- Initial efforts in treating anal fissures should concentrate on conservative measures such as sitz baths, fiber supplementation, and increased fluid intake.
- Obliteration of the internal opening is key to the successful resolution of an anal fistula.
- Sphincter-sparing methods should be the first line of treatment for fistula-in-ano patients with fecal incontinence.
- Anorectal abscesses are treated with drainage with adjuvant antibiotic therapy reserved for immunocompromised patients or patients with indwelling hardware.
- For herpes simplex virus and human papillomavirus, infectivity is not isolated to symptomatic outbreaks.

References

1. Siddiqi S, Vijay V, Ward M, Mahendran R, Warren S. Pruritus ani. Ann R Coll Surg Engl. 2008;90(6):457–63.
2. Markell KW, Billingham RP. Pruritus ani: etiology and management. Surg Clin North Am. 2010;90(1):125–35.
3. Lonsdale-Eccles A, Carmichael AJ. Treatment of pruritus associated with systemic disorders in the elderly: a review of the role of new therapies. Drugs Aging. 2003;20(3):197–208.
4. Potts RO, Buras Jr EM, Chrisman Jr DA. Changes with age in the moisture content of human skin. J Invest Dermatol. 1984;82(1):97–100.
5. Weismann K, Sand Petersen C, Roder B. Pruritus ani caused by beta-haemolytic streptococci. Acta Derm Venereol. 1996;76(5):415.
6. Kahlke V, Jongen J, Peleikis HG, Herbst RA. Perianal streptococcal dermatitis in adults: its association with pruritic anorectal diseases is mainly caused by group B streptococci. Colorectal Dis. 2013;15(5):602–7.
7. Paradisi M, Cianchini G, Angelo C, Conti G, Puddu P. Perianal streptococcal dermatitis: two familial cases. Cutis. 1994; 54(5):341–2.
8. Sheth S, Schechtman AD. Itchy perianal erythema. J Fam Pract. 2007;56(12):1025–7.
9. Baral J. *Pruritus ani* and *Staphylococcus aureus*. J Am Acad Dermatol. 1983;9(6):962.
10. Gordon PH, Nivatvongs S. Principles and practice of surgery of colon, rectum, and anus. 3rd ed. New York: Informa Healthcare; 2006.
11. Bowyer A, McColl I. Erythrasma and pruritus ani. Acta Derm Venereol. 1971;51(6):444–7.
12. Smith LE, Henrichs D, McCullah RD. Prospective studies on the etiology and treatment of pruritus ani. Dis Colon Rectum. 1982;25(4):358–63.
13. Bowyer A, McColl I. A study of 200 patients with pruritus ani. Proc R Soc Med. 1970;63(Suppl):96–8.
14. Laube S, Farrell AM. Bacterial skin infections in the elderly: diagnosis and treatment. Drugs Aging. 2002;19(5):331–42.
15. Dodi G, Pirone E, Bettin A, Veller C, Infantino A, Pianon P, et al. The mycotic flora in proctological patients with and without pruritus ani. Br J Surg. 1985;72(12):967–9.
16. Lochridge Jr E. Pruritus ani--perianal psoriasis. South Med J. 1969;62(4):450–2.
17. Bruynzeel DP. Dermatological causes of pruritus ani. BMJ. 1992;305(6859):955.
18. Hanno R, Murphy P. Pruritus ani. Classification and management. Dermatol Clin. 1987;5(4):811–6.
19. Virgili A, Lauriola MM, Mantovani L, Corazza M. Vulvar lichen sclerosus: 11 women treated with tacrolimus 0.1% ointment. Acta Derm Venereol. 2007;87(1):69–72.
20. Saunders NA, Haefner HK. Vulvar lichen sclerosus in the elderly: pathophysiology and treatment update. Drugs Aging. 2009;26(10):803–12.
21. Oskay T, Sezer HK, Genc C, Kutluay L. Pimecrolimus 1% cream in the treatment of vulvar lichen sclerosus in postmenopausal women. Int J Dermatol. 2007;46(5):527–32.
22. Jorizzo JL. The itchy patient. A practical approach. Prim Care. 1983;10(3):339–53.
23. Caplan RM. The irritant role of feces in the genesis of perianal itch. Gastroenterology. 1966;50(1):19–23.
24. Nix D, Haugen V. Prevention and management of incontinence-associated dermatitis. Drugs Aging. 2010;27(6):491–6.
25. Murie JA, Sim AJ, Mackenzie I. The importance of pain, pruritus and soiling as symptoms of haemorrhoids and their response to haemorrhoidectomy or rubber band ligation. Br J Surg. 1981;68(4):247–9.
26. Lysy J, Sistiery-Ittah M, Israelit Y, Shmueli A, Strauss-Liviatan N, Mindrul V, et al. Topical capsaicin--a novel and effective treatment for idiopathic intractable pruritus ani: a randomised, placebo controlled, crossover study. Gut. 2003;52(9):1323–6.
27. Wolff BG, American Society of Colon and Rectal Surgeons. The ASCRS textbook of colon and rectal surgery. New York: Springer; 2007. p. xxiv, 810.
28. Thomson WH. The nature of haemorrhoids. Br J Surg. 1975;62(7):542–52.
29. Loder PB, Kamm MA, Nicholls RJ, Phillips RK. Haemorrhoids: pathology, pathophysiology and aetiology. Br J Surg. 1994;81(7):946–54.
30. Lohsiriwat V. Hemorrhoids: from basic pathophysiology to clinical management. World J Gastroenterol. 2012;18(17):2009–17.
31. Johanson JF, Sonnenberg A. The prevalence of hemorrhoids and chronic constipation. An epidemiologic study. Gastroenterology. 1990;98(2):380–6.
32. American Gastroenterological Association medical position statement. Diagnosis and treatment of hemorrhoids. Gastroenterology. 2004;126(5):1461–2.
33. Muller-Lissner S. General geriatrics and gastroenterology: constipation and faecal incontinence. Best Pract Res Clin Gastroenterol. 2002;16(1):115–33.
34. Struckmann JR, Nicolaides AN. Flavonoids. A review of the pharmacology and therapeutic efficacy of Daflon 500 mg in patients with chronic venous insufficiency and related disorders. Angiology. 1994;45(6):419–28.
35. Mentes BB, Gorgul A, Tatlicioglu E, Ayoglu F, Unal S. Efficacy of calcium dobesilate in treating acute attacks of hemorrhoidal disease. Dis Colon Rectum. 2001;44(10):1489–95.

36. Blaisdell PC. Office ligation of internal hemorrhoids. Am J Surg. 1958;96(3):401–4.

37. Barron J. Office ligation treatment of hemorrhoids. Dis Colon Rectum. 1963;6:109–13.

38. Madoff RD, Fleshman JW. American gastroenterological association technical review on the diagnosis and treatment of hemorrhoids. Gastroenterology. 2004;126(5):1463–73.

39. Bat L, Melzer E, Koler M, Dreznick Z, Shemesh E. Complications of rubber band ligation of symptomatic internal hemorrhoids. Dis Colon Rectum. 1993;36(3):287–90.

40. Lee HH, Spencer RJ, Beart Jr RW. Multiple hemorrhoidal bandings in a single session. Dis Colon Rectum. 1994;37(1):37–41.

41. O'Hara VS. Fatal clostridial infection following hemorrhoidal banding. Dis Colon Rectum. 1980;23(8):570–1.

42. Jutabha R, Jensen DM, Chavalitdhamrong D. Randomized prospective study of endoscopic rubber band ligation compared with bipolar coagulation for chronically bleeding internal hemorrhoids. Am J Gastroenterol. 2009;104(8):2057–64.

43. Arezzo A, Podzemny V, Pescatori M. Surgical management of hemorrhoids. State of the art. Ann Ital Chir. 2011;82(2):163–72.

44. Corman ML, Gravie JF, Hager T, Loudon MA, Mascagni D, Nystrom PO, et al. Stapled haemorrhoidopexy: a consensus position paper by an international working party - indications, contra-indications and technique. Color Dis. 2003;5(4):304–10.

45. Chen JS, You JF. Current status of surgical treatment for hemorrhoids--systematic review and meta-analysis. Chang Gung Med J. 2010;33(5):488–500.

46. Abcarian H. Anorectal infection: abscess-fistula. Clin Colon Rectal Surg. 2011;24(1):14–21.

47. Parks AG, Gordon PH, Hardcastle JD. A classification of fistula-in-ano. Br J Surg. 1976;63(1):1–12.

48. Billingham RP, Isler JT, Kimmins MH, Nelson JM, Schweitzer J, Murphy MM. The diagnosis and management of common anorectal disorders. Curr Probl Surg. 2004;41(7):586–645.

49. Blumetti J, Abcarian A, Quinteros F, Chaudhry V, Prasad L, Abcarian H. Evolution of treatment of fistula in ano. World J Surg. 2012;36(5):1162–7.

50. Thomson JP, Parks AG. Anal abscesses and fistulas. Br J Hosp Med. 1979;21(4):413–4, 8, 20–2.

51. Soltani A, Kaiser AM. Endorectal advancement flap for cryptoglandular or Crohn's fistula-in-ano. Dis Colon Rectum. 2010;53(4):486–95.

52. Rojanasakul A. LIFT procedure: a simplified technique for fistula-in-ano. Tech Coloproctol. 2009;13(3):237–40.

53. Deeba S, Aziz O, Sains PS, Darzi A. Fistula-in-ano: advances in treatment. Am J Surg. 2008;196(1):95–9.

54. Ramanujam PS, Prasad ML, Abcarian H. The role of seton in fistulotomy of the anus. Surg Gynecol Obstet. 1983;157(5):419–22.

55. Zaghiyan KN, Fleshner P. Anal fissure. Clin Colon Rectal Surg. 2011;24(1):22–30. Pubmed Central PMCID: 3140330.

56. Hananel N, Gordon PH. Re-examination of clinical manifestations and response to therapy of fissure-in-ano. Dis Colon Rectum. 1997;40(2):229–33.

57. Chong PS, Bartolo DC. Hemorrhoids and fissure in ano. Gastroenterol Clin North Am. 2008;37(3):627–44. ix.

58. Klosterhalfen B, Vogel P, Rixen H, Mittermayer C. Topography of the inferior rectal artery: a possible cause of chronic, primary anal fissure. Dis Colon Rectum. 1989;32(1):43–52.

59. Schouten WR, Briel JW, Auwerda JJ, De Graaf EJ. Ischaemic nature of anal fissure. Br J Surg. 1996;83(1):63–5.

60. Jenkins JT, Urie A, Molloy RG. Anterior anal fissures are associated with occult sphincter injury and abnormal sphincter function. Color Dis. 2008;10(3):280–5.

61. Nelson RL, Thomas K, Morgan J, Jones A. Non surgical therapy for anal fissure. Cochrane Database Syst Rev. 2012;2, CD003431.

62. Kennedy ML, Sowter S, Nguyen H, Lubowski DZ. Glyceryl trinitrate ointment for the treatment of chronic anal fissure: results of a placebo-controlled trial and long-term follow-up. Dis Colon Rectum. 1999;42(8):1000–6.

63. Carapeti EA, Kamm MA, McDonald PJ, Chadwick SJ, Melville D, Phillips RK. Randomised controlled trial shows that glyceryl trinitrate heals anal fissures, higher doses are not more effective, and there is a high recurrence rate. Gut. 1999;44(5):727–30. Pubmed Central PMCID: 1727506.

64. Maria G, Cassetta E, Gui D, Brisinda G, Bentivoglio AR, Albanese A. A comparison of botulinum toxin and saline for the treatment of chronic anal fissure. N Engl J Med. 1998;338(4):217–20.

65. Sajid MS, Vijaynagar B, Desai M, Cheek E, Baig MK. Botulinum toxin vs glyceryltrinitrate for the medical management of chronic anal fissure: a meta-analysis. Color Dis. 2008;10(6):541–6.

66. Arroyo A, Perez F, Serrano P, Candela F, Lacueva J, Calpena R. Surgical versus chemical (botulinum toxin) sphincterotomy for chronic anal fissure: long-term results of a prospective randomized clinical and manometric study. Am J Surg. 2005;189(4):429–34.

67. Eisenhammer S. The surgical correction of chronic internal anal (sphincteric) contracture. S Afr Med J. 1951;25(28):486–9.

68. Poh A, Tan KY, Seow-Choen F. Innovations in chronic anal fissure treatment: a systematic review. World J Gastrointest Surg. 2010;2(7):231–41. Pubmed Central PMCID: 2999245.

69. Bhardwaj R, Parker MC. Modern perspectives in the treatment of chronic anal fissures. Ann R Coll Surg Engl. 2007;89(5):472–8. Pubmed Central PMCID: 2048592.

70. Giordano P, Gravante G, Grondona P, Ruggiero B, Porrett T, Lunniss PJ. Simple cutaneous advancement flap anoplasty for resistant chronic anal fissure: a prospective study. World J Surg. 2009;33(5):1058–63.

71. CDC. HIV/AIDS Surveillance Report, 2005. Vol. 17. Rev ed. Atlanta: U.S. Department of Health and Human Services, CDC; 2007:1–54.

72. Health Protection Agency. Table 4: number of selected STI diagnoses made at genito-urinary medicine clinics by gender, sexual orientation and age-group, UK, England and English SHAs: 2000-09, 2010.

73. Poulos CS. Genital injuries in postmenopausal women after sexual assault. J Elder Abuse Negl. 2008;20:323–35.

74. Jena AB, Goldman DP, Kamdar A, Lakdawalla DN, Lu Y. Sexually transmitted diseases among users of erectile dysfunction drugs: analysis of claims data. Ann Intern Med. 2010;153(1):1–7. doi:10.1059/0003-4819-153-1-201007060-00003.

75. Satterwhite CL, Torrone E, Meites E, Dunne EF, Mahajan R, Ocfemia MC, et al. Sexually transmitted infections among US women and men: prevalence and incidence estimates, 2008. Sex Transm Dis. 2013;40(3):187–93.

76. Lee PK, Wilkins KB. Condyloma and other infections including human immunodeficiency virus. Surg Clin North Am. 2010;90(1):99–112.

77. Prevention CfDCa. Sexually transmitted disease surveillance 2011. Atlanta: U.S. Department of Health and Human Services; 2012.

78. Gilliland R, Wexner SD. Complicated anorectal sepsis. Surg Clin North Am. 1997;77(1):115–53.

79. Schofield JB, Winceslaus SJ. Anorectal manifestations of sexually transmitted infections. Color Dis. 2001;3(2):74–81.

80. Quinn TC, Goodell SE, Mkrtichian E, Schuffler MD, Wang SP, Stamm WE, et al. Chlamydia trachomatis proctitis. N Engl J Med. 1981;305(4):195–200.

81. Rompalo AM, Mertz GJ, Davis LG, Benedetti J, Critchlow C, Stamm WE, et al. Oral acyclovir for treatment of first-episode herpes simplex virus proctitis. JAMA. 1988;259(19):2879–81.

82. Chatis PA, Miller CH, Schrager LE, Crumpacker CS. Successful treatment with foscarnet of an acyclovir-resistant mucocutaneous

infection with herpes simplex virus in a patient with acquired immunodeficiency syndrome. N Engl J Med. 1989;320(5):297–300.
83. Stanberry L, Cunningham A, Mertz G, Mindel A, Peters B, Reitano M, et al. New developments in the epidemiology, natural history and management of genital herpes. Antiviral Res. 1999;42(1):1–14.
84. Dua RS, Wajed SA, Winslet MC. Impact of HIV and AIDS on surgical practice. Ann R Coll Surg Engl. 2007;89(4):354–8. Pubmed Central PMCID: 1963606.
85. Nadal SR, Manzione CR, Galvao VM, Salim VR, Speranzini MB. Healing after anal fistulotomy: comparative study between HIV+ and HIV- patients. Dis Colon Rectum. 1998;41(2):177–9.
86. Crosbie EJ, Kitchener HC. Human papillomavirus as a target for management, prevention and therapy. Int J Hyperthermia. 2012;28(6):478–88.
87. Delbello A, Colli C, Martinez Tdel R, Trevisan G. Anal canal and rectal condylomatosis: exhaustive proctological examination and STD patients. Acta Dermatovenerol Alp Panonica Adriat. 2010;19(1):13–6.
88. Stanley M. Pathology and epidemiology of HPV infection in females. Gynecol Oncol. 2010;117(2 Suppl):S5–10.
89. Sohn N, Robilotti Jr JG. The gay bowel syndrome. A review of colonic and rectal conditions in 200 male homosexuals. Am J Gastroenterol. 1977;67(5):478–84.

Index

© Springer Science+Business Media New York 2017
D.A. Gordon, M.R. Katlic (eds.), *Pelvic Floor Dysfunction and Pelvic Surgery in the Elderly*,
DOI 10.1007/978-1-4939-6554-0

Printed in the United States
By Bookmasters